AAOS

Refresher

Energency Care and Transportation of the Sick and Injured

American Academy of Orthopaedic Surgeons

Series Editor:
Andrew N. Pollak, MD, FAAOS

Editors:
Carol L. Gupton, BEMS, NRPM
Rhonda J. Beck, NREMT-P

JONES AND BARTLETT PUBLISHERS

Sudbury, Massachusetts

BOSTON   TORONTO   LONDON   SINGAPORE

Jones and Bartlett Publishers

World Headquarters
Jones and Bartlett Publishers
40 Tall Pine Drive, Sudbury, MA 01776
info@jbpub.com
www.EMSzone.com

Jones and Bartlett Publishers Canada
6339 Ormindale Way
Mississauga, Ontario L5V 1J2
Canada

Jones and Bartlett Publishers International
Barb House, Barb Mews
London W6 7PA
United Kingdom

Jones and Bartlett's books and products are available through most book-stores and online booksellers. To contact Jones and Bartlett Publishers directly, call 800-832-0034, fax 978-443-8000, or visit our website www.jbpub.com.

Substantial discounts on bulk quantities of Jones and Bartlett's publications are available to corporations, professional associations, and other qualified organizations. For details and specific discount information, contact the special sales department at Jones and Bartlett via the above contact information or send an email to specialsales@jbpub.com.

American Academy of Orthopaedic Surgeons

Editorial Credits
Chief Education Officer: Mark W. Wieting
Director, Department of Publications: Marilyn L. Fox, PhD
Managing Editor: Barbara A. Scotese

Board of Directors 2006
Richard F. Kyle, MD, President
James H. Beaty, MD
E. Anthony Rankin, MD
William L. Healy, MD
Gordon M. Aamoth, MD
Leslie L. Altick
Dwight W. Burney, III, MD
John T. Gill, MD
Joseph C. McCarthy, MD
Norman Otsuka, MD
Andrew N. Pollak, MD
Matthew S. Shapiro, MD
James P. Tasto, MD
Kristy L. Weber, MD
Stuart L. Weinstein, MD
Ken Yamaguchi, MD
Karen L. Hackett, FACHE, CAE (ex-officio)

Production Credits

Chief Executive Officer: Clayton Jones
Chief Operating Officer: Donald W. Jones, Jr.
President, Higher Education and Professional
    Publishing: Robert W. Holland
V.P., Sales and Marketing: William J. Kane
V.P., Production and Design: Anne Spencer
V.P., Manufacturing and Inventory Control: Therese Connell
Publisher, Public Safety: Kimberly Brophy
Associate Managing Editor: Janet Morris

Production Editor: Karen Ferreira
Photo Research Manager/Photographer: Kimberly Potvin
Director of Marketing: Alisha Weisman
Text Design: Anne Spencer
Composition: Omegatype Typography, Inc.
Text Printing and Binding: Courier Kendallville
Cover Printing: Courier Stoughton
Cover Photograph: Craig Jackson/IntheDarkPhotography.com

The procedures and protocols in this book are based on the most current recommendations of responsible medical sources. The American Academy of Orthopaedic Surgeons and the publisher, however, make no guarantee as to, and assume no responsibility for, the correctness, sufficiency, or completeness of such information or recommendations. Other or additional safety measures may be required under particular circumstances.

This textbook is intended solely as a guide to the appropriate procedures to be employed when rendering emergency care to the sick and injured. It is not intended as a statement of the standards of care required in any particular situation, because circumstances and the patient's physical condition can vary widely from one emergency to another. Nor is it intended that this textbook shall in any way advise emergency personnel concerning legal authority to perform the activities or procedures discussed. Such local determinations should be made only with the aid of legal counsel.

Notice: The patients described in "You are the Provider" and "Assessment in Action" throughout this text are fictitious.

ISBN-13: 978-0-7637-4229-4
ISBN-10: 0-7637-4229-5

Library of Congress Cataloging-in-Publication Data
Gupton, Carol L.
    Refresher : emergency care and transportation of the sick and injured / authors, Carol L. Gupton, Rhonda J. Beck ; editor, Andrew N. Pollak ; American Academy of Orthopaedic Surgeons.—2nd ed.
        p. ; cm.
    ISBN-13: 978–0-7637–4229–4
    ISBN-10: 0–7637–4229–5
    1. Medical emergencies. 2. Transport of sick and wounded. I. Beck, Rhonda J. II. Pollak, Andrew N. III. American Academy of Orthopaedic Surgeons.
    IV. Title. [DNLM: 1. Emergency Medical Services—methods. 2. Emergencies. 3. Emergency Medical Technicians. 4. Emergency Treatment.
    5. Transportation of Patients.   WX 215 G977r 2007]
RC86.7.A43 2007
616.02'5—dc22

                                                                                2006018663

6048

Printed in the United States of America
10 09 08 07 06   10 9 8 7 6 5 4 3 2 1

Brief Contents

The following material can be found online at www.Refresher.EMSzone.com.
- Response to Terrorism and Weapons of Mass Destruction
- BLS Review
- National Registry Skill Sheets

Contents

Resource Preview

The American Academy of Orthopaedic Surgeons is pleased to bring you *Refresher: Emergency Care and Transportation of the Sick and Injured, Second Edition*. It combines current content with dynamic features, interactive technology, and both instructor and student resources.

Refresher thoroughly addresses the objectives in the DOT EMT-Basic Refresher National Standard Curriculum, while also including a wealth of enhancements to enrich EMT-Basic education.

Chapter Resources

This text is the core of the teaching and learning system with features that reinforce and expand on essential information for the recertifying EMT-Basic and make information retrieval a snap. These features include:

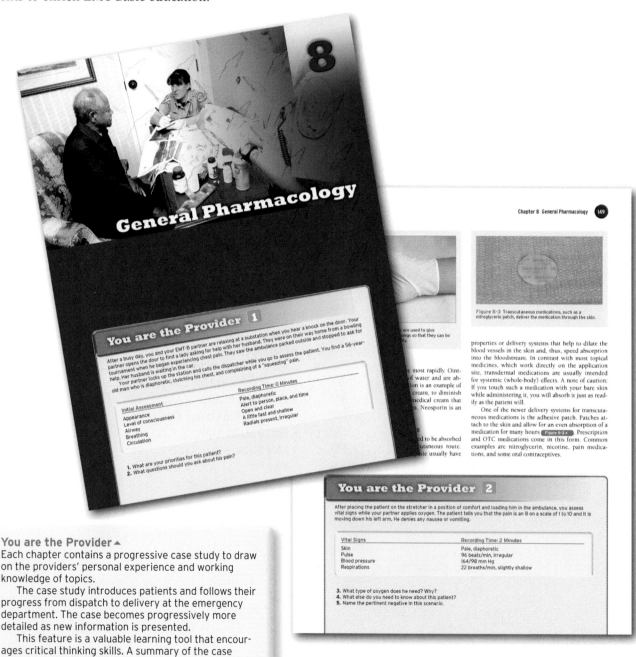

Figure 8-3 Transcutaneous medications, such as a nitroglycerin patch, deliver the medication through the skin.

You are the Provider ▲
Each chapter contains a progressive case study to draw on the providers' personal experience and working knowledge of topics.

The case study introduces patients and follows their progress from dispatch to delivery at the emergency department. The case becomes progressively more detailed as new information is presented.

This feature is a valuable learning tool that encourages critical thinking skills. A summary of the case study concludes the chapter.

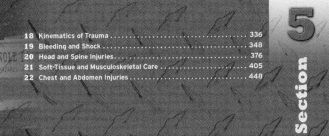

◀ **Section Objectives**
DOT EMT-Basic National Standard Curriculum objectives are provided for each section with corresponding page references.

Cognitive Objectives

1. Provide care to a patient with shock (hypoperfusion). (Chapter 19, p 366)
   ■ State methods of emergency medical care of external bleeding.
   ■ List signs and symptoms of shock (hypoperfusion).
   ■ State the steps in the emergency medical care of the patient with signs and symptoms of shock (hypoperfusion).
2. Provide care to a patient with suspected spinal injury. (Chapter 20, p 389)
   ■ State the signs and symptoms of a potential spine injury.
   ■ Describe how to stabilize the spine.
3. Provide care to a patient with a suspected head injury. (Chapter 20, p 384)
   ■ Relate mechanism of injury to potential injuries of the head and spine.
4. Provide care to a patient with a soft-tissue injury. (Chapter 21, p 00)
   ■ Describe the emergency medical care of the patient with a closed soft-tissue injury.
   ■ Describe the emergency medical care of the patient with an open soft-tissue injury.
5. Perform a rapid extrication of a trauma patient. (Chapter 20, p 386)
   ■ Describe the indications for the use of rapid extrication.
   ■ List steps in performing rapid extrication.

Affective Objectives

1. Explain the sense of urgency to transport patients that are bleeding and show signs of hypoperfusion. (Chapter 19, p 00)
2. Explain the rationale for splinting at the scene versus load and go. (Chapter 21, p 00)
3. Explain the rationale for using rapid extrication approaches only when they will make the difference between life and death. (Chapter 20, p 386)

Psychomotor Objectives

1. Demonstrate care of the patient experiencing external bleeding. (Chapter 19, p 00)
2. Demonstrate care of the patient exhibiting signs and symptoms of shock (hypoperfusion). (Chapter 19, p 366)
3. Demonstrate the steps in the care of open and closed soft-tissue injuries. (chest injuries, abdominal injuries, burns and amputations). (Chapters 21 and 22, pp 0)
4. Demonstrate the steps in the care of a patient with head or spine injury. (Chapter 20, p 385)
5. Demonstrate the procedure for rapid extrication. (Chapter 20, p 386)

Skill Drills ▶
Skill Drills provide written step-by-step explanations and visual summaries of important skills and procedures.

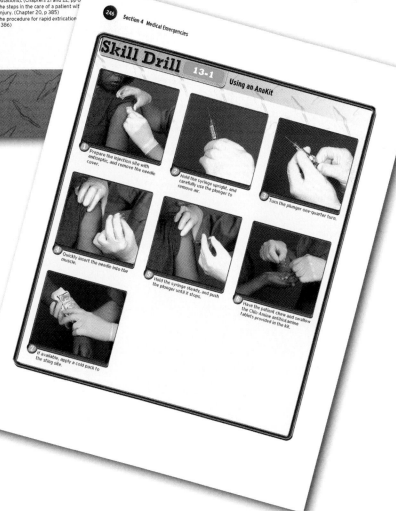

Skill Drill 13-1

Using an AnaKit

Prepare the injection site with antiseptic, and remove the needle cover.

Hold the syringe upright, and carefully use the plunger to remove air.

Turn the plunger one-quarter turn.

Quickly insert the needle into the muscle.

Hold the syringe steady, and push the plunger until it stops.

Have the patient chew and swallow the Chlo-Amine antihistamine tablets provided in the kit.

If available, apply a cold pack to the sting site.

EMT-B Safety

Regardless of the way the call is dispatched, you must always be alert for scene safety. Frightened family members, pets, and other seemingly innocuous situations can quickly become dangerous for rescuers.

administer supplemental oxygen. If necessary, provide assisted ventilation.

Circulation

Your assessment of the patient's circulation should begin with checking a pulse if the patient is unresponsive. If there is no pulse, follow your protocol for CPR and AED. If the patient is responsive, determine whether the pulse is fast or slow, weak or strong. Is the patient in shock? Oxygen administration is helpful for limiting the effects of hypoperfusion to the brain. Quickly assess for external bleeding based on the chief complaint. It is unlikely your stroke patient has experienced trauma, but you should consider the possibility and assess appropriately.

Transport Decision

Controversial evidence exists that new therapies, such as thrombolytics (clot dissolvers), may reverse stroke symptoms and even stop the stroke if given within 2 to 3 hours of the onset of symptoms. These therapies may not work for all patients, and they cannot be given to patients with bleeding-type (hemorrhagic) strokes. [...] hospital personnel will ultimately make the [...] decisions, you should

with a rapid physical exam and then obtain baseline vital signs and a SAMPLE history. A situation in which patients are unresponsive after AMS was noted is much more serious than when patients are awake but confused. Quickly looking for explanations (trauma, medical tags, track marks) for the AMS may help identify the cause of the unresponsiveness and, therefore, guide you to appropriate treatment more quickly.

When your rapid physical exam is complete, continue with obtaining the patient's vital signs and history. In a responsive medical patient, begin with a SAMPLE history, giving special attention to any information that may explain the patient's AMS. Perform a focused physical exam, and obtain the patient's baseline vital signs.

◀ **EMT-B Safety**
EMT-B safety reinforces safety concerns for both EMT-Bs and patients.

Teamwork Tips

While you are assessing the patient and coaching his or her breathing, your partner should set up the oxygen and talk to any family members or bystanders to obtain a history.

Teamwork Tips ▶
Teamwork tips offer practical advice and information on teamwork and communication with other health care providers.

affecting some 10% of the population at one time or another. The respirations of a person who is experiencing hyperventilation syndrome may be as high as more than 40 shallow breaths/min or as low as only 20 very deep breaths/min. The decision whether hyperventilation is being caused by a life-threatening illness or a panic attack should not be made outside the hospital. All patients who are hyperventilating should be given supplemental oxygen and transported to the hospital.

■ Assessment of the Patient in Respiratory Distress

Patients in respiratory distress are usually quite anxious. A calm and systematic assessment will help to decrease their anxiety level.

Scene Size-up

Body substance isolation precautions include gloves and, if you suspect a respiratory infection, a mask and [...] Scene safety may be as simple as

and tired? This initial impression will help you decide whether the patient's condition is stable or unstable.

At the same time, you should determine the patient's level of consciousness using the AVPU scale. If the patient is alert or responding to verbal stimuli, the brain is still receiving oxygen. If the patient is responsive to painful stimuli or unresponsive, the brain may not be oxygenated well and the potential for an airway or breathing problem is more likely. If the patient is alert or responding to verbal stimuli, what is the patient's chief complaint? Within seconds, you will be able to determine whether there are any immediate threats to life.

Airway and Breathing

Assess the airway. Is it patent? Is it adequate? Air must flow in and out of the chest easily for the airway to be considered patent and adequate. If snoring sounds are heard in an unresponsive patient, open the airway and insert an oral or nasal airway if necessary to maintain the airway. If you hear stridor, position the patient so he or she can breathe easily. If gurgling sounds are heard, suction as necessary.

If the airway is open and clear, you should next evaluate your patient's breathing. Is the patient breathing? Is the patient breathing adequately? If the patient is not breathing, give two ventilations immediately. As you ventilate, you need to evaluate if your ventilations are adequate.

1. Is the air going in?
2. Does the chest expand with each breath?
3. Does the chest fall after each breath?
4. Is the rate adequate for the patient's age?

[...] Chapter 5 for a review of ventilation [...] to continue

---

indicate underlying heart disease, even in the absence of pain or other symptoms.

■ Assessment of the Patient With Chest Pain

While en route, consider body substance isolation (BSI) precautions that will be needed. These precautions can be as simple as gloves when caring for a patient with chest pain or full BSI precautions for a patient in cardiac arrest. Remember, the patient's condition can change rapidly from the time you are dispatched.

Scene Size-up

Always ensure that the scene is safe for you, your partner, your patient, and bystanders. As you approach the scene, determine the nature of illness (NOI) and how many patients there are. From the nature of the call and first glance at your patient, determine whether you will need additional resources to assist in moving the patient. If you are in a tiered-response system, request that paramedics be dispatched to your location. You will need to assess the scene quickly to determine whether spinal stabilization is needed.

Initial Assessment

General Impression

All patient assessments begin by determining whether the patient is responsive. If the patient is not responsive, evaluate the ABCs (airway, breathing, and circu-

Documentation Tips

Document all findings including **pertinent negatives.** *Patient is complaining of substernal chest pain; denies any nausea or vomiting.* Also remember to use the patient's own words. *Patient states, "It feels like an elephant sitting on my chest."*

cardiac compromise may result in syncope (fainting) or dizziness. If either of these have occurred, be suspicious of spinal injuries from a fall. Assess and treat the patient as appropriate.

Assess the patient's breathing to determine whether the rate, depth, and effort are adequate. You should also listen to breath sounds. Some patients feel short of breath even though there are no obvious signs of respiratory distress. Apply oxygen with a nonrebreathing mask at 10 to 15 L/min. If the patient is not breathing or has inadequate breathing, ensure adequate breathing with bag-mask ventilation and 100% oxygen.

Circulation

Assess the patient's circulation. Determine the rate and quality of the patient's pulse. Is the pulse rhythm regular or irregular? Is it too fast or too slow? Pulses that are too fast, too slow, or irregular indicate abnor-

◀ **Documentation Tips**
Documentation tips provide advice on how to document patient care and highlight situations where documentation is especially crucial.

type of neurologic emergency that you encounter is AMS, which means that the patient is not thinking clearly or is incapable of being aroused. Patients with AMS can be alert but confused or may be unconscious. There are many causes of AMS, including hypoglycemia, hypoxemia, intoxication, drug overdose, unrecognized head injury, brain infection, and brain tumors.

Causes of AMS

Hypoglycemia

Patients with a low blood glucose level can have signs and symptoms that mimic stroke, and they can have seizures. Patients with hypoglycemia commonly, but not always, take medications that lower the blood glucose level. Check for and report medications, but remember that not all patients who have diabetes take insulin or other medications to lower the blood glucose level. Remember also that patients with a decreased level of consciousness should not be given anything by mouth.

Patients with hypoglycemia can also experience seizures, and you may arrive at the scene to find the patient in a postictal state. The mental status of a patient who has had a typical seizure is likely to improve; however, in a patient with hypoglycemia, the mental status is not likely to improve, even after several minutes. You should also consider hypoglycemia in a patient who has AMS after an injury such as a motor vehicle crash, even when there is the possi-

medications are also possible causes of AMS. A person who appears to have a psychological problem may also have an underlying medical condition. Infections are another possible cause of AMS, particularly those involving the brain or bloodstream. Infections in these areas are life threatening and need immediate attention. Patients may not demonstrate typical signs of infection, such as fever, particularly if they are very young or very old or have impaired immune systems.

Pediatric Needs

Children can have AMS caused by strokes, seizures, high or low blood glucose levels, infections (meningitis), poisoning, or tumors. Hemorrhagic strokes are usually caused by congenital defects in blood vessels; these defects are called berry aneurysms. Ischemic strokes can be due to disorders such as sickle cell anemia. However, children who have subarachnoid hemorrhages may not have a berry aneurysm; instead, they may have a congenital problem with the blood vessels in the brain. Children who have sickle cell anemia are at particularly high risk for ischemic stroke. Treat stroke and AMS in children the same way that you do in adults.

◀ Pediatric Needs
Highlight specific concerns and procedures for pediatric patients.

Geriatric Needs ▶
Highlight specific concerns and procedures for geriatric patients.

214   Section 4   Medical Emergencies

Geriatric Needs

When you are called to care for a geriatric patient with an AMS, consider the possibility of a stroke or transient ischemic attack (TIA). At the scene of a motor vehicle crash involving an older driver, consider a stroke or TIA as the precipitating factor in the crash. Be alert of altered mental status or unusual pupil responses (ie, constricted pupils in dim light, unequal pupils).

is usually in a postictal state. You must obtain as much information as possible from family or bystanders to verify that a seizure occurred and to obtain a description of the way the seizure developed.

Scene Size-up

Dispatchers are frequently given information about a seizure from the caller. Even if the caller has never seen a seizure before, the description often indicates a seizure is taking place. Although this may be an obvious nature-of-illness (NOI) problem as reported by bystanders, a mechanism of injury (MOI) may still be present. Consider the need for spinal precautions based on dispatch information and your assessment of the scene as you approach the patient. Ensure the scene is safe, and use appropriate BSI precautions. Gloves and eye protection, at a minimum, should be worn. ALS is not typically needed for a simple seizure; however,

threatening condition of status epilepticus may be present. If the patient is in the postictal stage of the seizure, he or she may be unresponsive or starting to regain awareness of the surroundings.

Airway, Breathing, and Circulation

As with any other situation, you should focus on the patient's ABCs on arrival. Bystanders may have tried to put objects in the patient's mouth to prevent the patient from swallowing his or her tongue. Assess the patient for adequate ventilation. Even if ventilation is adequate, administer high-flow oxygen at 15 L/min via nonrebreathing mask. Seizures will use up oxygen quickly and cause patients to be hypoxic. Breathing and circulation should be confirmed as normal or treated as necessary. Again, in the immediate postictal state following a major seizure, you should anticipate rapid, deep respirations and an accompanying fast heart rate due to the stress of the seizure. However, respirations and heart rate should begin to slow to normal rates after several minutes.

Transport Decision

Make sure that before packaging you have assessed the patient for trauma and have taken appropriate spinal precautions, if indicated. Never attempt to restrain a patient during a seizure because injury could result. Use soft materials for padding, and move any objects out of the way that may harm your patient.

Not every patient who has a seizure wants to be transported. It is usually in the b...

198   Section 4   Medical Emergencies

199   Chapter 10   Cardiovascular Emergencies

NOTE: While the steps below are widely accepted, be sure to consult and follow your local protocol.

	Chest Pain	Cardiac Arrest
Scene Size-up	Use BSI precautions. Ensure scene safety. Determine NOI from patient and/or bystanders. Request additional resources if needed. Determine if spinal stabilization is needed.	Use BSI precautions. Ensure scene safety. Bring AED. Determine NOI/MOI. Determine if spinal stabilization is needed.
Initial Assessment		
■ General impression	Determine if patient is responsive. If so, ask about chief complaint. If not, evaluate ABCs. If patient has lost consciousness and possibly fallen, consider spinal stabilization.	Determine patient's LOC and chief complaint. If patient is unresponsive and pulseless, prepare to defibrillate.
■ Airway	Ensure that the airway is patent.	
■ Breathing	If patient is short of breath or in respiratory distress, provide oxygen via nonrebreathing mask at 10-15 L/min. If patient is not breathing, provide bag-mask ventilation and 100% oxygen.	Check scene safety—do not defibrillate a patient in pooled water.
■ Circulation	Assess the pulse and skin. Place patient in position of comfort. Provide reassurance.	
■ Transport decision	Transport patients with chest pain immediately in gentle, stress-relieving manner.	
Focused History and Physical Exam	NOTE: The order of the steps in the focused history and physical exam differs depending on whether the patient is conscious or unconscious. The order below is for a conscious patient. For an unconscious patient, perform a rapid physical exam, obtain vital signs, and obtain the history.	
■ SAMPLE history	If patient is conscious, take brief SAMPLE history and ask OPQRST questions. Specifically, ask if the patient has had: ■ a previous heart attack? ■ heart problems? ■ risk factors: smoking, high blood pressure, high stress? ■ medications?	Not applicable to a cardiac arrest patient. See emergency care table on opposite page for summary of AED procedure.
■ Focused physical exam	Perform a focused physical exam, focusing on the cardiovascular and respiratory systems. Assess skin color, temperature, and condition. Is cyanosis present? Are neck veins distended? Check	

Chest Pain	Cardiac Arrest
Depending on local protocol, prepare to administer baby aspirin and assist with prescribed nitroglycerin. Check condition of medication(s) and expiration date(s).	**Defibrillation** For witnessed, confirmed adult cardiac arrest, immediately apply and use the AED. For unwitnessed adult cardiac arrest:
Aspirin Administer according to protocols.	1. Arrive on scene and perform your initial assessment. Verify patient is unresponsive, apneic, and pulseless. If the patient is responsive, do not apply the AED.
Nitroglycerin 1. Obtain permission from medical control.	2. If there is no pulse, perform CPR for 2 minutes (5 cycles of 30 compressions to 2 breaths).
2. Take patient's blood pressure. Continue only if systolic pressure greater than 100 mm Hg.	3. Prepare to use the AED. Power on the AED unit.
3. Check that you have the right medication, right patient, and right delivery route.	4. Remove any clothing from the patient's chest area if not already done. Apply the pads to the chest: one to the right of the sternum just below the clavicle, the other on the lower left chest wall (top of pad 2" to 3" below the armpit).
4. Question patient about last dose and effects. Ensure patient understands route of administration. Prepare to have the patient lie down to prevent fainting.	5. Stop CPR. Make sure that no one is touching the patient and loudly call "clear."
5. Ask patient to lift his or her tongue. Place tablet underneath tongue or spray under tongue if medication is in spray form. Have patient keep mouth closed until dissolved or absorbed.	6. Push the analyze button, if there is one, and wait for the AED unit to analyze.
6. Recheck blood pressure within 5 minutes. Record medication and time of administration. If chest pain persists and systolic blood pressure is greater than 100 mm Hg, repeat the dose every 5 minutes as authorized by medical control.	7. If a shock is not indicated, perform CPR for 2 minutes and then reassess pulse and analyze cardiac rhythm. If a shock is advised, make sure that no one is touching the patient. When the patient and the area around the patient are clear, push the shock button. Resume CPR, starting with compressions, immediately after the shock has been delivered.
Reevaluate transport decision. Do not delay transport to assist with nitroglycerin.	8. After 2 minutes of CPR, check for a pulse and analyze the cardiac rhythm. If the patient has a pulse, check the patient's breathing. If the patient is breathing adequately, give oxygen via non-rebreathing mask and transport. If the patient is...

Assessment and Emergency Care Summary Charts ▲
Each medical and trauma chapter concludes with two tables, one summarizing the assessment process and the other summarizing emergency care for the emergencies discussed in the chapter.

Chapter 8 General Pharmacology 163

Prep Kit

Ready for Review

- Patients having a medical emergency that requires medication administration are often anxious and scared. Recognize and respect your patient's feelings.
- Medications come in many forms: tablets and capsules, solutions and suspensions, metered-dose inhalers, topical medications, transdermal medications, gels, and gases.
- Medications may be administered through several routes: intravenous, intramuscular and subcutaneous injection, oral, sublingual, intraosseous, transcutaneous, by inhalation, and rectally.
- In all but the intravenous injection route, the medication is absorbed into the bloodstream through various body tissues. These routes of administration often determine the speed with which the medication takes effect.
- Three medications are typically carried on the EMS unit: oxygen, oral glucose, and activated charcoal. Two medicines have recently been added to the EMT-B list by some states and services: aspirin and epinephrine.
- There are three additional medications that you may help the patient self-administer: metered-dose inhaler medications, nitroglycerin, and epinephrine. Remember, though, that the administration of the medications may differ depending on local protocol.
- The administration of any medication requires approval by medical control, through direct orders given online or standing orders that are part of the local protocols.
- The steps to follow in administering medications are:
    - Obtain an order from medical control
    - Verify the proper medication
    - Verify the dose and route
    - Check the expiration date of the medication
    - Reassess vital signs and the patient's response to the medication
    - Accurately document the care you provided

Vital Vocabulary

absorption The process by which medications travel through body tissues until they reach the bloodstream.

action The therapeutic effect of a medication on the body.

contraindications Conditions that make a particular medication or treatment inappropriate, for example, a condition in which a medication should not be given because it would not help or may actually harm a patient.

dose The amount of medication given on the basis of the patient's size and age.

generic name The original chemical name of a medication (in contrast with one of its "trade names"); the name is not capitalized.

indications The therapeutic uses for a specific medication.

inhalation Breathing into the lungs; a medication delivery route.

intramuscular (IM) injection An injection into a muscle; a medication delivery route.

intraosseous (IO) Into the bone; a medication delivery route.

intravenous (IV) injection An injection directly into a vein; a medication delivery route.

metered-dose inhaler (MDI) A miniature spray canister through which droplets or particles of medication may be inhaled.

oral By mouth; a medication delivery route.

per os (PO) Through the mouth; a medication delivery route; same as oral.

per rectum (PR) Through the rectum; a medication delivery route.

pharmacology The study of the properties and effects of medications.

side effects Any effects of a medication other than the desired ones.

subcutaneous (SC) injection Injection into the tissue between the skin and muscle; a medication delivery route.

sublingual (SL) Under the tongue; a medication delivery route.

trade name The brand name that a manufacturer gives a medication; the name is capitalized.

transcutaneous Through the skin; a medication delivery route.

transdermal medications Medications that are designed to be absorbed through the skin (transcutaneously).

Techn

Interactivities
Vocabulary Ex
Anatomy Rev
Web Links
Online Revi

164

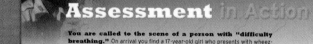

Assessment in Action

You are called to the scene of a person with "difficulty breathing." On arrival you find a 17-year-old girl who presents with wheezing and peripheral cyanosis. She has an albuterol metered-dose inhaler but has not used it.

1. An EMT-B can assist with all of the following medications EXCEPT:
    - **A.** albuterol in a metered-dose inhaler.
    - **B.** insulin.
    - **C.** nitroglycerin.
    - **D.** an EpiPen.

2. Before assisting with any medication, you should:
    - **A.** obtain permission from medical control to assist with the medication.
    - **B.** ensure that the prescription is for the patient.
    - **C.** check the expiration date.
    - **D.** all of the above.

3. What side effects do you expect after assisting with the metered-dose inhaler?
    - **A.** bradycardia
    - **B.** diaphoresis
    - **C.** tachycardia
    - **D.** hemoptysis

4. What is the next step after assisting with any medication?
    - **A.** Ask the patient about any allergies.
    - **B.** Call medical control.
    - **C.** Recheck the expiration date of the medication.
    - **D.** Monitor the patient.

5. What is the therapeutic effect of a medication?
    - **A.** any side effect
    - **B.** a contraindication
    - **C.** the action of the medication
    - **D.** the dose

6. What is the desired effect of albuterol?
    - **A.** tachycardia
    - **B.** bronchodilation
    - **C.** bronchoconstriction
    - **D.** tachypnea

Challenging Questions

7. Albuterol is a beta-2 selective sympathomimetic drug. What does this mean?

Prep Kit ▲
This engaging end-of-chapter material contains a bulleted summary of the chapter's main points, "Vital Vocabulary," and "Assessment in Action," an additional case study with multiple-choice questions.

Instructor Resources

Instructor's ToolKit CD-ROM

ISBN: 0-7637-4272-4

Preparing for class is easy with the resources found on this CD-ROM, including:

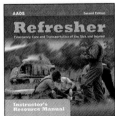

- PowerPoint Presentations, providing you with a powerful way to make presentations that are both educational and engaging. Slides can be modified and edited to meet your needs.
- Lecture Outlines, providing you with complete, ready-to-use lessons plans that outline all of the topics covered in the text. Lesson plans can be modified and edited to fit your course.
- Electronic Test Bank, containing multiple-choice and scenario-based questions, allows you to originate tailor-made classroom tests and quizzes quickly and easily by selecting, editing, organizing, and printing a test along with an answer key, that includes page references to the text.
- Image and Table Bank, providing you with many of the images and tables found in the text. You can use them to incorporate more images into the PowerPoint presentations, make handouts, or enlarge a specific image for further discussion.
- Skill Sheets, allowing you to track students' skills and conduct skill proficiency exams.

The resources found on the Instructor's ToolKit CD-ROM have been formatted so that you can seamlessly integrate them into the most popular course administration tools. Please contact Jones and Bartlett Publishers technical support at any time with questions.

Instructor's Resource Manual

ISBN: 0-7637-4273-2

The Instructor's Resource Manual is your guide to the entire teaching and learning system. This indispensable CD contains:

- Detailed lesson plans that are keyed to the PowerPoint presentations with sample lectures, quizzes, and teaching strategies.
- Teaching tips and ideas to enhance your classroom presentation.

- Answers to all end-of-chapter student questions found in the text.
- Skill Drill evaluation sheets.

Technology Resources

A key component to the teaching and learning system are interactivities and simulations to help EMT-Basics become even better providers.

www.Refresher.EMSzone.com

Make full use of today's teaching and learning technology with www.Refresher.EMSzone.com. This site has been specifically designed to complement *Refresher* and is regularly updated. Some of the resources available include:

- Chapter Pretests, prepare EMT-Basics for training. Each chapter has a pretest and provides instant results, feedback on incorrect answers, and page references for further study.
- Interactivities, allow EMT-Basics to experiment with the most important skills and procedures.
- Anatomy Review, provides interactive anatomical figure labeling exercises to reinforce EMT-Basics knowledge of human anatomy.
- Vocabulary Explorer, is a virtual dictionary where EMT-Basics can review key terms, test their knowledge of key terms through flashcards, and complete crossword puzzles.

The web site also provides:

- Response to Terrorism and Weapons of Mass Destruction enhancement chapter
- BLS Review enhancement chapter
- National Registry Skill Sheets
- Skill Evaluation Sheets

Acknowledgments

Series Editor

Andrew N. Pollak, MD, FAAOS
Medical Director, Baltimore County Fire Department
Associate Professor, University of Maryland School
of Medicine
Baltimore, Maryland

Authors

Carol L. Gupton, BEMS, NRPM
EMS Faculty
Omaha Fire Department
Omaha, Nebraska

Rhonda J. Beck, NREMT-P
Central Georgia Technical College
Macon, Georgia
Houston Healthcare EMS
Warner Robins, Georgia

Contributors

The AAOS and Jones and Bartlett Publishers wish to
thank the contributors of *Emergency Care and Transportation of the Sick and Injured, Ninth Edition.*

Reviewers

Brenda Beasley, RN, BS, EMT-P
Calhoun Community College
Wedowee, Alabama

Anne Beckle, BA, EMT-B
Cheyenne, Wyoming

Kim Bemenderfer, BS, NREMT-I
North Memorial EMS Education
Robbinsdale, Minnesota

Jerry Blaquiere, EMT-B
Wheatland County Ambulance
Harlowton, Montana

Mike Bova, EMS Instructional Chair
Milwaukee Area Technical College
Oak Creek, Wisconsin

Jeb Burress, EMT-B
Butler Community College
Andover, Kansas

Julie Chase, EMS Training Officer
Loudoun County Fire and Rescue
Leesburg, Virginia

Amanda J. Cotter, MS, NREMT-P
Greenville Technical College
Greenville, South Carolina

Robert B. Doyle, EMS I/C
Northeastern University, Institute for EMS
Burlington, Massachusetts

Phil Ester, BS, NREMT-P, CCEMT-P
Program Coordinator
Red Carpet Emergency Medical Training Consortium
Woodward, Oklahoma

Ryan P. Frandsen, BS
South Davis Metro Fire EMT
Bountiful, Utah

Robert Hawkes, BS, NREMT-P
Southern Maine Community College
South Portland, Maine

Kurt Klunder, NREMT-P, CCEMT-P
Rapid City Department of Fire & Emergency Services
Rapid City, South Dakota

Kris Krogstad, NREMT-P
NJ EMT Instructor
Montague, New Jersey

John E. Leighton, Jr., EMT-I, I/C
Southern Maine EMS
South Portland, Maine

William Matthews, BS, NREMT-P
Delaware Technical & Community College
Dover, Delaware

Tamara L. Meyers, BS, NREMT-P, EMSI
Southeast Community College
Lincoln, Nebraska

Scott Meagher, NREMT-P, REMT-B I/C
Safety Program Consultants, Inc.
Taunton, Massachusetts

Norajean Miles, Certification Administrator
Division of Health Services
Arkansas

Dave McDonald, AHS, NR/CCEMT-P
Oconee Memorial Hospital EMS
Seneca, South Carolina

Steve Monsam, BS, NREMT-P
Community Ambulance of Minot
Minot, South Dakota

Deborah L. Petty, BS, EMT-P
Paramedic Training Officer
St. Charles County Ambulance District
St. Peter's, Missouri

Alice Quiroz, USAFR, NC
EMT Program Manager
PHTLS Affiliate Faculty
Travis AFB, California

Stephen J. Rahm, NREMT-P
EMS Professions Educator
Bulverde-Spring Branch EMS
Spring Branch, Texas

John Rinard, BBA
WMD EMS Program Supervisor
Texas Engineering Extension Service
College Station, Texas

Louie Robinson, Flight Team Leader, Program Specialist
Charleston Area Medical Center
Charleston, West Virginia

Jay Reeves, NREMT-P
US Army MEDDAC Fort Knox
Fort Knox, Kentucky

Jose Salazar, MPH, NREMT-P
Loudoun County Fire and Rescue
Leesburg, Virginia

Tammy Samarripa, EMT-LP, AAS
Central Texas College
Killeen, Texas

Thom Seeber, CCEMPT-P
EMS Training and Education Coordinator
American Medical Response—Houston
Houston, Texas

Joseph T. Schnell, NREMT-I/IC
Emergency Training Associates of South Dakota
Lake Preston, South Dakota

Steve Simpson, BSBA, NREMT-P
Southern Union State Community College
Opelika, Alabama

Gary Shirley
Mississippi Gulf Coast Community College
Gulfport, Mississippi

Teresa Stoller, BS, NREMT-P
Assistant Professor, Prince George's Community College
Largo, Maryland

Michael Sanford, NREMT-P
North Memorial EMS Education
Crystal, Minnesota

Janet Schulte, BS, AS, NRCCEMT-P
St. Charles County Ambulance District Training Center
St. Peter's, Missouri

Kenneth E. Schaaf Jr., EMT-P
University of Texas Health Science Center San Antonio
International Emergency Preparedness Academy
McAllen, Texas

Geoffrey Smith, BS, NREMT-P, LP
Instructor, University of Texas Health Science Center
San Antonio
San Antonio, Texas

Brenda Voshalike, NREMT-P
Rochester Community Technical College
Cannon Falls, Minnesota

Laura Walker
Regional EMS Education Coordinator
Tidewater EMS Council
Norfolk, Virginia

Dean Williams, EMT-B
Salt Lake Tooele Applied Technology College
Salt Lake City, Utah

Sebastian Wong, EMT-P
Las Positas College
Livermore, California

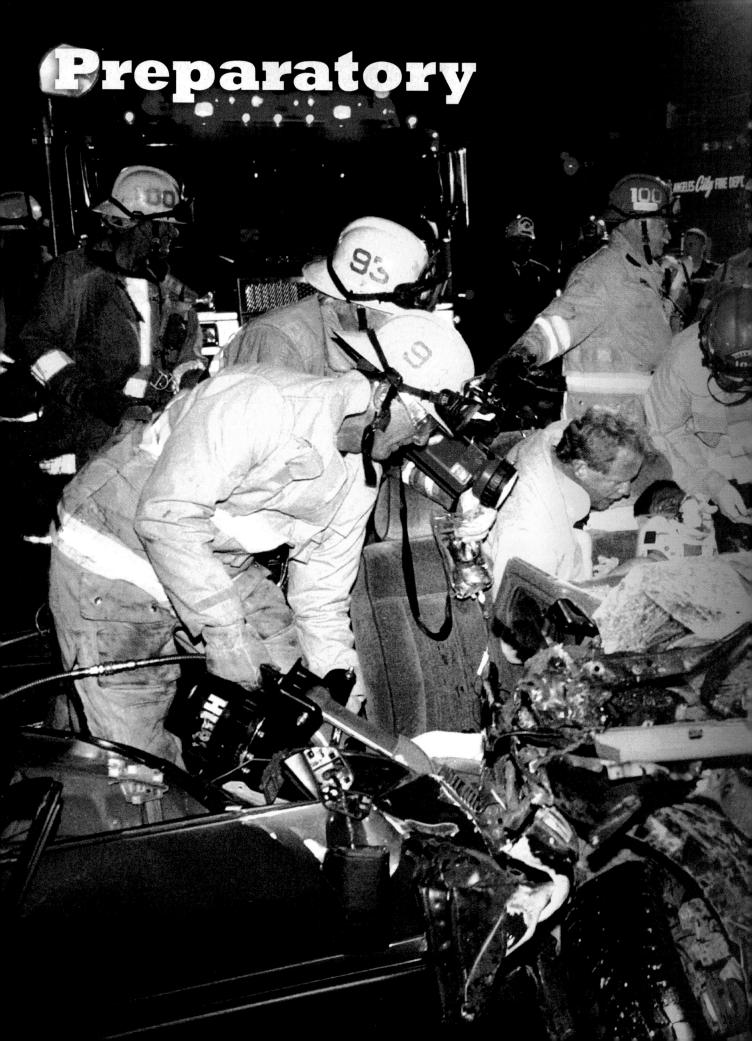

Preparatory

Section 1

Cognitive Objectives

1. Provide for safety of self, patient, and fellow workers. (Chapter 2, p 13)
   - Discuss the importance of body substance isolation (BSI).
   - Describe the steps the EMT-Basic should take for personal protection from airborne and bloodborne pathogens.
2. Identify the presence of hazardous materials. (Chapter 2, p 22)
   - Break down the steps to approaching a hazardous situation.
3. Participate in the quality improvement process. (Chapter 1, p 3)
   - Define quality improvement and discuss the EMT-Basic's role in the process.
4. Use physician medical direction for authorization to provide care. (Chapter 1, p 3)
   - Define medical direction and discuss the EMT-Basic's role in the process.
5. Use body mechanics when lifting and moving a patient. (Chapter 4, p 41)
   - Relate body mechanics associated with patient care and its impact on the EMT-Basic.
6. Use methods to reduce stress in self, a patient, bystanders, and coworkers. (Chapter 2, p 9)
   - Recognize the signs and symptoms of critical incident stress.
   - State possible steps that the EMT-Basic may take to help reduce or alleviate stress.
7. Obtain consent for providing care. (Chapter 3, p 31)
   - Define consent and discuss the methods for obtaining consent.
   - Discuss the implications for the EMT-Basic in patient refusal of transport.
   - Discuss the importance of Do Not Resuscitate {DNR} (advance directives) and local or state provisions regarding EMS application.
8. Assess and provide care to patients and families involved in suspected abuse or neglect. (Chapter 3, p 35)
   - Discuss the special considerations for assessing and managing a patient with suspected abuse or neglect.

Affective Objectives

1. Assess areas of personal attitude and conduct of the EMT-Basic. (Chapter 1)
2. Explain the rational for serving as an advocate for the use of appropriate protection equipment. (Chapter 2, p 15)
3. Explain the role of EMS and the EMT-Basic regarding patients with DNR orders. (Chapter 3, p 33)
4. Explain the rationale for properly lifting and moving patients. (Chapter 4, p 41)

Psychomotor Objectives

1. Working with a partner, move a simulated patient from the ground to a stretcher and properly position the patient on the stretcher. (Chapter 4, p 4)
2. Working with a partner, demonstrate the technique for moving a patient secured to a stretcher to the ambulance and loading the patient into the ambulance. (Chapter 4, p 46)

The Quality Improvement Process

You are the Provider 1

You are on the scene of a "person down" at a laundromat with two patients. You are caring for an 84-year-old woman with dyspnea, while your partner and the first responders are caring for her husband, a 90-year-old man in cardiac arrest. You have already called for two ALS units for backup.

Initial Assessment: 84-year-old woman	Recording Time: 0 Minutes
Appearance	Pale, diaphoretic
Level of consciousness	Alert and oriented
Airway	Open and clear
Breathing	A little fast and shallow
Circulation	Radials present, irregular

1. What are your priorities for this patient?
2. What questions should you ask about her history?

Introduction

As you know by now, being an EMT-B is a challenging and rewarding profession. You are faced with many different situations that demand good decision-making skills in order to provide quality patient care. Your initial education provided the foundation for the knowledge and abilities you have to provide quality care. Your continued experience and dedication to continuing education will build on this foundation.

The decisions you make in the field are based on your education and experience and are guided by your medical director and your agency. In this chapter, we will review medical direction and control and discuss your role in the quality improvement process.

Medical Direction and Control

As an EMT-B, the legal responsibility for you to provide medical care and perform patient care skills in the field is allowed or authorized by your physician medical director. This unique system allows you to care for patients in the prehospital setting without a physician being physically present at the scene. The medical director is the main contact between the hospitals, the medical community, and the EMTs. The medical director also helps determine and approve the continuing education and training programs that are required.

The medical director authorizes EMTs to provide medical care in the field by way of medical control. The medical director is responsible for the development and approval of protocols. Protocols, or standing orders, are written guidelines that outline the appropriate patient care to be delivered in the field. These guidelines are based on the patient's signs and

Documentation Tips

Any orders received from online medical control should be carefully documented and depending on local protocol, consider obtaining a signature from the physician who issued the order.

symptoms, injury, condition, or illness that the EMT determines by performing a patient assessment.

Medical control is either off-line (indirect) or on-line (direct). Online medical control consists of direction given over the phone or radio directly from the medical director or designated physician at the receiving facility. In this type of medical control, instructions for patient care are communicated directly to the EMT in the field. Off-line medical control refers to patient care guidelines (protocols and/or standing orders) that are authorized by the medical director. One of your responsibilities in the medical control process is to know and follow the protocols, policies, and procedures established by your medical director. Another responsibility of the EMT-B is to adhere to and to be involved with your agency's quality assurance program.

Quality Improvement (QI)

It is important to note that quality improvement programs are not intended to get providers into trouble. QI programs are necessary to ensure public safety, to validate and confirm your level of care, and to identify areas needing improvement. Traditionally, EMS providers have looked at QI programs in a negative light. To be a competent provider, you should look forward to and appreciate how you can participate in the program. Every medical profession uses a QI program. If you or a family member are being treated by a doctor for a significant injury or illness, you want assurances that the doctor is making the right decisions and is providing the most appropriate care. The

Teamwork Tips

Spend time with your partner during downtime critiquing each other's reports. This impromptu quality improvement can result in more thorough, accurate documentation.

You are the Provider 2

Bystanders tell your partner that the man clutched his chest and then slumped over in a chair. They assisted him to the floor and called 9-1-1.

Initial Assessment: 90-year-old man	Recording Time: 0 Minutes
Appearance	Pale, diaphoretic
Level of consciousness	Unresponsive
Airway	Open and clear
Breathing	Apneic
Circulation	Pulseless

3. What are the first steps in assessing this patient?
4. What equipment do you need?

public expects the same from the EMS providers who respond to them in their moment of need.

It is highly encouraged that you participate in and strongly support your agency's QI program. Most of the time, these programs and the results of the process help to make change, and justify and reaffirm your commitment to EMS.

Although ultimately, the responsibility of a quality control program for an EMS service lies with the medical director, all EMS providers in the agency contribute to and benefit from the program. The most successful EMS quality assurance programs involve all members of the agency in processes of development,

implementation, and policymaking. Continuous quality improvement (CQI) is a system of continuous internal and external reviews and audits that examine all aspects of an EMS call. This process includes run reviews, data collection, and reporting. Run reviews are used to identify significant strengths and weaknesses within the system. Positive feedback should always be included to reinforce the strengths of the EMT-Bs and to validate quality patient care. CQI programs and run reviews are not established to provide negative feedback and to only identify weaknesses—identifying strengths and reaffirming patient care decisions are just as important.

You are the Provider 3

Your patient has a history of asthma and has a metered-dose inhaler that she is having problems using. You call medical control on your portable radio to request orders to assist her with her medication.

Reassessment: 84-year-old woman	Recording Time: 3 Minutes
Pulse	96 beats/min, irregular
Blood pressure	164/98 mm Hg
Respirations	26 breaths/min, shallow
Breath sounds	Wheezing bilaterally
Pulse oximetry	92% on oxygen via nonrebreathing mask

5. What type of consent is used to treat this patient?
6. What type of medical control is used?
7. Who authorizes EMTs to provide medical care in the field by way of medical control?

You are the Provider 4

Your partner and the first responders are performing CPR on the second patient. Your partner attaches an AED and prepares to shock the patient. The AED analyzes and states that a shock is advised. Your partner charges the AED, clears the patient, and delivers the first shock.

Reassessment: 90-year-old man	Recording Time: 3 Minutes
Pulse	Pulseless
Respirations	Apneic
Airway	Open and clear
Pulse oximetry	Will not read

8. What type of consent is used to treat this patient?
9. What type of medical control is used?

Special attention is usually given to adherence to protocol and thorough documentation on the patient care report. By design, the CQI process identifies areas of improvement. The medical director will decide if the identified areas should be addressed through continuing education and remediation programs, or if policies or procedures should be changed.

You are the Provider Summary

Care for patients in the field is improved through the use of online and off-line medical control. The medical director is the main contact between the hospitals, the medical community, and the EMTs. The medical director also helps determine and approve the continuing education and training programs that are required.

1. **What are your priorities for this patient?**
   ABCs.
2. **What questions should you ask about her history?**
   What type of medical history does she have? Does she take any medications? Has she had her medication?
3. **What are the first steps in assessing this patient?**
   Open the airway, assess the airway and breathing, initiate ventilations, assess for a pulse, start CPR.
4. **What equipment do you need?**
   Personal protective equipment, a bag-valve-mask to ventilate, an oxygen cylinder, an AED, etc.
5. **What type of consent is used to treat this patient?**
   Expressed or informed consent. The patient is alert and able to make a decision regarding treatment.
6. **What type of medical control is used?**
   Online or direct medical control. You are talking directly to medical control.
7. **Who authorizes EMTs to provide medical care in the field by way of medical control?**
   The medical director.
8. **What type of consent is used to treat this patient?**
   Implied consent.
9. **What type of medical control is used?**
   Off-line or indirect medical control. Your partner is treating the patient based on standard operating procedures or standing orders.

Prep Kit

Ready for Review

- The legal responsibility for you to provide medical care and perform patient care skills in the field is allowed or authorized by your physician medical director.
- The medical director is responsible for the development of protocols, written guidelines that outline the appropriate patient care to be delivered in the field.
- Online medical control consists of direction given over the phone or radio directly from the medical director or designated physician at the receiving facility. Off-line medical control refers to patient care guidelines that are authorized by the medical director.
- Quality improvement programs are necessary to ensure public safety, to validate and confirm your level of care, and to identify areas needing improvement.

Vital Vocabulary

continuous quality improvement (CQI) A system of ongoing internal and external reviews and audits of all aspects of an EMS system.

medical control Physician instructions that are given directly by radio (online/direct) or indirectly by protocol/guidelines (off-line/indirect), as authorized by the medical director.

medical director The physician who authorizes or delegates the authority to perform medical care in the field.

off-line medical control Patient care guidelines that are authorized by the medical director.

online medical control Direct verbal communication, by radio or telephone, with an emergency department physician or a person designated by the physician.

quality control The responsibility of the medical director to ensure that the appropriate medical care standards are met by EMT-Bs on each call.

Technology

- Interactivities
- Vocabulary Explorer
- Anatomy Review
- Web Links
- Online Review Manual

Assessment in Action

Quality improvement is a major part of any EMS service. It is important to remember that quality improvement programs are not intended to get providers into trouble; they are designed to improve the care provided by your service.

1. By design, the CQI process identifies areas of _____.
   - **A.** feedback
   - **B.** improvement
   - **C.** development
   - **D.** review

2. Quality improvement programs are necessary to:
   - **A.** ensure public safety.
   - **B.** validate and confirm your level of care.
   - **C.** identify areas needing improvement.
   - **D.** all of the above.

3. The most successful EMS quality assurance programs involve all members of the agency in processes of:
   - **A.** development.
   - **B.** implementation.
   - **C.** policymaking.
   - **D.** all of the above.

4. The responsibility of a quality control program for an EMS service lies with _____.
   - **A.** the medical director
   - **B.** the EMS director
   - **C.** the training officer
   - **D.** none of the above

5. What is the purpose of run reviews?
   - **A.** to determine heavily populated call areas
   - **B.** to provide a demographic profile
   - **C.** to identify strengths and weaknesses
   - **D.** all of the above

Challenging Questions

6. What is continuous quality improvement (CQI)?

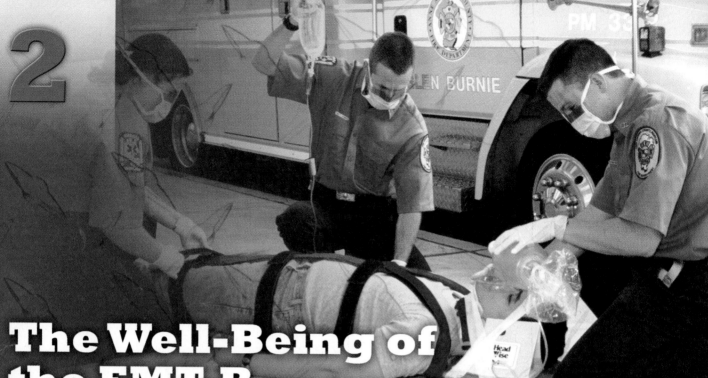

2

The Well-Being of the EMT-B

You are the Provider 1

A call comes in for a distressed person in front of the emergency department. You arrive on scene to find another EMT from your department sitting on the curb with his head in his hands. He tells you that he just can't take it any more. He is tired of dealing with the abuse at the local nursing homes, the politics at work, and the lack of caring that he has to see on a daily basis.

To make matters worse, earlier in the day he had to transport an intoxicated person who wanted a ride into town and he was only seconds away from a cardiac arrest of a 2-year-old child. Because he could not abandon the patient in his ambulance, the cardiac arrest had to wait for the next closest unit. The child was pronounced dead when the crew arrived at the emergency department.

Initial Assessment	Recording Time: 0 Minutes
Appearance	Visibly upset
Level of consciousness	Alert and oriented
Airway	Open and clear
Breathing	A little fast and shallow
Circulation	Radials present, rapid

1. What problem is this EMT experiencing?
2. What physical signs might you expect to see?
3. What would you suggest to him?

The Well-Being of the EMT-B

The personal health, safety, and well-being of all EMT-Bs are vital to all EMS systems. In caring for the critically ill and injured, there are many factors and situations that may interfere with the EMT-B's ability to treat the patient. Physical and mental issues and challenges must be dealt with in order to provide quality patient care. These issues include your own emotional well-being, scene safety issues such as hostile and violent environments, communicable diseases, and your ability to cope with high-stress situations. This chapter will review the challenges an EMT-B faces and will give you a greater understanding on how to be better prepared to maintain your own well-being.

Emotional Aspects of Emergency Care

At times, even the most experienced EMS providers have difficulty overcoming personal reactions and proceeding with patient care without hesitation. Tragedies involving children, dead patients, and patients with severe, physically altering injuries can stress the most experienced EMS provider. In all of these situations, you have to remain calm and in control of your emotions to carry out your responsibilities as an EMT-B. It is important to remember that even though you have to keep your personal emotions under control in order to do your job, having these feelings is normal. Every EMT-B who has been in these situations and others like them have had these feelings. The struggle to remain calm in the face of horrible circumstances contributes to the emotional stress of being an EMT-B.

Stressful Situations

Many situations, such as mass-casualty scenes, fatal or near-fatal motor vehicle crashes, pediatric trauma, amputations, abuse, or the death of a coworker or other public safety personnel, will be stressful for everyone involved. During stressful situations, you should always present a professional demeanor by exercising care in your words and your actions. Comments you only intend for a coworker to hear may be heard by the patient or a bystander. Words you say as a joke to someone else may be misinterpreted and taken as unprofessional or hurtful. Conversations at the scene must be professional. Avoid saying, "Everything will be all right," or "There is nothing to worry about." Reassure the patient with your calm and caring approach to the emergency situation. Patients expect you to bring some sense of order and stability to the chaos that they are experiencing   Figure 2-1 ▼ .

Stress Warning Signs and the Work Environment

EMS is a high-stress job. Understanding the causes of stress and knowing how to deal with them are critical to your job performance, health, and interpersonal relationships. To prevent stress from affecting your life negatively, you need to understand what stress is, how

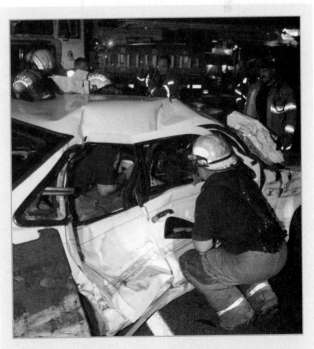

Figure 2-1 Let the patient know immediately that you are there to help.

Technology

Interactivities

Vocabulary Explorer

Anatomy Review

Web Links

Online Review Manual

Refresher.EMSzone.com

it affects you physically, and what you can do to minimize these effects.

Stress is the impact of stressors on your physical and mental well-being. Stressors include emotional, physical, and environmental situations or conditions that may cause a variety of physiologic, physical, and psychological responses. The body's response to stress begins with an alarm response, followed by a stage of reaction and resistance, and then recovery or, if the stress is prolonged, exhaustion.

This three-stage response is referred to as the general adaptation syndrome. The physiologic responses involve the chemical and physical reactions commonly known as the fight-or-flight response. Positive stress, such as exercise, as well as negative forms of stress, such as shift work, long hours, or the frustration of losing a patient, all have the same physiologic manifestations (Table 2-1 ▼).

Stress may also have physical symptoms such as fatigue, changes in appetite, gastrointestinal problems, or headaches. Stress may cause insomnia, irritability, inability to concentrate, hyperactivity, or underactivity. Additionally, stress may manifest itself in psychological reactions such as fear, dull or nonresponsive behavior, depression, guilt, anger, irritability, and frustration. Often, today's fast-paced lifestyles compound these effects by not allowing a person to rest and recover after periods of stress. Prolonged or excessive stress has been proven to be a strong contributor to heart disease, hypertension, cancer, alcoholism, and depression.

Critical Incident Stress

Many people are subject to cumulative stress, in which small, insignificant stressors grow into a larger stress-related problem. In the emergency services environment (EMS, fire fighters, police), stressors may also be

Table 2-1 Physiologic Responses to Stress
Increased respirations and heart rate
Increased blood pressure
Dilated venous vessels near the skin surface (cool, clammy skin)
Dilated pupils
Tensed muscles
Increased blood glucose levels
Perspiration
Decreased blood flow to the gastrointestinal tract

EMT-B Safety

Understanding the causes of stress and knowing how to deal with them are critical to your job performance, health, and interpersonal relationships. Find what methods of stress relief work for you—exercise, meditation, reading, etc.

sudden and more severe. Some events are unusually stressful or emotional, even by emergency services standards. These acute severe stressors result in what is referred to as critical incident stress. A critical incident is any event that causes anxiety and mental stress to emergency workers. Events that can trigger critical incident stress include the following:

- Mass-casualty incidents
- Serious injury or traumatic/sudden death of a child
- Crash with injuries, caused by an emergency services provider while responding to or from a call
- Death or serious injury of a coworker in the line of duty

You may be called to a situation so tragic that you find it difficult to organize your thoughts and respond as you were trained. You may have an immediate or delayed negative response to the incident. Do not be ashamed of such feelings; almost all responders have had the same reaction at one time or another. Remember that if you have these feelings, your partner and other members of the team may be experiencing them as well. Keep an eye on other members of your team. Confirm that they are under control and acting appropriately.

After a stressful run or a disaster, there may be an emotional letdown. This letdown is often overlooked. A process called critical incident stress management (CISM) has been developed to address acute stress situations after such an incident. The process theoretically confronts the responses to critical incidents and defuses them, directing the emergency services personnel toward physical and emotional stability. The most common form of CISM is peer defusing, when a group informally discusses events that they experienced together.

CISM can also occur as a debriefing for those who were on scene. This more formal component is called critical incident stress debriefing (CISD). CISD is a

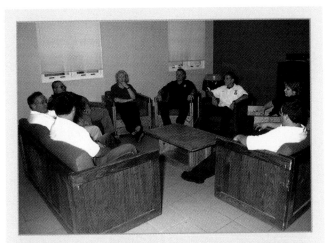

Figure 2-2 CISD sessions are sometimes used to assist providers in managing their stress.

Table 2-2 Strategies to Manage Stress
Change or eliminate stressors.
Change partners to avoid a negative or hostile personality.
Change work hours and cut back on overtime.
Change your attitude about the stressor.
Don't waste energy complaining or worrying about things that you cannot change, such as relapsing alcoholics and possible abuse situations. Focus on delivering high-quality care.
Try to adopt a more relaxed, philosophical outlook.
Expand your social support system apart from your coworkers.
Maintain friends and interests outside of EMS.
Minimize the physical response to stress by employing various techniques, including: ■ A deep breath to settle an anger response   ■ Stretching   ■ Slow, deep breathing   ■ Regular physical exercise   ■ Progressive muscle relaxation

program in which severely stressful job-related incidents are discussed. The purpose of CISD is to relieve personal and group anxieties and stress. CISD teams consist of peers and mental health professionals. The CISD session is conducted in strict confidence and within 24 to 72 hours of the incident Figure 2-2 ▲ . CISD teams can be located by calling your state EMS office or through your EMS agency.

Additionally, CISM can also be provided at the scene of a major emergency in the following circumstances:

- When personnel are assessed for signs and symptoms of distress while resting
- Before re-entering the scene
- During a scene demobilization in which personnel are educated about the signs of critical incident stress and given a buffer period to collect themselves before leaving

Stress Management

There are many methods for handling stress. Some are positive and healthy; others are harmful or destructive. Americans consume more than 20 tons of aspirin per day, and doctors prescribe muscle relaxants, tranquilizers, and sedatives more than 90 million times per year to patients in the United States. Although these medications have legitimate uses, they do nothing to effectively manage stress.

The term "stress management" refers to the tactics that have been shown to alleviate or eliminate stress reactions. These tactics may involve changing a few habits, changing your attitude, and perseverance Table 2-2 ▶ . A clue to the management of stress comes from the fact that it is not the event itself but the individual's reaction to it that determines how much it will strain the body's resources. Remember that stress is defined as anything that you perceive as a threat to your equilibrium. Stress is an undeniable and unavoidable part of our everyday life. By understanding how it affects you physiologically, physically, and psychologically, you can more successfully manage it. It is critical that you recognize the signs of stress so that it does not interfere with your work or life away from work, including your family life. The following sections provide some suggestions on how to better manage your stress.

Lifestyle Changes

Your well-being is of primary importance to effective EMS operations. The effectiveness and efficiency with which you do your job depend on your ability to stay in shape and avoid the risk of personal injury. Burnout is a condition of chronic fatigue and frustration that results from mounting stress over time. To avoid burnout, you need to be in good physical and mental health. Be aware of the potential hazards in emergency medical care and keep yourself physically and mentally prepared.

Nutrition

To perform efficiently, you must eat nutritious food. Food is the fuel that makes the body run. The physical exertion and stress that are a part of your job require a high energy output. If you do not have a ready source of fuel, your performance may be less than satisfactory. This can be dangerous for you, your partner, and your patient. Therefore, it is important for you to learn about and follow the rules of good nutrition.

Try eating several small meals throughout the day to keep your energy resources at constant high levels. Remember, however, that overeating may reduce your physical and mental performance. After a large meal, the blood that is needed for the digestive process is not available for other activities. You must also make sure that you maintain an adequate fluid intake Figure 2-3 ▶ . Hydration is important for proper functioning. Fluids can be easily replenished by drinking any nonalcoholic, noncaffeinated fluid. Water is generally the best fluid available. The body absorbs it faster than any other fluid. Avoid fluids that contain high levels of sugar. These can actually slow the rate of fluid absorption by the body and can also cause abdominal discomfort.

Exercise

A regular program of exercise enhances the benefits of maintaining good nutrition and adequate hydration. When you are in good physical condition, you can handle job stress more easily. A regular program

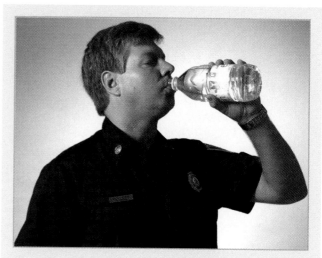

Figure 2-3 Maintain an adequate fluid intake by drinking plenty of water or other nonalcoholic, caffeine-free fluids.

of exercise increases your strength and endurance and reduces the chances of injury.

Balancing Work, Family, and Health

As an EMS provider, you are often dispatched on runs at any time of the day or night. Unfortunately, there is no rhyme or reason to the timing of these calls. Volunteer EMT-Bs are often called away from family or friends during social activities. Shift workers may be required to be apart from loved ones for long periods of time. You should never let the job interfere exces-

You are the Provider 2

He tells you that he just wants to go home and that he is not sure if he will ever come back. He feels like there is no reason to continue in this profession because "we just don't make a difference." He has been working extra shifts and feels like he has not slept in a month.

Vital Signs	Recording Time: 2 Minutes
Skin	Cool, clammy
Pulse	108 beats/min, regular
Blood pressure	158/86 mm Hg
Respirations	22 breaths/min

4. What do the vital signs tell you?
5. What is the body's first response to stress?
6. If not corrected, what will this lead to?

sively with your own needs. Find a balance between work and family; you owe it to yourself and to them. It is important to make sure that you have the time that you need to relax with family and friends.

It is also important to realize that coworkers, family, and friends often may not understand the stress caused by responding to EMS calls. As a result of a "bad call," you might not feel like going out to a movie or attending a family event that has been planned for some time. In these situations, help from a critical incident stress debriefing team or information sessions conducted by the EMS unit's employee assistance program may assist you in resolving these problems.

When possible, rotate your schedule to give yourself time off. If your EMS system allows you to move from station to station, rotate to reduce or vary your call volume. Take vacations to provide for your good health so that you will be able to respond the next time you are needed. If at any point you feel that the stress of work is more than you can handle, seek help. You may want to discuss your stress informally with your family or coworkers. Help from more experienced team members can be invaluable. You also may wish to get help from peer counselors or other professionals.

■ Scene Safety and Personal Protection

The steps you take to preserve personal safety should be automatic by now. The personal safety of yourself, your team members, the patient(s), and bystanders is your first priority. A second accident at the scene or an injury to you or your partner can create more challenging situations, delay emergency medical care of patients, increase the burden on other EMS personnel, and may result in unnecessary injury or death.

You should begin protecting yourself as soon as you are dispatched. Before you leave for the scene, prepare yourself both mentally and physically. Make sure you wear seat belts and shoulder harnesses en route to the scene. Wear seat belts and shoulder harnesses at all times, unless patient care makes it impossible Figure 2-4 ▶ . Many EMS agencies have mandatory seat-belt policies for the driver at all times, for all EMT-Bs during transit to the scene, and for anyone who is riding with a patient.

Protecting yourself at the scene is also very important. A second accident may damage the ambulance and may result in injury to you, your partner, or additional injury to the patient. The scene must be well

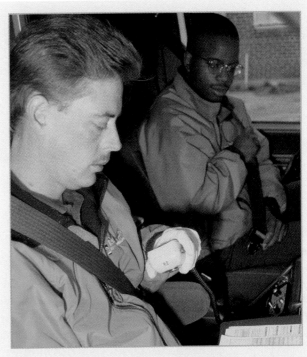

Figure 2-4 Always wear seat belts and shoulder harnesses.

marked. If law enforcement has not already done so, you should make sure that proper warning devices are placed at a sufficient distance from the scene Figure 2-5 ▼ . Park the ambulance at a safe but convenient distance from the scene. Before attempting to access patients who are trapped in a vehicle, check the vehicle's stability. Initiate any necessary measures to secure it. Do not rock or push on a vehicle to find out

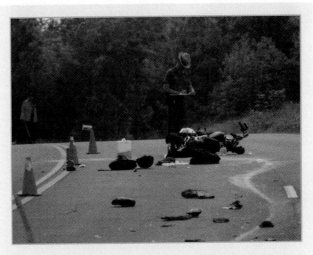

Figure 2-5 For continued safety, make sure the scene is well marked to decrease the chance of a second crash.

whether it will move. If you are uncertain about the safety of a crash scene, wait for appropriately trained individuals to arrive to assist you.

As you may have experienced, when working at night, you must have plenty of light. Poor lighting increases the risk of injury to both you and the patient. It also can result in poor emergency medical care. Reflective emblems or clothing helps to make you more visible at night and decreases your risk of injury Figure 2-6 ▾ .

■ Communicable Diseases

As an EMT-B, you are called on to treat and transport patients with a variety of communicable or infectious diseases. Most of these diseases are much harder to catch than is commonly believed. In addition, there are many immunizations, protective techniques, and devices that can help minimize your risk of infec-

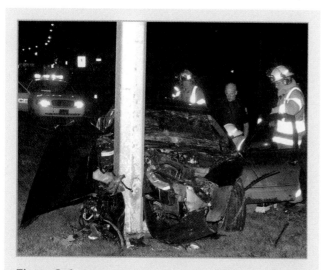

Figure 2-6 To improve your safety and visibility in the dark, wear reflective clothing.

tion. When these protective measures are used, your risk of contracting a serious communicable disease is negligible.

Risk Reduction and Prevention
Universal Precautions and Body Substance Isolation

The <u>Occupational Safety and Health Administration (OSHA)</u> develops and publishes guidelines for reducing risk in the workplace. It is also responsible for enforcing these guidelines. OSHA requires all EMT-Bs to be trained in the handling of bloodborne pathogens and in approaching the patient who may have a communicable or infectious disease. Training must also be provided for issues including blood and body fluid precautions, airborne precautions, and contamination precautions.

Because health care workers are exposed to so many different kinds of infections, the Centers for Disease Control and Prevention (CDC) developed a set of <u>universal precautions</u> for health care workers to use in treating patients. These protective measures are designed to prevent workers from coming into direct contact with germs carried by patients. <u>Direct contact</u> is the exposure or transmission of a communicable disease from one person to another by physical touching. <u>Exposure</u> is contact with blood, body fluids, tissues, or airborne droplets by direct or indirect contact. <u>Indirect contact</u> is exposure or transmission of a disease from one person to another by contact with a contaminated object.

The goal of universal precautions is to interrupt the transmission of germs by decreasing the chance that you will come into contact with them. Universal precautions are not universal in the sense that they will help to protect you against all infectious diseases. Instead, the word "universal" is meant to remind you to apply precautions in all situations in which you have direct patient contact. It is impossible to tell whether an individual is free from a communicable disease, even if he or she appears healthy.

You can also reduce your risk of exposure by following <u>body substance isolation (BSI)</u> precautions. BSI is the preferred infection control concept for EMS and fire personnel. BSI differs from universal precautions in that it is designed to approach all body fluids as being potentially infectious. In observing universal precautions, you assume that only blood and certain body fluids pose a risk for transmission of hepatitis B and human immunodeficiency virus (HIV). In 1988, the CDC removed many body fluids, such as sweat, tears, saliva, urine, feces, vomit, nasal secretions, and sputum, from the risk category unless these fluids contain visible blood. However, in the dark, you may not be able to see any blood. Therefore, EMS follows the BSI concept rather than the CDC's universal precautions.

Proper Hand Washing

Proper hand washing is perhaps one of the simplest yet most effective ways to control disease transmission. Always wash your hands before and after contact with a patient, regardless of whether you wear gloves. The longer the germs remain with you, the greater their chance of getting through your barriers. Although soap and water are not protective in all cases, in certain situations their use provides excellent protection against further transmission from your skin to others. If no running water is available, you may use waterless hand-washing substitutes. If you use a waterless substitute in the field, make sure that you wash your hands once you arrive at the hospital. The proper procedure for hand washing is as follows:

1. Use soap and warm water.
2. Rub your hands together for at least 10 to 15 seconds to work up a lather. Pay particular attention to your fingernails.
3. Rinse your hands, and dry them with a paper towel.
4. Use the paper towel to turn off the faucet.

Gloves and Eye Protection

Gloves and eye protection are the minimum standard for all patient care if there is any possibility for exposure to blood or body fluids. Both vinyl and latex gloves provide adequate protection. (Some individuals are allergic to latex. If you suspect that you are allergic, consult your supervisor for options.) Change latex gloves if they have been exposed to motor oil,

gasoline, or any petroleum-based product. Do not use petroleum jelly with latex gloves. Double glove if there is substantial bleeding or you anticipate that you will be exposed to large volumes of other body fluids. Be sure to change gloves if you are treating more than one patient at a time. For cleaning and disinfecting the unit or equipment, use heavy-duty utility gloves. You should never use lightweight latex or vinyl gloves for cleaning. Removing used latex or vinyl gloves after patient care is complete requires a methodical technique to avoid contaminating yourself

Skill Drill 2-1 ▶ .

1. **Begin by partially removing one glove.** With the other gloved hand, pinch the first glove at the wrist—being certain to touch only the outside of the first glove—and start to roll it back off the hand, inside out. Leave the exterior of the fingers on that first glove exposed (**Step 1**).
2. **Use the still-gloved fingers** of the first hand to pinch the wrist of the second glove and begin to pull it off, rolling it inside-out toward the fingertips as you did with the first glove (**Step 2**).
3. **Continue pulling the second glove off** until you can pull the second hand free (**Step 3**).
4. **With your now-ungloved second hand,** grasp the exposed inside of the first glove and pull it free of your first hand and over the now-loose second glove. Be sure that you touch only clean, interior surfaces with your ungloved hand (**Step 4**).

Gloves are the most common type of personal protective equipment (PPE). In many EMS rescue operations, you must also protect your hands and wrists from injury. You may wear puncture-proof leather gloves, with latex gloves underneath. This combination will allow you free use of your hands with added protection from blood and body fluids. Remember that latex or vinyl gloves are considered medical waste and must be disposed of properly. Leather gloves must be treated as contaminated material until they can be properly decontaminated.

Wearing protective eyewear is important to prevent exposure to blood or body fluids that may splatter in your eyes. Eye protection should shield the front of the eyes and also protect from any splashes that may enter from the side. Prescription glasses are acceptable as eye protection, but you must add removable side shields when on duty. Contact lenses are not considered protective eyewear.

EMT-B Safety

> Proper hand washing is one of the simplest yet most effective ways to control disease transmission.

Skill Drill   2-1   Removing Gloves

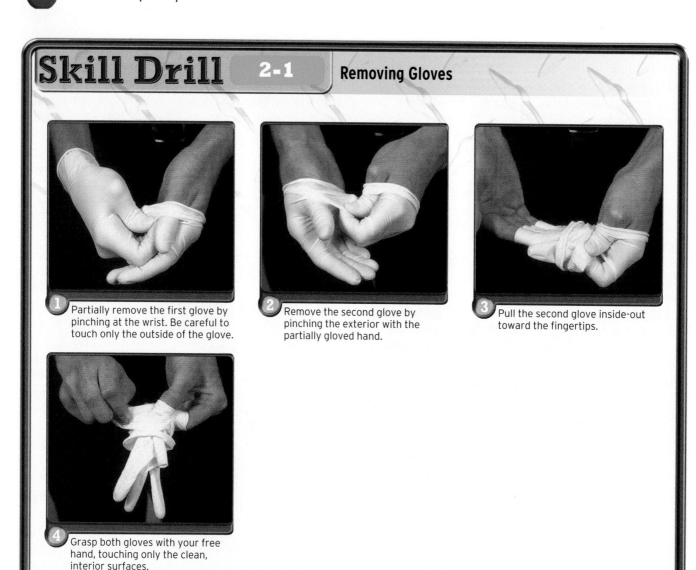

1. Partially remove the first glove by pinching at the wrist. Be careful to touch only the outside of the glove.

2. Remove the second glove by pinching the exterior with the partially gloved hand.

3. Pull the second glove inside-out toward the fingertips.

4. Grasp both gloves with your free hand, touching only the clean, interior surfaces.

Gowns

Gowns provide protection from extensive blood spatter. Gowns may be worn in situations such as childbirth or major trauma. However, wearing a gown may not be practical in many situations. If your uniform is significantly contaminated with blood or body fluid, a complete change of uniform is usually preferred. Follow your department's policies on the wearing of gowns and decontaminating uniforms.

Masks, Respirators, and Barrier Devices

The use of masks is a complex issue, especially in light of OSHA and CDC requirements regarding protection from tuberculosis. You should wear a standard surgical mask if blood or body fluid spatter is a pos-

sibility. If you suspect that a patient has an airborne disease, you should place a surgical mask on the patient. However, if you suspect that the patient has tuberculosis, place a surgical mask on the patient and a High-Efficiency Particulate Air (HEPA) respirator on yourself   Figure 2-7 ▶ . If the patient needs oxygen, use a nonrebreathing mask instead of a surgical mask on the patient. Do not place a HEPA respirator on the patient; it is unnecessary and uncomfortable. A simple surgical mask will reduce the risk of transmission of germs from the patient into the air. Use of a HEPA respirator should comply with OSHA standards, which state that facial hair, such as long sideburns or a mustache will prevent a proper fit.

With proper preparation, mouth-to-mouth resuscitation is rarely necessary in the EMS setting. Use a

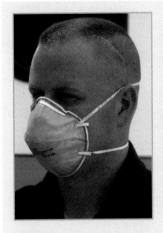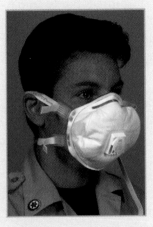

Figure 2-7 Wear a HEPA respirator if you are treating a patient with suspected tuberculosis (TB).

bag-mask device when possible. Although there are no documented cases of disease transmission to providers as a result of performing unprotected mouth-to-mouth resuscitation on a patient, you should always use a barrier device if you have to ventilate a patient without a bag-mask device or pocket mask.

Remember that the equipment you use is considered contaminated after it has been exposed to the patient. You must make sure that gloves, masks, gowns, and all other items that have been exposed to infectious processes or blood are properly disposed of according to local guidelines. If you are stuck by a needle, get blood or body fluids in your eye, or have any body fluid contact with the patient, report the incident to your supervisor immediately.

Proper Disposal of Sharps

Use caution when handling needles and other sharp items. The spread of HIV and hepatitis in the health care setting can usually be traced to careless handling of sharps. Do not recap, break, or bend needles. Even the most careful individuals may stick themselves accidentally. Dispose of all sharp items that have been in contact with human secretions in approved closed, rigid containers **Figure 2-8 ▶**.

You are the Provider 3

You and your partner try talking to him and offer to go with him to the supervisor. He says he is not sure he wants to try anything and will just turn in his resignation. His wife is not happy with the hours that he is working and he can't seem to make ends meet. He says that his marriage is not going to last if it keeps on. He has not been able to go to any of his son's baseball games and he feels guilty about that too.

Reassessment	Recording Time: 5 Minutes
Pulse	114 beats/min, regular
Blood pressure	172/94 mm Hg
Respirations	24 breaths/min
Breath sounds	Clear bilaterally
Pulse oximetry	97% on room air

7. What type of negative stressors is he experiencing?
8. What might help with his problems?
9. Has he had any events that could trigger critical incident stress?
10. Name a positive stressor that may help.

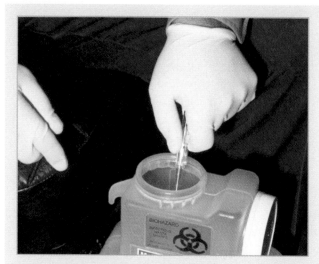

Figure 2-8 Properly dispose of sharps in a closed, marked container.

Employer Responsibilities

Your department cannot guarantee a 100% risk-free environment. The risk of exposure to a communicable disease is a part of your job. You have a right to know about diseases that may pose a risk to you. Remember, though, that your risk for infection is not high; however, OSHA regulations, especially for private and federal agencies, require that all employees be offered a workplace environment that reduces the risk for exposure.

In addition to OSHA guidelines, other national guidelines and standards, including those from the CDC and the National Fire Protection Agency (NFPA) Infection Control Standard 1581, address reducing the risk for exposure to bloodborne pathogens and airborne diseases. These agencies set a standard of care for all EMS and fire personnel and apply whether you are a paid EMT-B or a volunteer.

Personal Protective Equipment

Personal protective equipment (PPE) blocks entry of an organism into the body. OSHA requires that the following PPE be made available to you:

- Vinyl or latex gloves for patient care duties
- Heavy-duty gloves for cleaning
- Protective eyewear
- Masks (including a HEPA respirator)
- Cover gowns
- Devices for respiratory assistance

The proper PPE for each task is selected according to the way in which a communicable disease is transmitted. For example, transmission of an airborne disease can be blocked by a mask. Blood spatter into the eye can be prevented by wearing protective eyewear. The recommendations for PPE use should be followed; however, OSHA recognizes that there are times when these procedures cannot be performed. There is an exception statement in the OSHA regulation that states that when you believe that taking the time to use PPE will delay delivery of care to the patient or will pose a risk to your personal safety, you may choose not to use PPE. Risk to personal safety refers to the likelihood of being attacked by a person or an animal, not to concern over acquiring a communicable disease. If you choose not to use PPE, you may have to justify this action. It is your responsibility to follow the rules in a reasonable, prudent manner.

Exposure Control Plan

Another way to reduce your exposure risk is to follow your department's exposure control plan. This comprehensive plan incorporates CDC guidelines, OSHA regulations, NFPA Infection Control Standard 1581, and other applicable state and local regulations 〔 Table 2-3 ▸ 〕.

■ Diseases of Special Concern

HIV Infection

Exposure to the HIV virus, which causes AIDS, is the most feared infection risk for EMTs. There is no vaccine to protect against HIV, and despite great progress in drug treatments, AIDS is still fatal. Fortunately, the HIV virus is not easily transmitted in the EMS environment. HIV is far less contagious than hepatitis B. HIV is a potential hazard only when deposited on a mucous membrane or directly into the bloodstream. Therefore, the real risk of infection is limited to exposure to an infected patient's blood.

Many patients who are infected with HIV do not show any symptoms. This is the basis for the BSI requirement that health care workers wear gloves any time they are likely to come into contact with secretions or blood from any patient. Put on gloves before leaving the ambulance to care for a patient. Also take great care in handling and disposing of needles and sharps to avoid inadvertently exposing yourself or others to a needlestick. Finally, cover any small cuts or abrasions on your own skin while you are on the job.

If you have any reason to think that a patient's blood or secretions may have entered your system,

Table 2-3 Components of an Exposure Control Plan

Determination of Exposure

- Determines who is at risk for ongoing contact with blood and other body fluids
- Creates a list of tasks that pose a risk for contact with blood or other body fluids
- Includes personal protective equipment (PPE) required by OSHA

Education and Training

- Explains why a qualified individual is required to answer questions about communicable diseases and infection control, rather than relying on packaged training materials
- Includes availability of an instructor able to train EMTs regarding bloodborne and airborne pathogens, such as hepatitis B and C, HIV, syphilis, and tuberculosis
- Ensures that the instructor provides appropriate education, which is the best means for correcting many myths surrounding these issues

Hepatitis B Vaccine Program

- Spells out the vaccine offered, its safety and efficacy, record keeping, and tracking
- Addresses the need for postvaccine antibody titers to identify individuals who do not respond to the initial three-dose vaccination series

Personal Protective Equipment (PPE)

- Lists the PPE offered and why it was selected
- Lists how much equipment is available and where to obtain additional PPE
- States when each type of PPE is to be used for each risk procedure

Cleaning and Disinfection Practices

- Describes how to care for and maintain vehicles and equipment
- Identifies where and when cleaning should be performed, how it is to be done, what PPE is to be used, and what cleaning solution is to be used
- Addresses medical waste collection, storage, and disposal

Tuberculin Skin Testing/Fit Testing

- Addresses how often employees should undergo skin testing
- Addresses how often fit testing should be done to determine the proper size mask to protect the EMT from tuberculosis
- Addresses all issues dealing with HEPA respirator masks

Postexposure Management

- Identifies whom to notify when exposure may have occurred, forms to be filled out, where to go for treatment, and what treatment is to be given

Compliance Monitoring

- Addresses how the service or department evaluates employee compliance with each aspect of the plan
- Ensures that employees understand what they are to do and why it is important
- States that noncompliance should be documented
- Indicates what disciplinary action should be taken in the face of continued noncompliance

Record Keeping

- Outlines all records that will be kept, how confidentiality will be maintained, and how records can be assessed and by whom

follow your department's exposure control policy and seek medical advice as soon as possible. Physicians often recommend immediate treatment if the exposure involves a patient with known HIV infection. If the patient's HIV status is unknown or the physician considers the patient to be at low risk for HIV infection, testing for both the patient and responder is usually recommended before treatment is started. As further research concerning HIV is conducted, testing and treatment recommendations may change. It is important that you immediately see your doc-

tor or your program's designated physician every time you are potentially exposed to a communicable disease.

Hepatitis

Hepatitis is an inflammation (and often infection) of the liver. Symptoms of hepatitis include fever, loss of appetite, jaundice, and fatigue. It can be caused by a number of different viruses and toxins. There is no sure way for EMS providers to tell which patients with hepatitis have a contagious form of the disease.

Hepatitis A can be transmitted only from a patient who has an acute infection, whereas hepatitis B and C can also be transmitted from chronic carriers who have no signs of illness. A <u>carrier</u> is a person (or animal) in whom an infectious organism has taken up permanent residence, although it may not be causing any active disease. Carriers may never know that they harbor the organism.

Hepatitis A is transmitted orally via oral/fecal <u>contamination.</u> This generally means that you must eat or drink something contaminated with the virus. The organisms that cause hepatitis B and C may enter the body through a transfusion or needlestick with infected blood; the latter puts health care workers at high risk for contracting hepatitis B, the most virulent member of this disease category.

<u>Virulence</u> is the strength or ability of a pathogen to produce disease. Hepatitis B is far more contagious than HIV. For this reason, hepatitis B vaccination is important for all EMS providers. Not everyone who is vaccinated develops immediate immunity. Sometimes, but not always, an additional dose (booster) is necessary to provide immunity. EMS providers should be tested after receiving the hepatitis B shot series to determine immunity status.

Meningitis

<u>Meningitis</u> is an inflammation of the meningeal coverings of the brain. Patients with meningitis will have signs and symptoms such as fever, headache, stiff neck, skin rash, and altered mental status. It is an uncommon but severe disease. Meningitis can be caused by viruses or bacteria, and most cases are not contagious. However, one form, meningococcal meningitis, is highly contagious. The meningococcal bacterium colonizes the human nose and throat and only rarely causes an acute infection. When it does, it can be fatal. Patients with this kind of infection often have a rash that resembles red blotches on their skin.

Use universal precautions and follow BSI techniques when caring for a patient with suspected meningitis. The use of gloves and a mask is crucial in preventing the patient's airborne pathogens from entering your nose and mouth.

Tuberculosis

Most patients who are infected with *Mycobacterium tuberculosis* (the tubercle bacillus) are well most of the time. In the United States, <u>tuberculosis</u> is a chronic disease that usually attacks the lungs. Except in infants, it

is not usually serious. After the primary infection, the tubercle bacillus is rendered dormant by the immune system. However, even after decades of lying dormant, the germ can reactivate. Reactivated tuberculosis is common and can be much more difficult to treat due to the increasing number of tuberculosis strains that have grown resistant to many drug treatments.

Tuberculosis patients who pose the highest contagious risk almost always have a cough. You can consider respiratory tuberculosis to be the only contagious form because it is the only one that is spread by airborne transmission. The droplets produced by coughing are not the real threat of exposure. The real problem is the droplet nuclei—what remains of the droplets after excess water has evaporated. These particles are tiny enough to be totally invisible and can remain suspended in the air for long periods of time. The EMT-B may be at risk by simply entering a closed room that the patient left long ago. Droplet nuclei are too small to be stopped by routine surgical masks. Inhaled, they are carried directly to the alveoli of the lungs where the bacteria may begin to grow. Under normal circumstances, however, tuberculosis transmission is not very efficient, and it typically causes no illness in a new host. Many patients with tuberculosis do not even transmit the infection to family members. In crowded environments with poor ventilation, however, the disease spreads relatively easily.

If you are exposed to a patient who has pulmonary tuberculosis, you will be given a tuberculin skin (Mantoux) test. A positive result means that infection has occurred; it does not mean that you have active tuberculosis. It takes at least 6 weeks for the bacteria to show up in a laboratory test. Most tuberculosis transmissions occur silently, without the health care worker even knowing that an exposure has occurred. This is why health care workers, including EMS providers, receive tuberculin skin tests on a regular basis (usually annually). If the infection is found before the individual becomes ill, preventive therapy is almost 100% effective.

Newly Recognized Diseases

Newly recognized diseases, such as those caused by Hantavirus or enteropathogenic *Escherichia coli,* are being reported. These diseases are not transmitted from person to person directly; rather, they are carried by a vehicle, such as food, or a vector, such as rodents. Although not a newly discovered illness, West Nile virus has caused some concern recently. This virus' vector is the mosquito, and it affects humans and birds. The virus is actually tracked by tests done on birds suspected of being killed by the virus. These diseases are not communicable and do not pose a risk to you during patient care.

There is also significant concern of late with SARS (severe acute respiratory syndrome) and the avian flu (bird flu). SARS is a serious, potentially life-threatening viral infection caused by a recently discovered family of viruses best known as the second most common cause of the common cold. SARS usually starts with flu-like symptoms, which may progress to pneumonia, respiratory failure, and, in some cases, death. The SARS virus strain probably spread from Guangdong province in southern China to Hong Kong, Singapore, and Taiwan. Canada has had a significant outbreak in the Toronto area. SARS is thought to be primarily transmitted by close person-to-person contact. Most cases have involved persons who lived with or cared for a person with SARS or who had exposure to contaminated secretions from a SARS patient.

Avian flu occurs naturally in the bird population. This flu is highly contagious among birds and is spread between the birds after contact with contaminated secretions (saliva, nasal secretions, or feces). The stronger form of the virus spreads quickly among the bird population and has a significant mortality rate. The virus occurs primarily among bird populations and does not typically infect people. In early 2004, avian flu (H5N1) killed over 100 million birds in eight Asian countries. New outbreaks have been reported in Europe and Asia (none in the United States) and have caused concern for leaders worldwide.

The CDC also has a growing concern over the potential infection of this virus in the human population. Since 1997, there have been over 100 cases of avian flu infection in humans. Most of these cases are the result of the person having contact with an infected bird or a contaminated surface from an infected bird's secretions. There are only a few cases of documented transmission of the virus from person to person.

There are many forms of the avian flu. Human infection of the H5N1 form in Europe and Asia has caused over a 50% mortality rate. The spread of this form of avian flu has not continued after one person-to-person contact; however, experts are concerned that mutation of the virus could result in a version of the bird flu that would spread easily and quickly between people, resulting in a pandemic or worldwide outbreak.

Scientists continue to track and study this virus. There is no current vaccine available for avian flu, but studies are underway to develop an effective vaccine and treatment options for the disease. EMS providers are encouraged to visit the CDC web site for updates.

General Postexposure Management

In many instances, you will not know that a patient has an airborne or bloodborne disease, and you may be exposed without knowing it. The Ryan White Law requires that the hospital notify your department's designated officer, the individual in the department who is charged with the responsibility of managing exposures and infection control issues, within 48 hours of the time the hospital identifies the patient's disease. In the event of possible exposure, there should be a protocol in place to obtain information from your local hospital or other medical resource. You should be screened and given information about the necessity of medical follow-up. Treatment depends on the disease. Your designated officer will assist you with the necessary information.

If you experience a needlestick injury or some other unprotected exposure to blood, you must notify your department's designated officer as soon as possible and complete an incident report. The designated officer can contact the hospital for information and the hospital has 48 hours to report back to the designated officer. Depending on your state laws and whether it is possible, patient testing is completed, followed by baseline testing on you. Because there are many diseases for which there are no outward signs of infection, your best protection lies in the use of PPE and/or prompt reporting of exposure. Be familiar with the postexposure protocols outlined in your department's exposure control plan.

Infection Control Routine Review

Infection control includes the safe practices and procedures to reduce infection in health care providers and patients. These practices should be established by policy as part of your regular, daily work routine. Remember the following steps on every call:

1. En route to the scene, make sure that all equipment is out and available.
2. On arrival, make sure the scene is safe to enter, perform a quick visual assessment of the patient, noting whether any blood or body fluid is present.
3. Select the proper PPE according to the tasks you are likely to perform.

4. Change gloves and wash hands between patients; do not unnecessarily delay treatment for use of PPE. Remove gloves and other gear after contact with the patient, unless you are in the patient compartment. Remember that good hand washing is always necessary.

5. Limit the number of providers in contact with the patient at significantly contaminated scenes (large amounts of blood) and with patients known or highly suspected to have an infectious disease.

6. If you or your partner is exposed while providing care, try to relieve one another as soon as possible so that you can seek care. Notify the designated officer and report the incident. This will also help to maintain confidentiality. Be sure to routinely clean the ambulance after each run and on a daily basis.

Cleaning is an essential part of the prevention and control of communicable diseases and will remove surface organisms that may remain in the unit. Clean your unit as quickly as possible so that you can return to service. Address the high-contact areas, including surfaces that were in direct contact with the patient's blood or body fluids or surfaces that you touched while caring for the patient.

You can use a solution of bleach and water at a 1:10 dilution to clean the unit. A hospital-approved disinfectant that is effective against *M tuberculosis* can also be used. Do not use alcohol or aerosol spray products to clean your unit. Pay attention to disinfectant directions. Some need to remain on the surface for a few minutes to work effectively. Review the regulations defining medical waste in your area. The disposal of infectious waste, such as sharps and heavily soiled dressings, may vary.

Scene Hazards

As an EMT-B, you are at risk for many different types of scene hazards. Unfortunately, some of these situations can be a threat to life. You should always be aware of the potential for scene hazards and take action to properly protect yourself or to avoid the hazard completely.

Hazardous Materials

Your safety is the most important consideration at a hazardous materials incident. On arrival at a potential HazMat scene, you should first try to read labels and identification numbers. All hazardous materials should be marked with safety placards, although this policy is not always followed. These placards are marked with colored diamond-shaped labels Figure 2-9 . Although it is important for you to

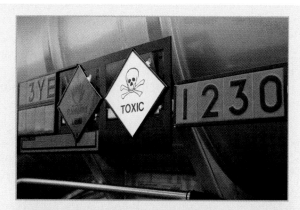
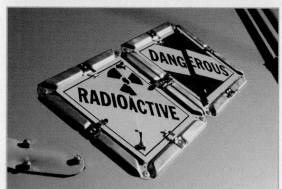

Figure 2-9 Hazardous materials safety placards are marked with colored, diamond-shaped labels.

You are the Provider 4

He finally agrees to go with you to the supervisor. He is enrolled in an employee assistance program and goes through several CISM sessions. He learns how to change his attitude about the things that he cannot change and how to manage his time more wisely to include family time. He is started on a new diet and exercise program and is back at work after two weeks off.

obtain information from the placards, you should never approach any object marked with a placard.

It is useful to carry binoculars so that you can read placards from a safe distance. A specially trained and equipped hazardous materials team will be called to handle disposal of materials and removal of patients. Do not begin to care for patients until they have been moved away from the scene and are decontaminated or the scene is declared safe for you to enter.

The DOT's 2004 *Emergency Response Guidebook* is an important resource ⬤Figure 2-10 ▾. It lists most hazardous materials and the proper procedures for scene control and emergency care of patients. A copy of the guidebook and other information relevant to your area should be available in your unit or at the dispatch center. You should be able to begin proper emergency management as soon as the hazardous material is identified. Again, do not go into an area and risk exposure to yourself. Do not enter the area unless you are absolutely sure that no hazardous spill has occurred.

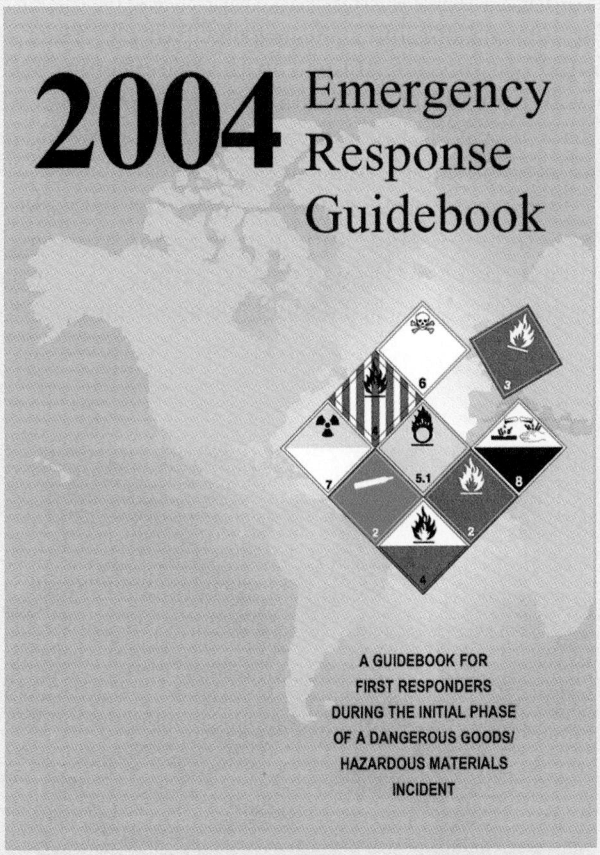

Hazardous materials are classified according to toxicity levels, which dictate the level of protection required. The toxicity levels—0, 1, 2, 3, 4—measure the risk the substance poses to an individual. The higher the number, the greater the toxicity and the greater the protection needed ⬤Table 2-4 ▾. It is important to remember the potential risks you face at a hazardous materials situation. Do not enter the scene unless it is safe.

Electricity

Electrical shock can be produced by human-made sources (power lines) or natural sources (lightning). No matter what the source, evaluate the risk to you and to the patient before you begin patient care.

Power Lines

The amount of current that is involved greatly affects the level of risk for injury. Your local power company may offer training to evaluate the risks involved with electrical emergencies and procedures you should follow when dealing with power lines.

Energized, or "live" power lines, especially high-voltage lines, behave in unpredictable ways. You need

Figure 2-10 The DOT's 2004 *Emergency Response Guidebook* lists many hazardous materials and the proper procedures for scene control and emergency care of patients.

Table 2-4 Toxicity Levels of Hazardous Materials

Level	Hazard	Protection Needed
0	Little to no hazard	None
1	Slightly hazardous	Self-contained breathing apparatus only (level C suit)
2	Slightly hazardous	Self-contained breathing apparatus only (level C suit)
3	Extremely hazardous	Full protection, with no exposed skin (level A or B suit)
4	Minimal exposure causes death	Special HazMat gear (level A suit)

in depth training to be able to handle the equipment that is used in an electrical emergency. The equipment also has specific storage needs and requires careful cleaning. Dirt or other contaminants can make this equipment useless or dangerous.

At the scene of a motor vehicle crash, above-ground and below-grade power lines may become hazards. Disrupted overhead wires are usually a visible hazard. Always use caution even if you do not see sparks coming from the lines. Visible sparks are not always present in charged wires. The area around downed power lines is always a danger zone. This danger zone extends well beyond the immediate accident scene.

Use the utility poles as landmarks for establishing the perimeter of the danger zone. The danger zone must be a restricted area. Remember, the safety zone is one span of the power pole's distance. Only emergency personnel, equipment, and vehicles are allowed inside this area. Do not approach downed wires or touch anything that downed wires have come in contact with until qualified personnel have concluded that no risk of electrical injury exists. This may mean that you are unable to access a severely injured victim of a motor vehicle crash even though you can see and talk to him or her.

If you must enter this type of situation, be sure to wear the proper protective equipment according to the type of incident. A helmet and turnout gear are typically called for, though you cannot count on turnout gear for protection from electrical hazards.

Lightning

Lightning is a complex natural phenomenon. You are unwise to think that "lightning never strikes in the same place twice." If the right conditions remain, a repeat strike in the same area can occur. Lightning is a threat in two ways: through a direct hit and through ground current. After the lightning bolt strikes, the current drains along the earth, following the most conductive pathway. Although you should avoid high ground to avoid a direct strike, to avoid being injured by a ground current, stay away from drainage ditches, moist areas, small depressions, and wet ropes. Recognize the warning signs that occur just before a lightning strike. As your surroundings become charged, you may feel a slight tingling sensation on your skin, or your hair may even stand on end. In this situation, a strike may be imminent. Move immediately to the lowest possible area.

If you are caught in an open area, try to make yourself the smallest possible target for a direct hit or for ground current. To keep from being hit by the initial strike, stay away from projections from the ground, such as a single tree. Drop all equipment, particularly metal objects that project above your body. Avoid fences and other metal objects. These can transmit current from the initial strike over a long distance. Position yourself in a low crouch. This position exposes only your feet to the ground current. If you sit, both your feet and your buttocks are exposed. Place an object made of nonconductive material, such as a blanket, under your feet. Get inside a car or your unit, if possible, as vehicles will protect you from lightning.

Fire

EMT-Bs are often dispatched to the scene of a fire. There are five common hazards in a fire:

1. Smoke
2. Oxygen deficiency
3. High ambient temperatures
4. Toxic gases
5. Building collapse

Smoke is made up of particles of tar and carbon. These particles irritate the respiratory system on contact. Most smoke particles are trapped in the upper respiratory system, but many smaller particles enter the lungs. You must be trained in the use of appropriate airway protection, such as a self-contained breathing apparatus (SCBA) or a disposable short-term device, and have it available at all fire scenes **Figure 2-11▼**.

Fire consumes oxygen. Particularly in a closed space, such as a room, fire may consume most of the available oxygen. This will make breathing difficult for anyone in that space. The high ambient temperatures

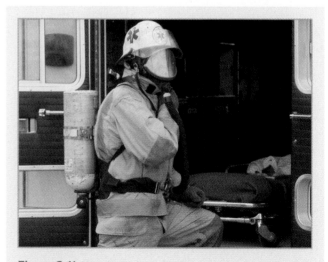

Figure 2-11 You should be trained in SCBA use and have it available if you may be working near fire scenes.

in a fire can result in thermal burns and damage to the respiratory system. Breathing air that is heated above 120°F (49°C) can damage the respiratory system.

A typical building fire emits a number of toxic gases, including carbon monoxide and carbon dioxide. Carbon monoxide is a colorless, odorless gas that is responsible for more fire deaths each year than any other byproduct of combustion. Carbon monoxide combines with the hemoglobin in your red blood cells about 200 times more readily than oxygen does. It blocks the ability of the hemoglobin to transport oxygen to your body tissues. Carbon dioxide is also a colorless, odorless gas. Exposure causes increased respirations, dizziness, and sweating. Breathing concentrations of carbon dioxide greater than 10% to 12% will result in death within a few minutes.

During and after a fire, there is always a possibility that all or part of the burned structure will collapse. Often, there are no warning signs. As an EMS provider, you should never enter a burning building without proper breathing apparatus and the approval of the incident commander at the scene. Hasty entry into a burning structure may result in serious injury and possibly death. Once inside a burning building, you are subject to an uncontrolled, hostile environment. Fires are not selective about their victims. You must be extremely cautious whenever you are near a burning structure or one in which a fire has just been placed under control. At any fire scene, follow the instructions of the incident commander and safety officer and never undertake any task (ie, enter a burning structure or initiate search and rescue) unless you have been properly trained to do so.

Fuel and fuel systems of vehicles that have been involved in crashes are also a hazard. Although this rarely happens, any leaking car fuel may ignite under the right conditions. If you see or smell a fuel leak, or if people are trapped in the vehicle, you must coordinate appropriate fire protection. Gasoline and other auto fluids are considered hazardous materials.

Make sure that you are properly protected if there is or has been a fire in the vehicle. Wear appropriate respiratory protection and thermal protection, as the smoke from a vehicle fire contains many toxic by-products. The use of appropriate protective gear at a crash scene can reduce your risk of injury. Avoid using oxygen in or near a vehicle that is smoking, smoldering, or leaking fuel.

■ Violent Situations

The safety of you and your team is of primary concern. Civil disturbances, domestic disputes, and crime scenes, especially those involving gangs, can create many hazards for EMS personnel. Large gatherings of hostile or potentially hostile people are also dangerous. Several agencies will respond to large civil disturbances. In these instances, it is important for you to know who is in command and controlling the scene. However, you and your partner may be on your own when a group of people seems to grow larger and become increasingly hostile. In these cases, you should call law enforcement immediately if they are not already present. You may need to wait for law enforcement to arrive before you can begin treatment or safely approach a patient.

Remember that you and your partner must be protected from the dangers at the scene before you can provide patient care. Law enforcement must make sure the scene is safe before you and your partner enter. A crime scene often poses potential problems for EMS personnel. If the perpetrator is still somewhere on the scene, this person could reappear and threaten you and your partner or attempt to further injure the patient you are treating. Bystanders who are trying to be helpful may interfere with your emergency medical care. Family members may be very distraught and not understand what you are doing when you attempt to splint an injured extremity and the patient cries out in pain. Be sure that you have adequate assistance from the appropriate public safety agency in these situations.

There is a potential that you will be at a scene where a dangerous situation is underway, such as a hostage situation or riot. In these instances, it may be necessary for EMS personnel to be protected from projectiles such as bullets, bottles, and rocks. Law enforcement personnel will ordinarily provide for concealment or cover of personnel who are involved in the response to the incident. Cover and concealment involve the tactical use of an impenetrable barrier for protection. EMT-Bs should not be placed in a position that will endanger their lives or safety during such incidents. Do not depend on someone else for your safety.

Remember that your personal safety is of the utmost importance. You must thoroughly understand the risks of each environment you enter. Whenever

Teamwork Tips

Set up a staging area away from the fire and wait for fire fighters to bring the patients to you.

you are in doubt about your safety, do not put yourself at risk. Never enter an unstable environment, such as a shooting, a fight, a hostage situation, or a riot. Always evaluate the scene for the potential for violence during your scene size-up. If violence is a possibility, call for additional resources. Failure to do so may put you and your partner at serious risk. When appropriate, allow law enforcement personnel to secure the scene before you approach; they have the necessary experience and expertise in handling these situations.

Other Considerations

Remember to attempt to maintain the chain of evidence at any potential crime scene. Do not disturb the scene unless it is absolutely necessary in caring for the patient. Animals, such as dogs, can also present a hazard. Reasonable requests to secure an animal with a leash or place an animal in another room are usually well received by those at the scene.

As an EMT-B, you know that issues of scene safety and personal protection are of the utmost importance to your own well-being. Protect yourself from the risk present at every scene—infectious disease—by following proper BSI precautions. Know and follow your department's infectious disease control policy. Protect yourself and your partner from potential hazards with awareness and early recognition of hazardous materials and potential scenes of violence. Remember that your safety is your number one priority. Never hesitate to request additional help and resources.

You are the Provider Summary

EMS is a high-stress job. To prevent stress from affecting your life negatively, you need to understand what stress is, how it affects you physically, and what you can do to minimize these effects. Your personal well-being is an integral part of how you perform your duties as an EMT-B. Learn the warning signs and seek treatment early.

1. **What problem is this EMT experiencing?**

   Stress.

2. **What physical signs might you expect to see?**

   Increased respirations, heart rate, and blood pressure
   Cool, clammy skin
   Dilated pupils
   Tensed muscles
   Perspiration

3. **What would you suggest to him?**

   He needs to seek treatment. CISM or counseling may be helpful.

4. **What do the vital signs tell you?**

   That he is experiencing the physiologic responses to stress.

5. **What is the body's first response to stress?**

   An alarm response followed by a stage of reaction and resistance.

6. **If not corrected, what will this lead to?**

   Exhaustion and burnout.

7. **What type of negative stressors is he experiencing?**

   Nursing home abuse, death of a child, repeat ambulance abuse, problems at home, guilt, apathy, long work hours

8. **What might help with his problems?**

   Counseling, proper nutrition and exercise, more time off, expanding his social network, etc.

9. **Has he had any events that could trigger critical incident stress?**

   Yes, the death of the child. Even though the child was not under his care, he still felt responsible.

10. **Name a positive stressor that may help.**

    Exercise is great because it stresses the body and makes it healthier.

Prep Kit

Ready for Review

- When signs of stress such as fatigue, anxiety, anger, feelings of hopelessness, worthlessness, or guilt, and other such indicators manifest themselves, behavioral problems can develop.
- Recognizing the signs of stress is important for all EMT-Bs.
- Every patient encounter should be considered to be potentially dangerous. It is essential that you take all available precautions to minimize exposure and risk to scene hazards and infectious and communicable diseases.
- Even if you are exposed to an infectious disease, your risk of becoming ill is low.
- Whether or not an acute infection occurs depends on several factors, including the amount and type of infectious organism and your resistance to that infection.
- You can take several steps to protect yourself against exposure to infectious diseases, including:
  - keeping up-to-date with recommended vaccinations
  - using universal precautions
  - following BSI precautions at all times
  - handling all needles and other sharp objects with great care
- Because it is often impossible to tell which patients have infectious diseases, you should avoid direct contact with the blood and body fluids of all patients.
- If you think you may have been exposed to an infectious disease, see your physician (or your department's designated physician) immediately.
- You should know what to do if you are exposed to an airborne or bloodborne disease. Your department's designated officer will be able to assist.
- Infection control should be an important part of your daily routine. Be sure to follow the proper steps when dealing with potential exposure situations.
- Scene hazards include potential exposure to:
  - Hazardous materials
  - Electricity
  - Fire
- At a hazardous materials incident, your safety is the most important consideration. Never approach an object labeled with a hazardous materials placard. Use binoculars to read the placards from a safe distance.
- Do not begin caring for patients until they have been moved away from the scene and decontaminated by the hazardous materials team or the scene has been made safe for you to enter.
- Electrical shock can be produced by power lines or by lightning.
- There are five common hazards in a fire:
  - Smoke
  - Oxygen deficiency
  - High ambient temperatures
  - Toxic gases
  - Building collapse
- Violent situations such as civil disturbances, domestic disputes, and crime scenes can create many hazards for EMS personnel.
- If you see the potential for violence during a scene size-up, call for additional resources.

Vital Vocabulary

body substance isolation (BSI) An infection control concept and practice that assumes that all body fluids are potentially infectious.

burnout A condition of chronic fatigue and frustration that results from mounting stress over time.

carrier An animal or person who is infected with and may transmit an infectious disease but may not display any symptoms of it; also known as a vector.

contamination The presence of infectious organisms on or in objects such as dressings, water, food, needles, wounds, or a patient's body.

cover and concealment The tactical use of an impenetrable barrier to conceal EMS personnel and protect them from projectiles (eg, bullets, bottles, rocks).

critical incident stress debriefing (CISD) A confidential group discussion of a highly traumatic incident that usually occurs within 24 to 72 hours of the incident.

critical incident stress management (CISM) A process that confronts the responses to critical incidents and defuses them, directing the emergency services personnel toward physical and emotional equilibrium.

designated officer The individual in the department charged with the responsibility of managing exposures and infection control issues.

direct contact Exposure or transmission of a communicable disease from one person to another by physical touching.

exposure A situation in which a person has had contact with blood, body fluids, tissues, or airborne particles in a manner that suggests that disease transmission may occur.

Technology

- Interactivities
- Vocabulary Explorer
- Anatomy Review
- Web Links
- Online Review Manual

Refresher.EMSzone.com

exposure control plan   A comprehensive plan that helps employees reduce their risk of exposure to or acquisition of communicable diseases.

general adaptation syndrome   The body's three-stage response to stress. First, stress causes the body to trigger an alarm response, followed by a stage of reaction and resistance, and then recovery, or if the stress is prolonged, exhaustion.

hazardous material   Any substance that is toxic, poisonous, radioactive, flammable, or explosive, and may cause injury or death with exposure.

hepatitis   Inflammation of the liver, usually caused by a viral infection, that causes fever, loss of appetite, jaundice, fatigue, and altered liver function.

indirect contact   Exposure or transmission of disease from one person to another by contact with a contaminated object.

infection control   Procedures to reduce transmission of infection among patients and health care personnel.

meningitis   An inflammation of the meningeal coverings of the brain and spinal cord; it is usually caused by a virus or a bacterium.

Occupational Safety and Health Administration (OSHA)   The governmental agency that develops, publishes, and enforces guidelines concerning safety in the workplace, including infectious diseases and minimum training requirements.

personal protective equipment (PPE)   Protective equipment worn by EMS providers to prevent injury or disease transmission.

tuberculosis   A chronic bacterial disease, caused by *Mycobacterium tuberculosis*, that usually affects the lungs but can also affect other organs such as the brain or kidneys.

universal precautions   Protective measures that have been developed by the Centers for Disease Control and Prevention for use in dealing with objects, blood, body fluids, or other items which are associated with a risk of communicable disease.

virulence   The strength or ability of a pathogen to produce disease.

Assessment in Action

It has been a very busy day. You have delivered your fifth patient of the day to the emergency department and it is just past lunch. One of the nurses pulls you off to the side to tell you that one of the patients brought in earlier is being tested for possible TB. The patient was coughing a lot and said he had been treated a week ago for an upper respiratory infection that had been ongoing for several weeks.

1. What is the best protection for you when transporting a patient with possible TB?
    A. surgical mask
    B. HEPA respirator
    C. gown and goggles
    D. face shield

2. How is tuberculosis transmitted?
    A. direct contact
    B. indirect contact
    C. vector borne
    D. airborne

3. Tuberculosis patients who pose the highest contagious risk almost always have _____.
    A. hemoptysis
    B. a rash
    C. a cough
    D. a resistance to drugs

4. If you have an exposure, when should you notify your department's designated officer?
    A. within 24 hours
    B. within 48 hours
    C. after the disease has been identified
    D. immediately

5. What is the most common type of personal protective equipment?
    A. masks
    B. goggles
    C. gloves
    D. boots

6. What is the preferred infection control concept for EMS and fire personnel?
    A. PPE
    B. BSI
    C. universal precautions
    D. CDC

Challenging Questions

7. Why do health care workers receive tuberculin skin tests on a regular basis even if no known exposure has occurred?

8. What is a carrier?

Medical and Legal Issues

You are the Provider 1

You are assessing a 34-year-old man who fell from the top of a scaffold approximately 15' high. He presents with multiple contusions and abrasions, including a golf ball-sized hematoma above his left eye. He tells your partner that he may have passed out and he was slightly light-headed, but he drank some water and he feels better. He is not sure he wants to be "checked out."

Initial Assessment	Recording Time: 0 Minutes
Appearance	Warm, diaphoretic
Level of consciousness	Alert and oriented
Airway	Open and clear
Breathing	Rapid and deep
Circulation	Radials present, bounding

1. What must you do before touching the patient?
2. What is the charge for touching without consent?
3. How will you convince him that he needs medical treatment?

Introduction

A basic principle of emergency care is to do no further harm. Simply stated, your goal should be to deliver the patient to the receiving facility in the same or better condition as you found him or her. A health care provider who acts in good faith and is following the standard of care will rarely be involved in any legal actions. However, as EMS has become more involved in our health care system and the profession has progressed to include more complex treatments and skills, public expectation has increased. For this reason and others, we have seen an increase in lawsuits involving EMS personnel.

Even when you provide the proper care to a patient, there are times when you may be sued by a patient or their family. There are also state EMS agency regulations that you must follow. Failure to do so may result in your EMT-B license or certificate being suspended or revoked. Do Not Resuscitate orders, patient confidentiality, and possible abuse situations also have legal and ethical implications that EMT-Bs should understand.

Consent

Under most circumstances, consent is required from every conscious, mentally competent adult before care can be started. A person receiving care must give permission, or consent, for treatment. An injured or sick adult that is in control of his or her actions has a legal right to refuse your care. You cannot treat these patients. An EMT-B who provides care to a person who has refused treatment may face both criminal and civil action, such as assault and battery. Consent can be

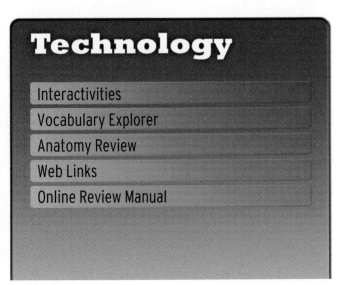

Technology

Interactivities

Vocabulary Explorer

Anatomy Review

Web Links

Online Review Manual

Refresher.EMSzone.com

Documentation Tips

When transporting a minor or mentally incompetent patient without consent from a parent or guardian, thoroughly document your reasons for transport.

- Significant mechanism of injury
- Unstable vital signs
- Compromise of airway, breathing, or circulation, etc.

Transporting without proper cause or poor documentation could result in charges of kidnapping.

---

actual or implied and can involve the care of a minor or a mentally incompetent patient.

Expressed Consent

Expressed consent is consent in which the patient speaks or acknowledges that he or she wants you to provide care. This type of consent must be informed consent, which means that the patient has been told of the potential risks, benefits, and alternatives to treatment and has agreed to the treatment. The legal concept is that the patient has a right to determine what is done to his or her body. The patient must be of legal age and able to make a rational decision.

Implied Consent

When a person is unconscious and unable to give consent or when an immediate threat to life exists, the law assumes that the patient would consent to care and transport to a medical facility ◖ Figure 3-1 ▶ ◗. This implied consent is limited to life-threatening emergency situations and is appropriate when the patient is unconscious, delusional, unresponsive as a result of drug or alcohol use, or otherwise unable to give expressed consent. In most instances, the law allows the spouse or another close relative to give consent for a patient who is unable to do so.

Minors and Consent

Because a minor might not have the wisdom, maturity, or judgment to give valid consent, the law requires that a parent or legal guardian give consent for treatment or transport. However, in some states, a minor can give consent to receive medical care, depending

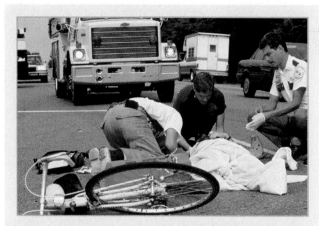
Figure 3-1 When an immediate threat to life exists and the patient is unconscious and unable to give consent, the law assumes that the patient would consent to care and transport to a medical facility.

on age and maturity. Many states also allow emancipated, married, or pregnant minors to be treated as adults for the purposes of consenting to medical treatment. Obtain consent from a parent or legal guardian whenever possible. If a true emergency exists and the parent or legal guardian is not available, the consent to treat the minor is implied, just as with an adult.

Mentally Incompetent Adults

Providing care for patients who are mentally ill, suffering from a behavioral emergency, under the influence of drugs or alcohol, or are developmentally delayed is complicated. An adult patient who is mentally incompetent is not able to give informed consent. This situation, from a legal perspective, is similar to treating minors. Try to obtain consent from someone with legal responsibility for the patient, such as a guardian or conservator. In most situations, however, such permission will not be readily obtainable. Many states have protective custody statutes allowing for these types of patients to be taken to a medical facility under law enforcement authority. Review the laws in your area. Remember that when a life-threatening emergency exists, you can assume that implied consent exists.

Forcible Restraint

Forcible restraint is the act of physically preventing an individual from any physical action. Restraining a mentally disturbed patient may be required before emergency care can be rendered. If you believe that a patient will injure him/herself or others, you can legally restrain the patient. You must follow your lo-

cal protocol—whether by standing orders, contacting medical control, or involving law enforcement to restrain the patient. In some states, only a law enforcement officer may forcibly restrain an individual Figure 3-2 ▼.

Your department should have clearly defined protocols to deal with situations involving restraints. Unless the restraints pose a risk to the patient, do not remove the restraints once they have been applied, even if the patient promises to behave.

Remember that if the patient is conscious and the situation is not urgent, consent is required. Adults who appear to be in control of their senses cannot be forced to accept your care or transport to a medical facility. Adults are not legally required to make "correct" decisions, or to agree with medical advice.

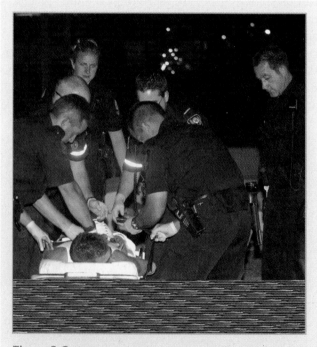
Figure 3-2 Know your local protocol regarding restraining a patient. In some states, only a law enforcement officer has the authority to restrain a patient.

■ The Right to Refuse Treatment

Mentally competent adults have the right to refuse treatment or withdraw from treatment at any time. If a patient refuses treatment or transport, you must make sure that he or she understands (is informed about) the potential risks, benefits, treatments, and alternatives to treatment—encourage the patient to ask questions. Remember that competent adults who refuse specific treatment for themselves based on religious reasons generally have a legal right to do so. Document all refusals according to your department's policy.

When a patient refuses treatment, you must assess whether the patient's mental condition is impaired. If the patient refusing treatment is confused or delusional, you cannot assume that the refusal is an informed refusal. When in doubt, it is always best to provide care. Providing treatment is a much more defensible position than failing to treat, which may be considered negligence. Do not place yourself in danger to provide care. Use law enforcement to ensure your own safety in these situations.

You may also be faced with a situation in which a parent refuses to allow you to treat an ill or injured child. You must consider the emotional impact of the emergency on the parent's judgment. In this and virtually all cases of refusal, you can usually resolve the situation with patience and calm persuasion. You may also need the help of others, such as medical control or law enforcement.

As you have probably already experienced, there are times when you are not able to persuade the patient, guardian, or parent of a minor or mentally incompetent patient to allow you to provide treatment. In this situation, obtain the signature of the individual who is refusing care on an official release form that acknowledges the refusal. Document any assessment findings and emergency care that you provide. Also, obtain a signature from a witness to the refusal. In addition to the release form, be sure to document the refusal on the patient care report and keep the two forms together. If the patient refuses to sign the refusal form, follow your department's policy. This typically requires you to document the situation and the patient's refusal to sign on the patient care report.

■ Advance Directives

Occasionally, you may respond to a call in which a patient is dying from an illness. When you arrive on scene, you may find that family members present do not want you to try to resuscitate the patient. Without valid written documentation from a physician, such as an advance directive or a Do Not Resuscitate (DNR) order (also known as a "Do Not Attempt Resuscitation" order or a "no code"), this type of request places you in a difficult position. An <u>advance directive</u> is a written document, from a competent patient, that specifies medical treatment should he or she become unable to make health care decisions. An advance directive is also commonly called a living will. There are

You are the Provider 2

You explain to him the potential for injury based on the way he presents and the mechanism of injury. He says that he is sure he passed out but does not want to spend the rest of the day at the hospital. He thinks he will just wait and go later if he feels worse.

Vital Signs	Recording Time: 2 Minutes
Skin	Warm, diaphoretic
Pulse	98 beats/min, strong
Blood pressure	132/84 mm Hg
Respirations	22 breaths/min, deep

4. What might you offer other than transport?

5. If he still refuses, what should you do?

6. What are the potential consequences of trying to restrain this patient "for his own good"?

several types of advance directives. Not all advance directives are directions from the patient to withhold all medical care. For example, a comfort care order is an advance directive that specifies care a person should receive in the event that he or she becomes incompetent and is unable to make health care decisions.

DNR orders allow you *not* to attempt resuscitation when you otherwise would. Although laws differ from state to state, there are some general guidelines regarding DNR orders. DNR orders:

- Should clearly state the patient's medical problem(s)
- Be signed by the patient or legal guardian
- Be signed by a physician

In some states, the DNR order must have an expiration date (usually within the past year to be valid). However, some states do not require an expiration date—you should be familiar with the laws in your area. Even in the presence of a valid DNR, you are still obligated to provide supportive measures (oxygen, pain relief, and comfort) to a patient who is not in cardiac arrest. Each EMS agency, in consultation with its medical director and legal counsel, must develop a protocol to follow in these circumstances.

EMT-Bs are dealing with these situations on a more frequent basis due to increased numbers of patients in nursing homes and hospice and home health care programs. As previously stated, laws and guidelines vary from state to state regarding advance directives and DNR orders; however, the following statements are general guidelines and are a good review:

1. **Patients have the right to refuse treatment,** including resuscitative efforts, provided that they are able to communicate their wishes.

Documentation Tips

When documenting a competent patient's refusal, be sure to include the following:

- All assessment findings
- Any care given
- Your explanation to the patient of potential risks associated with refusal of care
- Witness signatures
- That the patient was advised to call EMS back if needed

2. **A written order from a physician is required** for DNR orders to be valid in a health care facility.
3. **You should periodically review** state and local protocols and legislation regarding advance directives.
4. **When you are in doubt** or the written orders are not present, you have an obligation to resuscitate.

■ Confidentiality

Communication between you and the patient is considered confidential and generally cannot be disclosed without permission from the patient or a court order. Confidential information includes the patient history, assessment findings, and treatment provided. If you disclose information regarding a patient's condition or treatment without the patient's consent, you may find yourself liable for breach of confidentiality.

In certain situations, you may release confidential information to designated individuals. In most states, records may be released when a legal subpoena is presented or the patient signs a written release. The patient must be mentally competent and fully understand the nature of the release.

Another means for disclosing information is with an automatic release, which does not require a written release from the patient. This type of release allows you to share information with other health care providers so that they may continue caring for the patient.

In many states, you do not need a written release to report information about cases of rape or abuse to the proper authorities. Third-party payment billing forms may also be completed without written consent.

HIPAA

HIPAA stands for the Health Insurance Portability and Accountability Act of 1996. The original goals of this law included improving the portability and continuity of health insurance coverage and combating waste and fraud in health insurance and medical care. HIPAA standards affect EMS primarily relating to patient privacy. The aim of this section was to strengthen laws for the protection of the privacy of health care information and to safeguard patient confidentiality. As such, it provides guidance on what type of information is protected, the responsibility of health care providers regarding that protection, and penalties for breaching that protection.

In some areas, the law has limited the ability of EMS providers to obtain follow-up information about patients they treat and the degree to which they may have been exposed to a communicable disease as a result of a patient encounter.

Most personal health information is protected and should not be released without the patient's permission. If you are not sure, do not give any information to anyone other than those directly involved in the care of the patient. EMS agencies that meet the definition of a "covered entity" must have specific HIPAA policies and procedures that address patient confidentiality, release of information, and how personal health information is handled and secured by the agency. EMS agencies are also required to designate a HIPAA compliance officer and a HIPAA security officer (oftentimes this is the same person). Consult with your supervisor for any specific questions regarding HIPAA and your department; as always, you should know and follow your department's policies and procedures.

■ Special Reporting Requirements

Abuse of Children, the Elderly, and Others

As an EMT, you have probably had at least one experience involving the abuse or neglect of a child or an elderly person. Every state has laws that protect abused children, and some have added other protected groups such as the elderly and "at-risk" adults. Most states have a mandatory reporting obligation for certain individuals such as EMS providers, nurses, and physicians. You must be aware of the requirements of the law in your state. Such statutes frequently grant immunity from liability for libel, slander, or defamation of character to the individual who makes the report regardless of the final outcome as long as the reports are made in good faith.

Injury During the Commission of a Felony

Many states have laws requiring the reporting of any injury that is likely to have occurred during the commission of a crime such as gunshot wounds, knife wounds, or poisonings.

Drug-Related Injuries

In some instances, drug-related injuries must be reported. It should be noted that the US Supreme Court has ruled that drug addiction, in contrast to drug possession or sale, is an illness and not a crime. Therefore, an injury as a result of a drug overdose may not be within the definition of an injury resulting from a crime.

You are the Provider 3

He allows you to take his vital signs and your partner to apply a bandage to a large abrasion on his right forearm. He agrees to go to the hospital but refuses to be immobilized. He tells you that he is capable of walking and does not want to be carried.

A police officer arrives on scene to file an incident report since the patient was doing work for someone else. He asks for a copy of your patient care report (PCR) to put with his report.

Reassessment	Recording Time: 5 Minutes
Pulse	108 beats/min, strong
Blood pressure	136/92 mm Hg
Respirations	20 breaths/min, deep
Breath sounds	Clear bilaterally
Pulse oximetry	95% on room air

7. How should you handle the patient's request?

8. What type of consent is used to treat him?

9. Can you give the officer a copy of the PCR? Why or why not?

10. What should you do if the patient changes his mind en route to the hospital and refuses care?

Some states, by statute, specifically establish confidentiality and excuse certain individuals from reporting drug cases, either to a government agency or to a minor's parents, if, in the opinion of those individuals, withholding reporting is necessary for the proper treatment of the patient. You must be familiar with the legal requirements in your state.

Childbirth

Many states require that anyone who attends a live birth in any place other than a licensed medical facility report the birth. Again, you must be familiar with state requirements.

Other Reporting Requirements

Other reporting requirements may include attempted suicides, animal bites, certain communicable diseases, assaults, and rapes. Most EMS agencies require that all exposures to infectious diseases be reported. Check with your supervisor and be familiar with the policies on the reporting requirements for your department.

Crime Scenes

If there is evidence at a scene that a crime may have been committed, and law enforcement is not on scene, notify the dispatcher immediately so that law enforcement can respond. You should not stop providing lifesaving medical care; however, your safety is a priority, so you must ensure that the scene is safe to enter. You may have to transport the patient to the hospital before law enforcement arrives.

While providing care, be careful not to disturb the scene of the crime any more than is absolutely necessary. Notes and drawings should be made of the position of the patient when you first found him or her and of the presence and position of any weapons or other items that may be valuable to the investigating officers. If possible, do not cut through holes in clothing that were caused by a weapon or a gunshot.

In some states, EMT-Bs do not have the authority to pronounce a patient dead. If the patient is obviously dead and you are at a potential crime scene, do not move the body or disturb the scene. As before, it is a good idea to review your local protocol regarding this issue.

You are the Provider 4

The patient signs the refusal for immobilization and will not ride on the stretcher. He is secured to the bench seat with seat belts where he remains for the duration of the trip. He is treated at the hospital for a mild concussion and told to stay home from work for the rest of the week.

You are the Provider Summary

Not all patients will agree to treatment, even when they need it. Regardless of how you try and convince them, a competent patient can still refuse care. To protect yourself, you must provide thorough, accurate documentation that is properly signed and witnessed. Always tell any patient who is refusing care that he or she can always change his or her mind.

1. **What must you do before touching the patient?**

   Obtain consent from the patient.

2. **What is the charge for touching without consent?**

   Battery.

3. **How will you convince him that he needs medical treatment?**

   Explain to him that he has a significant mechanism of injury with great potential coupled with the loss of consciousness and the hematoma. He could have a head injury.

4. **What might you offer other than transport?**

   Assess his vital signs to see if they are within normal limits. If not, that may be a convincing factor for him to agree to transport.

5. **If he still refuses, what should you do?**

   Explain to him why he should go, what possible injuries he may have sustained, any assessment findings, and the ramifications of not seeking treatment. Have him sign a refusal and have it witnessed by law enforcement, a neighbor, etc.

6. **What are the potential consequences of trying to restrain this patient "for his own good"?**

   Restraining an alert and oriented patient against his will can result in the EMT-B being charged with assault, battery, and kidnapping.

7. **How should you handle the patient's request?**

   You should explain why you feel he needs to be immobilized and if he still refuses, document thoroughly the refusal and have him sign along with a witness.

8. **What type of consent is used to treat him?**

   Informed. You have explained the possible risks and benefits and he has agreed to treatment.

9. **Can you give the officer a copy of the PCR? Why or why not?**

   No. This would constitute a breach of confidentiality. If it turned into a lawsuit, the trip report could be subpoenaed for evidence.

10. **What should you do if the patient changes his mind en route to the hospital and refuses care?**

    Try to convince him to go, but if all else fails, document thoroughly and have him sign the refusal. Release him from the ambulance with the understanding that he can still call if he changes his mind.

Prep Kit

Ready for Review

- You must obtain consent from a patient before providing care. A conscious, rational adult patient can give you expressed consent. Expressed consent must also be informed consent.
- When a patient is unconscious and unable to give consent, the law assumes implied consent. You should try to obtain consent from a parent or guardian when your patient is a minor.
- Mentally competent patients have the right to refuse care. In these instances, have the patient sign a refusal form.
- An advance directive is a written document that specifies medical treatment in the event that a mentally competent patient becomes unable to make a health care decision.
- You should never withhold lifesaving care unless a valid DNR order is present.
- DNR orders give you permission to not attempt resuscitation in the event of cardiac arrest. You should be familiar with your department's protocols regarding advance directives and DNR orders.
- Communication between you and the patient is confidential and should not be disclosed without permission from the patient or a court order.
- HIPAA stands for the Health Insurance Portability and Accountability Act of 1996. Its intent is to protect the patient's personal health information.
- You should know what the special reporting requirements are in your department involving child and elder abuse, injuries related to crimes, childbirth, animal bites, and drug-related injuries.

Vital Vocabulary

advance directive Written documentation that specifies medical treatment for a competent patient should the patient become unable to make decisions; also called a living will.

consent Granting permission to another to render care.

do not resuscitate (DNR) orders Written documentation giving permission to medical personnel not to attempt resuscitation in the event of cardiac arrest.

expressed consent A type of consent in which a patient gives expressed authorization for provision of care or transport.

implied consent Type of consent in which a patient who is unable to give consent is given treatment under the legal assumption that he or she would want treatment.

informed consent Permission for treatment given by a competent patient after the potential risks, benefits, and alternatives to treatment have been explained and are understood.

Technology

Interactivities

Vocabulary Explorer

Anatomy Review

Web Links

Online Review Manual

Assessment in Action

During the course of each shift, an EMT-B can be exposed to numerous medical and legal challenges. Your actions in any given situation may result in legal action against you and/or the service for which you work. A good understanding of legal issues and providing proper patient care are your best protection.

1. An emancipated minor is one who is:
   A. married.
   B. pregnant.
   C. in the military.
   D. all of the above.

2. During a life-threatening emergency, minors or mentally incompetent adults are treated under what type of consent?
   A. expressed
   B. implied
   C. informed
   D. legal

3. What should you do when a patient is in cardiac arrest and family members tell you there are DNR orders but cannot produce them?
   A. Do nothing.
   B. Begin resuscitation.
   C. Wait for the family to find the orders before proceeding.
   D. Transport the patient to the morgue.

4. Which of the following is considered confidential information?
   A. patient history
   B. assessment findings
   C. treatment provided
   D. all of the above

5. _____ consent means that the risks, benefits, and alternatives to treatment have been explained.
   A. expressed
   B. implied
   C. informed
   D. legal

Challenging Questions

6. What is the proper procedure when a competent patient refuses treatment?

7. What is the difference between an advance directive and a DNR order?

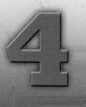

Lifting and Moving Patients

You are the Provider 1

You and your partner are on the second floor of an apartment building with a patient who needs to be transported. The patient is a 57-year-old woman with congestive heart failure who is in mild respiratory distress. She is propped up in her bed on several pillows. She is a large woman and you and your partner do not feel comfortable carrying her. An engine company is on the way to assist you.

Initial Assessment	Recording Time: 0 Minutes
Appearance	Flushed
Level of consciousness	Alert and oriented
Airway	Open and clear
Breathing	A little fast and shallow
Circulation	Radials present, irregular

1. What are your priorities for this patient?
2. What are your primary considerations for moving her?

■ Introduction

In your experience as an EMT-B, you have undoubtedly faced many challenges in lifting, moving, and carrying patients in and out of difficult places. You know that during the course of the call, you have to move a patient several times to provide care and transport to the hospital. Many EMS providers have been injured while lifting, moving, or carrying patients. It is important to review safety precautions and lifting guidelines for your own personal health and safety, and for those who work with you.

Lifting and carrying are dynamic processes. To reduce the risk of injury to yourself, your team members, or the patient, you must know where to position your team members and how to direct everyone so that all parties act in unison. This chapter will cover lifting, carrying, and reaching techniques as well as principles of moving patients that include emergency, urgent, and nonurgent moves.

■ Body Mechanics

When standing upright, the weight of anything lifted and carried in the hands is distributed to the shoulder girdle, spinal column, pelvis, and then to the legs Figure 4-1▼. If your body is aligned properly when you lift, the line of force exerted on the spine occurs in an essentially straight line down the vertebrae Figure 4-2▶. In this way, the strong stacked vertebrae support the lift, very little strain occurs in the muscles and ligaments that keep the spinal column in alignment, and significant weight can be lifted and carried without injury to the back. However, you may injure your back if you lift with your back curved Figure 4-3▶. Two key rules of lifting are to always keep the back in a straight, upright position and to lift without twisting.

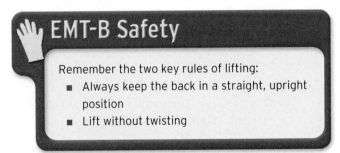

EMT-B Safety

Remember the two key rules of lifting:
- Always keep the back in a straight, upright position
- Lift without twisting

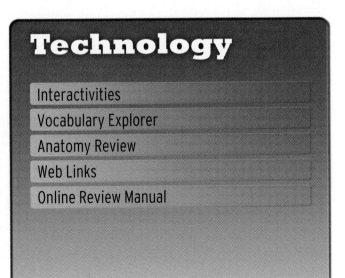

Technology

Interactivities

Vocabulary Explorer

Anatomy Review

Web Links

Online Review Manual

Refresher.EMSzone.com

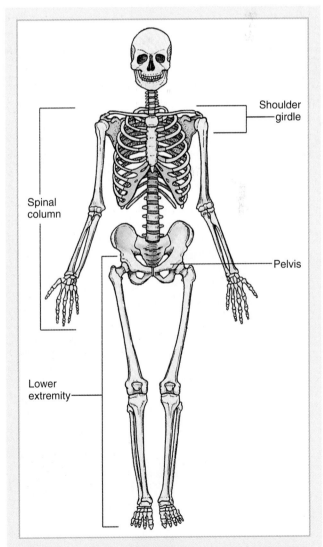

Figure 4-1 When you are standing upright, the weight of anything that you lift and carry in your hands is borne by the shoulder girdle, the spinal column, the pelvis, and the legs.

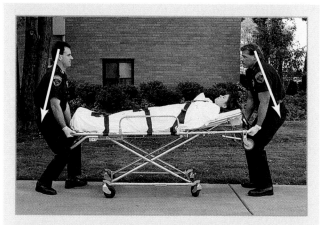

Figure 4-2 If your body is properly aligned when you lift, the line of force exerted against the spine occurs in an essentially straight line down the vertebrae. In this way, the vertebrae support the lift.

When lifting, you should spread your legs about 15" apart (shoulder width) and place your feet so that your center of gravity is balanced properly between them. Then, with the back held upright, bring your upper body down by bending the legs. Once you have properly grasped the patient or cot and made any necessary adjustments in the location of your feet, lift

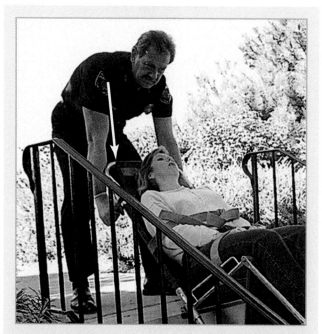

Figure 4-3 You may be injured if you lift with your back curved, as the lifting force is exerted primarily across, rather than down, the spinal column. When this occurs, the muscles of the back, not the vertebrae, are supporting the lift.

EMT-B Safety

When pulling, never extend your arms more than 15" to 20" in front of your torso. Pull by slowly flexing your arms and then reposition before continuing the move.

by raising your upper body and arms and straightening your legs until you are again standing. Lifting by extending the properly placed flexed legs is also the most powerful and safest way to lift. This method is called a power lift. To lift safely with the power lift, follow these steps Skill Drill 4-1 ▶ :

1. **Tighten your back in its normal upright position** and use your abdominal muscles to lock it in a slight inward curve.
2. **Position your feet about 15" apart** (shoulder width) and bend your legs to lower your torso and arms.
3. **Grasp the stretcher or backboard with your hands held palms up** and just in front of you.
4. **Adjust your position** until the weight is balanced and centered between both arms (**Step ①**).
5. **With your arms extended down,** lift by straightening your legs until you are standing. Make sure your back is locked in and that your upper body comes up before your hips. Always keep the weight that you are lifting as close to your body as possible and avoid bending at the waist or twisting (**Steps ② and ③**).

Power Grip

You should use the power grip to get the maximum force from your hands whenever you are lifting Figure 4-4 ▶ . You have the greatest lifting strength when your hands are facing palm up. When you grasp a backboard or a stretcher, keep your hands at least 10" apart. Each hand should be inserted under the handle with the palm facing up. To maintain the power grip, make sure that the underside of the handle is fully supported on your curved palm with only the fingers and thumb preventing it from being pulled sideways or upward out of the palm. If you must lift the object higher once you have lifted by extending your legs, you will be able to "curl" the object higher by using your biceps to flex the arms while maintaining the power grip. Table 4-1 ▶ outlines the general principles of lifting.

Skill Drill 4-1 Power Lift

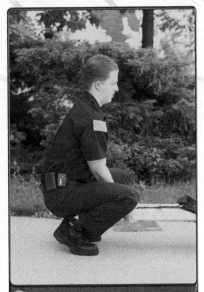

1 Position your feet about 15" apart (shoulder width) and bend your legs to lower your torso and arms. Grasp the backboard, palms up. Balance and center the weight between your arms.

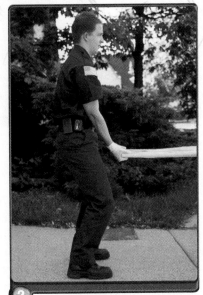

2 Lift by straightening your legs until you are standing. Make sure your back is locked in and that your upper body comes up before your hips.

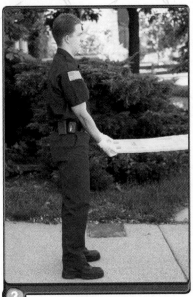

3 Keep the weight as close to your body as possible and avoid bending at the waist or twisting.

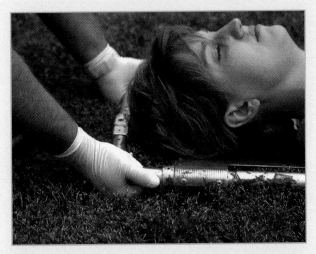

Figure 4-4 To perform the power grip, grasp the handle with your palms up. Make sure your hands are about 10" apart and that your fingers are all at the same angle.

Table 4-1 General Principles of Lifting

Be aware of your own physical abilities and limitations.

Always consider the patient's weight. Call for additional help if necessary.

Bend at your knees, not at your waist.

Use your legs, not your back, to lift.

Keep the weight as close to your body as possible.

Maintain your back in its normal curvature position. Lift without twisting.

Keep your feet properly positioned and balanced to maintain your center of gravity.

Communicate clearly and frequently with your partner.

Evenly distribute the weight.

■ Carrying

Whenever possible, you should use a device that can be rolled to move a patient. When a wheeled device is not available, you and your team will have to carry the patient on a backboard or similar device. If a patient is on a backboard or sitting or lying on a cot, his or her weight is not equally distributed between the two ends of the device. Between 68% and 78% of the body weight of a patient in a horizontal position is in the torso. Therefore, more of the patient's weight rests on the head half of the device than on the foot half. A patient on a backboard or cot should be lifted and carried by four rescuers in a <u>diamond carry</u>, with one EMT-B at the head of the device, one at the foot end, and one at each side of the patient's torso `Figure 4-5 ▶` .

You should use a <u>stair chair</u> instead of a backboard or stretcher, whenever possible, to carry a patient down stairs or other significant inclines `Skill Drill 4-2 ▶` .

1. **Secure the patient to the stair chair with straps.** At a minimum, use a lap belt at the hips and a strap around the chest. You should also strap the arms and hands if possible (**Step ①**).
2. **Position team members at the head and foot of the chair.** The EMT-B at the head will give directions to coordinate the lift and carry (**Step ②**).
3. **A third rescuer should precede the two carrying the stair chair** to help direct and guide the movements and to serve as a safety back-up (**Step ③**).

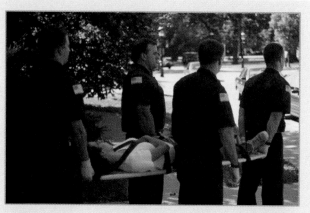

Figure 4-5 The diamond carry requires four EMT-Bs, one at the head, one at the feet, and one on each side of the patient.

4. **When you reach a landing or other flat interval,** lower the chair to the ground and roll it rather than carrying it. When you reach the cot, roll the chair into position next to the cot to transfer the patient (**Step ④**).

When you must use a backboard or stretcher, be sure that the patient is secured to the device so that he or she cannot slide significantly when the stretcher is at an angle `Skill Drill 4-3 ▶` .

1. **Apply a strap** tightly across the upper torso and through each armpit (but not over the arms) leaving the arms free. Secure the strap to the side handles to prevent the patient from sliding (**Step ①**).

You are the Provider 2

The stairs take a 90-degree turn halfway down making it impossible to use the stretcher. The fire department engine company has arrived and you have plenty of lifting assistance. You have placed her on a nonrebreathing mask at 15 L/min and she seems to be breathing a little easier. You ask if she can stand with assistance and her husband tells you that she cannot.

Vital Signs	Recording Time: 2 Minutes
Skin	Flushed
Pulse	102 beats/min, irregular
Blood pressure	172/108 mm Hg
Respirations	22 breaths/min, slightly shallow

3. How should you move the patient from the bed?
4. What might you use to move this patient down the stairs?
5. How should the rescuers be positioned for carrying the patient down the stairs?

Skill Drill   4-2   Using a Stair Chair

1 Secure the patient to the stair chair with straps.

2 Position team members at the head and foot of the chair.

3 A third rescuer "backs up" the EMT-B at the foot end.

4 Lower the chair to roll it on landings and for the transfer to the cot.

2. **When you carry the patient down stairs** or an incline, carry the backboard or stretcher with the foot end first so that the head end is elevated higher than the foot end. The straps should be secured to prevent the patient from sliding down or off the backboard (**Step 2**).

3. **When you carry a patient up stairs** or an incline, the elevated head end of the backboard or stretcher should go first (**Step 3**).

Always remember to keep your back in a locked-in position and to flex at the hips, not the waist. You should also bend at the knees and keep the patient's weight and your arms as close to your body as possible. Twisting while carrying or moving a patient will increase the risk of injury. Try to avoid any unnecessary lifting and carrying of the patient. If an assist, log

roll, or body drag will not harm or jeopardize the patient, use one to move the patient onto the backboard or cot.

■ Principles of Safe Reaching and Pulling

When you use a body drag to move a patient, the same basic body mechanics and principles apply as when lifting and carrying. Your back should always be locked and straight, not curved or bent laterally, and you should avoid any twisting. When you are reaching overhead, avoid hyperextending your back. When you are pulling a patient who is on the ground, you should always kneel to minimize the distance that

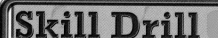

Skill Drill   4-3   Carrying a Patient on Stairs

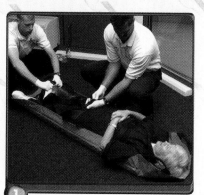

1 Strap the patient securely. Make sure one strap is across the upper torso and under the arms. Secure the strap to the side handles to prevent the patient from sliding.

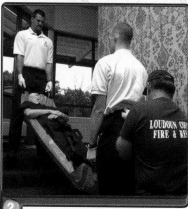

2 Carry the patient down the stairs with the foot end first, head elevated.

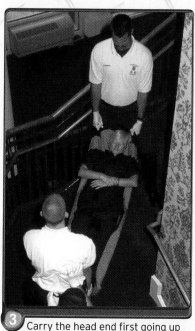

3 Carry the head end first going up stairs, always keeping the head elevated.

you will have to lean over Figure 4-6 A ▶. To keep your reach within the recommended distance, reach forward and grasp the patient so that your elbows are just in front of your chest Figure 4-6 B ▶. When you are pulling a patient who is at a different height from you, bend your knees until your hips are just below the height across from which you will be pulling the patient. When you are pulling, you should extend your arms no more than 15" to 20" in front of your torso. Reposition your feet (or knees, if kneeling) so that the force of the pull will be centered and balanced equally between both of your arms Figure 4-6 C ▶. Pull the patient by slowly flexing your arms. When you can pull no farther because your hands have reached the front of your torso, stop and move back another 15" to 20". When you are properly repositioned, repeat the steps.

◼ Moving and Positioning the Patient

Moving a patient should normally be done in an orderly, planned, and unhurried fashion. This approach will protect both you and the patient from further injury and reduce the risk of worsening the patient's condition when he or she is moved. On most calls you will have to lift and carry the patient to the cot, move the cot and patient to the ambulance, and load the cot into the patient compartment.

Emergency Moves

You should use an <u>emergency move</u> to move a patient before initial assessment and care are provided when there is potential danger, and you and the patient must move to a safe place to avoid serious harm or death.

Documentation Tips

If you must perform an emergency move, carefully document the reason for the move as well as an exact account of how the move was accomplished.

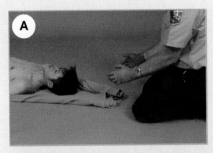
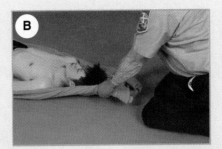
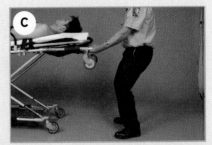

Figure 4-6 A-C Reaching and pulling safely. **A.** Kneel to pull a patient who is on the ground. **B.** When pulling, your elbows should be just in front of your chest. **C.** Bend your knees to pull a patient who is at a different height than you are. Position your feet to balance the force of the pull.

The presence of fire, explosives, or hazardous materials and your inability to protect the patient from harm or gain access to others that need lifesaving care are all situations in which you should use an emergency move.

The only other time you should use an emergency move is if you cannot properly assess the patient or provide immediate critical emergency care because of the patient's location or position. If you are alone and danger at the scene makes it necessary for you to use an emergency move, regardless of a patient's injuries, you should use a drag to pull the patient along the long axis of the body Figure 4-7 ▶. This will help keep the spinal column in line as much as possible. When performing an emergency move, one of your primary concerns is the danger of aggravating an existing spinal injury. Remember that it is impossible to remove a patient quickly from a vehicle while providing as much protection to the spine as you would give by using an immobilization device. However, if you follow certain guidelines during the move, you can usually move a patient from a life-threatening situation without causing further injury to the patient.

If you are alone and must remove an unconscious patient from a car, you should first move the patient's legs so they are clear of the pedals. Then rotate the patient so that his or her back is positioned toward the open car door. Next, place your arms through the armpits and support the patient's head against your body. While supporting the patient's weight, drag the

You are the Provider 3

The patient is lifted from the bed by four rescuers using a draw sheet. She is placed in a stair chair and the straps are secured in preparation for moving the patient down the stairs. She is scared that she may be dropped.

Reassessment	Recording Time: 5 Minutes
Pulse	112 beats/min, irregular
Blood pressure	172/108 mm Hg
Respirations	20 breaths/min, not quite as shallow
Breath sounds	Rales bilaterally
Pulse oximetry	96% on oxygen via nonrebreathing mask

6. What should you do before moving the patient?
7. Where should the stretcher be placed?
8. How should your hands be positioned when lifting to ensure maximum strength?
9. In what position should your back be kept when lifting?
10. Lifting and carrying are dynamic processes—what is meant by this?

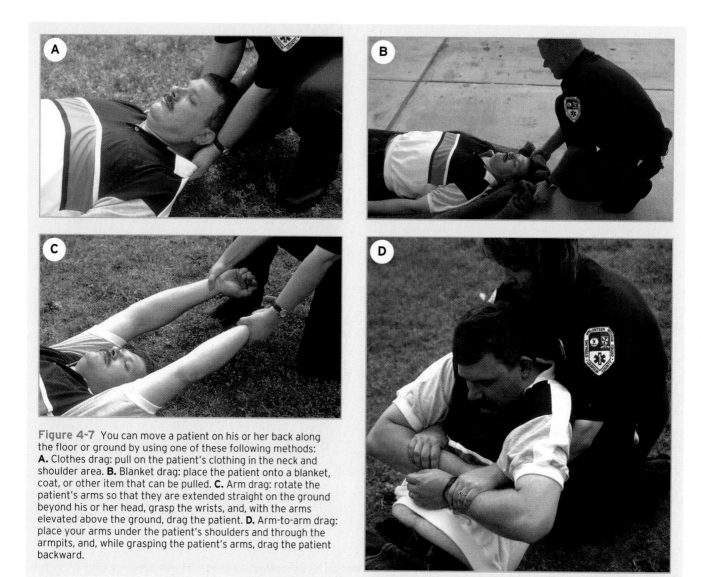

Figure 4-7 You can move a patient on his or her back along the floor or ground by using one of these following methods: **A.** Clothes drag: pull on the patient's clothing in the neck and shoulder area. **B.** Blanket drag: place the patient onto a blanket, coat, or other item that can be pulled. **C.** Arm drag: rotate the patient's arms so that they are extended straight on the ground beyond his or her head, grasp the wrists, and, with the arms elevated above the ground, drag the patient. **D.** Arm-to-arm drag: place your arms under the patient's shoulders and through the armpits, and, while grasping the patient's arms, drag the patient backward.

patient from the seat. If the legs and feet do not clear the car easily, you can slowly lower the patient until he or she is lying on his or her back next to the car, clear the legs from the vehicle, and, as previously described, use a long-axis body drag to move the patient a safe distance from the vehicle (Figure 4-8 ▶).

Urgent Moves

An urgent move may be necessary for moving a patient with an altered mental status, inadequate ventilation, or shock (hypoperfusion). An extreme weather condition may also make an urgent move necessary. In some cases, patients must be urgently moved from the location or position in which they are found. When a patient who is in a vehicle must be urgently moved, you should use the rapid extrication technique.

(Table 4-2 ▶) describes the situations in which you should use the rapid extrication technique.

In such cases, the delay that occurs in applying an extrication-type vest or half-board is contraindicated. However, the manual support and immobilization that you provide when using the rapid extrication technique produce a greater risk of spine movement. You should not use the rapid extrication technique if there is not an urgent reason to do so. To perform rapid extrication, follow the steps in (Skill Drill 4-4 ▶).

1. **First EMT-B provides in-line manual support** of the head and cervical spine from behind. Support may be applied from the side, if necessary, by reaching through the door (**Step 1**).
2. **Second EMT-B applies a cervical collar** and performs the initial assessment (**Step 2**).

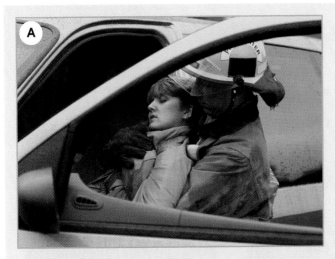
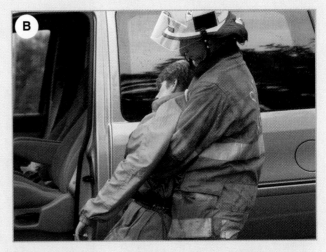

Figure 4-8 One-person technique for moving an unconscious patient from a car. **A.** Grasp the patient under the arms. **B.** Pull the patient out into a supine position.

3. **Second EMT-B provides continuous support** of the patient's torso until the patient is supine on the backboard.

4. **Third EMT-B is responsible for rotating the patient's legs and feet** as the torso is turned, ensuring that they are free of the pedals and any other obstruction. After the third EMT-B moves the legs together, the legs should be moved as a unit (**Step ③**).

5. **The patient is rotated** so that his or her back is facing out the driver's door and the feet are on the front passenger's seat. This coordinated movement is done in three or four short, quick turns. Hand position changes should be made between moves.

6. **The first EMT-B supports the head and neck** while the second and third EMT-Bs lower the patient onto the backboard. If the first EMT-B is unable to support the head and neck, another available

EMT-B or bystander must take over support (**Step ④**).

7. **As soon as the patient has been rotated** and the backboard is in place, second and third EMT-Bs lower the patient onto the board while supporting the head and torso so that neutral alignment is maintained. First EMT-B holds the backboard until the patient is secured (**Step ⑤**).

8. **Fourth EMT-B maintains manual cervical immobilization** and takes over giving the commands. Second EMT-B stands with his or her back to the door, facing the rear of the vehicle. The backboard should be immediately in front of the third EMT-B. Second EMT-B grasps the patient's shoulders or armpits. On command, the two EMT-Bs slide the patient 6" to 12" along the backboard, repeating this slide until the patient's hips are firmly on the backboard (**Step ⑥**).

9. **Third EMT-B gets out of the vehicle** and moves to the opposite side of the backboard, across from second EMT-B. Third EMT-B now takes control at the shoulders and the second EMT-B controls the hips. The patient can then be slid until placed fully on the board (**Step ⑦**).

10. **Cervical immobilization is maintained** and the EMT-Bs grasp the backboard and carry the patient away from the vehicle (**Step ⑧**).

Rapid extrication must be considered as a general procedure to be adapted as needed. Two-door cars differ from four-door models. Larger cars differ from smaller compact models, pickup trucks, and full-size

Table 4-2 Rapid Extrication Situations

The vehicle or scene is unsafe.

The patient cannot properly be assessed before being removed from the car.

The patient needs immediate intervention that requires a supine position.

The patient's condition requires immediate transport.

The patient blocks the EMT-B's access to another seriously injured patient.

Skill Drill 4-4   Rapid Extrication Technique

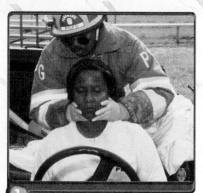

1 First EMT-B provides in-line manual support of the head and cervical spine.

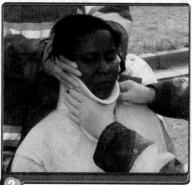

2 Second EMT-B applies a cervical collar and performs the initial assessment.

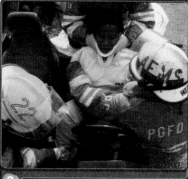

3 Second EMT-B supports the torso. Third EMT-B frees the patient's legs and moves the legs together, without moving the pelvis or spine.

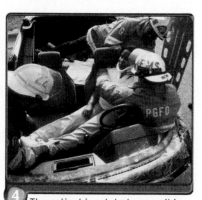

4 The patient is rotated as a unit in several short, coordinated moves. The patient's head and neck are continuously supported.

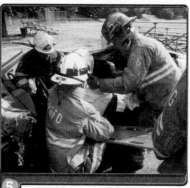

5 The backboard is placed into position.

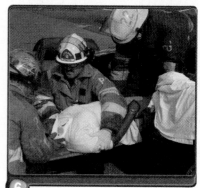

6 The patient is slid along the backboard in coordinated moves until the hips rest on the backboard.

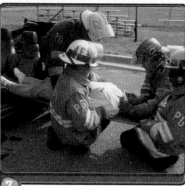

7 The EMT-Bs move into position to slide the patient fully on to the backboard.

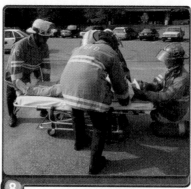

8 Cervical immobilization is maintained and the patient is carried away from the vehicle.

sedans and four-wheel-drive vehicles. You will handle a large, heavy adult differently from a small adult or child. Your resourcefulness and ability to adapt are necessary elements to perform successfully the rapid extrication technique.

Nonurgent Moves

When both the scene and the patient are stable, you should plan carefully how to move the patient. If your patient move is rushed or not well planned, it may result in discomfort or injury to the patient, you, or your crew. Before you attempt any move, the team leader must be sure that there are enough personnel, any obstacles have been identified or removed, the proper equipment is available, and the procedure and path to be followed have been clearly identified and discussed. In nonurgent situations, you and your team will choose the most effective and safe method to lift and carry the patient.

■ Geriatrics

Many individuals transported by EMS are geriatric patients. For many older patients, the fear of illness and disability is ever present, and being transported to the hospital can be a terrifying experience. In addition, there are physiologic changes that occur with aging that require special attention when lifting and moving a geriatric patient.

Skeletal changes such as brittle bones (osteoporosis) and spinal curvatures (kyphosis and spondylosis) present special challenges in packaging and moving

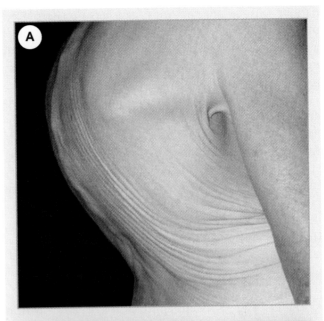

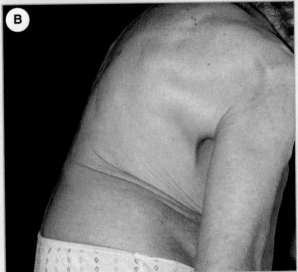

Figure 4-9 **A.** Kyphosis **B.** Spondylosis

older patients Figure 4-9 ▲ . Many patients cannot lie supine on a backboard without causing additional injury or discomfort. Special care and creativity must be used in immobilizing such patients. For example, a

You are the Provider 4

The patient is carried down the stairs and placed on the stretcher in a position of comfort. She feels much more at ease and is able to relax en route to the hospital. Her breathing is easier and she commends you and the other rescuers for your professional teamwork.

patient with spinal curvature may have to be placed on his or her side and immobilized in place with towel and blanket rolls. Consult your local protocols and medical direction about alternative immobilization techniques.

Many elderly patients have a lot of fear and anxiety when they have to access the EMS system. A sympathetic and compassionate approach can go a long way to calm them. Imagine how frightening being strapped to a cot and carried down a flight of stairs can be to an individual who lives in constant fear of falls and broken bones. Slow down and explain everything to the patient. This can go a long way in gaining their cooperation and decreasing their anxiety.

■ Bariatrics

Estimates suggest that approximately 100 million adults in the United States are overweight or obese. About 35% of women and 31% of men older than 19 years are obese or overweight. The numbers among children are even more significant. Approximately 20% to 25% of children are either overweight or obese. Conservative estimates suggest that the management of obesity consumes approximately $100 billion yearly.

Americans are becoming so large that a new field of medicine has been named for the care of the obese. Bariatrics is the branch of medicine concerned with the management (prevention or control) of obesity and associated diseases. It comes from the Greek words *baros*, weight, and *iatreia*, medical treatment. There is a direct correlation between degree of obesity and frequency and severity of health problems. The larger the patient, the more likely he or she is to need emergency treatment and transportation. This problem is taking an increasing toll on the health and functioning of EMS providers, as back injuries account for the largest number of missed days of work and both temporary and permanent disability.

Although ambulance cot and equipment manufacturers are producing equipment with ever higher weight capacities, this does not address the danger to the users of that equipment. European ambulance manufacturers regularly install mechanical lifts on their units, but these are not as common in the United States.

As an EMS provider, you should take great care in the proper lifting and moving techniques in order to reduce the risk of injury. Always use the resources available to you, review lifting techniques on a regular basis, and maintain your physical condition.

You are the Provider Summary

To provide the safest, easiest move for both the patient and your team, the move should be well planned prior to lifting the patient. Make sure you have adequate personnel to support the patient's weight. Use a series of coordinated moves, stopping as needed to reposition.

1. **What are your priorities for this patient?**

   ABCs; applying oxygen.

2. **What are your primary considerations for moving her?**

   The patient needs to be kept in an upright position to support her breathing. You also need additional assistance before attempting the move.

3. **How should you move the patient from the bed?**

   Since she cannot stand, she should be lifted with a draw sheet. This helps to prevent injury to the patient from pulling her by her extremities. It also protects the rescuers.

4. **What might you use to move this patient down the stairs?**

   A stair chair would be easier to maneuver down the stairs and would also keep the patient upright.

5. **How should the rescuers be positioned for carrying the patient down the stairs?**

   There should be one rescuer at the back of the stair chair and one at the feet. If there are enough, rescuers should also be positioned behind the two who are carrying the chair to help steady them.

6. **What should you do before moving the patient?**

   Reassure her that there are enough of you to move her safely. Make sure all straps are secure.

7. **Where should the stretcher be placed?**

   At the base of the stairs but out of the way of moving the stair chair onto the landing.

8. **How should your hands be positioned when lifting to ensure maximum strength?**

   Your palms should face up in a power grip for maximum power.

9. **In what position should your back be kept when lifting?**

   Keep your back locked in an upright position with a slight inward curve.

10. **Lifting and carrying are dynamic processes—what is meant by this?**

    Moves should be coordinated prior to lifting and allowances made for repositioning as needed. Dynamic means constantly changing and the move should be planned accordingly.

Prep Kit

Ready for Review

- Key rules of lifting are always to keep your back in an upright position and lift without twisting.
- The power lift is the safest and most efficient way to lift.
- The safety of you, your team, and the patient depends on the use of proper lifting techniques and maintaining a firm hold when lifting or carrying a patient.
- Pushing is better than pulling.
- It is always best to move a patient on a device that can be rolled.
- You must constantly coordinate your moves with your team members and make sure that you communicate with them.
- When lifting a cot, you must make sure that all team members use correct lifting techniques.
- If you must carry a patient on a backboard or cot up or down stairs or an incline, be sure that the patient is tightly secured to prevent the patient from sliding.
- Be sure to carry the backboard or cot foot end first so that the patient's head is elevated higher than the feet when going down an incline.
- Team members must anticipate and understand every move and execute it in a coordinated manner.
- You should know how much you can comfortably and safely lift and not attempt to lift more than this amount.
- Do not hesitate to call for additional help to lift and carry.
- The same basic body mechanics apply for safe reaching and pulling as for lifting and carrying.
- Keep your back locked and straight, and avoid twisting.
- Do not hyperextend your back when reaching overhead.
- You should normally move a patient with nonurgent moves, in an orderly, planned, and unhurried fashion.
- Select methods that involve the least amount of lifting and carrying.
- At times, you have to use an emergency move to maneuver a patient before providing care.
- You should use an urgent move if a patient has an altered mental status, inadequate ventilation, or is in shock.
- You should practice lifting and moving techniques with your team members often so that you are able to perform the moves quickly, safely, and efficiently.

Vital Vocabulary

diamond carry A carrying technique in which one EMT-B is located at the head, one at the foot, and one at each side of the patient, all facing forward as they walk.

emergency move A move in which the patient is dragged or pulled from a dangerous scene before initial assessment and care are provided.

power grip A technique in which the litter or backboard is gripped by inserting each hand under the handle with the palm facing up and the thumb extended, fully supporting the underside of the handle on the curved palm with the fingers and thumb.

power lift A lifting technique in which the EMT-B's back is held upright, with legs bent, and the patient is lifted when the EMT-B raises his or her upper body and arms and straightens his or her legs.

rapid extrication technique A technique that was developed to move a patient from a sitting position inside a vehicle to a supine position on a backboard in less than 1 minute.

stair chair A lightweight folding device that is used to carry a conscious, seated patient up or down stairs.

Technology

- Interactivities
- Vocabulary Explorer
- Anatomy Review
- Web Links
- Online Review Manual

Assessment in Action

You are on scene with an obese patient complaining of dyspnea. The patient is over 500 pounds. The fire department is also there to provide assistance.

1. Which of the following is considered the most powerful and safest way to lift?
   - **A.** power grip
   - **B.** power lift
   - **C.** curls
   - **D.** stair chair

2. Which of the following is considered proper body mechanics when using a body drag?
   - **A.** Keep your back locked and straight.
   - **B.** Avoid any twisting.
   - **C.** Avoid hyperextending your back.
   - **D.** All of the above.

3. When there is potential danger, which of the following methods should be used to move a patient before initial assessment and care are provided?
   - **A.** alternate move
   - **B.** emergency move
   - **C.** nonurgent move
   - **D.** rapid extrication technique

4. When transporting a geriatric patient, one concern is brittle bones or _____.
   - **A.** osteoporosis
   - **B.** kyphosis
   - **C.** spondylosis
   - **D.** none of the above

5. What branch of medicine is concerned with the management of obesity and associated diseases?
   - **A.** Osteorthotics
   - **B.** Bariatrics
   - **C.** Iatrogenics
   - **D.** Obstetrics

Challenging Questions

6. Lifting and moving are *dynamic* processes. What is meant by this?

7. What is the purpose of pulling a patient along the long axis of the body when you must perform an emergency move?

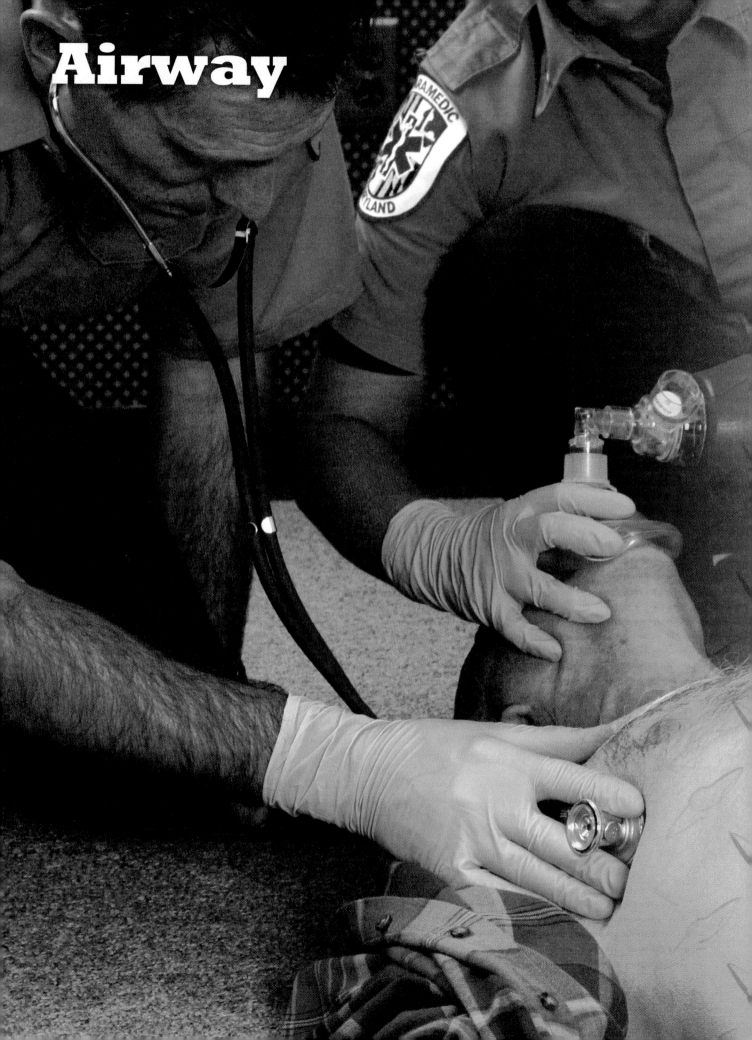

Airway

Cognitive Objectives

1. Perform techniques to ensure a patent airway. (p 63)
   - Describe the steps to perform the head tilt–chin lift.
   - Describe the steps to perform the jaw thrust.
   - Describe the techniques of suctioning.
   - Describe how to measure and insert an oropharyngeal (oral) airway.
   - Describe how to measure and insert a nasopharyngeal (nasal) airway.
2. Provide ventilatory support for a patient. (p 73)
   - Describe the steps to perform the skill of artificially ventilating a patient with a bag-valve mask for one and two rescuers.
   - Describe the steps to artificially ventilate a patient with a flow-restricted, oxygen-powered ventilation device.
3. Use oxygen delivery system components (nasal cannula, face mask, etc). (p 72)
   - Identify a nonrebreathing face mask and state the oxygen flow requirements needed for its use.
   - Identify a nasal cannula and state the flow requirements needed for its use.

Affective Objectives

1. Explain the rationale for basic life support artificial ventilation and airway protection skills taking priority over most other life support skills. (p 61)
2. Explain the rationale for providing oxygenation through high-inspired oxygen concentrations to patients who, in the past, may have received low concentrations. (p 72)

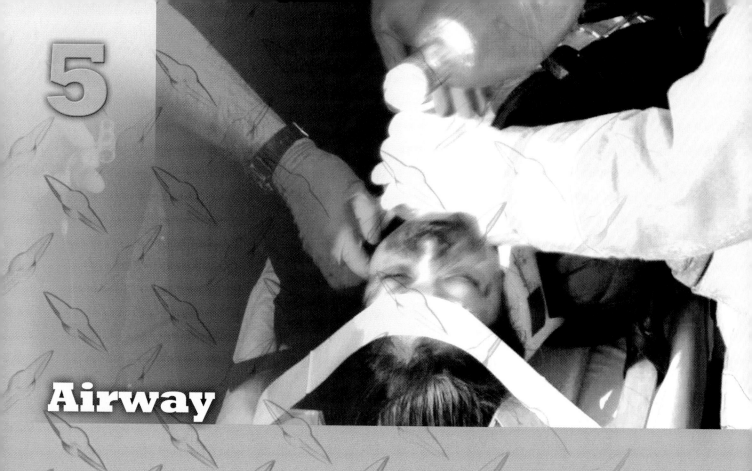

5

Airway

You are the Provider 1

You and your EMT-B partner have just delivered a patient to a local dialysis center located in a strip mall shopping center. As you are returning to the ambulance, you are suddenly summoned by a frantic shopper in front of a nearby store. She is yelling about a woman not breathing. Your partner grabs the jump bag from the side door and you both rush toward the shopper. On the way your partner radios the dispatcher to alert her of the situation and your position.

When you enter the dress shop you note that there are several women gathered near the back and all of them are talking excitedly. On reaching them you see a woman lying supine outside a dressing room.

Initial Assessment	Recording Time: 0 Minutes
Appearance	Pale, circumoral cyanosis
Level of consciousness	Pain responsive
Airway	Snoring respirations
Breathing	Slow and shallow
Circulation	Radial pulse present

1. What is your first priority for this patient?
2. What is the most common cause of snoring respirations in an unresponsive person?
3. What factors might alter your initial care?
4. What questions should you ask of bystanders?
5. What assistance might you request?

Introduction

Managing the airway is the most important step in caring for any patient—you must make sure that the patient is breathing adequately. The patient who cannot breathe effectively is not delivering oxygen to body tissues and cells, which need a constant supply of oxygen to survive. Within seconds of being deprived of oxygen, vital organs such as the heart and brain may not function normally.

Oxygen reaches body tissues and cells through two separate but related processes: breathing and circulation. As we inhale, oxygen moves from the atmosphere into our lungs, then passes from the air sacs in the lungs into the capillaries to oxygenate the blood. At the same time, carbon dioxide, produced by cells in the tissues of the body, moves from the blood into the air sacs. The blood, enriched with oxygen, travels through the body by the pumping action of the heart. Carbon dioxide then leaves our bodies as we exhale. EMT-Bs must be able to locate the parts of the respiratory system, understand how the system works, and be able to recognize which patients are breathing adequately and which ones are breathing inadequately.

This chapter will review the anatomy and physiology of the respiratory system. It will also review how to assess patients quickly to determine their airway and ventilation status. The equipment, procedures, and guidelines that you will need to manage a patient's airway and breathing are described in detail. Because airway management equipment can be dangerous if used improperly, the chapter will thoroughly discuss airway adjuncts, oxygen therapy devices, and artificial ventilation methods.

Refresher.EMSzone.com

Technology

Interactivities

Vocabulary Explorer

Anatomy Review

Web Links

Online Review Manual

Anatomy of the Respiratory System

The respiratory system consists of all the structures that make up the airway and help us breathe, or ventilate. Structures that help us breathe include the diaphragm, the muscles of the chest wall, accessory muscles of breathing, and the nerves from the brain and spinal cord to those muscles. Ventilation is the exchange of air between the lungs and the environment. The diaphragm and muscles of the chest wall are responsible for the regular rise and fall of the chest that accompanies normal breathing.

Structures of the Airway

The airway is divided into the upper and lower airways Figure 5-1 ▶. The upper airway consists of the nose, mouth, throat (pharynx), and the epiglottis. The epiglottis is a leaf-shaped structure located above the larynx that prevents food and liquid from entering the larynx during swallowing. The portion of the throat behind the nose is called the nasopharynx; the portion behind the mouth is the oropharynx.

The lower airway consists of the larynx, trachea, main bronchi, bronchioles, and alveoli. The lower airway begins with the larynx (vocal cords). The cricoid cartilage is a firm cartilage ring that forms the lower part of the larynx. The trachea is connected to the larynx. The main bronchi and bronchioles branch off from the trachea, extending into each lung. The bronchioles eventually end in the alveoli. The alveoli are small sacs where the actual exchange of oxygen and carbon dioxide occurs.

The chest (thoracic cage) contains the lungs Figure 5-2 ▶. The lungs hang freely within the chest cavity. The mediastinum is the space between the lungs. This space contains the heart, the great vessels, the esophagus, the trachea, the major bronchi, and many nerves.

Structures of Breathing

As you remember, breathing is both voluntary and automatic. The automatic stimulus to breathe is initiated by a control center in the brain stem that continually monitors the levels of carbon dioxide and pH (a measurement of acid and base balance) in the blood. The stimulus to breathe is initiated by recognition of high levels of carbon dioxide by chemoreceptors found in aortic and carotid bodies. To initiate breathing, nerve impulses travel through the spinal cord to the diaphragm and intercostal muscles (muscles between

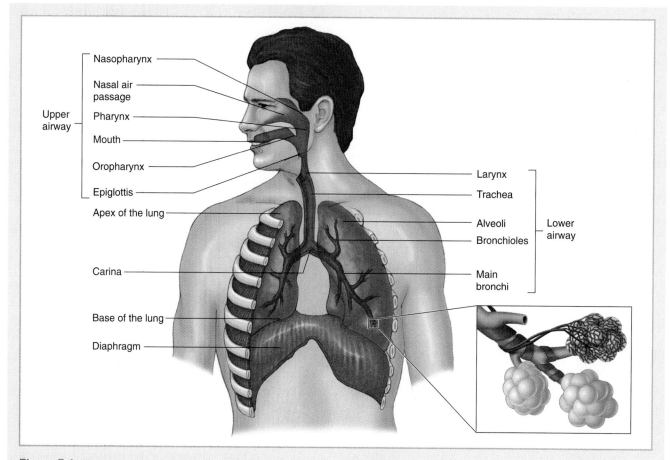

Figure 5-1 The upper and lower airways contain the structures that help us breathe.

Figure 5-2 The thoracic cage contains anatomic structures for respiration, including the lungs, the heart, the great vessels, the trachea, and the major bronchi.

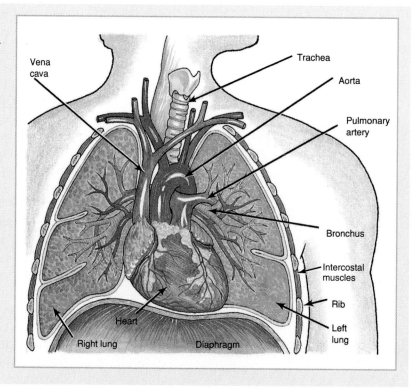

the ribs), stimulating contraction. When the body senses a rise in the concentration of carbon dioxide in the blood, the brain stem signals you to breathe. The lungs, because they have no muscle tissue, cannot move on their own. They need the help of other structures to be able to expand and contract. The ability of the lungs to function properly is dependent on the movement of the chest and supporting structures. These structures include the thorax, the thoracic cage (chest), the diaphragm, the intercostal muscles, and the accessory muscles of breathing.

The diaphragm is a skeletal muscle that is the primary muscle of breathing. It separates the thoracic cavity from the abdominal cavity. The diaphragm is considered a specialized muscle because it functions as a voluntary and an involuntary muscle. It acts as a voluntary muscle whenever we take a deep breath, cough, or hold our breath. However, unlike other skeletal or voluntary muscles, the diaphragm also performs an automatic function. Breathing continues while we sleep and at all other times. Even though we can hold our breath or temporarily increase or decrease our breathing, we cannot continue these variations indefinitely.

Inhalation

The active, muscular part of breathing is called <u>inhalation</u>. As we inhale, air enters the body through the trachea. This air travels to and from the lungs, filling and emptying the alveoli. During inhalation, the diaphragm and intercostal muscles contract. When the diaphragm contracts, it moves down and enlarges the thoracic cage from top to bottom. When the intercostal muscles contract, they lift the ribs up and out. These combined actions enlarge the thorax in all directions.

The air pressure outside the body (atmospheric pressure) is normally higher than the air pressure within the thorax. As we inhale and the thoracic cage expands, the air pressure within the thorax decreases, creating a slight vacuum. This pulls air in through the trachea, causing the lungs to fill. When the air pressure outside of the thorax equals the air pressure inside, air stops moving. Gases, such as oxygen, move from an area of high pressure to an area of lower pressure until the pressures are equal.

<u>Tidal volume</u>, a measure of the depth of breathing, is the amount of air in milliliters (mL) that is moved into or out of the lungs during a single breath. The average tidal volume for a male is approximately 500 mL. <u>Minute volume</u> is the amount of air moved through the lungs in 1 minute and is calculated by multiplying the tidal volume and the respiratory

> ## Documentation Tips
>
> A patient's respiratory status can be reported in terms of rate and depth such as "18 and shallow" or "16 and deep". It can also be noted by referring to the patient's ability to talk. Use phrases such as "talking in complete sentences" or "presents with 2- to 3-word dyspnea," meaning the patient cannot complete sentences without gasping for breath.

rate. Therefore, if a patient is breathing at a rate of 12 breaths/min and has a tidal volume of 500 mL per breath, his minute volume would be 6,000 mL (6 L). It is important to note that variations in tidal volume, respiratory rate, or both, will affect minute volume. For example, if a patient is breathing at a rate of 12 breaths/min, but the tidal volume is reduced (shallow breathing), the minute volume will decrease. Likewise, if a patient is breathing at a rate of 12 breaths/min and the tidal volume is increased (deep breathing), the minute volume will increase.

Exhalation

<u>Exhalation</u> is a passive process that normally does not require muscular effort. During exhalation, the diaphragm and the intercostal muscles relax, the thorax decreases in size, and the ribs and muscles assume a normal resting position. When the size of the thoracic cage decreases, air in the lungs is compressed into a smaller space. The air pressure within the thorax then becomes higher than the pressure outside, and air is pushed out through the trachea.

Remember that air can only get into the lungs if it travels through the trachea. This is why clearing and maintaining an open airway are so important. Clearing the airway means removing obstructing material, tissue, or fluids from the nose, mouth, or throat. Maintaining the airway means keeping the airway <u>patent</u> so that air can enter and leave the lungs freely.

■ Physiology of the Respiratory System

All living cells need energy to survive. Cells take energy from nutrients through a series of chemical processes. The name given to these processes as a whole is <u>metabolism</u>. During metabolism, each cell combines nutrients and oxygen and produces energy and waste products, primarily water and carbon dioxide.

Each living cell in the body requires a supply of oxygen and a regular means of disposing of waste (carbon dioxide). The body provides these through respiration. Some cells need a constant supply of oxygen to survive. Other cells in the body can tolerate short periods without oxygen and still survive. For example, after 4 to 6 minutes without oxygen, brain cells and cells in the nervous system may be severely or permanently damaged and may even die. Dead brain cells can never be replaced. However, cells in the kidney may be without oxygen for 45 minutes or more and still survive. Normally, the air that we breathe contains 21% oxygen and 78% nitrogen. Small amounts of other gases make up the remaining 1%.

The Exchange of Oxygen and Carbon Dioxide

As blood travels through the body, it supplies oxygen and nutrients to various tissues and cells. Oxygen passes from blood in the arteries through the capillaries to tissue cells, while carbon dioxide and cell waste pass in the opposite direction: from tissue cells through capillaries and into the veins.

Each time we inhale, the alveoli receive a supply of oxygen-rich air. The alveoli are surrounded by a network of tiny pulmonary capillaries. These capillaries are located in the walls of the alveoli. This means that the air in the alveoli and the blood in the capillaries are separated only by two very thin layers of tissue. Each time we exhale, the carbon dioxide from the bloodstream travels across the same two layers of tissue to the alveoli and is expelled into the atmosphere.

Oxygen and carbon dioxide pass rapidly across the walls of the alveoli and the capillaries through diffusion. Diffusion is a passive process in which molecules move from an area of higher concentration to an area of lower concentration. Oxygen molecules move from the alveoli into the blood because there are fewer oxygen molecules in the pulmonary capillaries. In the same way, molecules of carbon dioxide move from the blood into the alveoli because there are fewer carbon dioxide molecules in the alveoli.

The alveoli normally produce a chemical, called surfactant, that helps keep the alveoli open. By keeping the alveoli open, diffusion is more efficient. Anything that removes or destroys surfactant (such as water from drowning) will cause acute respiratory distress.

The Control of Breathing

The area of the brain stem that controls breathing is deep within the skull, in one of the best-protected parts of the nervous system. The nerves in this area act as sensors, reacting primarily to the level of carbon dioxide in the arterial blood. If the levels of carbon dioxide become too high or too low, the brain automatically adjusts breathing accordingly. This happens very quickly, after every breath. In a healthy person, this stimulus to breathe is referred to as the primary respiratory drive.

When the level of carbon dioxide becomes too high, the brain stem sends nerve impulses down the spinal cord that cause the diaphragm and the intercostal muscles to contract. This increases our breathing, or respirations. The higher the level of carbon dioxide in the blood, the stronger the impulse is to breathe. Once the carbon dioxide returns to an acceptable level, the strength and frequency of respirations decrease.

Hypoxia

Hypoxia is an extremely dangerous condition in which the body's tissues and cells do not have enough oxygen. Patients may die in a matter of moments if this condition is not reversed. Hypoxia develops quickly in the vital organs of patients who are not breathing or who are breathing inadequately. Inadequate breathing means that the person cannot move enough air into the lungs with each breath to meet the body's metabolic needs. Hypoxia can have a profound effect on breathing. If the brain senses that there is not enough oxygen in the blood, it will send messages via the spinal cord to the diaphragm and respiratory muscles to increase the patient's respiratory rate and depth.

Patients with chronic respiratory diseases (such as COPD, emphysema) maintain a low oxygen level and chronic high levels of carbon dioxide in their blood. The sensors in the brain become accustomed to these levels. Unlike a healthy person whose primary respiratory drive is triggered by increased carbon dioxide levels in the blood, the primary stimulus to breathe for a patient with a chronic respiratory disease is a low oxygen level in the blood, a condition called the hypoxic drive.

Patients who are breathing inadequately will show varying signs and symptoms of hypoxia. The onset and the degree of tissue damage caused by hypoxia often depend on the quality of ventilations. Early signs of hypoxia include restlessness, irritability, apprehension, fast heart rate (tachycardia), and anxiety. Late signs of hypoxia include mental status changes, a weak (thready) pulse, and cyanosis. Conscious patients will report shortness of breath (<u>dyspnea</u>) and may not be able to talk in complete sentences. The best time to give a patient oxygen is before any signs and symptoms of hypoxia appear.

The following conditions are commonly associated with hypoxia:

- **Heart attack (myocardial infarction).** Ischemia within the heart muscle from myocardial infarction occurs when there is inadequate circulation of oxygen-carrying blood to the tissues of the heart. The weakened heart then pumps oxygenated blood to the remainder of the body less efficiently, resulting in systemic hypoxia.
- **Pulmonary edema.** Fluid accumulates in the lungs, making the exchange of oxygen and carbon dioxide in the alveoli less efficient.
- **Overdoses** (narcotic or sedative). Respirations may become decreased and shallow (reduced tidal volume).
- **Inhalation of smoke and/or toxic fumes.** These substances cause pulmonary edema and destroy lung tissue, causing problems with gas exchange.
- **Stroke** (cerebrovascular accident). The cause of hypoxia in a stroke may be due to facial paralysis leading to potential airway compromise or poor control of respirations if the respiratory center in the brain is affected.
- **Chest injury.** Pain interferes with full chest wall expansion, thus limiting effective ventilation. Lung damage itself, secondary to pulmonary contusion, can also prevent efficient gas exchange.
- **Shock** (hypoperfusion). Shock often occurs as a result of injuries that affect the circulatory system. When the circulatory system fails to deliver adequate amounts of oxygen, the tissues begin to die.
- **Chronic obstructive pulmonary disease** (COPD; for example, chronic bronchitis and emphysema). Chronic irritation of the lungs and air passages produces alveolar damage and poor gas exchange.
- **Asthma.** Narrowing of respiratory passages and buildup of mucus causes air trapping and poor gas exchange.

All hypoxic patients, whatever the cause of their condition, should be treated with high-flow supplemental oxygen. The method of oxygen delivery depends on the severity of the hypoxia and the adequacy of breathing.

■ Patient Assessment

Recognizing Adequate Breathing

Breathing should appear easy, not labored. Normal (adequate) breathing has the following characteristics:

- A normal rate ⬛ Table 5-1 ▾
- A regular pattern of inhalation and exhalation
- Clear and equal lung sounds on both sides of the chest (bilateral)
- Regular and equal chest rise and fall
- Adequate depth (tidal volume)

Recognizing Inadequate Breathing

As an EMT-B, you know that an adult patient who is awake, alert, and talking to you generally has no immediate airway or breathing problems. However, you should always have supplemental oxygen and a bag-mask device or pocket mask close at hand to assist with breathing if necessary. An adult who is breathing normally has respirations of 12 to 20 breaths/min. The adult patient who is breathing slower (fewer than 12 breaths/min) or faster (more than 20 breaths/min) than normal should be evaluated for inadequate breathing by assessing the depth of respirations. A patient with shallow respirations (reduced tidal volume) may require assisted ventilations, even if his or her respiratory rate is within normal limits.

A patient with inadequate breathing may appear to be working hard to breathe. This type of breathing pattern is called <u>labored breathing</u>. It requires effort and, especially among children, may involve the use of accessory muscles. Accessory muscles are secondary muscles of respiration and include the neck muscles (sternocleidomastoid), the chest (pectoralis major) muscles, and the abdominal muscles ⬛ Figure 5-3 ▸ . These muscles are not used during normal breathing. Signs of inadequate breathing in adult patients are as follows:

- Respiratory rate of less than 12 breaths/min or more than 20 breaths/min
- Irregular rhythm, such as a patient taking a series of deep breaths followed by periods of <u>apnea</u>, or lack of spontaneous breathing.

Table 5-1 Normal Respiratory Rates

Adults	12 to 20 breaths/min
Children	15 to 30 breaths/min
Infants	25 to 50 breaths/min

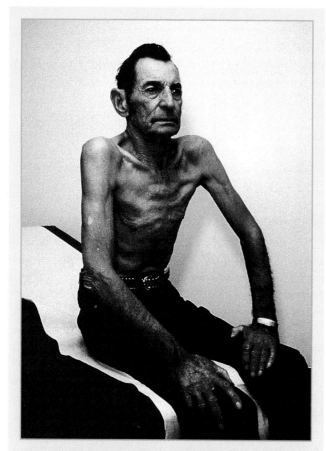

Figure 5-3 The accessory muscles of breathing can be seen in a patient with difficulty breathing.

- Auscultated breath sounds that are diminished, absent, or noisy
- Unequal or inadequate chest expansion—resulting in reduced tidal volume
- Increased effort of breathing—use of accessory muscles
- Shallow depth (reduced tidal volume)
- Skin that is pale, cyanotic, cool, or moist (clammy)
- Skin pulling in around the ribs or above the clavicles during inspiration (<u>retractions</u>)

As an experienced EMT-B, you may also have observed occasional, gasping respirations in a patient whose heart has stopped. These are called <u>agonal respirations</u> and they occur when the respiratory center in the brain continues to send signals for the body to breathe.

Some patients may have irregular respiratory breathing patterns that are related to a specific condition. For example, Cheyne-Stokes respirations are

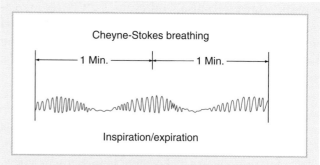

Figure 5-4 Cheyne-Stokes breathing has irregular respirations followed by a period of apnea.

often seen in patients with a stroke and patients with severe head injuries **Figure 5-4 ▲**. Cheyne-Stokes respirations consist of an irregular respiratory pattern in which the patient breathes with an increasing rate and depth of respiration that is followed by a period of apnea or lack of spontaneous breathing, followed again by a pattern of increasing rate and depth of respiration. Severe head injuries may also cause changes in the normal respiratory rate and pattern of breathing. The result may be irregular, ineffective respirations that may or may not have an identifiable pattern (<u>ataxic respirations</u>). Rapid, deep respirations (Kussmaul's) in the presence of an acetone odor may be sign of a diabetic emergency (diabetic ketoacidosis).

Though you initially learned the signs and symptoms of inadequate breathing, you now know that these signs and symptoms tend to present in certain patterns when you see these patients in the field. A specific pattern may not contain all items in the list, but these patterns are often quite distinctive. Learning to recognize them is a big part of the contribution that your experience makes to the quality of the care you provide.

Patients with inadequate breathing have inadequate minute volume and need to be treated immediately. This is most easily recognized in patients who are unable to speak in complete sentences when at rest or who have a fast or slow respiratory rate, both of which may result in a reduction in tidal volume. Emergency medical care includes airway management, supplemental oxygen, and ventilatory support.

■ Opening the Airway

Emergency medical care begins with ensuring an open airway. The patient's airway and breathing status are the first steps in your initial assessment for a very good reason: unless you can immediately open and maintain a patent airway, you cannot provide effective patient care. Regardless of the patient's condition, the airway must remain patent at all times.

When you respond to a call and find an unconscious patient, you need to assess and determine immediately whether the patient has an open airway and breathing is adequate. To most effectively open the airway and assess breathing, the patient should be in the supine position. However, if your patient is in a position that delays placement in a supine position (for example, entrapped in the vehicle), the patient's airway must be opened and assessed in the position in which you find the patient. If your patient is found in the prone position, he or she must be repositioned to allow for assessment of airway and breathing and to begin CPR should it become necessary. The patient should be log rolled as a unit so the head, neck, and spine all move together without twisting. Unconscious patients, especially when there are no witnesses who can rule out trauma, should be moved as a unit because of the potential for spinal injury.

In an unconscious patient, the most common airway obstruction is the patient's own tongue, which falls back into the throat when the muscles of the throat and tongue relax. Dentures, blood, vomitus, mucus, food, and other foreign objects may also create an airway obstruction. Therefore, you should always be prepared to help clear and maintain a patent (open) airway.

Head Tilt–Chin Lift Maneuver

Opening the airway to relieve an obstruction can often be done quickly and easily with a head tilt–chin lift maneuver. For patients who have not sustained trauma, this simple maneuver is sometimes all that is needed for the patient to resume breathing.

To perform the head tilt–chin lift maneuver, follow these steps (Skill Drill 5-1 ▶):

1. **With the patient in a supine position,** position yourself beside the patient's head. **Place one hand on the patient's forehead,** and apply firm backward pressure with your palm to tilt the patient's head back. This extension of the neck will move the tongue forward, away from the back of the throat, and clear the airway if the tongue is blocking it (**Step 1**).
2. **Place the tips of the fingers of your other hand under the lower jaw** near the bony part of the chin. Do not compress the soft tissue under the chin, as this may block the airway (**Step 2**).

You are the Provider 2

Your partner opens her airway with a head tilt-chin lift maneuver and inserts an oropharyngeal airway. She tolerates this without a problem. He notes that she has dentures and that her airway is clear. You tell him to go ahead and initiate ventilations via a bag-mask device attached to 100% oxygen while you call for the nearest fire rescue for additional help.

You assess her vital signs and do a quick head-to-toe survey. During the survey you note some slightly distended neck veins and +3 pedal edema.

Vital Signs	Recording Time: 2 Minutes
Skin	Pale, dry
Pulse	122 beats/min, regular
Blood pressure	158/84 mm Hg
Respirations	6 breaths/min without ventilations

6. What questions should your partner consider about her airway?
7. What is significant about your assessment findings?
8. What else should you assess based on these findings?

Skill Drill   5-1   Head Tilt-Chin Lift Maneuver

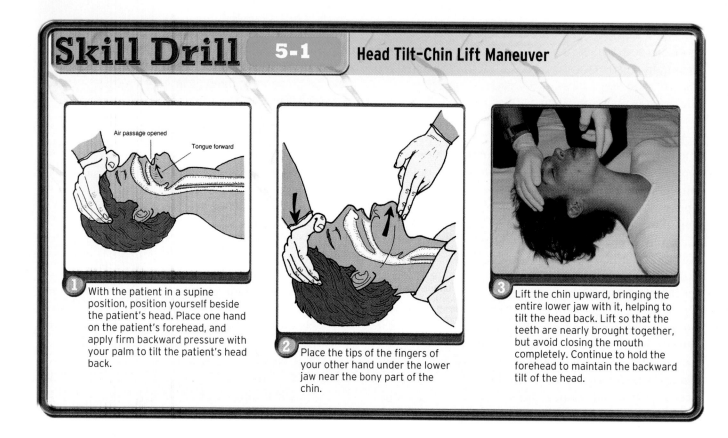

1. With the patient in a supine position, position yourself beside the patient's head. Place one hand on the patient's forehead, and apply firm backward pressure with your palm to tilt the patient's head back.

2. Place the tips of the fingers of your other hand under the lower jaw near the bony part of the chin.

3. Lift the chin upward, bringing the entire lower jaw with it, helping to tilt the head back. Lift so that the teeth are nearly brought together, but avoid closing the mouth completely. Continue to hold the forehead to maintain the backward tilt of the head.

3. **Lift the chin upward,** bringing the entire lower jaw with it, helping to tilt the head back. Do not use your thumb to lift the chin. Lift so that the teeth are nearly brought together, but avoid closing the mouth completely. Continue to hold the forehead to maintain the backward tilt of the head (**Step** ③).

Jaw-Thrust Maneuver

The head tilt–chin lift maneuver will open the airway in most patients. If you suspect a cervical spine injury, the method of choice is the jaw-thrust maneuver. The jaw-thrust maneuver is a technique to open the airway by placing the fingers behind the angle of the jaw and lifting the jaw upward. Since maintaining an open airway is a priority, you should use the head tilt–chin lift if the jaw-thrust maneuver does not adequately open the airway in an unresponsive trauma patient with a suspected cervical spine injury.

To perform the jaw-thrust maneuver, follow these steps (Skill Drill 5-2 ▶):

1. **Position yourself at the patient's head.** Place your fingers behind the angles of the lower jaw, and

move the jaw upward. Use your thumbs to help position the lower jaw to allow breathing through the mouth and the nose (**Step** ①).

2. **Use your thumbs to open the patient's mouth** to allow breathing through the mouth as well as the nose. The completed maneuver should open the airway with the mouth slightly open and the jaw jutting forward (**Step** ②).

3. Once the airway has been opened, the patient may start to breathe on his or her own. Assess whether breathing has returned by using the look, listen, and feel technique.

4. With a severe airway obstruction, there will be no movement of air. Regular chest wall movement indicates a respiratory effort is present. If there is no movement of air, the patient is not breathing and you must begin artificial ventilation immediately.

■ Basic Airway Adjuncts

The primary function of an airway adjunct is to prevent obstruction of the upper airway by the tongue and allow the passage of air and oxygen to the lungs.

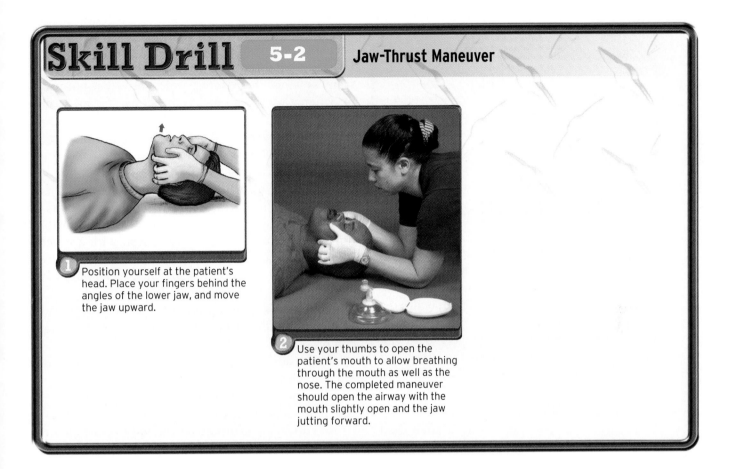

Skill Drill 5-2 | Jaw-Thrust Maneuver

1. Position yourself at the patient's head. Place your fingers behind the angles of the lower jaw, and move the jaw upward.

2. Use your thumbs to open the patient's mouth to allow breathing through the mouth as well as the nose. The completed maneuver should open the airway with the mouth slightly open and the jaw jutting forward.

Oropharyngeal Airways

An oropharyngeal (oral) airway has two principal purposes. The first is to keep the tongue from blocking the upper airway. The second is to make it easier to suction the oropharynx if necessary. Suctioning is possible through an opening down the center or along either side of the oropharyngeal airway. This type of airway is often used in conjunction with bag-mask ventilation. An oropharyngeal airway should be inserted promptly in unconscious patients who have no gag reflex, whether or not they are breathing on their own.

Indications for the oropharyngeal airway include the following:

- Unconscious patients without a gag reflex
- Any apneic patient being ventilated with a bag-mask device

Contraindications for the oropharyngeal airway include the following:

- Conscious patients
- Any patient who has an intact gag reflex

The gag reflex is a protective reflex mechanism that prevents food and other particles from entering the airway. If you try to insert an oral airway in a patient with a gag reflex, the result may be vomiting or a spasm of the vocal cords. If the patient gags while you are attempting to insert an oral airway, immediately remove the oral airway and be prepared to suction the oropharynx, should vomiting occur. The use of an oral airway may make manual airway maneuvers such as the head tilt–chin lift and the jaw-thrust easier to maintain; however, manual maneuvers are often still needed to ensure that the airway remains patent. If your patient becomes responsive and regains a gag reflex after you have inserted the oral airway, gently remove the airway by pulling it out along the normal curvature of the tongue.

If the oropharyngeal airway is too large, it may actually push the tongue back into the pharynx, blocking the airway. Conversely, an oral airway that is too small may block the airway directly, just like any other foreign body obstruction. To insert an oral airway, follow these steps Skill Drill 5-3 ▶ :

1. **Select the proper sized airway** by measuring from the patient's earlobe or angle of the jaw to the corner of the mouth on the side of the face (**Step ①**).

Pediatric Needs

In children, the alternative method of inserting an oral airway, using a tongue blade to hold the tongue down while inserting the oral airway, is the only acceptable method. Because the airways of children are not as developed as the adult patient, rotating an oral airway in the posterior pharynx may cause damage.

2. **Open the patient's mouth with the cross-finger technique.** Hold the airway upside down with your other hand. Insert the airway with the tip facing the roof of the mouth until it touches the roof of the mouth (**Step ②**).
3. **Rotate the airway 180°.** The flange should rest against the lips or teeth, with the other end opening into the pharynx (**Step ③**).

Nasopharyngeal Airways

A <u>nasopharyngeal (nasal) airway</u> is most often used in patients who have an intact gag reflex but are not able to maintain an airway (Figure 5-5 ▶). You may have used this airway in patients with an altered mental status or those who have just had a seizure. In many systems, the nasopharyngeal airway is not used in patients with head or facial trauma. If a nasal airway is accidentally pushed through the hole caused by a fracture of the base of the skull, it may penetrate the cranium and enter the brain. As always, check and follow your local protocol.

This type of airway is usually better tolerated by patients who have an intact gag reflex. It is not as likely as the oropharyngeal airway to cause vomiting. You should coat the airway well with a water-soluble lubricant before it is inserted. Be aware that slight bleeding may occur even when the airway is inserted properly. Never force the airway into place, or it may cause a significant posterior nasal bleed, which will be very difficult to control and may cause airway compromise.

Indications for the nasopharyngeal airway include the following:

- Semiconscious or unconscious patients with an intact gag reflex
- Patients who otherwise will not tolerate an oropharyngeal airway

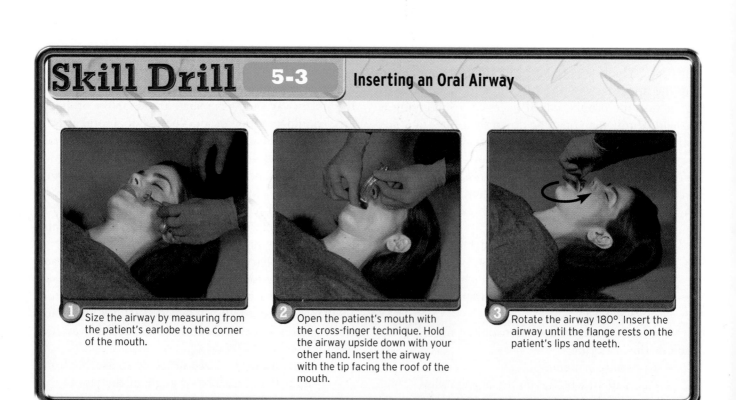

Skill Drill   5-3   Inserting an Oral Airway

① Size the airway by measuring from the patient's earlobe to the corner of the mouth.

② Open the patient's mouth with the cross-finger technique. Hold the airway upside down with your other hand. Insert the airway with the tip facing the roof of the mouth.

③ Rotate the airway 180°. Insert the airway until the flange rests on the patient's lips and teeth.

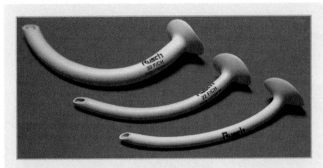

Figure 5-5 A nasal airway is better tolerated than an oral airway by patients who have an intact gag reflex.

Contraindications for the nasopharyngeal airway include the following:

- Severe head injury with blood draining from the nose
- History of fractured nasal bones

To insert a nasal airway, follow the steps in **Skill Drill 5-4**:

1. **Select the proper sized airway** by measuring from the tip of the nose to the earlobe. Coat the tip with a water-soluble lubricant. In almost all individuals, one nostril is larger than the other (**Step 1**).
2. **The airway should be placed** in the larger nostril, with the curvature of the device following the curve of the floor of the nose. If using the right nostril, the bevel should face the septum (**Step 2**). If using the left nostril, insert the airway with the tip of the airway pointing upward, which will allow the bevel to face the septum.
3. **Advance the airway gently** (**Step 3**). If using the left nostril, insert the airway until resistance is met. Then rotate the nasal airway 180° into position. This rotation is not required if using the right nostril.
4. **When completely inserted,** the flange rests against the nostril. The other end of the airway opens into the posterior pharynx (**Step 4**). If the patient becomes intolerant of the nasal airway, you may have to remove it. Gently withdraw the airway from the nasal passage.

Suctioning

You must keep the airway clear so that you can ventilate the patient properly. Once the airway is open, check for the presence of dentures (false teeth), blood, vomitus, mucus, food, or other foreign objects. You should always have a suction device available to help open and maintain the airway. If the airway is not clear, you will force the fluids and secretions into the lungs and possibly cause a complete airway obstruction. If a patient has foreign material in their oral cavity (such as broken teeth, food, or vomitus), it must be removed before ventilation. If you have any doubt about the situation, remember this rule: If you hear gurgling, the patient needs suctioning!

Suctioning Equipment

Portable, hand-operated, and fixed (mounted) suctioning equipment is essential for resuscitation **Figure 5-6**. A portable suctioning unit must provide enough vacuum pressure and flow to allow you to suction the mouth and nose effectively. Hand-operated suctioning units with disposable chambers are reliable, effective, and relatively inexpensive. A fixed suctioning unit should generate airflow of more than 40 L/min and a vacuum of more than 300 mm Hg when the tubing is clamped.

A Yankauer or tonsil-tip catheter is the best kind of catheter for suctioning the oropharynx in adults and is preferred for infants and children. The plastic tips have a large diameter and are rigid, so they do not collapse **Figure 5-7**. Soft plastic, nonrigid catheters, sometimes called French or whistle-tip catheters, are used to suction the nose and liquid secretions in the back of the mouth and in situations in which you cannot use a rigid catheter, such as for a patient with a stoma **Figure 5-8**. French catheters are also used to suction an endotracheal tube. Before you insert any catheter, make sure to measure for the proper size. Use the same technique as you would use when measuring for an oropharyngeal airway. Be careful not to touch the back

Skill Drill 5-4   Inserting a Nasal Airway

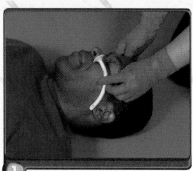

1 Size the airway by measuring from the tip of the nose to the patient's earlobe. Coat the tip with a water-soluble lubricant.

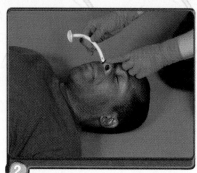

2 Insert the airway into the larger nostril with the curvature following the floor of the nose.

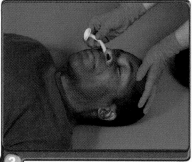

3 Gently advance the airway. If using the left nostril, insert the airway until resistance is met. Then rotate the nasal airway 180° into position. This rotation is not required if using the right nostril.

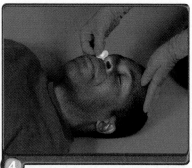

4 Continue inserting until the flange rests against the nostril. If you feel any resistance, remove the airway and attempt to insert it in the other nostril.

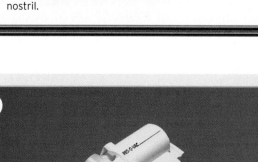

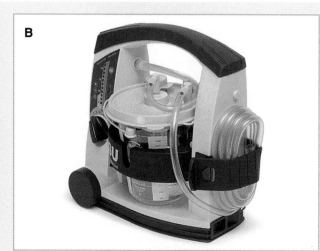

Figure 5-6 Suction equipment is essential for resuscitation. **A.** Hand-operated unit. **B.** Portable unit.

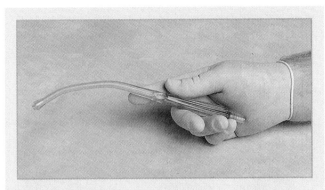

Figure 5-7 Yankauer (tonsil-tip) catheters are the best for suctioning because they have wide diameter tips and are rigid.

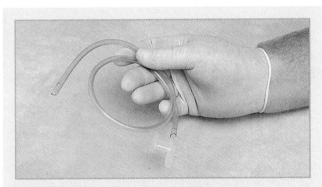

Figure 5-8 French (whistle-tip) catheters are used in situations in which rigid catheters cannot be used, such as patients whose teeth are clenched or those that have a stoma. French catheters are also used to suction an endotracheal tube.

of the airway with a suction catheter. This can activate the gag reflex, cause vomiting, and increase the possibility of <u>aspiration</u>.

Techniques of Suctioning

You should inspect your suctioning equipment regularly to make sure it is in proper working condition. Turn on the suction, clamp the tubing, and make sure that the unit generates a vacuum of more than 300 mm Hg. Check that a battery-charged unit has charged batteries.

Never suction the mouth or nose for more than 15 seconds at one time for adult patients, 10 seconds for children, and 5 seconds for infants. Suctioning removes oxygen from the airway and can result in hypoxia. Rinse the catheter and tubing with water to prevent clogging of the tube with dried vomitus or

other secretions. Repeat suctioning only after the patient has been adequately ventilated and reoxygenated.

You should use extreme caution when suctioning a conscious or semiconscious patient. Put the tip of the suction catheter in only as far as you can visualize. Be aware that suctioning may induce vomiting in these patients.

To suction a patient, follow the steps in Skill Drill 5-5 ▶ :

1. Turn on the assembled suction unit. **Measure the catheter** to the correct depth by measuring the catheter from the corner of the patient's mouth to the edge of the earlobe or angle of the jaw (**Step ①**).
2. **Open the patient's mouth** using the cross-finger technique or tongue-jaw lift, and insert the tip of the catheter to the depth measured (**Step ②**).
3. **Apply suction in a circular motion as you withdraw the catheter.** Do not suction an adult for more than 15 seconds (**Step ③**).

At times, a patient may have secretions or vomitus that cannot be suctioned quickly and easily, and some suction units cannot effectively remove solid objects such as teeth, foreign bodies, and food. In these cases, you should remove the catheter from the patient's mouth, log roll the patient to the side, and then clear the mouth carefully with your gloved finger. A patient may also produce frothy secretions as quickly as you can suction them from the airway. In this situation, you should suction the patient's airway for 15 seconds (less time in infants and children), and then ventilate the patient for 2 minutes. This alternating pattern of suctioning and ventilating should continue until all secretions have been cleared from the patient's airway. Continuous ventilation is not appropriate if vomitus or other particles are present in the airway. You should clean and decontaminate your suctioning equipment after each use according to the manufacturer's guidelines.

Maintaining the Airway

The <u>recovery position</u> is used to help maintain a clear airway in a patient who is not injured and is breathing on his or her own with a normal rate and adequate tidal volume Figure 5-9 ▶ . Once patients have resumed spontaneous breathing after being resuscitated, the recovery position will help to prevent aspiration. However, this position is not appropriate for patients with suspected spinal trauma, nor is it adequate for patients who are unconscious and require ventilatory assistance. You must reposition such patients to

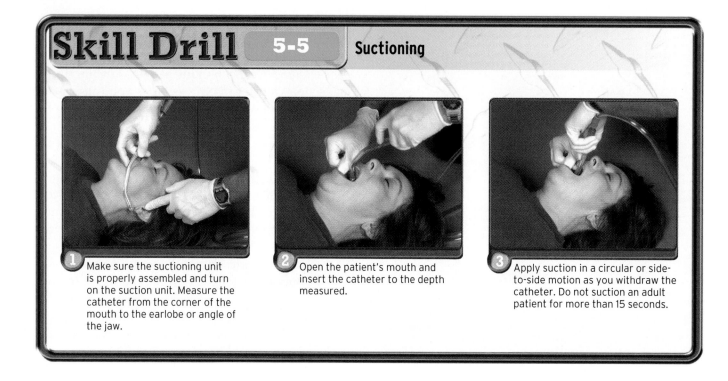

Skill Drill   5-5   Suctioning

1. Make sure the suctioning unit is properly assembled and turn on the suction unit. Measure the catheter from the corner of the mouth to the earlobe or angle of the jaw.

2. Open the patient's mouth and insert the catheter to the depth measured.

3. Apply suction in a circular or side-to-side motion as you withdraw the catheter. Do not suction an adult patient for more than 15 seconds.

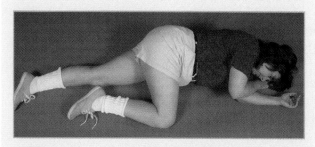

Figure 5-9 In the recovery position, the patient is rolled onto the left side.

provide adequate access to the airway while maintaining appropriate spinal immobilization.

▇ Supplemental Oxygen

You should always give supplemental oxygen to patients who are not breathing on their own, are hypoxic, or are not breathing well enough to deliver adequate oxygen to the tissues and cells of the body. Never withhold oxygen from any patient who is in need. Your experience has taught you to use high-concentration oxygen in any cardiac or respiratory arrest situation. These patients need as much oxygen as possible. Do not worry about problems resulting from too much oxygen; these develop only after several days of more than 50% inspired oxygen delivered at higher than normal pressures. COPD patients are the only concern for high concentrations of oxygen. You should never withhold oxygen from them if they are in need of it, as evidenced by signs and symptoms. However, you should be aware that a small percentage of these patients are true carbon dioxide retainers and may stop breathing when given a high concentration of oxygen. This can occur in as little as 15 minutes. Therefore it is important to be prepared to ventilate with a bag-mask device in the event of respiratory arrest.

Oxygen Delivery Equipment

Depending on local protocol, the oxygen delivery equipment that is generally used in the field is limited to nonrebreathing masks, bag-mask devices, and nasal cannulas. However, you may encounter other devices during transports between medical facilities.

Nonrebreathing Mask

The nonrebreathing mask is the preferred way of giving oxygen in the prehospital setting to patients who are breathing adequately but are suspected of having or are showing signs of hypoxia. With a good mask-to-face seal, it is capable of providing up to 90% inspired oxygen.

The nonrebreathing mask is a combination mask and reservoir bag system. Oxygen fills a reservoir bag that is attached to the mask by a one-way valve. The system is called a nonrebreathing mask because the exhaled gas escapes through flapper valve ports at the cheek areas of the mask. These valves prevent the patient from rebreathing exhaled gases.

You must be sure that the reservoir bag is full before the mask is placed on the patient. Adjust the flow rate so that the bag does not fully collapse when the patient inhales, to about two thirds of the bag volume, or 10 to 15 L/min. Use a pediatric nonrebreathing mask, which has a smaller reservoir bag, with infants and children, as they will inhale a smaller volume.

Nasal Cannula

A nasal cannula delivers oxygen through two small tube-like prongs that fit into the patient's nostrils. This device can provide 24% to 44% inspired oxygen when the flow meter is set at 1 to 6 L/min. For the comfort of your patient, flow rates above 6 L/min are not recommended with the nasal cannula.

The nasal cannula delivers dry oxygen directly into the nostrils, which, over prolonged periods, can cause dryness or irritate the mucous membrane lining of the nose. Therefore, when you anticipate a long transport time, you should consider the use of humidification.

A nasal cannula has limited use in the prehospital care setting. Always try to give high-flow oxygen through a nonrebreathing mask. In your experience you may have found patients who did not tolerate this device. In these cases, the patient may find a nasal cannula more comfortable. Also consider that a patient with COPD who requires transport and has no significant signs or symptoms of hypoxia or difficulty breathing may only need 1 to 2 liters by cannula. As always, a good assessment of your patient will guide your decision.

■ Assisted and Artificial Ventilation

Obviously, a patient who is not breathing needs artificial ventilation and 100% supplemental oxygen.

You are the Provider 3

You are told by the dress shop staff that the woman was "feeling faint" and they tried to sit her down. When her knees buckled, several of the women helped to lay her down on the floor.

There is a fire station just down the street and they arrive on scene just as you are finishing your survey. Two of the fire fighters have brought the stretcher in from your ambulance and they assist you in lifting the patient onto the stretcher while your partner continues to ventilate her.

One of the women has checked her purse and tells you that she has found two pill bottles—one labeled nitroglycerin and one labeled furosemide. She also has an albuterol metered-dose inhaler.

Reassessment	Recording Time: 6 Minutes
Skin	Pale, dry
Pulse	116 beats/min, regular
Blood pressure	158/84 mm Hg
Respirations	6 breaths/min without ventilations
Breath sounds	Diffuse rales/crackles in the lower lobes

9. Is c-spine immobilization necessary? Why or why not?
10. Where else might you obtain a history?
11. Why do you think her pulse rate has dropped?
12. What do the rales/crackles signify?

Patients who are breathing inadequately, such as those who are breathing too fast or too slow with reduced tidal volume, are unable to speak in complete sentences, or have an irregular pattern of breathing, will also require artificial ventilation to assist them in maintaining adequate minute volume. Keep in mind that fast, shallow breathing can be as dangerous as very slow breathing. Fast, shallow breathing moves air primarily in the larger airway passages (dead air space) and does not allow for adequate exchange of air and carbon dioxide in the alveoli. Patients with inadequate breathing require assisted ventilations with some form of positive-pressure ventilation. Remember to follow body substance isolation (BSI) precautions as needed when managing the patient's airway.

Once you determine that a patient is not breathing or is breathing inadequately, you should begin artificial ventilation immediately. The methods that an EMT-B may use to provide artificial ventilation include mouth-to-mask ventilation, bag-mask ventilation (one- or two-person), and the flow-restricted, oxygen-powered ventilation device.

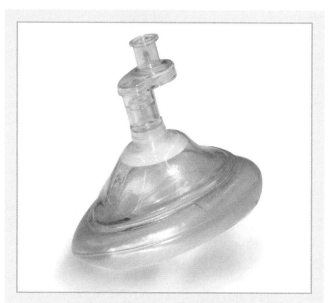

Figure 5-10 Barrier devices such as a plastic shield or a pocket mask with a one-way valve provide adequate BSI. Photo is of the Laerdal® PocketMask.

Mouth-to-Mask Ventilation

As you know, mouth-to-mouth ventilations are now routinely performed with a barrier device, such as a mask or face shield. A barrier device is a protective item that features a plastic barrier placed on a patient's face with a one-way valve to prevent the backflow of secretions, vomitus, and gases. Barrier devices provide adequate BSI (Figure 5-10 ▶). Mouth-to-mouth ventilations without a barrier device should be provided only in extreme conditions. Performing mouth-to-mask ventilations with a pocket mask with a one-way valve is a safer method of ventilation to prevent possible disease transmission.

A mask with an oxygen inlet provides oxygen during mouth-to-mask ventilation to supplement the air from your own lungs. Remember that the gas you exhale contains 16% oxygen. With the mouth-to-mask system, however, the patient gets the additional benefit of significant oxygen enrichment with inspired air. This system also frees both your hands to help keep the airway open and helps you to provide a better seal between the mask and the face, thus delivering adequate tidal volume. To perform mouth-to-mask ventilation, follow the steps in (Skill Drill 5-6 ▶):

1. **Position yourself at the patient's head.** Open the airway using the head tilt–chin lift maneuver or the jaw-thrust maneuver if indicated. Insert an

oral or nasal airway. Connect the one-way valve to the face mask. Place the mask on the patient's face. Make sure the top is over the bridge of the nose and the bottom is in the groove between the lower lip and the chin. Hold the mask in position by placing your thumbs over the top part of the mask and your index fingers over the bottom half. Grasp the lower jaw with the remaining three fingers on each hand. Make an airtight seal by pulling the lower jaw into the mask. Maintain an upward and forward pull on the lower jaw with your fingers to keep the airway open. This method of securing the mask to the patient's face is known as the EC clamp method (**Step ①**).

2. **Take a normal breath in and exhale** through the open port of the one-way valve. Exhale into the patient's mask for 1 second and observe for adequate chest rise (**Step ②**).

3. **Remove your mouth,** and watch for the patient's chest to fall during passive exhalation (**Step ③**).

You know that you are providing adequate ventilations if you see the patient's chest rise with each breath. Feel for resistance of the patient's lungs as they expand, and listen and feel for air escape as the patient exhales. Deliver the number of breaths/min appropriate for the patient's age. Do not deliver more breaths per minute than what is recommended. Remember, your breaths should not be forceful and

Skill Drill 5-6   Performing Mouth-to-Mask Ventilation

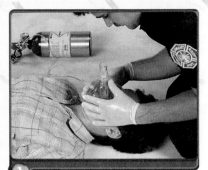

1 Once the patient's head is properly positioned and an airway adjunct is inserted, place the mask on the patient's face. Seal the mask to the face using both hands with the EC clamp method.

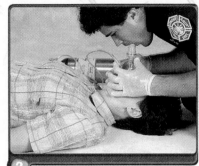

2 Exhale into the one-way valve for 1 second as you watch for the patient's chest to rise.

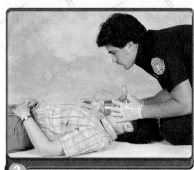

3 Remove your mouth and watch the patient's chest fall during exhalation.

only deep enough to cause the patient's chest to rise. Breaths that are too large of a volume or too forceful can result in gastric distention. To increase the oxygen concentration, administer high-flow oxygen at 15 L/min through the oxygen inlet valve of the mask. This, when combined with your exhaled breath, will deliver approximately 55% oxygen to the patient.

The Bag-Mask Device

With an oxygen flow rate of 15 L/min and an adequate mask-to-face seal, a bag-mask device with an oxygen reservoir can deliver nearly 100% oxygen. Most devices on the market today include modifications or accessories (reservoirs) that permit the delivery of oxygen concentrations approaching 100%. However, the device can deliver only as much volume as you can squeeze out of the bag by hand. The bag-mask device provides less tidal volume than mouth-to-mask ventilation; however, it delivers a much higher oxygen concentration.

The bag-mask device is the most common method used to ventilate patients in the field. As an experienced EMT-B, you will be able to supply adequate tidal volumes with a bag-mask device. Be sure to practice on ventilation manikins on a regular basis to maintain your skill of using the bag-mask device on a patient. If you have difficulty adequately ventilating a

patient with the bag-mask device, you should immediately switch to an alternate method of ventilation, such as the mouth-to-mask technique.

A bag-mask device should be used when you need to deliver high concentrations of oxygen to patients who are not ventilating adequately. The device is also used for patients in respiratory arrest, cardiopulmonary arrest, and respiratory failure. The bag-mask device consists of a self-inflating bag, one-way valve, face mask, and oxygen reservoir. The device may be used with or without oxygen. However, to ensure the highest concentration of delivered oxygen, you must attach supplemental oxygen and a reservoir. You should use an oral or nasal airway adjunct in conjunction with the bag-mask device.

The total volume in the bag of an adult bag-mask device is usually 1,200 to 1,600 mL. The pediatric bag contains 500 to 700 mL, and the infant bag holds 150 to 240 mL. The volume of air (oxygen) to deliver to the patient is based on one key observation—chest rise and fall. In most situations, you will be using the bag-mask device attached to high-flow oxygen (15 L/min). When using the device with high-flow oxygen, you should squeeze the bag for 1 second—just enough to cause visible chest rise. Ventilations that are too forceful or are given with too much volume should be avoided. Doing so will increase the chance of getting air in the stomach (<u>gastric disten-tion</u>) and the likelihood of vomiting. In the cardiac arrest patient, studies have also shown that ventilations with larger tidal volumes interfere with blood return to the heart, which makes chest compressions less efficient. Limiting the number of breaths per minute and the length of each breath or ventilation also reduces the time when chest compressions are not being delivered. The key is to watch for good chest rise and fall—let these observations determine the appropriate amount of volume to deliver.

Technique

Whenever possible, you and your partner should work together to provide ventilation using a bag-mask device. One EMT-B can maintain a good mask seal by securing the mask to the patient's face with two hands while the other EMT-B squeezes the bag. Ventilation using a bag-mask device is a challenging skill: it may be very difficult for one EMT-B to maintain a proper seal between the mask and the face with one hand while squeezing the bag efficiently enough to deliver an adequate volume to the patient. This skill can be difficult to maintain if you do not have many opportunities to practice. Effective one-person bag-mask device ventilation requires considerable experience. Follow these steps for the one-person technique **Skill Drill 5-7 ▼** :

1. **Position yourself at the patient's head.** The patient's head and neck should be positioned with a head tilt–chin lift or a jaw-thrust maneuver as indicated. You can use your knees to immobilize the head if needed. Suction as needed. Insert an oropharyngeal or nasopharyngeal airway to maintain an open airway (**Step ①**).
2. **Place a proper sized mask on the patient's face.** Make sure the top is over the bridge of the nose and the bottom is in the groove between the lower lip and the chin.
3. **Bring the lower jaw up to the mask** with the last three fingers of your hand. This will help to maintain an open airway. Make sure you do not grab the fleshy part of the neck, as you may compress structures and create an airway obstruction. Connect the bag to the mask if you have not already done so (**Step ②**).
4. **Hold your index finger over the lower part of the mask,** your thumb over the upper part of the mask, and then use your remaining fingers to pull the lower jaw into the mask. This is known

Skill Drill   5-7   Performing One-Person Bag-Mask Ventilation

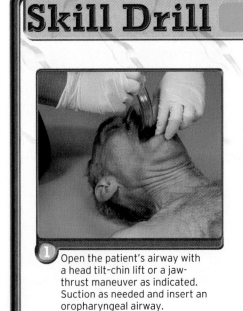

① Open the patient's airway with a head tilt-chin lift or a jaw-thrust maneuver as indicated. Suction as needed and insert an oropharyngeal airway.

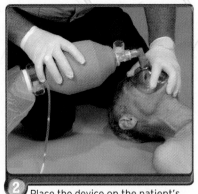

② Place the device on the patient's face. Make sure the top is over the bridge of the nose and the bottom is in the groove between the lower lip and the chin. Bring the lower jaw up to the mask with the last three fingers of your hand. Make sure you do not grab the fleshy part of the neck.

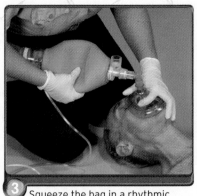

③ Squeeze the bag in a rhythmic manner that is not too forceful and only enough so that you see the patient's chest rise. Deliver ventilations to the adult patient at a rate of 10 to 12 breaths/min (about one breath every 5 to 6 seconds). Ventilate pediatric patients at a rate of 12 to 20 breaths/min (about one breath every 3 to 5 seconds).

as the C-clamp and will maintain an effective face-to-mask seal. Use the head tilt–chin lift maneuver to make sure the neck is extended. If a spinal injury is suspected, stabilize the patient's head in a neutral in-line position with your knees as you pull the patient's lower jaw into the mask.

5. **Squeeze the bag in a rhythmic manner** that is not too forceful and only enough so that you see the patient's chest rise. Deliver ventilations to the adult patient at a rate of 10 to 12 breaths/min (about one breath every 5 to 6 seconds). Ventilate pediatric patients at a rate of 12 to 20 breaths/min (about one breath every 3 to 5 seconds) (**Step ③**).

Follow these steps for the two-person bag-mask device technique (Skill Drill 5-8 ▾):

1. **Position yourself at the patient's head.** Your partner should be at the side of the head to bag the patient while you hold a seal between the mask and the patient's face with two hands. The patient's head and neck should be positioned with a head tilt–chin lift or a jaw-thrust maneuver as indicated. Suction as needed. Insert an oropharyngeal or nasopharyngeal airway to maintain an open airway (**Step ①**).

2. **Place a proper sized mask on the patient's face.** Hold the mask in position by placing the thumbs over the top part of the mask, and the index and middle fingers over the bottom half. Do not grab the fleshy part of the neck, as you may create an airway obstruction. Connect the bag to the mask and the oxygen tubing to the supplemental oxygen source if you have not already done so.

3. **Hold the mask in place** while your partner squeezes the bag with two hands until the chest rises. Deliver ventilations to the adult patient at a rate of 10 to 12 breaths/min (about one breath every 5 to 6 seconds). Ventilate pediatric patients at a rate of 12 to 20 breaths/min (about one breath every 3 to 5 seconds) (**Step ②**).

When you are using a bag-mask device to assist ventilations of a patient who is breathing too slowly (hypoventilation) with reduced tidal volume, squeeze the bag as the patient tries to breathe in. Then, for the next 5 to 10 breaths, slowly adjust the rate and volume of air delivered. To assist respirations of a patient who is breathing too fast (hyperventilation) with reduced tidal volume, you must first explain the procedure to the patient if the patient is coherent. Initially assist respirations at the rate at which the patient

Skill Drill 5-8 Performing Two-Person Bag-Mask Ventilation

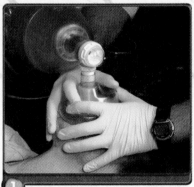

1 Position yourself at the patient's head. Your partner should be at the side of the head to bag the patient while you hold a seal between the mask and the patient's face with two hands.

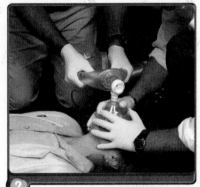

2 Hold the mask in place while your partner squeezes the bag with two hands until the chest rises. Deliver ventilations to the adult patient at a rate of 10 to 12 breaths/min (about one breath every 5 to 6 seconds). Ventilate pediatric patients at a rate of 12 to 20 breaths/min (about one breath every 3 to 5 seconds).

has been breathing, squeezing the bag each time the patient inhales. Then, for the next 5 to 10 breaths, slowly adjust the rate and the delivered tidal volume until an adequate minute volume is achieved.

When you are using a bag-mask device, evaluate the effectiveness of your delivered ventilations. You will know that artificial ventilation is not adequate if the patient's chest does not rise and fall with each ventilation, the rate at which you are ventilating is too slow or too fast, or the heart rate does not return to normal. If the patient's chest does not rise and fall, you may need to reposition the head, use an airway adjunct, or use cricoid pressure.

You should use caution when ventilating a patient to avoid causing gastric distention, inflation of the stomach with air, in the patient. To prevent or alleviate distention, you should do the following: (1) ensure that the patient's airway is appropriately positioned, (2) ventilate the patient at the appropriate rate and not forcefully, and (3) ventilate the patient with the appropriate volume. If an additional rescuer is available, use the Sellick maneuver Figure 5-11 ▼. To perform the Sellick maneuver, apply cricoid pressure on the patient by placing the thumb and index finger on either side of the cricoid cartilage (at the inferior border of the larynx) and press down. By occluding the esophagus, this will (1) inhibit the flow of air into the stomach, thus reducing gastric distention, and (2) reduce the chance of aspiration by helping to block the regurgitation of gastric contents from the esophagus. Cricoid pressure should be performed only on unconscious patients.

If the patient's stomach appears to be distending, you should reposition the head and use cricoid pressure. Make sure you are not ventilating too forcefully

or with too much volume—remember to only ventilate enough to make the patient's chest rise. If too much air is escaping from under the mask, reposition the mask for a better seal. If the patient's chest still does not rise and fall after you have made these corrections, check for an airway obstruction. If an obstruction is not present, you should attempt ventilations using an alternate method, such as the mouth-to-mask technique.

Advanced airway techniques are beneficial when a good seal is difficult to maintain, the patient has a cervical spine injury, or the patient's condition warrants. These techniques are described in Chapter 28, Advanced Airway Management. The bag-mask device may also be used in conjunction with an endotracheal tube or with other advanced airway devices such as the esophageal-tracheal Combitube, the pharyngeotracheal lumen airway, and the laryngeal mask airway.

Flow-Restricted, Oxygen-Powered Ventilation Devices

Another method of providing artificial ventilation is with flow-restricted, oxygen-powered ventilation devices Figure 5-12 ▼. These devices are widely available and have been used in EMS for several years. However, recent findings suggest that they should not be used routinely because of the high incidence of gastric distention and possible damage to structures within the chest cavity. Flow-restricted, oxygen-powered devices should not be used on infants and children or on patients with COPD or suspected cervical spine or

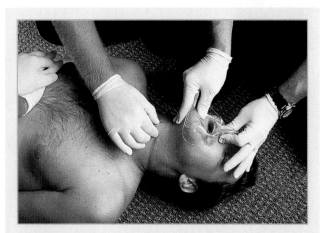

Figure 5-11 The Sellick maneuver will help prevent gastric distention when artificial ventilations are being performed.

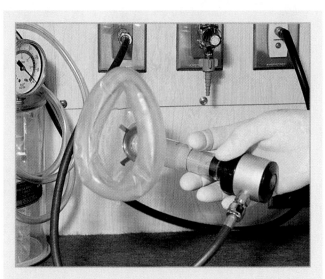

Figure 5-12 A flow-restricted, oxygen-powered ventilation device.

chest injuries. Cricoid pressure must be maintained whenever flow-restricted, oxygen-powered ventilation devices are used to ventilate a patient. This will help to reduce the amount of gastric distention, the most common and significant complication of the device.

Components

Flow-restricted, oxygen-powered ventilation devices should have the following components:

- A peak flow rate of 100% oxygen at up to 40 L/min
- An inspiratory pressure safety release valve that opens at approximately 60 cm of water and vents any remaining volume to the atmosphere or stops the flow of oxygen
- An audible alarm that sounds whenever you exceed the relief valve pressure
- The ability to operate satisfactorily under normal and varying environmental conditions
- A trigger (or lever) positioned so that both of your hands can remain on the mask to provide an airtight seal while supporting and tilting the patient's head and keeping the jaw elevated

Technique

As with bag-mask devices, ensure an airtight fit between the patient's face and mask, and be alert for gastric distention. Pressures that are too great can injure a lung. Always follow local protocols carefully when you use this device. To ventilate with a flow-restricted, oxygen-powered device, follow these steps.

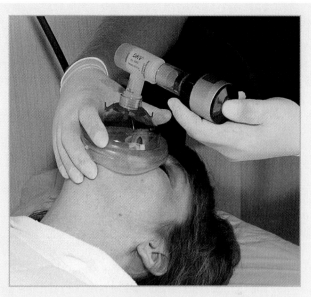

Figure 5-13 Open the patient's airway, and suction as needed. Insert an oral or nasal airway.

1. **Open the patient's airway,** and suction as needed. Insert an oral or nasal airway Figure 5-13 ▲ .
2. **Place the face mask** on the patient and establish a good seal.
3. **Trigger the device's demand valve** until the patient's chest rises, and ventilate at the appropriate rate.
4. If the chest does not rise, the patient is not being ventilated effectively. Consider the possible causes and act accordingly.

You are the Provider 4

Once the patient is loaded into the ambulance, your partner turns the ventilations over to one of the firefighters so that he can drive to the hospital. You consider a paramedic rendezvous, but the hospital is only about 2 miles away so you decide a rapid transport is the best course of action. You continue to monitor her airway, checking patency frequently, and prepare to turn her over to the emergency department staff.

At the hospital she is treated aggressively for exacerbation of congestive heart failure and has a good prognosis for a rapid recovery.

You are the Provider Summary

Recognizing associated signs and symptoms can lead you in the right direction for treating a patient. Early, aggressive airway management can mean the difference between life and death.

1. **What is your first priority for this patient?**

   After ensuring personal safety, your first concern for the patient is to open and assess the airway.

2. **What is the most common cause of snoring respirations in an unresponsive person?**

   The tongue falling back over the airway is the most common cause of snoring respirations in a patient with an altered mental status. It is easily remedied by opening the airway with a head tilt-chin lift or modified jaw-thrust maneuver.

3. **What factors might alter your initial care?**

   Does this patient need c-spine control? If so, managing the airway may require an extra set of hands to hold the c-spine while opening the airway with a modified jaw-thrust maneuver.

4. **What questions should you ask of bystanders?**

   The first question should be whether or not the woman fell. Secondly, does anyone know if she has any type of medical history?

5. **What assistance might you request?**

   The fire department or rescue can provide the extra hands needed to ventilate the patient en route to the hospital as well as provide any lifting assistance.

6. **What questions should your partner consider about her airway?**

   Do her dentures fit snugly? If not, they should be removed so as not to hinder ventilation efforts by creating an obstruction. Is there any need for suctioning?

7. **What is significant about your assessment findings?**

   Distended neck veins and pedal edema are indicative of right-sided heart failure. Cardiac problems and respiratory problems often go hand in hand.

8. **What else should you assess based on these findings?**

   Since right-sided heart failure often follows left-sided heart failure, you should assess for pulmonary edema by auscultating breath sounds bilaterally.

9. **Is c-spine immobilization necessary? Why or why not?**

   No. The woman did not fall. Bystanders lowered her to the floor.

10. **Where else might you obtain a history?**

    Look for any medic alert bracelets, necklaces, etc.

11. **Why do you think her pulse rate has dropped?**

    The more hypoxic the patient becomes, the more her pulse rises in an attempt to circulate what little oxygen is there. When she is ventilated with 100% oxygen, she becomes less hypoxic and her heart rate drops.

12. **What do the rales/crackles signify?**

    Pulmonary edema. Since this is not treatable on an EMT-B level, rapid transport to the closest, most appropriate facility is the best option for this patient. If the transport time was longer, a paramedic rendezvous would be beneficial.

Prep Kit

Ready for Review

- Clearing the airway means removing obstructing material; maintaining the airway means keeping it open.
- Patients who are breathing inadequately show signs of hypoxia, a dangerous condition in which the body's tissues and cells do not have enough oxygen.
- Patients with inadequate breathing need to be treated immediately. Emergency medical care includes airway management, supplemental oxygen, and ventilatory support.
- Basic techniques for opening the airway include the head tilt–chin lift maneuver or, if trauma is suspected, the jaw-thrust maneuver. If the jaw thrust maneuver does not adequately open the patient's airway, carefully perform the head tilt–chin lift maneuver.
- One basic airway adjunct is the oropharyngeal or oral airway, which keeps the tongue from blocking the airway in unconscious patients with no gag reflex. If the oral airway is not the proper size or is inserted incorrectly, it can actually cause an obstruction.
- Another basic airway adjunct is the nasopharyngeal or nasal airway, which is usually used with patients who have a gag reflex and is better tolerated than the oral airway.
- Suctioning is the next priority after opening the airway. Rigid tonsil-tip catheters are the best catheters to use when suctioning the pharynx; soft plastic catheters are used to suction the nose and liquid secretions in the back of the mouth.
- The recovery position is used to help maintain the airway in patients without traumatic injuries who are unconscious and breathing adequately.
- You must provide immediate artificial ventilations with supplemental oxygen to patients who are not breathing on their own. Patients with inadequate breathing may also require artificial ventilations to maintain effective tidal volume.
- Nasal cannulas and nonrebreathing masks are used most often to deliver oxygen in the field.
- The methods of providing artificial ventilation include mouth-to-mask ventilation, two-person bag-mask ventilation, flow-restricted, oxygen-powered ventilation device, and one-person bag-mask ventilation.
- Gentle, non-forceful breaths and the use of cricoid pressure during artifical ventilation can help to minimize the incidence of gastric distention.

■ Vital Vocabulary

agonal respirations Occasional, gasping breaths that occur after the heart has stopped.

airway The upper airway, which includes the nose, mouth, and throat, and the lower airway, which consists of the larynx, trachea, main bronchi, bronchioles, and alveoli.

apnea A period of not breathing.

aspiration The introduction of vomitus or other foreign material into the lungs.

ataxic respirations Irregular, ineffective respirations that may or may not have an identifiable pattern.

bag-mask device A device with a one-way valve and a face mask attached to a ventilation bag; when attached to a reservoir and connected to oxygen, delivers more than 90% supplemental oxygen.

barrier device A protective item, such as a pocket mask with a valve, that limits exposure to a patient's body fluids.

cricoid pressure Pressure on the cricoid cartilage; applied to occlude the esophagus in order to inhibit gastric distention and regurgitation of vomitus in the unconscious patient.

diffusion A process in which molecules move from an area of higher concentration to an area of lower concentration.

dyspnea Difficulty breathing.

exhalation The passive part of the breathing process in which the diaphragm and the intercostal muscles relax, forcing air out of the lungs.

gag reflex A normal reflex mechanism that causes retching and is activated by touching the soft palate or the back of the throat.

gastric distention A condition in which air fills the stomach, often as a result of high volume and pressure during artificial ventilation.

head tilt–chin lift maneuver A technique to open the airway that combines tilting back the forehead and lifting the chin.

hypoxia A dangerous condition in which the body tissues and cells do not have enough oxygen.

hypoxic drive A condition in which chronically low levels of oxygen in the blood stimulate the respiratory drive; seen in patients with chronic lung diseases.

inhalation The active, muscular part of breathing that draws air into the airway and lungs.

jaw-thrust maneuver A technique to open the airway in which your fingers are placed behind the angles of the patient's lower jaw and the jaw is moved forcefully forward.

Technology

- Interactivities
- Vocabulary Explorer
- Anatomy Review
- Web Links
- Online Review Manual

labored breathing   Breathing that requires greater than normal effort; may be slower or faster than normal and usually requires the use of accessory muscles.

metabolism   The biochemical processes that result in production of energy from nutrients within the cells.

minute volume   The volume of air moved through the lungs in 1 minute; calculated by multiplying tidal volume and respiratory rate.

nasal cannula   An oxygen delivery device in which oxygen flows through two small, tube-like prongs that fit into the patient's nostrils.

nasopharyngeal (nasal) airway   Airway adjunct inserted into the nostril of a conscious patient who is not able to maintain a natural airway.

nonrebreathing mask   A mask and reservoir bag system that is the preferred way to give oxygen in the prehospital setting; delivers up to 90% inspired oxygen.

oropharyngeal (oral) airway   Airway adjunct inserted into the mouth to keep the tongue from blocking the upper airway and to make suctioning the airway easier.

patent   Open, clear of obstruction.

recovery position   A side-lying position used to maintain a clear airway in unconscious patients without injuries who are breathing adequately.

retractions   Movements in which the skin pulls in around the ribs during inspiration.

Sellick maneuver   A technique that is used to prevent gastric distention in which pressure is applied to the cricoid cartilage; also referred to as cricoid pressure.

tidal volume   The amount of air that is exchanged with each breath.

ventilation   Exchange of air between the lungs and the air of the environment, either spontaneously by the patient or with assistance from an EMT-B.

Assessment in Action

After a busy morning and no breakfast, you and your partner stop for lunch. Just as you sit down to begin your meal you notice a middle-aged gentleman at the next table clutching his throat in the universal sign for choking. After asking the man, "Are you choking?" to which he nods affirmatively, you proceed to administer the Heimlich maneuver. A piece of hamburger is dislodged and he begins breathing spontaneously. However, he is now unresponsive.

1. What is your first step in caring for this patient?
   - **A.** Check his airway.
   - **B.** Lower him to the ground.
   - **C.** Assist ventilations.
   - **D.** Place him back in his chair.

2. Once you have lowered him to the floor, you hear gurgling from his airway. What should you do?
   - **A.** Call medical control and ask what you should do.
   - **B.** Initiate ventilations with a bag-mask device and 100% oxygen.
   - **C.** Suction immediately.
   - **D.** Call for an ALS unit.

3. What is the maximum time limit for suctioning this patient?
   - **A.** 5 seconds
   - **B.** 10 seconds
   - **C.** 15 seconds
   - **D.** 20 seconds

4. What is the next step after suctioning and ensuring that the airway is clear?
   - **A.** Ventilate with a bag mask at a rate of 12 to 20 breaths/min.
   - **B.** Apply oxygen via a nonrebreathing mask.
   - **C.** Check for radial pulses.
   - **D.** Assess breathing.

5. You determine that the patient's rate of breathing is 16 times per minute and shallow. What type of oxygen does he need?
   - **A.** nasal cannula at 5 L/min
   - **B.** nonrebreathing mask at 8 L/min
   - **C.** nonrebreathing mask at 15 L/min
   - **D.** ventilate with a bag-mask device attached to 100% oxygen

Challenging Questions

6. When ventilating a patient, it is important to use either an oral or nasal airway. What are the contraindications of each?

7. Since you were eating lunch and were not actually dispatched, should you call for another unit to transport the patient, or should you and your partner transport the patient? Why?

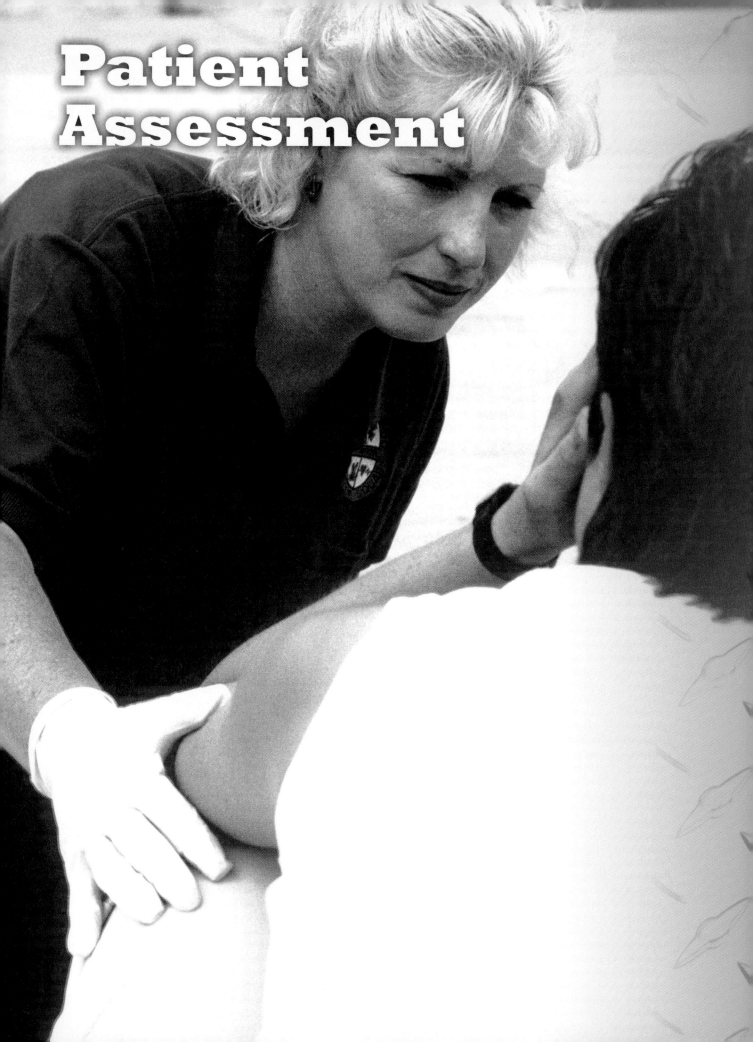

Patient Assessment

3

Section

Cognitive Objectives

1. Assess scene safety. (Chapter 6, p 91)
   - Recognize hazards/potential hazards.
   - Describe common hazards found at the scene of a trauma and a medical patient.
   - Determine if the scene is safe to enter.
2. Assess the need for additional resources at the scene. (Chapter 6, p 93)
   - Explain the reason for identifying the need for additional help or assistance.
3. Assess mechanism of injury. (Chapter 6, p 92)
4. Assess nature of illness. (Chapter 6, p 92)
   - Discuss common mechanisms of injury/nature of illness.
5. Perform an initial patient assessment and provide care based on initial assessment findings. (Chapter 6, p 97)
   - Summarize the reasons for forming a general impression of the patient.
   - Discuss methods of assessing altered mental status.
   - Discuss methods of assessing the airway in the adult, child, and infant patient.
   - Describe methods used for assessing if a patient is breathing.
   - Differentiate between a patient with adequate and inadequate breathing.
   - Distinguish between methods of assessing breathing in the adult, child, and infant patient.
   - Describe the methods used to obtain a pulse.
   - Describe normal and abnormal findings when assessing skin color, temperature, and condition.
   - Explain the reason for prioritizing a patient for care and transport.

6. Obtain a **SAMPLE** history (Signs and Symptoms of the present illness/injury, Allergy, Medications, Past medical history, Last oral intake, Events leading to present illness/injury). (Chapter 6, p 105)
   - Identify the components of a **SAMPLE** history
7. Perform a rapid trauma assessment and provide care based on assessment findings. (Chapter 6, p 111)
   - State the reasons for performing a rapid trauma assessment.
   - Recite examples and explain why patients should receive a rapid trauma assessment.
8. Perform a history and physical examination focusing on the specific injury and provide care based on assessment findings. (Chapter 6, p 105)
   - Discuss the reason for performing a focused history and physical examination.
9. Perform a history and physical examination focusing on a specific medical condition and provide care based on assessment findings. (Chapter 6, p 113)
   - Differentiate between the history and physical examination that are performed for responsive patients with no known prior history and responsive patients with a known history.
   - Differentiate between the assessment that is performed for a patient who is unresponsive or has an altered mental status and other medical patients requiring assessment.
10. Perform a detailed physical examination and provide care based on assessment findings. (Chapter 6, p 116)
    - State the areas of the body that are evaluated during the detailed physical examination.
    - Explain what additional care should be provided while performing the detailed physical examination.

11. Perform ongoing assessments and provide care based on assessment findings. (Chapter 6, p 121)
    - Discuss the reasons for repeating the initial assessment as part of the ongoing assessment.
    - Describe the components of the ongoing assessment.
12. Complete a prehospital care report. (Chapter 7, p 136)
    - Apply the components of the essential patient information in a written report.
13. Communicate with the patient, bystanders, other health care providers and patient family members while providing patient care. (Chapter 7, p 130)
    - Discuss the communication skills that should be used to interact with the patient.
    - Discuss the communication skills that should be used to interact with the family, bystanders, individuals from other agencies while providing patient care and hospital personnel, and the difference between skills used to interact with the patient and those used to interact with others.
14. Provide a report to medical direction of assessment findings and emergency care given. (Chapter 7, p 127)
    - Explain the importance of effective communication of patient information.

Affective Objectives

1. Explain the value of performing each component of the prehospital patient assessment. (Chapter 6, p 89)
2. Recognize and respect the feelings that patients might experience during assessment. (Chapter 6, p 97)
3. Explain the rationale for providing efficient and effective radio and written patient care reports. (Chapter 7, p 129)

Psychomotor Objectives

1. Demonstrate the steps in performing a scene size-up. (Chapter 6, p 91)
2. Demonstrate the steps in performing an initial assessment. (Chapter 6, p 97)
3. Demonstrate the rapid trauma assessment that should be used to assess a patient based on mechanism of injury. (Chapter 6, p 107)
4. Demonstrate the steps in performing a focused history and physical on a medical and a trauma patient. (Chapter 6, p 109)
5. Demonstrate the skills involved in performing a detailed physical examination. (Chapter 6, p 116)
6. Demonstrate the skills involved in performing an ongoing assessment. (Chapter 6, p 121)
7. Complete a prehospital care report. (Chapter 7, p 136)

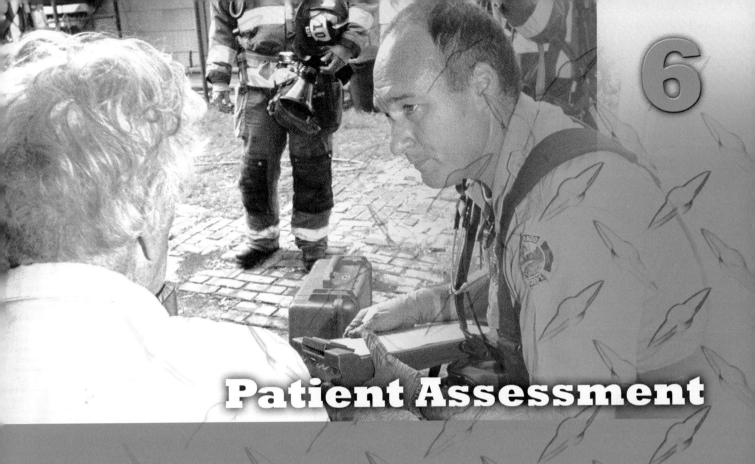

Patient Assessment

You are the Provider 1

You are called to the scene of a motor vehicle crash. There is a small pickup resting against a power pole and lines are down across the vehicle and the highway. There is fluid leaking from the rear of the vehicle. Law enforcement has been dispatched but is not yet on scene. Other motorists are driving over the downed lines seemingly unaware of the situation.

 The driver, who looks to be a male, is slumped over the steering wheel and does not appear to be aware of his surroundings. You can see that the windshield is spider-webbed and that the driver is not wearing a shoulder belt. There is blood on the windshield.

Initial Assessment	Recording Time: 0 Minutes
Appearance	Unable to tell—bleeding
Level of consciousness	Appears unresponsive
Airway	Unknown
Breathing	Unknown
Circulation	Unknown

1. What is your first course of action?
2. What hazards are present?
3. What is your general impression of the patient?

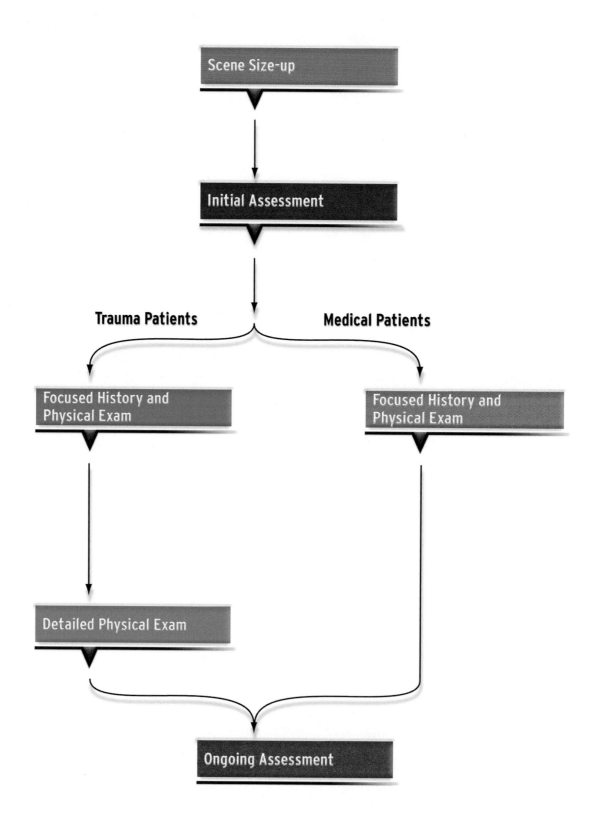

■ Introduction

As an EMT-B, you are aware of the significance of patient assessment. Good assessment skills are critical in the evaluation and treatment of your patients. This chapter reviews the assessment process and will provide a clear and comprehensive approach to patient assessment. A flowchart has been developed to provide a quick visual reference to guide you through the patient assessment process. The chapter has been divided into six sections. Every section is color-coded and numbered for easy reference. The Patient Assessment Flowchart is repeated at every section to show you "at a glance" where you are in the patient assessment process.

Special care has been taken to reflect the current EMT-B National Standard Curriculum (1994), but enhancement information will prepare you for your work in the field. You will also find the special patient assessment needs of pediatric patients in Chapter 24 and of geriatric patients in Chapter 26.

Patient Assessment

From a practical point of view, prehospital emergency care is simply a series of decisions about treatment and transport. The process that guides decision making in EMS is based on your patient assessment findings. For you to make good decisions about how to most effectively care for your patient, you must be able to perform a thorough and accurate patient assessment. Your assessment findings will determine the patient care you provide and the urgency with which you provide it. The patient assessment process includes the following components:

- Size up the scene to identify safety threats and prepare for the call.
- Identify initial threats to the patient's life and treat them. Identify life-threatening conditions and treat them.
- Perform a physical exam of the patient, looking for signs of illness or injury.
- Obtain vital signs to determine how your patient is tolerating the problem.
- Gather history that may help to explain the physical findings and abnormal vital signs if present.
- Prepare the patient for transport and continuously assess for changes in his or her condition.

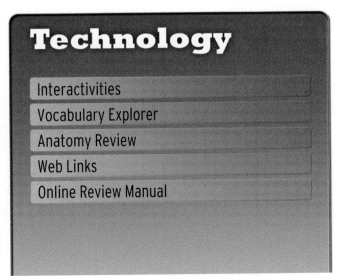

Refresher.EMSzone.com

Technology

Interactivities

Vocabulary Explorer

Anatomy Review

Web Links

Online Review Manual

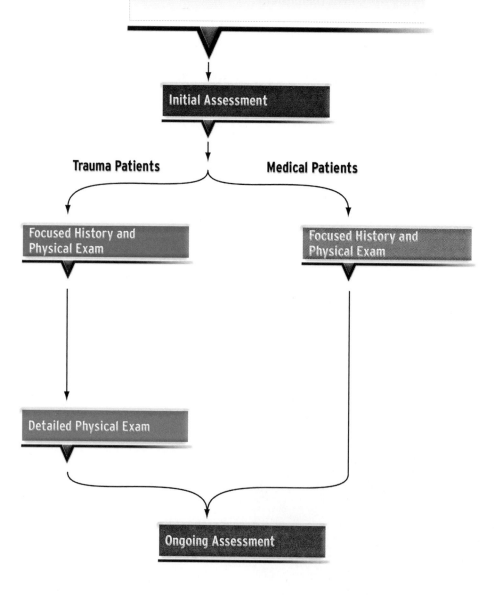

■ Scene Size-up

When you are dispatched to an emergency call, the dispatcher will provide you with some basic information about the call. Your scene size-up begins here. The scene size-up is how you prepare for a specific situation. From the moment you are called into action until you finally reach your patient, you must consider a variety of things that will have an impact on how you begin to care for your patient. The scene size-up includes dispatch information and must be combined with an inspection of the scene to help you identify scene hazards, safety concerns, mechanisms of injury, the natures of illness, and the number of patients you may have, as well as additional resources you might need to care safely and effectively for the patient.

Body Substance Isolation

Personal safety requires you to protect yourself. This includes wearing the proper protective equipment needed to reduce your risk of exposure to communicable disease. Personal protective equipment (PPE) also reduces your risk for injury or illness. The type of PPE you wear depends a great deal on your specific job responsibilities as an EMT. For example, fire fighters wear turnout gear to protect them from injury. Hazardous material technicians wear more sophisticated PPE. As a medical responder, responsible primarily for patient care, you will need to use body substance isolation (BSI) precautions. This is the most effective way to reduce your risk of exposure to potentially infectious substances. The concept of BSI assumes that all body fluids pose a potential risk for infection whether a known infection exists or not.

You should be using BSI precautions when you step out of the vehicle and before you enter the scene. If you have not taken the appropriate BSI precautions when you first approach your patient, the excitement of the call may cause you to begin providing care without the proper protection. Gloves are always indicated. Eye protection and masks should be used when blood or fluids may become airborne by coughing or splattering. Masks will protect you from some airborne diseases.

The use of BSI, including gloves, gowns, masks, and eye protection, may be dictated by your local protocol. If a situation requires additional PPE, you must be appropriately trained in the use of that PPE in those specific situations. If you are not appropriately trained, you should not approach the scene and should call for additional help.

EMT-B Safety

Scene safety is the first step on **ANY** call. You must ensure safety for yourself, your partner, and any bystanders before approaching the patient.

Scene Safety

Every scene can potentially cause injury to you, your team, your patients, and bystanders. You will need to evaluate for potential or actual hazards as you approach the scene. Information provided by dispatch may help in determining potential hazards. For example, a call to an industrial site may have chemicals involved or a private residence may have animals that pose a threat. You should be open to many possible risks, ranging from complex hazardous materials spills to slippery grass. If you become injured at the scene, you will not be able to provide appropriate help to your patient. In fact, you may take important resources away from the original patients.

Personal Protection

Ensuring your personal protection begins by looking for possible dangers as you approach the scene and before you step out of the vehicle:

- Oncoming traffic
- Unstable surfaces (eg, wet or icy patches, loose gravel, slopes)
- Leaking fluids and fumes (eg, gasoline, diesel fuel, battery acid, transmission fluids)
- Broken utility poles and downed electrical wires
- Aggravated or hostile bystanders with a potential for violence
- Smoke or fire
- Possible hazardous or toxic materials (eg, propane, hydrogen chloride)
- Crash or rescue scenes with unstable elements such as unsecured vehicles
- Crime scenes and scenes with a potential for violence

You should consider your ambulance a safe haven for you to care for your patient. Park your unit in a

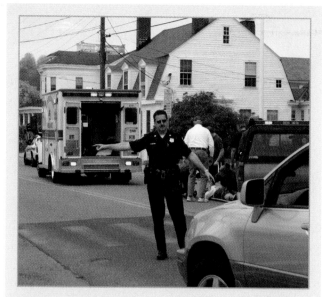

Figure 6-1 Park your unit in a place that allows you the greatest safety but also gives you rapid access to your patient and your equipment.

place that provides you and your partner the greatest safety but allows you rapid access to your patient and your equipment **Figure 6-1▲**. In many instances, law enforcement will be on scene before you arrive. You should talk to them prior to entering the scene to ensure the scene is safe. Follow local protocol if it is a crime scene. As you enter, stop briefly and take a mental note of where the victim is, where the weapon is, if appropriate, and the presence of unusual objects and their location. Careful documentation of these facts may be helpful later if you are asked to testify in a case, but your initial concern must be your own safety. Ask for law enforcement to accompany you if the victim is a suspect in a crime.

Making an Unsafe Scene Safe

If the scene is not safe, you should make it safe before you enter. Occasionally you and your partner will not be able to enter a scene safely. The scene may not be safe to enter because of the need for extrication, possible hazardous conditions, such as toxic substances or unstable surfaces, or scenes of crime and violence. These situations make it difficult to provide medical care, but your safety and that of your partner must remain your primary concern. If the hazard presents a real risk to your health and safety, you should request the appropriate assistance. Do not hesitate to ask for it. Be as specific as possible when requesting assis-

tance. To keep time on your side, request additional resources as soon as the need is identified.

On other occasions, you may be working at a scene that appears safe and then becomes unsafe. If you have the appropriate training and PPE to make the scene safe, you should make it safe. If not, extricate yourself and your patient as quickly as possible, protecting him or her from injury as best you can.

Consider Mechanism of Injury/ Nature of Illness

As you are aware, there are standard questions to ask and consider on most calls. Depending on the answers to these questions, you usually ask other questions and follow other leads. This information-gathering system begins in the scene size-up stage. Although you may not routinely and consciously review the steps in the scene size-up on every call, your awareness of the importance of BSI and scene safety issues automatically keeps you focused on protecting yourself, your crew, and the bystanders and patient at the scene.

Once you have decided that a scene is safe and taken BSI precautions, your next decision is to consider the mechanism of injury (MOI) and/or the nature of illness (NOI). For trauma patients, you will evaluate the mechanism of injury. You can use the MOI as a guide to predict possible injuries and their severity by evaluating three factors: the amount of force applied to the body, the length of time the force was applied, and the areas of the body involved.

For medical patients, you must examine the nature of the illness (NOI). There are similarities between the mechanism of injury and the nature of illness. Both require you to search for clues regarding how the incident occurred. You must make an effort to determine the general type of illness, which is often best described by the patient's chief complaint: the reason EMS was called. In order to determine quickly the nature of the illness, talk with the patient, family, or bystanders about the problem. Common signs and symptoms of illness include chest pain, difficulty breathing, diabetic reactions, seizures, and altered mental status.

Considering the MOI or NOI early can be of value in preparing to care for your patient. For example, when you begin to gather equipment from the unit to treat your patient, what would you take for an older patient complaining of chest pain? How would that equipment differ from the equipment used for a pedestrian struck by a vehicle? The appearance of the scene may also guide you in your preparation. Family members, bystanders, or even law enforcement personnel may also provide important trauma or medical information to help you prepare as you approach the patient.

You may be tempted to categorize your patient immediately as a trauma or medical patient as you begin your assessment and care. Remember, the fundamentals of a good patient assessment are the same despite the unique aspects of trauma and medical care. If an unconscious patient is found at the bottom of a ladder, did he fall off the ladder, strike his head, and become unconscious, or did he climb down the ladder and then lose consciousness? Early in the assessment, it can be difficult to identify with absolute certainty whether the problem is of a traumatic or medical origin. Although further assessment is needed to come to a conclusion, considering the MOI or NOI early will help you prepare for the rest of your assessment.

Determine the Number of Patients

As part of the scene size-up, it is essential that you accurately identify the total number of patients. This evaluation is critical in determining your need for additional resources. When there are multiple patients you should establish incident command, call for additional units, and then begin triage **Figure 6-2 ▶**.

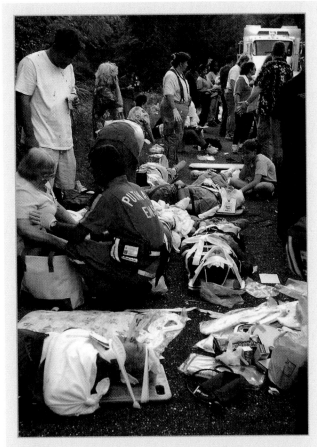

Figure 6-2 With multiple patients, you should establish incident command, call for additional resources, and then begin triage.

Triage is the process of sorting patients based on the severity of each patient's condition.

Once all the patients have been triaged, you can begin to establish treatment and transport priorities. This process will help you allocate your personnel, equipment, and resources to provide the most effective care to everyone. When a large number of patients are present, or if patient needs are greater than your available resources, you should put your mass casualty plan into action based on your local protocols. You should be familiar with the Incident Management System and understand your local protocols regarding responsibilities for establishing and transferring incident command.

Consider Additional Resources

Some trauma or medical situations may simply require more ambulances, while others may have needs for specific additional help. Basic life support (BLS)

Teamwork Tips

When assessing a critical patient, have another rescuer assess the MOI in more detail while you focus on the patient. For example, at an MVC (motor vehicle crash), the rescuer should walk around the outside of the vehicle and lift airbags and other structures, noting any damage.

units may be all that are needed for some patients; however, advanced life support (ALS) should be requested for patients with severe injuries or complex medical problems depending on available resources and local protocols. ALS may be provided by EMT-Is or EMT-Ps, depending on how your EMS system is set up. Air medical support is another good resource for ALS. Follow your local protocols in requesting ALS resources.

Many resources in addition to fire suppression are often available through the fire department, including high-angle rescue, hazardous materials management, complex extrication from motor vehicle crashes, water rescue, or other specific types of rescue, such as swift water rescue. Search and rescue teams can be helpful in finding, packaging, and transporting pa-

tients over long distances or through unusual terrain. Law enforcement also may be needed to control traffic or intervene in domestic violence situations. Knowing how your EMS system is organized will help you determine what additional resources may be required. The sooner these resources are identified, the sooner they can be requested.

Consider C-Spine Immobilization

If an injury is suspected, consider early spinal immobilization. This is an important step, as moving such a patient without proper spinal immobilization can have serious implications. When you are uncertain whether spinal immobilization is necessary, err on the side of caution and immobilize the patient.

You are the Provider 2

You call for the power company. The dispatcher tells you that they are already en route and should arrive momentarily. Law enforcement arrives and takes over traffic control. First responders are on scene and are standing by waiting for your instructions.

The power company arrives and secures the downed lines. As you approach the scene, you hear snoring respirations. Your partner takes c-spine control and opens the patient's airway with a modified jaw-thrust maneuver. This alleviates the snoring and you begin your initial assessment.

Vital Signs	Recording Time: 2 Minutes
Skin	Pale, diaphoretic—bleeding from the forehead is minimal
Pulse	104 beats/min, weak
Blood pressure	108/62 mm Hg
Respirations	22 breaths/min, slightly shallow

4. What else do you need to look at other than the patient?
5. Should you do a focused exam or a rapid trauma assessment?
6. What type of PPE do you need for this patient?

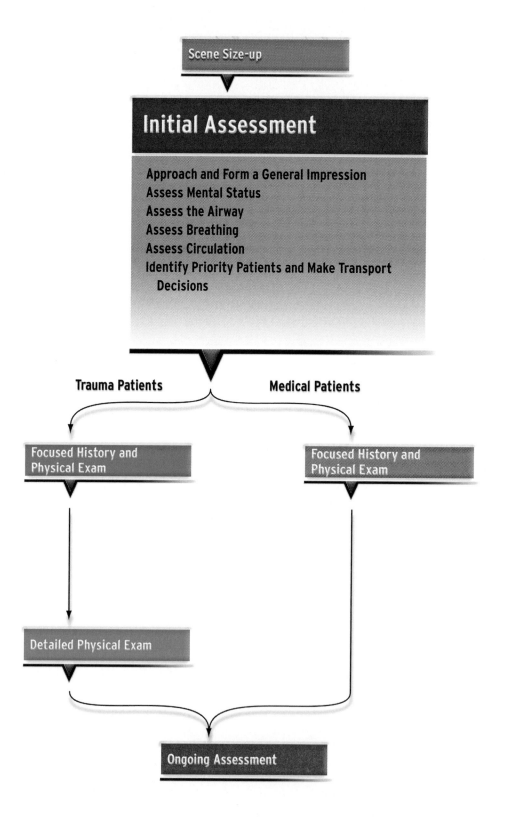

Initial Assessment

The <u>initial assessment</u> has a single, critical, all-important goal: to identify and initiate treatment of immediate or potential life threats. Information concerning life-threatening conditions can be obtained from the visual appearance of the patient, how the patient's complaints relate to the current MOI or NOI, and obvious problems with the patient's airway, breathing, and circulation (ABCs). In all cases, your assessment of the patient's ABCs will determine the extent of your treatment at the scene. Always give priority to the ABCs to ensure lifesaving treatment.

General Impression

As you approach the scene and the patient, begin to form an impression as to the severity and significance of the patient's situation (Figure 6-3 ▶). The <u>general impression</u> is based on the immediate assessment of the environment and the patient's chief complaint upon initial patient contact. This impression immediately directs the priority of care in deciding if the patient is "sick" or "not sick." General impressions tend to set the tone and the pace of the call. You know when you first approach a patient if the call appears to be a critical or a noncritical situation.

Check to see whether the patient is moving or still, awake or unconscious, and/or bleeding or not bleeding when you first approach. Look for the mechanism of injury or the nature of the illness. Listen to the patient and bystanders. Take note of the patient's age, race, and gender.

Answer the following questions to begin forming your general impression:

- Does the patient appear to have a life-threatening emergency? Clues include unconsciousness, obvious difficulty breathing, and either cyanotic (blue) or very pale skin color. If you suspect a life-threatening condition, provide immediate care and transport.
- Was trauma involved? On the basis of the MOI, would you expect the patient to be severely injured? If so, or if you are not sure, assume the worst and begin treatment, including spinal immobilization. If no trauma is suspected, cervical immobilization is not necessary.
- Does the patient appear coherent and able to answer questions? If not, you will rely more heavily on your own assessment skills and the information you can learn from others.

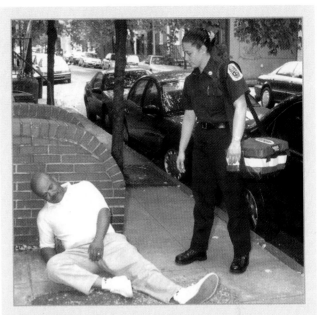

Figure 6-3 As you approach the patient, form a general impression of his or her overall condition.

Determine the Chief Complaint

As part of the assessment process, you should determine the patient's <u>chief complaint</u>. This may be done by simply asking, "What happened?" or "How may I help you?" The chief complaint is the most serious thing that the patient is concerned about and is usually expressed in the patient's own words (symptoms); however, it may be something observable by the EMT-B (signs). In unresponsive patients, their chief complaint is often expressed as being "unresponsive." Keep in mind the chief complaint expressed by the patient may not be the most serious thing that is wrong; however, it is a good place to start. For example, a patient with difficulty breathing from a chronic lung condition may complain about leg problems from poor perfusion. Your responsibility is to determine what is more important—the leg problem or the difficulty breathing. The chief complaint gives you a reference point to begin with during your assessment process.

As an EMT-B you are called on to treat an almost infinite number of different problems. The chief complaint will help you narrow down the MOI or NOI information gathered in the scene size-up. Evaluating how a person was injured may help predict the types of injuries the person may have. If you suspect a potential for a spinal injury, manually stabilize the

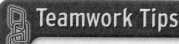

Teamwork Tips

While one EMT is assessing and packaging the patient with the help of first responders/fire fighters, the second EMT should interview family members or bystanders to gain as much history about the patient and/or the incident as possible.

patient's head. You know that it is not always easy to determine whether a patient is a medical or trauma patient until you have completed a more in-depth assessment. This should not prevent you from providing stabilization to a patient with a suspected spinal injury. In many situations, medical emergencies and trauma go hand in hand.

For this reason, the initial assessment does not encourage you to differentiate immediately between medical and trauma patients. Rather, the assessment process begins by assuming that all patients may have both medical and trauma aspects to their condition. This approach is both simpler and safer than an approach that starts with an unsupported assumption that the patient is either ill or injured. One way to evaluate "the big picture" is to obtain a general impression of the patient before focusing in on specific concerns.

Assess Mental Status

Assessing the patient's mental status is your best way to evaluate the functioning of your patient's brain. Many conditions, medical or trauma, may alter brain function and therefore the patient's level of consciousness. Mental status and level of consciousness can be evaluated in just a few seconds by using two separate tests: responsiveness and orientation.

In EMS we use the <u>AVPU</u> scale to assess how well a patient responds to external stimuli, including verbal stimuli (sound), and painful stimuli (such as pinching the patient's earlobe). The AVPU scale is based on the following criteria:

- Alert. The patient's eyes open spontaneously as you approach, and the patient appears aware of you and responsive to the environment. The patient appears to follow commands, and the eyes visually track people and objects.
- Responsive to Verbal Stimulus. The patient's eyes do not open spontaneously. However, the

patient's eyes do open to verbal stimuli, and the patient is able to respond in some meaningful way when spoken to.

- Responsive to Pain. The patient does not respond to your questions but moves or cries out in response to painful stimulus. There are appropriate and inappropriate methods of applying painful stimulus based a great deal on personal preference Figure 6-4 ▶. Be aware that some methods may not give an accurate result if a spinal cord injury is present.
- Unresponsive. The patient does not respond spontaneously or to verbal or painful stimulus. These patients usually have no cough or gag reflex and lack the ability to protect their airway. If you are in doubt about whether a patient is truly unresponsive, assume the worst and treat appropriately.

For a patient who is alert and responsive to verbal stimuli, you should next evaluate orientation. Orientation tests mental status by checking a patient's memory and thinking ability. The most common test evaluates a patient's ability to remember four things:

- Person. The patient is able to remember his or her name.
- Place. The patient is able to identify his or her current location.
- Time. The patient is able to tell you the current year, month, and approximate date.
- Event. The patient is able to describe what happened (the MOI or NOI).

These questions were not selected at random. They evaluate long-term memory (person and place),

⚠ Pediatric Needs

Mental status may be difficult to evaluate in children. First, determine whether the child is alert. Even infants should be alert to your presence and should follow you with their eyes (a process called "tracking"). Ask the parent whether the child is behaving normally, particularly in regards to alertness. Most children older than 2 years should know their own name and the names of their parents and siblings. Evaluate mental status in school-age children by asking about holidays, recent school activities, or teachers' names.

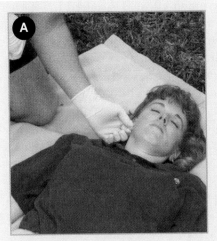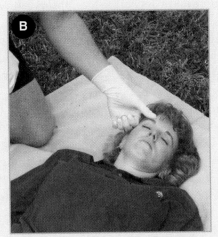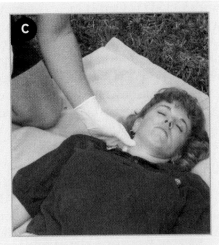

Figure 6-4 **A.** Gently but firmly pinch the patient's earlobe. **B.** Press down on the bone above the eye. **C.** Pinch the muscles of the neck.

intermediate memory (place and time when asking year or month), and short-term memory (time when asking approximate date and event). If the patient knows these facts, the patient is said to be "alert and fully oriented" or "alert and oriented to person, place, time, and event." If a patient does not know these facts, he or she is considered less than fully oriented.

An altered mental status may be caused by a variety of conditions, including head trauma, hypoxemia, hypoglycemia, stroke, cardiac problems, or drug use. If the patient has an altered mental status, you should rapidly complete the initial assessment, provide high-flow supplemental oxygen, consider spinal immobilization if trauma is suspected, and initiate transport. Support the ABCs and continually reassess for changes in the patient's condition.

Assess the Airway

As you perform the initial assessment, you must always be alert for signs of respiratory compromise or airway obstruction. Regardless of the cause, a partial or complete airway obstruction will result in inadequate or absent air flow into and out of the lungs. To prevent permanent damage to the brain, heart, and lungs, or even death, you must determine if the airway is open (patent) and adequate.

Responsive Patients

Patients of any age who are responsive and talking or crying have an open airway. Watching and listening to how patients speak, particularly those with respiratory problems, may provide important clues about the adequacy of their airway and breathing status.

If you identify an airway problem, stop and provide airway management. Use the head tilt–chin lift or jaw-thrust maneuver to maintain the airway. Clear the airway of any fluids, secretions, or foreign objects. Although airway and breathing problems are not the same, the signs and symptoms often overlap. A patient who can speak only two to three words without pausing to take a breath, a condition known as two-to three-word dyspnea, is in respiratory distress. The presence of retractions or the use of accessory muscles or nasal flaring also indicates severe respiratory distress. Any of these may be signs of an immediate or pending airway or breathing problem. Be prepared to manage the airway, administer supplemental oxygen, assist ventilation, and initiate transport.

Unresponsive Patients

With an unresponsive patient or a patient with an altered mental status, you should immediately assess the patency of the airway. If it is clear, you can continue your assessment. If the airway is not clear, your next priority is to open it using the head tilt–chin lift or jaw-thrust maneuver. An airway obstruction in an

Documentation Tips

When documenting level of consciousness, you may use the abbreviation AOX4: The patient is alert and oriented to person, place, time, and event.

unconscious patient is most commonly due to relaxation of the tongue muscles. Dentures, blood clots, vomitus, mucus, food, or other foreign objects may also create an obstruction. Signs of airway obstruction in an unconscious patient include the following:

- Obvious trauma, blood, or other obstruction
- Noisy breathing, such as snoring, bubbling, gurgling, crowing, or other abnormal sounds (Normal breathing is quiet.)
- Extremely shallow or absent breathing

If the airway is not patent, you should open it using the head tilt–chin lift or jaw-thrust maneuver, suction as necessary, and use an airway adjunct as necessary. The body will not have the necessary oxygen needed to survive if the airway is not managed quickly and efficiently.

Assess Breathing

A patient's breathing status is directly related to the adequacy of his or her airway. Make sure the patient's airway is open, and then make sure the patient's breathing is present and adequate. As you assess a patient's breathing, look, listen, and feel for the presence of breathing and then assess the adequacy of breathing. A normal respiratory rate varies widely in adults, ranging from 12 to 20 breaths/min. Children breathe at even faster rates. However, taking the time to actually count respirations may distract you from assessing more life-threatening problems. With practice, you should be able to estimate the rate and note whether it is too fast or too slow. At times it may be important to actually count the number of respirations in your initial assessment. Remember, the goal of your initial assessment is to identify and treat airway, breathing, and circulation problems as quickly as possible. Measuring vital signs more exactly is accomplished later on in the assessment process.

Observe how much effort is required for the patient to breathe. Normal respirations are not usually shallow or excessively deep. Shallow respirations can be identified by little movement of the chest wall (reduced tidal volume). Deep respirations cause a great deal of chest rise and fall. The presence of retractions or the use of <u>accessory muscles</u> of respiration is also a sign of inadequate breathing. Nasal flaring and see-saw breathing in pediatric patients indicate inadequate breathing. A patient who can only speak two or three words without pausing to take a breath has a serious breathing problem. As you assess the patient's breathing, you should ask yourself the following questions:

- Does the patient appear to be choking?
- Is the respiratory rate too fast or too slow?
- Are the patient's respirations shallow or deep?
- Is the patient cyanotic (blue)?
- Do you hear abnormal sounds when listening to the lungs?
- Is the patient moving air into and out of the lungs on both sides?

It may be helpful to listen to <u>breath sounds</u> early in the initial assessment **Figure 6-5 ▼**. This can help identify the adequacy of air movement in both lungs. Normal breath sounds should be equal and clear. Decreased or absent breath sounds on one side of the chest or that are not clear indicate inadequate breathing.

If a patient seems to develop difficulty breathing after your initial assessment, you should immediately reassess the airway. If the airway is open and breathing is present and adequate, you should consider placing the patient on supplemental oxygen. If breathing

⚠ Pediatric Needs

You can feel the pulse of a child at the carotid artery, as in an adult. However, palpating the pulse in an infant may present a problem. Because an infant's neck is often very short and fat, and its pulse is often quite fast, you may have a hard time finding the carotid pulse. Therefore, in infants younger than 1 year, you should palpate the brachial artery to assess the pulse.

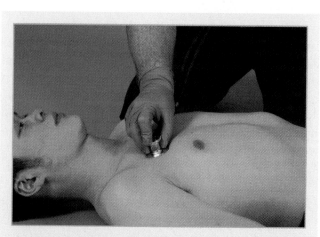

Figure 6-5 Listen to breath sounds on each side of the patient's chest.

is present and inadequate because respirations are too fast (generally more than 20 breaths/min), too shallow, or too slow (generally less than 12 breaths/min), you should place the patient on supplemental oxygen and consider providing positive pressure ventilations.

Any patient with a decreased level of consciousness, respiratory distress, or poor skin color should receive high-flow oxygen. If there is no risk of spinal injury, the patient should remain in a comfortable position that supports breathing; this is usually sitting up with the legs dangling or even a high Fowler's position (sitting up at almost a 90° angle). In any patient with a possible spinal injury, you should immobilize the cervical spine, ensuring that respirations are not compromised. Remember that airway takes priority. If you are unable to maintain the airway with a jaw-thrust, use a head tilt–chin lift maneuver.

Oxygen should be delivered to patients using a nonrebreathing mask at 15 L/min. Any patient identified as having potential airway or breathing problems or immediate airway or breathing problems should be given supplemental oxygen and observed for inadequate breathing. Do not withhold oxygen from any patient at the scene.

Assess Circulation

Assessing circulation helps you to evaluate how well blood is circulating to the major organs, including the brain, lungs, heart, kidneys, and the rest of the body. A variety of problems can impair circulation, including blood loss, shock, and conditions that affect the heart and major blood vessels. Circulation is evaluated by assessing the rate and quality of the pulse, identifying external bleeding, and evaluating the skin.

Assess the Pulse

The first goal in assessing circulation is to determine if the patient's pulse is present and adequate. Assess the pulse by feeling for the radial artery. If a pulse cannot be felt at the radial artery, check the carotid artery. If you cannot palpate a pulse in an unresponsive patient, begin CPR and prepare to use the AED. The AED is indicated for use on patients who have been assessed to be unresponsive, not breathing, and pulseless. You should use an AED with pediatric pads (if available) on patients between the ages of 1 and 7 years old who are unresponsive, not breathing, and pulseless. Follow your local protocol.

If the patient has a pulse but is not breathing, provide ventilations at a rate of 10 to 12 breaths/min for

adults and 12 to 20 breaths/min for a child or infant. Continue to monitor the pulse to evaluate the effectiveness of your ventilations. If at any time the pulse is lost, start CPR and apply the AED.

After determining that a pulse is present, next determine its adequacy. Assess the rate, rhythm, and strength of the pulse. Although the normal pulse rate varies depending on the patient's underlying physical conditions, a rate of 60 to 100 beats/min is normal in most adults. In pediatrics, generally the younger the patient, the faster the pulse rate. The actual number of pulsations per minute is not as important as obtaining a sense of whether the rate is too slow, in the normal range, or too fast. This will help to speed up your initial assessment and allow you to focus on finding potentially life-threatening problems. A pulse that is too slow or too fast may change decisions related to transporting your patient. The pulse should be easily felt at the radial or carotid artery and have a regular pattern. If it is difficult to feel or irregular, the patient may have problems with his or her circulatory system that may need further evaluation later in your assessment.

Assess and Control External Bleeding

The next step is to identify any major external bleeding. In some instances blood loss can be very rapid and can quickly result in shock or even death. Therefore, this step demands your immediate attention as soon as the patient's airway is patent and breathing has been stabilized. Signs of blood loss include active bleeding from wounds and/or evidence of bleeding such as blood on the clothes or near the patient. When you evaluate an unconscious patient, do a sweep for blood quickly and lightly by running your gloved hands from head to toe, pausing periodically to see if your gloves are bloody.

Controlling external bleeding is often very simple. Initially, direct pressure with your gloved hand and soon thereafter, a sterile bandage over the wound will control bleeding in most instances. Most often, bleeding can be adequately controlled by using direct

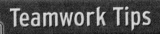

Teamwork Tips

Do not suspend your initial assessment to control bleeding when you have additional assistance. Instruct another rescuer to manage bleeding while you continue with the assessment.

pressure, along with elevating the extremity if bleeding is from the arms or legs. When direct pressure and elevation are not successful, you may apply pressure directly over arterial pressure points.

Assess Perfusion

Assessing the skin is one of the most important and most readily accessible ways of evaluating circulation. A normally functioning circulatory system will perfuse the skin with oxygenated blood. A lack of perfusion or hypoperfusion will result in hypoxia of the brain, lungs, heart, and kidneys. In most situations hypoperfusion is caused by shock. Perfusion is assessed by evaluating a patient's skin color, temperature, and moisture.

Color

Skin color depends on pigmentation, blood oxygen levels, and the amount of blood circulating through the vessels of the skin. For this reason, skin color is a valuable assessment tool. The normal skin color of lightly pigmented people is pinkish. Deeply pigmented skin may hide skin color changes that result from injury or illness. Therefore, you should look for changes in color in areas of the skin that have less pigment: the fingernail beds, the sclera (white of the eye), the conjunctiva (lining of the eyelid), and the mucous membranes of the mouth. Normal skin color, particularly of the conjunctiva and mucous membranes, is pinkish. Skin colors that should alert you to possible medical problems include cyanosis (blue), flushed (red), pale (white), and jaundice (yellow). Cyanosis and pale skin colors indicate a lack of perfusion.

Temperature

The skin has many functions. It helps maintain the water content of the body, acts as insulation and protection from infection, and also plays a role in regulating body temperature by changing the amount of blood circulating through the surface of skin. With poor perfusion, the body pulls blood away from the surface of the skin and diverts it to the core of the body. The result is cool, pale, clammy skin—a good indication in your initial assessment of hypoperfusion and inadequacy of circulatory system function (shock).

Condition

Assessing the condition of the skin is really assessing the presence of moisture on the skin. The skin is nor-

Documentation Tips

Document not only the respiratory rate but also the quality and degree of distress. Include any treatment and response to treatment.

For example: Respirations—14 and shallow with intercostal retractions. Pt ventilated with bag-mask attached to 100% oxygen and oxygen saturation increased to 97%.

mally warm and dry. Skin that is cool or cold, moist, or clammy suggests shock (hypoperfusion). Again, these characteristics are important findings in your initial assessment because hypoperfusion can lead to serious consequences if treatment is delayed or ignored.

Capillary Refill

Another way to assess perfusion is to check capillary refill. This method is most accurate in children younger than 6 years. Although capillary refill is a quick and very general way to evaluate perfusion, it is important to remember that other conditions, not related to the body's circulation, may also slow capillary refill. These conditions include, but are not limited to, the patient's age as well as exposure to a cold environment (hypothermia), frozen tissue (frostbite), and vasoconstriction. Injuries to bones and muscles of the extremities may cause local circulatory compromise resulting in hypoperfusion of an extremity rather than hypoperfusion of the body in general.

Identify Priority Patients and Make Transport Decisions

As you complete your initial assessment, you have to make some decisions about patient care. You should have already identified and begun treatment of life-threatening injuries and illnesses. Now you should identify the priority status of your patient. Would you consider your patient a high priority or a medium or low priority for transport? Priority designation is used to determine if your patient needs immediate transport or will tolerate more time on scene. Patients with any of the following conditions are examples of high-priority patients and should be transported immediately:

- Difficulty breathing
- Poor general impression

- Unresponsive with no gag or cough reflexes
- Severe chest pain, especially when the systolic blood pressure is less than 100 mm Hg
- Pale skin, or other signs of poor perfusion
- Complicated childbirth
- Uncontrolled bleeding
- Responsive, but unable to follow commands
- Severe pain in any area of the body
- Inability to move any part of the body

A high-priority patient should be transported as quickly as possible. The decision to transport should be made at this point in the assessment, and preparations for packaging and transport initiated. Protecting the patient's spine and identifying fractured extremities are an integral part of packaging for transport. These injuries can be made worse if you neglect to assess and treat them before moving the patient.

Recognizing the need to transport critical trauma patients is of such importance that you may hear colleagues refer to the <u>Golden Hour</u>. This refers to the time from injury to definitive care. After the first 60 minutes, the body has increasing difficulty in compensating for shock and traumatic injuries. For this reason you should spend as little time as possible on scene with patients who have sustained significant or severe trauma. Aim to assess, stabilize, package, and begin transport to the appropriate facility within 10 minutes after arrival on scene whenever possible (a difficult or complex extrication may obviously limit possibilities).

Some patients may benefit from remaining on scene and receiving continuing care. For example, an older patient with chest pain may be better served on scene by being administered nitroglycerin and waiting for an ALS vehicle than by immediate transport. ALS should be called for if not already en route to the scene, and depending on the travel distance, can be met while transporting the critical patient. If ALS is delayed or farther away, coordinating a rendezvous may be a better decision for your high-priority patient. Your decision to stay on scene or transport immediately will be based on your patient's condition, the availability of more advanced help, the distance you must transport, and your local protocols.

Correct identification of high-priority patients is an essential aspect of the initial assessment and helps to improve patient outcome. While initial treatment is important, it is essential to remember that immediate transport is one of the keys to the survival of any high-priority patient. Transport should be initiated as soon as practical and possible.

From here, you proceed to the appropriate focused history and physical exam based on your assessment of whether the cause of the patient's problem is a result of trauma, medical emergency, or both.

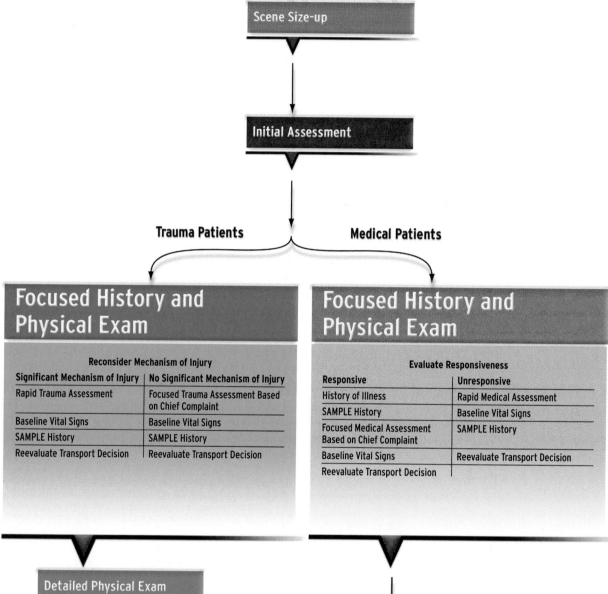

Focused History and Physical Exam

Take a moment to review a call you have been on. After ensuring scene safety, finding and treating any life threats, and making a transport decision, what did you do next? Depending on the circumstances of the call—trauma, medical, or a combination—did you proceed with your assessment based on that particular patient's circumstances? The decisions you make and the assessments you perform are based on two general conditions.

The first condition is the patient's level of responsiveness. If the patient is able to speak to you, you tend to guide your assessment with questions you ask and statements made by the patient. For the unresponsive patient, this information is not available. When the patient cannot tell you what's going on, you must complete a more thorough assessment to find out all the information needed to make treatment and transport decisions. Secondly, you will also consider whether the patient's condition is a result of trauma, a medical condition, or a combination of the two. Patient assessments vary based on this factor.

Unresponsive trauma patients and those with significant mechanisms of injury need a rapid trauma assessment. Responsive trauma patients and those with isolated injuries or injuries from minor MOIs may not need a complete head to toe exam. For these patients, your experience and information from the patient will guide your assessment and treatment.

The same is true for an unresponsive medical patient when the history and circumstances are unknown. This situation requires a more thorough assessment to obtain as much information as you can to properly treat the patient.

The focused history and physical exam will help you to identify specific problems. It is based on the patient's chief complaint (what happened to this patient) and has the following goals:

- Understand the specific circumstances surrounding the chief complaint. What key factors were associated with the event? Does the mechanism of injury put the patient at high risk for serious injuries?
- Obtain objective measurements of the patient's condition. Do these measurements validate the seriousness of this patient's condition? How well is the patient dealing with his or her injury or illness?

Documentation Tips

Thoroughly document all SAMPLE history findings:
- Signs and symptoms
- Allergies
- Medications
- Pertinent past history
- Last oral intake
- Events leading up to the injury or illness

- Direct further physical examination. What physical clues help us to identify problems?

The focused history and physical exam has three components to meet these goals: an evaluation of the patient's medical history, obtaining baseline vital signs, and performing a physical exam based on the patient's complaint, or, in the case of a critical patient, the MOI or NOI.

For some EMT-Bs, taking the patient's history seems to be a bewildering series of questions that seem to bear little or no relationship to the patient's need for help. This becomes worse with patients who have had many medical problems; taking their history is time consuming and may yield little or no information that is useful to you. However, this does not need to be the case. The patient's history can help to tie together your findings from the physical exam and the vital signs. We will review how the focused history and physical exam applies to medical and trauma patients, and how to question patients and obtain a SAMPLE history and a focused history of specific problems using the OPQRST Table 6-1 mnemonic.

The baseline vital signs provide useful information about the overall functions of the patient. They

Table 6-1 The OPQRST Mnemonic

Onset
Provoking factors
Quality of pain
Radiation of pain
Severity
Time

Documentation Tips

Document baseline vital signs and all subsequent vital signs to note any trends.

Remember:

Every 5 minutes for critical patients

Every 15 minutes for stable patients

are an important part of your assessment if your patient appears to have problems related to blood loss, circulation, or breathing. In other patients, you may simply document the vital signs as baseline information. If the patient's condition is stable, you should reassess vital signs every 15 minutes until you reach the emergency department. If the patient is unstable you should reassess at a minimum of every 5 minutes, or as often as the situation permits.

Do not be falsely reassured by apparently normal vital signs. The body has amazing abilities to compensate for severe injury or illness, especially in children and young adults. Even patients with severe medical or traumatic conditions may initially present with fairly normal vital signs. However, the body may eventually lose its ability to compensate (decompensated shock), and the vital signs may deteriorate rapidly, especially in children. In fact, this tendency for the vital signs to fall rapidly as the patient decompensates is the reason that it is important to frequently recheck and record vital signs. Treating a patient for shock before obvious signs of shock appear would help to reduce the overall effects of decompensated shock and therefore potentially increase your patient's survival rate.

There are two types of physical exams performed in this part of the assessment: a rapid physical exam or a focused physical exam. Either one is performed on a medical or a trauma patient depending on the circumstances surrounding the illness or injury.

Rapid Physical Exam

A rapid physical exam is a quick head-to-toe exam to identify any Deformities, Contusions, Abrasions, Punctures/Penetrations, Burns, Tenderness, Lacerations, and Swelling, among other signs, that may indicate a problem. This can be remembered with the mnemonic DCAP-BTLS. This exam is performed in as

quickly as 60 to 90 seconds. The goal of a rapid physical exam is to quickly identify the potential for hidden injuries or identifiable causes that may not have been easily found in the initial assessment. It is usually performed on a trauma patient with a significant MOI or an unresponsive medical patient. Follow these steps for a Rapid Physical Exam **Skill Drill 6-1 ▶** :

1. **Assess the head,** looking and feeling for DCAP-BTLS and crepitus, the grinding that is often felt when two ends of a broken bone rub together. (**Step ①**).
2. **Assess the neck,** looking and feeling for DCAP-BTLS, jugular venous distention, tracheal deviation, and crepitus (**Step ②a**). In trauma patients you should now apply a cervical collar (**Step ②b**).
3. **Assess the chest,** looking and feeling for DCAP-BTLS, paradoxical motion, and crepitus. You should also listen to breath sounds on both sides of the patient's chest (**Step ③**).
4. **Assess the abdomen,** looking and feeling for DCAP-BTLS, rigidity (firm or soft), and distention (**Step ④**).
5. **Assess the pelvis,** looking for DCAP-BTLS. If there is no pain, gently compress the pelvis downward and inward for instability or crepitus (**Step ⑤**).
6. **Assess all four extremities,** looking and feeling for DCAP-BTLS. Also assess bilaterally for distal pulses, motor, and sensory function (**Step ⑥**).
7. **Assess the back** and buttocks, looking and feeling for DCAP-BTLS. In all trauma patients you should maintain in-line stabilization of the spine while rolling the patient on his or her side in one motion (**Step ⑦**).

Focused Physical Exam

A focused physical exam uses specific assessment techniques to evaluate the patient's chief complaint. The exam generally focuses on the location or body system related to the chief complaint. For example, in a person complaining of a headache, you should carefully assess the head and/or the neurologic system. A person with a laceration to the arm may need only that arm evaluated. The goal of a focused assessment is to focus your attention on the immediate problem. It is usually performed on a trauma patient without a significant mechanism of injury or a responsive

Skill Drill 6-1   Performing a Rapid Physical Exam

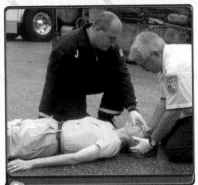

1 Assess the head. Have your partner maintain in-line stabilization.

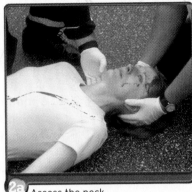

2a Assess the neck.

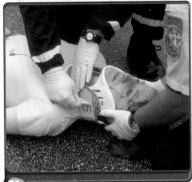

2b Apply a cervical spinal immobilization device on trauma patients.

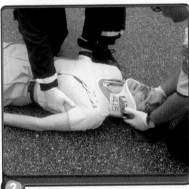

3 Assess the chest. Listen to breath sounds on both sides of the chest.

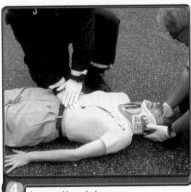

4 Assess the abdomen.

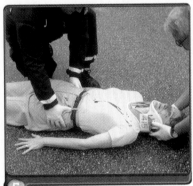

5 Assess the pelvis. If there is no pain, gently compress the pelvis downward and inward.

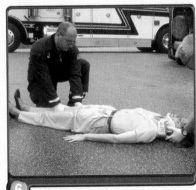

6 Assess all four extremities. Assess pulse, motor, and sensory function.

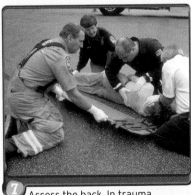

7 Assess the back. In trauma patients, roll the patient in one motion.

medical patient. To review the Focused Physical Exam (only use the relevant steps for what is related to the patient's chief complaint), follow this procedure Skill Drill 6-2 ▶ :

1. **Head, neck, and cervical spine.** Assess the head, neck, and cervical spine. Gently palpate the head and back of the neck for any pain, deformity, tenderness, crepitus, and bleeding (**Step ①**). Ask a responsive patient if he or she feels any pain or tenderness. Check the neck for signs of trauma, swelling, or bleeding. Palpate the neck for subcutaneous emphysema (**Step ②**). In patients where spinal injury is not suspected, you may inspect for pronounced or distended jugular veins with the patient sitting at a 45° angle.

2. **Chest and breath sounds.** Expose as needed and assess the chest. Palpate the chest for injury or signs of trauma, including bruising, tenderness, or swelling (**Step ③**). Watch for equal chest rise and fall. Look for signs of inadequate breathing, including retractions or paradoxical motion. Feel for crepitus. Palpate the chest for subcutaneous emphysema. Auscultate breath sounds.

3. **Abdomen.** Assess the abdomen for any obvious injuries, bruising, and bleeding (**Step ④**). Palpate both the front and back of the abdomen, evaluating for tenderness and bleeding.

4. **Pelvis.** Assess for any obvious signs of injury, bleeding, or deformity (**Step ⑤**). If the patient reports no pain, gently press downward and inward on the pelvic bones.

5. **Extremities.** Assess for DCAP-BTLS (**Step ⑥**). Check for pulses and motor and sensory function.

6. **Back.** Feel the back for tenderness, deformity, and open wounds (**Step ⑦**). Carefully palpate the spine from the neck to the pelvis for tenderness or deformity, and look under clothing for obvious injuries, including bruising and bleeding.

Here are some suggestions for assessing some common chief complaints. Remember that you will also be assessing history and vital signs with each of these.

- **Chest pain:** Look for trauma to the chest and listen for breath sounds. Obtain a set of vital signs, including skin vitals.
- **Shortness of breath:** Look for signs of airway obstruction, as well as trauma to the neck or chest. Listen to breath sounds and assess for signs of inadequate breathing. Obtain vital signs. Because the location of this complaint is the chest, ask the patient if he or she is having any chest pain as well.
- **Abdominal pain:** Look for trauma to the abdomen or distention. Palpate the abdomen for tenderness, rigidity, and patient guarding.
- **Any pain associated with bones or joints:** Expose the area and check the pulse, motor, and sensory function adjacent to and below the affected area.
- **Dizziness:** Assess the patient's mental status (AVPU). Check vitals—changes in blood pressure, heart rate, and skin condition may be the result of hypoperfusion.

Steps in a Focused History and Physical Exam

At this point in the assessment, the focused history and physical exam guides you to take actions that will stabilize or relieve the patient's problems. It will always have three components: baseline vital signs, SAMPLE history, and a rapid or focused physical exam. The physical exam will tell you what is happening outside the body, the vital signs will tell you what is happening inside the body, and the history will help make sense out of the two by guiding your assessment and treatment. The order in which you will perform these three components will depend on whether your patient is a trauma or a medical patient. The order also depends on the type of trauma or the type of medical patient you encounter.

The next four sections describe how to perform the focused history and physical exam on four types of patients: trauma with significant MOI; trauma without significant MOI; responsive medical patients; and unresponsive medical patients.

Skill Drill 6-2 Focused Physical Exam

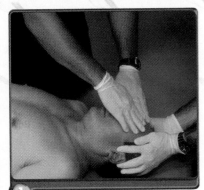

1 Gently palpate the head for any pain, deformity, tenderness, crepitus, and bleeding.

Ask a responsive patient if he or she feels any pain or tenderness.

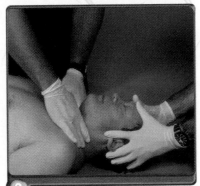

2 Gently palpate the back of the neck.

Ask a responsive patient if he or she feels any pain or tenderness.

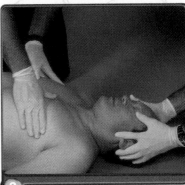

3 Inspect, visualize, and palpate over the chest area for injury or signs of trauma.

Auscultate breath sounds.

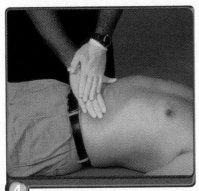

4 Palpate the abdomen, evaluating for tenderness and bleeding.

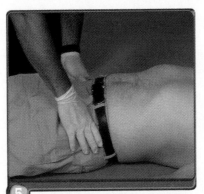

5 Inspect the pelvis for any obvious signs of injury, bleeding, or deformity.

If the patient reports no pain, gently press downward and inward on the pelvic bones.

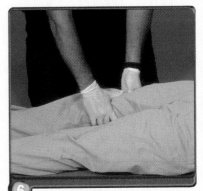

6 Inspect the extremities for open wounds, bruises, swelling, obvious injuries, and bleeding.

Palpate along each extremity for deformities.

Check for pulses and motor and sensory function.

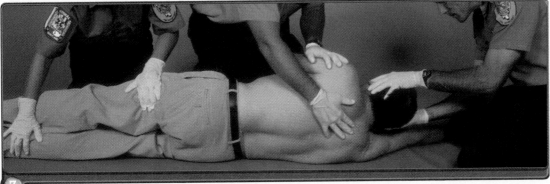

7 Feel the back for tenderness, deformity, and open wounds.

Carefully palpate the spine from the neck to the pelvis for tenderness or deformity.

Look under clothing for obvious injuries, including bruising and bleeding.

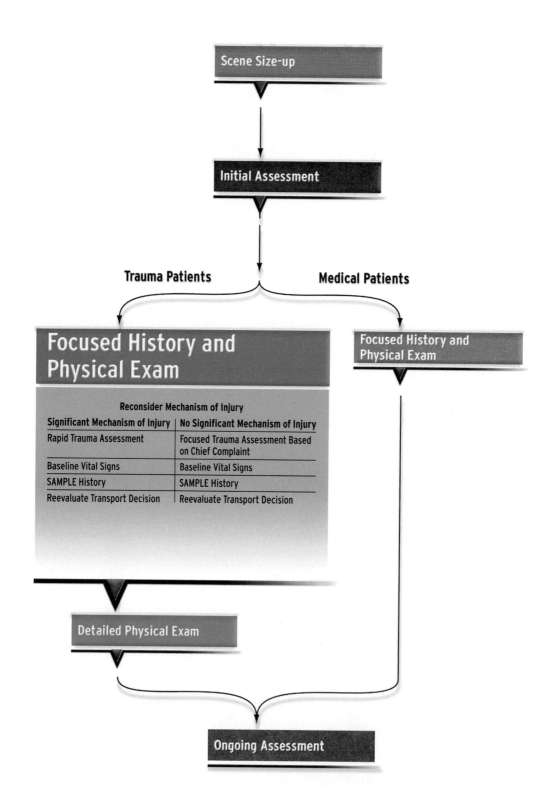

■ Focused History and Physical Exam: Trauma Patients

Trauma Patients With a Significant MOI

At this point in the assessment process, you should reconsider the MOI to ensure that you have not missed important information. Remember that significant mechanisms of injury for adults and children may include the following:

- Ejection from a vehicle
- Death of another occupant of the vehicle
- Fall greater than 15' to 20' or three times the patient's height
- Vehicle rollover
- High-speed vehicle collision
- Vehicle-pedestrian collision
- Motorcycle or bicycle crash
- Unresponsive or altered mental status following trauma
- Penetrating trauma to the head, chest, or abdomen

Rapid Trauma Assessment

In a trauma patient with a significant MOI, you should begin with a rapid trauma assessment to identify both hidden and obvious injuries. This assessment will help you to identify and treat life threats that were not apparent in the initial assessment. Secondly, you will know better how to prepare your patient for packaging and rapid transport. Review Skill Drill 6-1 for the steps in the rapid physical exam.

Baseline Vital Signs

After the rapid trauma exam is complete, obtain your baseline vital signs. A good baseline set of vital signs will be useful as you continue to monitor changes in the patient's condition. These may be obtained in the ambulance if rapid transport is necessary.

SAMPLE History

In the trauma patient with a significant MOI, the patient's history is not as critical as performing a rapid physical exam or obtaining vital signs; however, it should not be ignored. Many of these patients are conscious and able to provide some history. A SAMPLE history should be obtained in case the patient becomes unresponsive and is unable to provide the emergency department with this important information. If your patient is unresponsive, continue to gather history from witnesses, bystanders, or from the environment.

Reevaluate Transport Decision

If transport is not yet under way, consider transporting the patient at this time.

Trauma Patients With No Significant MOI

Focused Trauma Assessment Based on Chief Complaint

After evaluating the MOI, you determine the patient has sustained only minor trauma—for example, a twisted ankle or a laceration on the arm. In this case, a focused physical exam guiding you to the specific injury would be appropriate. If your patient has multiple complaints—for example, neck pain, a twisted ankle, and a laceration on the arm—you may want to perform a focused exam on each of these areas.

Baseline Vital Signs

After evaluating each of the patient's complaints, obtain a complete set of vital signs. Assess the patient's pupils if there is any indication of a head injury. Remember your baseline vital signs help to evaluate any changes in the patient's condition during transport.

SAMPLE History

A SAMPLE history should be gathered to determine whether a medical problem may have caused the trauma. The mnemonic OPQRST is used to evaluate conditions such as chest pain and headaches; however, it may also be used to evaluate ankle or shoulder pain or pain related to trauma.

Reevaluate Transport Decision

If transport is not yet under way, consider transporting the patient at this time.

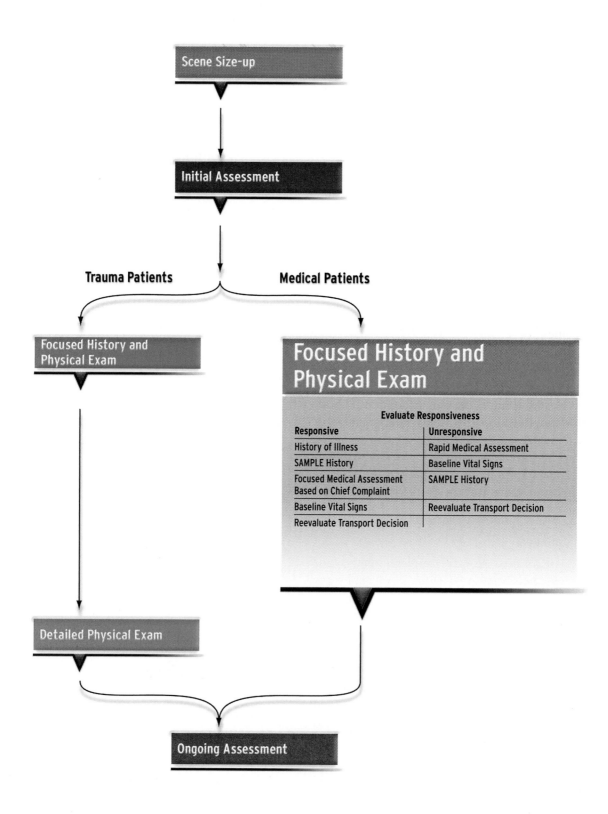

■ Focused History and Physical Exam: Medical Patients

Medical Patients Who Are Responsive

History of Illness

The patient's response to your questions about the chief complaint drives your assessment of the history of the present illness (focused history) and physical exam in the medical patient. You should take the time to listen to your patient to help you understand the patient's condition. In many cases, the chief complaint may not be obvious or the patient's real problem isn't related to the information you received when you were dispatched. The chief complaint will help you focus your questions to ask (focused history) and guide your physical exam of the patient. If the patient cannot tell you what is wrong, try to get the information from a family member or bystander or from your observations of the scene and patient actions.

SAMPLE History

Evaluate as many signs and symptoms as possible using the SAMPLE history. For example, a 50-year-old man with chest pain and dizziness may be having a heart attack. The same person with chest pain and a cough rather than dizziness may be having an asthma attack. As you listen to the patient, make some brief notes to aid your memory and assist with documentation after the call. You should attempt to record the chief complaint in a few of the patient's own words.

Focused Medical Assessment Based on Chief Complaint

After you have evaluated the chief complaint using OPQRST and have obtained a thorough SAMPLE history, you should perform a focused medical exam. The key to this exam is to emphasize the priorities you have learned during the history. Be logical and investigate problems that you identified during the initial assessment and history. As discussed earlier, you can focus on the region of the problem or the physiological system involved. For example, if the patient's history suggests congestive heart failure, you should look for peripheral edema (check feet and ankles) and listen to lung sounds.

Baseline Vital Signs

Although vital signs are obtained last in the focused history and physical exam of a responsive medical patient, they are important to establish a baseline for how your patient is compensating with regard to his or her chief complaint. In problems related to the cardiovascular system and respiratory system, the vital signs will also be a part of your focused physical exam.

Reevaluate Transport Decision

If transport is not yet under way, consider transporting the patient at this time.

Medical Patients Who Are Unresponsive

Rapid Medical Assessment

Since an unresponsive medical patient cannot tell you what is wrong or what happened to them, you will need to perform a rapid medical exam after your initial assessment and treatment for life threats. In 60 to 90 seconds, assess the patient from head to toe looking for problems and possible life threats that may be hidden or not found in your initial assessment.

Baseline Vital Signs

After performing a rapid physical exam, you should evaluate the patient's vital signs to determine if the person is tolerating the unresponsive state well and establish a baseline for your continuing assessment.

SAMPLE History

While packaging the patient for transport, gather what history you can from family, witnesses, and bystanders. Remember, the environment may provide important clues as to the patient's condition. For example, drug paraphernalia including syringes may indicate an overdose has occurred. A medical identification device (eg, MedicAlert Tag, Global Med Net Card, or Vial of Life Container) may also provide important medical history. Patient medication labels may also be used to help determine the patient's medical condition.

Reevaluate Transport Decision

If transport is not yet under way, consider transporting the patient at this time.

Tying It Together

The focused history and physical exam is the most complex step in the assessment process. This part of the assessment is based on whether your patient has been injured from trauma or is sick from a medical condition. Secondarily, it is based on whether the trauma (MOI) was significant and whether the patient is responsive or unresponsive. All patients, however, regardless of the cause, require the following exam: a focused or rapid physical exam, baseline vital signs, and SAMPLE history.

You are the Provider 3

You ask one of the first responders to insert an oral adjunct and ventilate the patient with a bag-mask device attached to 100% oxygen. You apply a cervical collar. A rapid extrication is performed and the patient is moved from the vehicle onto a backboard. Once he is secure on the board, he is loaded into the ambulance to prepare for transport.

Reassessment	Recording Time: 5 Minutes
Pulse	116 beats/min, weak
Blood pressure	94/60 mm Hg
Respirations	Ventilating at 12 breaths/min
Breath sounds	Clear bilaterally
Pulse oximetry	97% on oxygen via bag-mask device

7. What should you do next?
8. What are *baseline* vital signs?
9. What is the purpose of a focused history and physical exam?
10. During the rapid trauma assessment you assess for DCAP-BTLS. What is this?
11. How often should this patient be reassessed?
12. At what point should the abrasion on the forehead be treated?

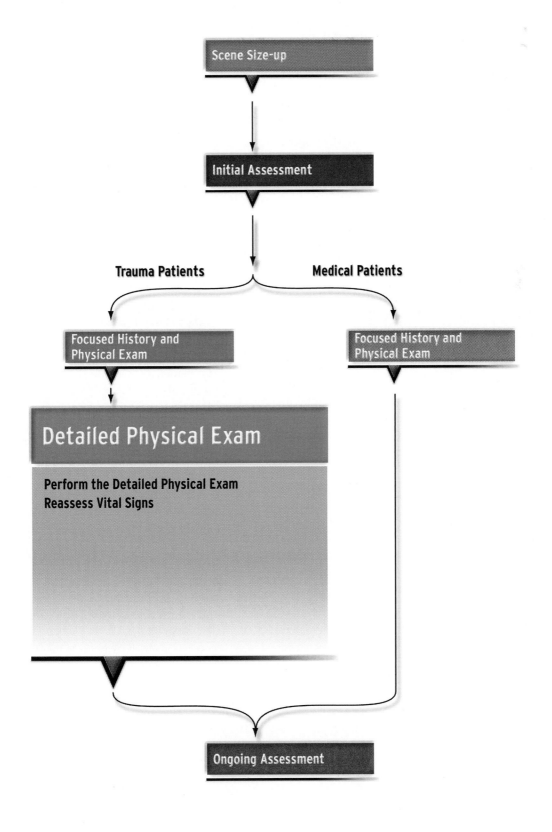

Detailed Physical Exam

The detailed physical exam is a more in-depth examination that extends the focused physical exam. The need for this exam will depend on the particular injury or condition. As you have seen, your patients do not always receive a detailed physical exam when it is unnecessary or impossible because of time constraints.

You have no doubt cared for patients with isolated problems that you were able to evaluate adequately early in the assessment process. Your identification and treatment of the problem made a more detailed physical exam of the entire body unnecessary. A few patients will have life-threatening conditions that are identified during the initial assessment. You may spend all of your time stabilizing ABCs with these patients and never have a chance to perform a detailed assessment.

In summary, you will perform detailed exams only on stable patients with problems that are not identified earlier in the assessment process. In most cases, these are minor or isolated problems. Regardless of the exact situation, the detailed physical exam is usually performed en route to the hospital since the problem may be time-consuming to identify. As you evaluate each area of the body, inspect and palpate to find evidence of injury, using DCAP-BTLS. Follow the steps in **Skill Drill 6-3 ▶**:

1. Look at the face for obvious lacerations, bruises, or deformities (**Step 1**).
2. Inspect the area around the eyes and eyelids (**Step 2**).
3. Examine the eyes for redness. Assess the pupils using a penlight (**Step 3**).
4. Look behind the patient's ear to assess for bruising (Battle's sign) (**Step 4**).
5. Use the penlight to look for drainage of spinal fluid or blood in the ears (**Step 5**).
6. Look for bruising and lacerations about the head. Palpate for tenderness, depressions of the skull, and deformities (**Step 6**).
7. Palpate the cheekbones (zygomas) for tenderness or instability (**Step 7**).
8. Palpate the upper and lower jaw (**Step 8**).
9. Assess the mouth and nose for cyanosis, foreign bodies (including loose teeth or dentures), bleeding, lacerations, or deformities (**Step 9**).
10. Check for unusual odors on the patient's breath (**Step 10**).
11. Look at the neck for obvious lacerations, bruises, and deformities (**Step 11**).
12. Palpate the front and the back of the neck for tenderness and deformity (**Step 12**).
13. Look for distended jugular veins. Note that distended neck veins are not necessarily significant in a patient who is lying down (**Step 13**).
14. Look at the chest for obvious signs of injury before you begin palpation. Be sure to watch for equal chest rise and fall (**Step 14**).
15. Gently palpate over the ribs for any tenderness or pain. Avoid pressing over obvious bruises or fractures (**Step 15**).
16. Listen for breath sounds over the midaxillary and midclavicular lines (**Step 16**).
17. Listen also at the bases and apices of the lungs (**Step 17**).
18. Look at the abdomen and pelvis for obvious lacerations, bruises, and deformities (**Step 18**).
19. Gently palpate the abdomen for tenderness (**Step 19**).
20. Gently compress the pelvis from the sides to assess for tenderness (**Step 20**).
21. Gently press the iliac crests to elicit instability, tenderness, or crepitus (**Step 21**).
22. Inspect all four extremities for lacerations, bruises, swelling, deformities, and medic alert anklets or bracelets. Also assess distal pulses and motor and sensory function in all extremities (**Step 22**).
23. Assess the back for tenderness or deformities. Remember, if you suspect a spinal cord injury, use spinal precautions as you log roll the patient (**Step 23**).

Skill Drill 6-3 Performing the Detailed Physical Exam

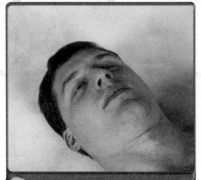

1 Assess the face.

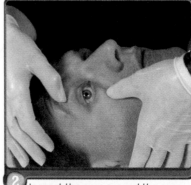

2 Inspect the area around the eyes and eyelids.

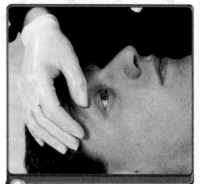

3 Examine the eyes for redness and contact lenses. Check pupil reaction.

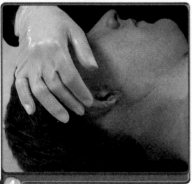

4 Look behind the ears for Battle's sign.

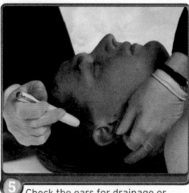

5 Check the ears for drainage or blood.

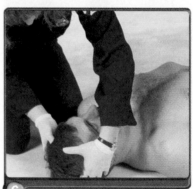

6 Observe and palpate the head.

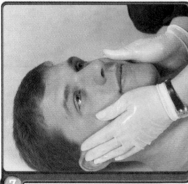

7 Palpate the cheekbones.

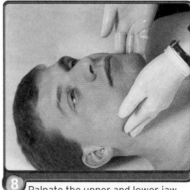

8 Palpate the upper and lower jaw.

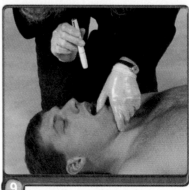

9 Assess the mouth and nose.

continued

Skill Drill   6-3   Performing the Detailed Physical Exam continued

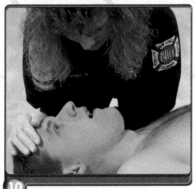

10 Check for unusual breath odors.

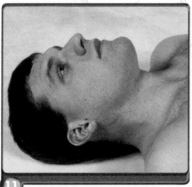

11 Inspect the neck.

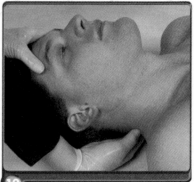

12 Palpate the front and back of the neck.

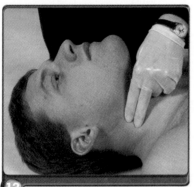

13 Assess for jugular vein distention.

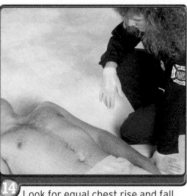

14 Look for equal chest rise and fall.

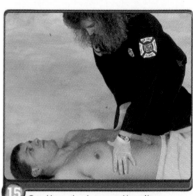

15 Gently palpate over the ribs.

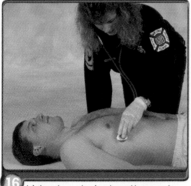

16 Listen to anterior breath sounds (midaxillary, midclavicular).

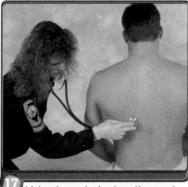

17 Listen to posterior breath sounds (bases, apices).

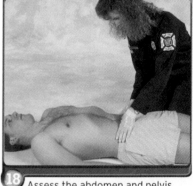

18 Assess the abdomen and pelvis.

continued

Skill Drill 6-3   Performing the Detailed Physical Exam continued

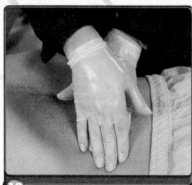
19 Gently palpate the abdomen.

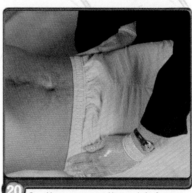
20 Gently compress the pelvis from the sides.

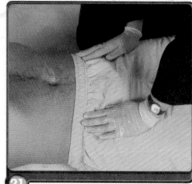
21 Gently press the iliac crests.

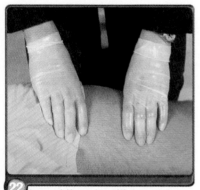
22 Inspect the extremities; assess distal circulation and motor sensory function.

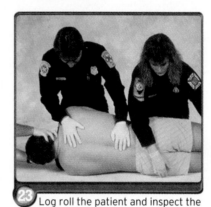
23 Log roll the patient and inspect the back.

You are the Provider 4

Once vital signs are taken your partner starts driving toward the hospital. A rapid trauma assessment is performed and you note that he has bilateral femoral fractures and angulation of his right forearm. The first responder is still ventilating the patient and his tidal volume is good. On arrival at the hospital he is rushed into surgery.

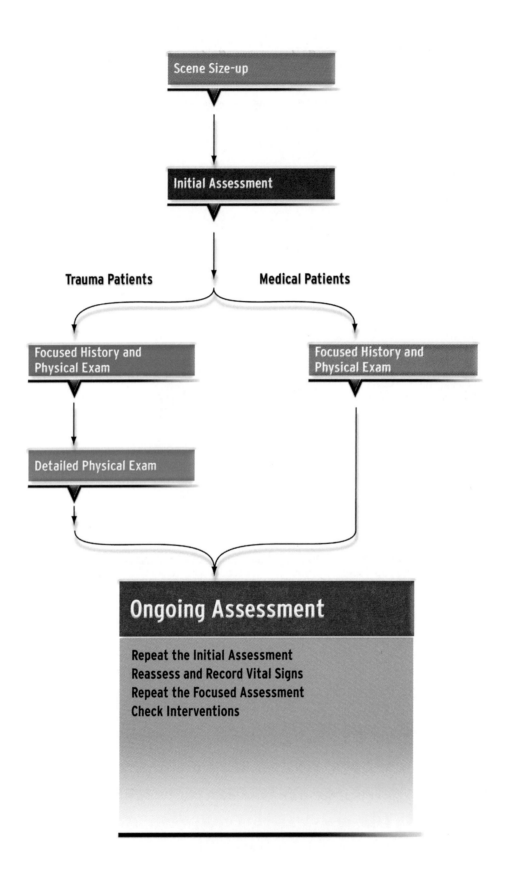

◼ Ongoing Assessment

Unlike the detailed physical exam, the <u>ongoing assessment</u> is performed on all patients during transport. Its purpose is to ask and answer the following questions:

- Is treatment improving the patient's condition?
- Has an already identified problem gotten better? Worse?
- What is the nature of any newly identified problems?

The ongoing assessment helps you to monitor changes in the patient's condition. If the changes are improvements, simply continue whatever treatment you are providing. However, in some instances, the patient's condition will deteriorate. When this happens, you should be prepared to modify treatment as appropriate and then begin new treatment on the basis of the problem identified.

The procedure for the ongoing assessment is simply to repeat the initial assessment and the focused assessment and to check your interventions. These steps should be repeated and recorded every 15 minutes for a stable patient and every 5 minutes for an unstable patient. Remember to use your judgment when timing the ongoing assessments. Some patients may require more frequent assessments.

The steps of the ongoing assessment are as follows:

1. Repeat the initial assessment.
   - Reassess mental status.
   - Maintain an open airway.
   - Monitor the patient's breathing.
   - Reassess pulse rate and quality.
   - Monitor skin color and temperature.
   - Reestablish patient priorities.
2. Reassess and record vital signs.
3. Repeat your focused assessment regarding patient complaint or injuries, including questions about the patient's history.
4. Check interventions.

Repeat the Initial Assessment

The first step is to repeat the initial assessment. If you have been treating the ABCs, you need to continue monitoring these essential functions. It is particularly important to reassess mental status; changes can be initially subtle and then rapidly decline.

Reassess and Record Vital Signs

Be sure that the patient's vital signs have not changed. Record these so that your documentation is accurate and complete. If the vital signs have changed, determine why they have changed and provide treatment if needed.

Repeat the Focused Assessment

As you transport your patient, remember to ask the patient about the chief complaint. Is the chest pain getting better or worse? Is leg pain improving with treatment or staying about the same? If you previously asked the patient to rate symptoms on a 0 to 10 scale, ask the patient for an updated rating for comparison.

Check Interventions

Reevaluate any interventions you started. Take a moment to make certain that the airway is still open, the bleeding has been controlled, the oxygen is still flowing, and the backboard straps are still tight.

You are the Provider Summary

The initial assessment is designed to find and treat all life threats. You must recognize early the need for definitive interventions and not waste time on scene. Any significant mechanism of injury or alteration in mental status or ABCs constitutes a load and go patient. Early recognition and transport is vital to patient care.

1. **What is your first course of action?**

   Ensure scene safety. Call for the power company to secure the lines and block traffic from continuing through the area. Ensure that, regardless of the patient's condition, no one approaches the vehicle until there is confirmation that the downed wires are not live electrical lines.

2. **What hazards are present?**

   Downed power lines, fluid leaking from the vehicle, traffic, blood, broken glass

3. **What is your general impression of the patient?**

   A male patient who appears to be unresponsive with a possible head injury. He has obviously struck the windshield and at least his upper body is unrestrained.

4. **What else do you need to look at other than the patient?**

   The vehicle. What type of damage do you see? Are any airbags deployed? Where was the impact? Is there an intrusion into the passenger compartment? If so, how much?

5. **Should you do a focused exam or a rapid trauma assessment?**

   Rapid trauma assessment. Based on the mechanism of injury and the altered mental status, he is a load-and-go patient.

6. **What type of PPE do you need for this patient?**

   Gloves are sufficient unless there is bleeding with splashing involved.

7. **What should you do next?**

   Baseline vital signs and SAMPLE history if possible, then begin the head-to-toe exam.

8. **What are _baseline_ vital signs?**

   Baseline vital signs are the first set taken. This gives a reference for each time vitals are reassessed. Without a baseline you miss trends, particularly whether the patient's condition improves or deteriorates.

9. **What is the purpose of a focused history and physical exam?**

   It helps to identify specific problems and is based on the patient's chief complaint.

10. **During the rapid trauma assessment you assess for DCAP-BTLS. What is this?**

    Deformities, contusions, abrasions, punctures/penetrations, burns, tenderness, lacerations, swelling

11. **How often should this patient be reassessed?**

    Every 5 minutes because he is unstable. Every 15 minutes for stable patients.

12. **At what point should the abrasion on the forehead be treated?**

    This is a secondary injury and should be managed after the head-to-toe exam has been performed.

Prep Kit

Ready for Review

- The assessment process begins with the scene size-up, which identifies real or potential hazards. The patient should not be approached until these hazards have been dealt with in a way that eliminates or minimizes risk to both the EMTs and the patient(s).
- The initial assessment is performed on all patients. It identifies any life-threatening conditions to the airway, breathing, and circulation (ABCs). Any life threats identified must be treated before moving on to the next step of the assessment.
- The focused history and physical exam includes vital signs, patient history, and a physical exam. The type of physical exam, rapid or focused, and the order of these three components depends on if your patient is a trauma or a medical patient.
- The detailed physical exam is performed on a select group of patients. It helps you to further understand problems that were identified during the focused exam and may also be used to evaluate problems that cannot be identified using the focused exam. The detailed physical exam should be performed en route to the hospital.
- The ongoing assessment is also performed on all patients. It gives you an opportunity to reevaluate problems that are being treated and to recheck treatments to be sure that they are still being delivered correctly. Information from the ongoing assessment may be used to change treatment plans.
- The assessment process is both systematic and dynamic. All patients will be evaluated by using these same steps. However, because the focused history and physical exam will focus your attention on the patient's major problems, each assessment you perform will be slightly different, depending on the needs of the patient. The result will be a process that will enable you to quickly identify and treat the needs of all patients, both medical and trauma.

Vital Vocabulary

accessory muscles The secondary muscles of respiration.

AVPU A method of assessing a patient's level of consciousness by determining whether a patient is Awake and alert, responsive to Verbal stimulus or Pain, or Unresponsive; used principally in the initial assessment.

body substance isolation (BSI) An infection control concept and practice that assumes that all body fluids are potentially infectious.

breath sounds An indication of air movement in the lungs, usually assessed with a stethoscope.

capillary refill A test that evaluates distal circulatory system function by squeezing (blanching) blood from an area such as a nail bed and watching the speed of its return after releasing the pressure.

chief complaint The reason a patient called for help; also, the patient's response to general questions such as "What's wrong?" or "What happened?"

crepitus A grating or grinding sensation caused by fractured bone ends or joints rubbing together; also air bubbles under the skin that produce a crackling sound or crinkly feeling.

cyanosis Bluish-gray skin color that is caused by reduced oxygen levels in the blood.

DCAP-BTLS A mnemonic for assessment in which each area of the body is evaluated for Deformities, Contusions, Abrasions, Punctures/Penetrations, Burns, Tenderness, Lacerations, and Swelling.

detailed physical exam The part of the assessment process in which a detailed area-by-area exam is performed on patients whose problems cannot be readily identified or when more specific information is needed about problems identified in the focused history and physical exam.

focused history and physical exam The part of the assessment process in which the patient's major complaints or any problems that are immediately evident are further and more specifically evaluated.

general impression The overall initial impression that determines the priority for patient care; based on the patient's surroundings, the mechanism of injury, signs and symptoms, and the chief complaint.

Golden Hour The time from injury to definitive care, during which treatment of shock or traumatic injuries should occur because survival potential is best.

initial assessment The part of the assessment process that helps you to identify any immediately or potentially life-threatening conditions so that you can initiate lifesaving care.

jaundice A yellow skin color that is seen in patients with liver disease or dysfunction.

mechanism of injury (MOI) The way in which traumatic injuries occur; the forces that act on the body to cause damage.

nature of illness (NOI) The general type of illness a patient is experiencing.

Technology

- Interactivities
- Vocabulary Explorer
- Anatomy Review
- Web Links
- Online Review Manual

Refresher.EMSzone.com

ongoing assessment   The part of the assessment process in which problems are reevaluated and responses to treatment are assessed.

OPQRST   The six pain questions: Onset, Provoking factors, Quality, Radiation, Severity, Time.

SAMPLE history   A key brief history of a patient's condition to determine Signs/Symptoms, Allergies, Medications, Pertinent past history, Last oral intake, and Events leading to the illness/injury.

scene size-up   A quick assessment of the scene and the surroundings made to provide information about its safety and the mechanism of injury or nature of illness, before you enter and begin patient care.

triage   The process of establishing treatment and transportation priorities according to severity of injury and medical need.

Assessment in Action

You are taking a Basic Trauma Life Support course and it is your turn to do your patient assessment. It has been a while since you have been in school and you are having a little problem remembering all of the mnemonics and the order of the assessment.

1. What is the first step in any patient assessment, regardless of the nature of the call?
   - **A.** LOC
   - **B.** c-spine control
   - **C.** PPE
   - **D.** general impression

2. What is the first step in assessing circulation?
   - **A.** Assess CRTs.
   - **B.** Check skin color, temperature, and moisture.
   - **C.** Check radial pulses.
   - **D.** Look for exsanguinating hemorrhage.

3. What are the functions of the skin?
   - **A.** maintains water content
   - **B.** insulates and protects
   - **C.** regulates temperature
   - **D.** all of the above

4. CRTs may be delayed by _____.
   - **A.** hyperthermia
   - **B.** vasoconstriction
   - **C.** hyperperfusion
   - **D.** all of the above

5. A patient who reports pain after a fall needs what type of assessment?
   - **A.** secondary assessment
   - **B.** focused assessment
   - **C.** rapid trauma assessment
   - **D.** delayed neurologic assessment

6. A patient with which of the following signs/symptoms is considered a priority patient?
   - **A.** poor general impression
   - **B.** complicated childbirth
   - **C.** severe pain
   - **D.** all of the above

Challenging Questions

7. What is the most common airway obstruction in an unresponsive patient?

8. What are the steps for controlling external bleeding?

Communications and Documentation

You are the Provider 1

You and your partner are on scene with a 57-year-old man who is experiencing chest pain. He is deaf and his wife is not at home. You have determined that his chest hurts, but that is all you could understand.

Initial Assessment	Recording Time: 0 Minutes
Appearance	Pale, diaphoretic
Level of consciousness	Alert to person, place, and time
Airway	Open and clear
Breathing	A little fast and shallow
Circulation	Radials present, irregular

1. What are your priorities for this patient?

2. How will you try to communicate?

▪ Introduction

Effective communication is an essential component of prehospital care. Radio and telephone communications link you and your team with other members of the EMS, fire, and law enforcement communities. This link helps the entire team to work together more effectively and provides an important layer of safety and protection for each member of the team. You must know what your system can and cannot do, and you must be able to use your system efficiently and effectively. You must be able to send precise, accurate reports about the scene, the patient's condition, and the treatment that you provide.

Verbal communication is a vital skill for EMT-Bs. Your verbal skills will enable you to gather information from the patient and bystanders. These skills also make it possible for you to effectively coordinate the variety of responders who are often present at the scene. Excellent verbal communications are also an integral part of transferring the patient's care to the nurses and physicians at the hospital. You must possess good listening skills to fully understand the nature of the scene and the patient's problem. You must also be able to organize your thoughts to quickly and accurately verbalize instructions to the patient, bystanders, and other responders. One of the most important aspects of verbal communications in EMS is the ability to communicate effectively by radio to the hospital staff—to "paint the picture" of the patient's presentation, condition, and the emergency care you have provided.

A written report is the portion of the EMT's patient care interaction that becomes part of the patient's permanent medical record. It serves many purposes, including demonstrating that the care delivered was appropriate and within your scope and practice. Adequate reporting and accurate records ensure the continuity of patient care. Complete patient records also guarantee proper transfer of responsibility, comply with the requirements of health departments and law enforcement agencies, and fulfill your organization's administrative needs. Reporting and record-keeping duties are an essential aspect of patient care, although they are performed only after the patient's condition has been stabilized. Documentation in the field drives both funding and research for EMS.

This chapter reviews the skills that you need to be an effective communicator. It begins with a review of standard radio operating procedures and protocols. Next, the roles of the Federal Communications Commission (FCC) in EMS are described. The chapter concludes with a discussion of a variety of effective methods of verbal communications and guidelines for appropriate written documentation of a patient care report.

▪ Radio Communications

All radio operations in the United States, including those used in EMS systems, are regulated by the Federal Communications Commission (FCC). The FCC has jurisdiction over interstate and international telephone and telegraph services and satellite communications—all of which may involve EMS activity. The FCC has five principal EMS-related responsibilities:

1. **Allocating specific radio frequencies for use by EMS providers.** Modern EMS communications began in 1974. At that time, the FCC assigned 10 MED channels in the 460- to 470-MHz (UHF) band to be used by EMS providers. These UHF channels were added to the several VHF frequencies that were already available for EMS systems. However, these VHF frequencies had to be shared with other "special emergencies" uses, including school buses and veterinarians. In 1993, the FCC created an EMS-only block of frequencies in the 220-MHz portion of the radio spectrum.

2. **Licensing base stations and assigning appropriate radio call signs for those stations.** An FCC license is usually issued for 5 years, after which time it must be renewed. Each FCC license is granted only for a specific operating group. Often, the longitude and latitude (locations) of the antenna and the address of the base station determine the call signs.

Technology

- Interactivities
- Vocabulary Explorer
- Anatomy Review
- Web Links
- Online Review Manual

3. **Establishing licensing standards and operating specifications for radio equipment used by EMS providers.** Before it can be licensed, each piece of radio equipment must be submitted by its manufacturer to the FCC for type acceptance, based on established operating specification and regulations.

4. **Establishing limitations for transmitter power output.** The FCC regulates broadcasting power to reduce radio interference between neighboring communications systems.

5. **Monitoring radio operations.** This includes making spot field checks to help ensure compliance with FCC rules and regulations.

Responding to the Scene

EMS communication systems may operate on several different frequencies and may use different frequency bands. Some EMS systems may even use different radios for different purposes. However, all EMS systems depend on the skill of the dispatcher.

Once EMS personnel have been alerted, they must be properly dispatched and sent to the incident **Figure 7-1 ▶**. Every EMS system should use a standard dispatching procedure. The dispatcher should give the responding unit(s) the following information:

- The nature and severity of the injury, illness, or incident
- The exact location of the incident
- The number of patients
- Responses by other public safety agencies
- Special directions or advisories, such as adverse road or traffic conditions, severe weather reports, or potential scene hazards
- The time at which the unit or units are dispatched

Your unit must confirm to the dispatcher that you have received the information and that you are en route to the scene. Local protocol will dictate whether it is the job of the dispatcher or your unit to notify other public safety agencies that you are responding to an emergency.

You should report any problems during your response to the dispatcher. You should also inform the dispatcher when you have arrived at the scene. The arrival report to the dispatcher should include any obvious details, such as hazards or specific instructions to reach the patient, that you see during scene size-up. This information is particularly useful if additional units are responding to the same scene.

All radio communications during dispatch, as well as other phases of operations, must be brief and eas-

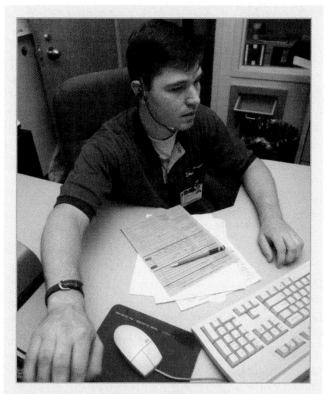

Figure 7-1 Dispatch assigns you to the scene.

ily understood. Although speaking in plain English is best, many areas find that 10 codes are shorter and simpler for routine communications. The development and use of such codes require strict discipline. When used improperly or not understood, codes create confusion rather than clarity.

Communicating With Medical Control and Hospitals

The principal reason for radio communication is to facilitate communication between you and medical control (and the hospital). Medical control may be located at the receiving hospital, another facility, or sometimes even in another city or state. You must, however, notify the hospital of an incoming patient, to request advice or orders from medical control, or to advise the hospital of special situations.

It is important to plan and organize your radio communication before you begin your transmission. Remember, a concise, well-organized report is the best method of accurately and thoroughly describing the patient and his or her medical condition to care providers who will be receiving the patient. It also demonstrates your competence and professionalism to all who hear your report.

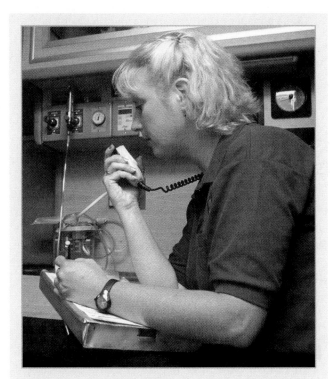
Figure 7-2 The patient report to the hospital should be professional, brief, and accurate.

Hospital notification is the most common type of communication between you and the hospital. The purpose of these calls is to notify the receiving facility of the patient's complaint and condition (Figure 7-2 ▲). On the basis of this information, the hospital is able to prepare staff and equipment appropriately to receive the patient.

Giving the Patient Report

The patient report follows a standard format established by your EMS system. The patient report commonly includes the following elements:

1. Your unit identification and level of services
2. The receiving hospital and your estimated time of arrival
3. The patient's age and gender
4. The patient's chief complaint or your perception of the problem and its severity
5. A brief history of the patient's current problem
6. A brief report of physical findings. This report should include level of consciousness, the patient's general appearance, pertinent abnormalities noted, and vital signs.
7. A brief summary of the care given and any patient response.

Be sure that you report all patient information in an objective, accurate, and professional manner. People with scanners are listening. You could be successfully sued for slander if you describe a patient in a way that injures his or her reputation.

The Role of Medical Control

The delivery of EMS involves an impressive array of assessments, stabilization, and treatments. In some cases, you may assist patients in taking medications. Intermediate and advanced EMTs go beyond this level by initiating medication therapy based on the patient's presenting signs. For logical, ethical, and legal reasons, the delivery of such sophisticated care must be done in association with physicians. For this reason, every EMS system needs input and involvement from physicians. One or more physicians, including your system or department medical director, will provide medical direction (medical control) for your EMS system. Medical control guides the treatment of patients in the system through protocols, direct orders and advice, and post-call review.

Depending on your local protocol, you may need to call medical control for direct orders (permission) to administer certain treatments, to determine the transport destination of patients, or to be allowed to stop treatment and/or not transport a patient. In these cases, the radio or cellular phone provides a vital link between you and the base physician.

To maintain this link 24 hours a day, 7 days a week, medical control must be readily available on the radio at the hospital or on a mobile or portable unit. In most areas, medical control is provided by the physicians who work at the receiving hospital. However, many variations have developed across the country. For example, some EMS units receive medical direction from one hospital even though they are taking the patient to another hospital. In other areas, medical direction may come from a free-standing center or even from an individual physician. Regardless of your system's design, your link to medical control is vital to maintain the high quality of care that your patient requires and deserves.

Calling Medical Control

You can use the radio in your unit or a portable radio to call medical control. A cellular telephone can also be used. Regardless of the type of communication, you should use a channel that is relatively free of other radio traffic and interference. Because of the large number of EMS calls to medical control, your radio report must be well organized and precise and contain only important information. In addition, because you need specific directions on patient care, the information that you provide to medical control must be accurate. Remember, the physician on the other end bases his or her instructions on the information that you provide.

You should never use codes when communicating with medical control unless you are directed by local protocol to do so. You should use proper medical terminology when giving your report. Never assume that medical control will know what a "10–50" or "Signal 70" means. Most medical control systems handle many different EMS agencies and will most likely not know your unit's special codes or signals.

To ensure complete understanding, once you receive an order from medical control, you must repeat the order back, word for word, and then receive confirmation. Whether the physician gives an order for medication or a specific treatment or denies a request for a particular treatment, you must repeat the order back word for word. This "echo" exchange helps to eliminate confusion and the possibility of poor patient care. Orders that are unclear or seem inappropriate or incorrect should be questioned. Do not blindly follow an order that does not make sense to you. The physician may have misunderstood or may have missed part of your report.

Standard Procedures and Protocols

You must use your radio communications system effectively from the time you acknowledge a call until you complete your run. Standard radio operating procedures are designed to reduce the number of misunderstood messages, to keep transmissions brief, and to develop effective radio discipline. Standard radio communications protocols help both you and the dispatcher to communicate properly. Protocols should include guidelines specifying a preferred format for transmitting messages, definitions of key words and phrases, and procedures for troubleshooting common radio communications problems.

Reporting Requirements

Proper use of the EMS communications system will help you to do your job more effectively. From acknowledgment of the call until you are cleared from the medical emergency, you will use radio communications. You must report in to dispatch at least six times during your run:

1. **To acknowledge the dispatch information** and to confirm that you are responding to the scene
2. **To announce your arrival at the scene**

3. **To announce that you are leaving** the scene and are en route to the receiving hospital. (At this point, you typically should also state the number of patients being transported, your estimated arrival time at the hospital, and the run status.)
4. **To announce your arrival at the hospital** or facility
5. **To announce that you are clear of the incident** or hospital and available for another assignment
6. **To announce your arrival back at headquarters** or other off-the-air location

While en route to and from the scene, you should report to the dispatcher any special hazards or road conditions that might affect other responding units. Report any unusual delay, such as roadblocks, traffic, or construction. Once you are at the scene, you may request additional EMS or other public safety assistance and then help to coordinate their response.

■ Verbal Communications

As an EMT-B, you have mastered many communication skills, including radio operations and written communications. Verbal communications with the patient, the family, and the rest of the health care team are also essential to high-quality patient care. Never forget that you are the vital link between the patient and the remainder of the health care team.

Communicating With Other Health Care Professionals

EMS is the first step in what is often a long and involved series of treatment phases. Effective communication between the EMT-B and health care professionals in the receiving facility is an essential cornerstone of efficient, effective, and appropriate patient care. Your reporting responsibilities do not end when you arrive at the hospital. The transfer of care officially occurs during your oral report at the hospital, not as a result of your radio report en route. Once you arrive at the hospital, a hospital staff member should promptly take responsibility for the patient from you Figure 7-3 ▶. Once a hospital staff member is ready to take responsibility for the patient, you must provide that person with a formal oral report of the patient's condition.

Giving a report is a longstanding and well-documented part of transferring the patient's care from one provider to another. Your oral report is usually given at the same time that the staff member is doing something for the patient. For example, a nurse or physician may be looking at the patient, beginning assessment, or helping you to move the patient from the

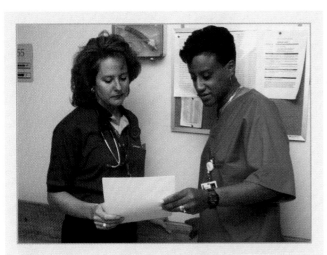

Figure 7-3 Once you arrive at the hospital, a staff member should promptly take responsibility for the patient from you.

stretcher to an examination table. Therefore, you must report important information in a complete, precise way. The following components should be included in the oral report:

1. **The patient's name** (if you know it) and the chief complaint, nature of illness, or mechanism of injury
2. **More detailed information** of what you gave in your radio report
3. **Any important history** that was not given already
4. **The patient's response to treatment** given en route. It is especially important to report any changes in the patient or the treatment provided since your radio report.
5. **The vital signs assessed** during transport and after the radio report
6. **Any other information** that you may have gathered that was not important enough to report sooner. Information that was gathered during transport, any patient medications you have

Teamwork Tips

A concise, well-organized report is the best method of accurately and thoroughly describing the patient and his medical condition to care providers who will be receiving the patient and can prepare staff and equipment appropriately to receive the patient.

brought with you, and any other details about the patient that was provided by family members or friends may be included.

Communicating With Patients

Your communication skills are put to the test when you communicate with patients and/or families in emergency situations. Remember that someone who is sick or injured is scared and might not understand what you are doing and saying. Therefore, your gestures, body movements, and attitude toward the patient are critically important in gaining the trust of both the patient and family. The following guidelines will help you to calm and reassure your patients:

1. **Make and keep eye contact** with your patient at all times. Give the patient your undivided attention. This will let the patient know that he or she is your top priority. Look the patient straight in the eye to establish rapport. Establishing rapport is building a trusting relationship with your patient. This will make the job of caring for the patient much easier for both you and the patient.
2. **Use the patient's proper name** when you know it. Ask the patient what he or she wishes to be called. Avoid using terms such as "Honey" or "Dear." Use a patient's first name only if the patient is a child or the patient asks you to use his or her first name. Rather, use a courtesy title, such as "Mr. Peters," "Mrs. Smith," or "Ms. Butler." If you do not know the patient's name, refer to him or her as "sir" or "ma'am."
3. **Tell the patient the truth.** Even if you have to say something very unpleasant, telling the truth is better than lying. Lying will destroy the patient's trust in you and decrease your own confidence. You might not always tell the patient everything, but if the patient or a family member asks a specific question, you should answer truthfully. A direct question deserves a direct answer. If you do not know the answer to the patient's question, say so.
4. **Use language that the patient can understand.** Do not talk up or down to the patient in any way. Avoid technical medical terms that the patient might not understand. For example, ask the patient whether he or she has a history of "heart problems." This will usually result in more accurate information than if you ask about "previous episodes of myocardial infarction" or a "history of cardiomyopathy."

5. **Be careful of what you say about the patient to others.** A patient might hear only part of what is said. As a result, the patient might seriously misinterpret (and remember for a long time) what was said. Therefore, assume that the patient can hear every word you say, even if you are speaking to others and even if the patient appears to be unconscious or unresponsive.

6. **Be aware of your body language** Figure 7-4 ▶ . Nonverbal communication is extremely important in dealing with patients. In stressful situations, patients may misinterpret your gestures and movements. Be particularly careful not to appear threatening. When practical, position yourself at a lower level than the patient. Remember that you should always conduct yourself in a calm, professional manner.

7. **Always speak slowly, clearly, and distinctly.** Pay close attention to your tone of voice.

8. **If the patient is hearing impaired, speak clearly,** and face the person so that he or she can read your lips. Do not shout at a person who is hearing impaired. Shouting will not make it any easier for the patient to understand you. Instead, it may frighten the patient and make it even more difficult for the patient to understand you. Never assume that an older patient is hearing impaired or otherwise unable to understand you. Also, never use "baby talk" with older patients or with anyone other than infants.

9. **Allow time for the patient to answer** or respond to your questions. Do not rush a patient unless there is immediate danger. Sick and injured people may not be thinking clearly and may need time to answer even simple questions. This is especially true in treating older patients.

10. **Act and speak in a calm, confident manner** while caring for the patient. Make sure that you attend to the patient's pains and needs. Try to make the patient physically comfortable and relaxed. Find out whether the patient is more comfortable sitting or lying down. Is the patient cold or hot? Does the patient want a friend or relative nearby? Patients literally place their lives in your hands. They deserve to know that you can provide medical care and that you are concerned about their well-being.

Communicating With Older Patients

According to US Census Data, almost 35 million individuals are older than 65 years. It is projected that by the year 2030, the geriatric population will be greater

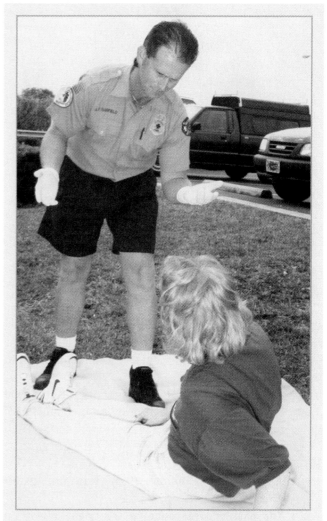

Figure 7-4 Watch your body language, as patients may misinterpret your gestures, movements, and stance.

than 70 million. A person's actual age might not be the most important factor in making him or her geriatric. It is more important to determine a person's functional age. The functional age relates to the person's ability to function in daily activities, the person's mental state, and activity pattern.

As an EMS provider, when you step onto a scene to care for an older patient, you are being asked to take control. You have been called because a person needs help. What you say and how you say it have an impact on the patient's perception of the call. You should present yourself as competent, confident, and concerned. You must take charge of the situation, but do so with compassion. You are there to listen, then act on what you learn. Don't limit your assessment to the obvious problem. Oftentimes, older patients who express that they are not well or who are overly concerned about their health or general condition are at risk for a serious decline in their physical, emotional, or psychological state. Most older people think clearly, can give you a clear medical history, and can answer your questions **Figure 7-5 ▼** . Do not assume that an older patient is senile or confused. Remember, though, that communicating with some older patients is extremely difficult. Some may be hostile, irritable, and/ or confused. Do not assume this is normal behavior for an older patient. These signs may be caused by a simple lack of oxygen (hypoxia), brain injury including a cerebrovascular accident (CVA), unintentional drug overdose, or even hypovolemia. Never attribute altered mental status simply to "old age."

Others may have difficulty hearing or seeing you. You need great patience and compassion when you are called upon to care for such a patient. Think of the patient as someone's grandmother or grandfather—or even as yourself when you reach that age.

Approach an older patient slowly and calmly. Allow plenty of time for the patient to respond to your questions. Watch for signs of confusion, anxiety, or impaired hearing or vision. The patient should feel confident that you are in charge and that everything possible is being done for him or her.

Older patients often do not feel much pain. An older person who has fallen or been injured may report no pain. In addition, older patients might not be fully aware of important changes in other body systems. As a result, be especially vigilant for objective changes—no matter how subtle—in their condition. Even minor changes in breathing or mental state may signal major problems.

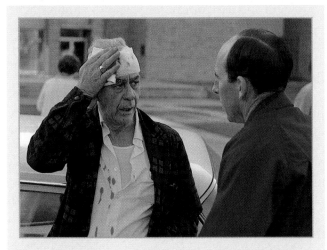

Figure 7-5 You need compassion and patience when caring for older patients. Do not assume that the patient is senile or confused.

Teamwork Tips

Have a second rescuer talk with family members to determine a baseline mental status when a patient appears to be impaired.

When possible (which is more often than you'd think), give the patient some time to pack a few personal items before leaving for the hospital. Be sure to get any hearing aids, glasses, or dentures packed before departure; it will make the patient's hospital stay much more pleasant. You should document on the prehospital care report that these items accompanied the patient to the hospital and were given to a specific staff person in the emergency department.

Communicating With Children

Everyone who is thrust into an emergency situation becomes frightened to some degree. However, fear is probably most severe and most obvious in children. Children may be frightened by your uniform, the ambulance, and the number of people who have suddenly gathered around. Even a child who says little may be very much aware of all that is going on.

Familiar objects and faces will help to reduce this fright. Let a child keep a favorite toy, doll, or security blanket to give the child some sense of control and comfort. Having a family member or friend nearby is also helpful. When not impractical due to the child's condition, it is often helpful to let the parent or an adult friend hold the child during your evaluation and treatment. However, you will have to make sure that this person will not upset the child. Sometimes, adult family members are not helpful because they become too upset by what has happened. An overly anxious parent or relative can make things worse.

Children can easily see through lies or deceptions, so you must always be honest with them. Make sure that you explain to the child over and over again what and why certain things are happening. If treatment is going to hurt, such as applying a splint, tell the child ahead of time. Also tell the child that it will not hurt for long and that it will help "make it better."

Respect a child's modesty. Little girls and little boys are often embarrassed if they have to undress or be undressed in front of strangers. This anxiety often intensifies during adolescence. When a wound or site of injury has to be exposed, try to do so out of sight of strangers. Again, it is extremely important to tell the child what you are doing and why you are doing it.

You should speak to a child in a professional yet friendly way. A child should feel reassured that you are there to help in every way possible. Maintain eye contact with a child, as you would with an adult, to let the child know that you are helping and that you can be trusted Figure 7-6 . It is helpful to position yourself at the child's level so that you do not appear to tower above the child.

Communicating With Hearing-Impaired Patients

Patients who are hearing impaired or deaf are usually not ashamed or embarrassed by their disability. Often, it is the people around a deaf or hearing-impaired person who have the problem coping. Remember that you must be able to communicate with hearing-impaired patients so that you can provide necessary or even lifesaving care.

Most hearing-impaired patients have normal intelligence. Hearing-impaired patients can usually understand what is going on around them, provided that you can successfully communicate with them. Most

patients who are hearing impaired can read lips to some extent. Therefore, you should place yourself in a position so that the patient can see your lips. Many hearing-impaired patients have hearing aids to help them communicate. Be careful that hearing aids are not lost during an accident or fall. Hearing aids may also be forgotten if the patient is confused or sick. Remember the following five steps to help you efficiently communicate with patients who are hearing impaired:

1. Have paper and a pen available. This way, you can write down questions and the patient can write down answers, if necessary. Be sure to print so that your handwriting is not a communications barrier.
2. If the patient can read lips, you should face the patient and speak slowly and distinctly. Do not cover your mouth or mumble. If it is night or dark, consider shining a light on your face.
3. Never shout.
4. Be sure to listen carefully, ask short questions, and give short answers. Remember that although many hearing-impaired patients can speak distinctly, some cannot.
5. Learn some simple phrases in sign language. For example, knowing the signs for "sick," "hurt," and "help" may be useful if you cannot communicate in any other way Figure 7-7 .

Communicating With Visually Impaired Patients

Like hearing-impaired patients, visually impaired and blind patients have usually accepted and learned to deal with their disability. Of course, not all visually impaired patients are completely blind. Many can perceive light and dark or can see shadows or movement. Ask the patient whether he or she can see at all. Also remember that, as with other patients who have disabilities, you should expect that visually impaired patients have normal intelligence.

When you care for a visually impaired patient, explain everything that you are doing in detail as you are doing it. Be sure to stay in physical contact with the patient as you begin your care. Hold your hand lightly on the patient's shoulder or arm. Try to avoid sudden movements. If the patient can walk to the ambulance, place his or her hand on your arm, taking care not to rush. Transport any mobility aids, such as a cane, with the patient to the hospital. A visually impaired person may have a guide dog. Guide dogs are easily identified by their special harnesses. They are trained not to leave their masters and not to respond to strangers.

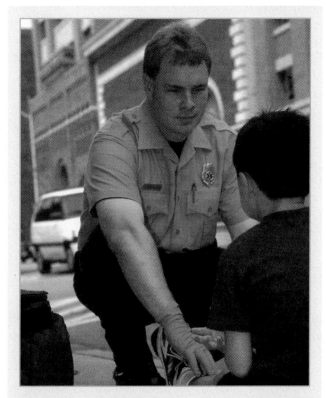

Figure 7-6 Maintain eye contact with a child to let him or her know that you are there to help.

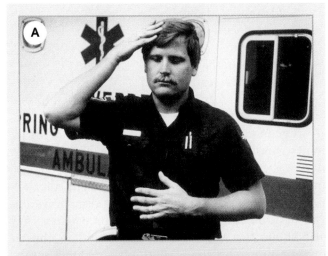

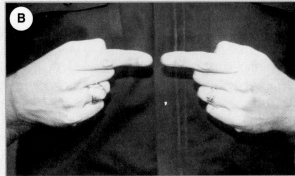

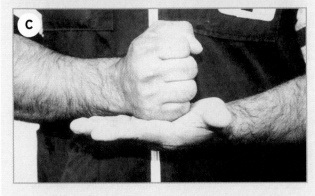

Figure 7-7 Learn simple phrases in sign language. **A.** Sick. **B.** Hurt. **C.** Help.

A visually impaired patient who is conscious can tell you about the dog and give instructions for its care. If circumstances permit, bring the guide dog to the hospital with the patient. If the dog has to be left behind, you should arrange for its care.

Communicating With Non-English-Speaking Patients

As part of the focused history and physical exam, you must obtain a medical history from the patient. You cannot skip this step simply because the patient does not speak English. Most patients who do not speak English fluently will still know certain important words or phrases.

Your first step is to find out how much English the patient can speak. Use short, simple questions and simple words whenever possible. Avoid difficult medical terms. You can help patients to better understand if you point to specific parts of the body as you ask questions. In many areas, particularly large urban centers, major segments of the population do not speak English. Your job will be much easier if you learn some common words and phrases in their language, especially common medical terms. Pocket cards are available that show the pronunciation of these terms. If the patient does not speak any English, find a family member or friend to act as an interpreter.

■ Written Communications and Documentation

Along with your radio report and verbal report, you must also complete a formal written report about the patient before you leave the hospital. You might be able to do the written report en route, if the trip is long enough and the patient needs minimal care. Usually, you will finish the written report after you have transferred the care of the patient to a hospital staff member. Be sure to leave the report at the hospital before you leave.

Data Collection

The information you collect during a call becomes part of the patient's medical record. The National EMS Information System (NEMSIS) has been collecting prehospital care information for research purposes since the early 1970s. NEMSIS has identified specific data points needed to enable communication and comparison of EMS runs between agencies, regions, and states. The minimum data set includes both narrative

Documentation Tips

Document on your PCR any items that were transported with the patient and whom they were turned over to at the hospital.

components and check-off boxes `Figure 7-8`. An example of information collected on a Prehospital Care Report (PCR) includes:

- Chief complaint
- Level of consciousness (AVPU) or mental status
- Systolic blood pressure for patients older than 3 years
- Capillary refill for patients younger than 6 years
- Skin color and temperature
- Pulse
- Respirations and effort

Examples of administrative information gathered in a PCR:

- The time that the incident was reported
- The time that the EMS unit was notified
- The time that the EMS unit arrived at the scene
- The time that the EMS unit left the scene
- The time that the EMS unit arrived at the receiving facility
- The time that patient care was transferred

Prehospital Care Report

Prehospital care reports help to ensure efficient continuity of patient care. This report describes the nature of the patient's injuries or illness at the scene and the initial treatment you provide. Although this report might not be read immediately at the hospital, it may be referred to later for important information. The prehospital care report serves the following six functions:

1. Continuity of care
2. Legal documentation
3. Education
4. Administrative
5. Essential research record
6. Evaluation and continuous quality improvement

A good prehospital care report documents the patient's condition on arrival at the scene and the care that was provided. It also documents any changes in the patient's condition upon arrival at the hospital. The information in the report also shows that you have provided proper care. In some instances, it also shows that you have properly handled unusual or uncommon situations. Both objective and subjective information is included in this report. It is critical that you document everything in the clearest manner possible. Should you ever be called to give testimony concerning patient care, you and your prehospital care report will be utilized to present evidence. As with your personal appearance, your prehospital care report will reflect a professional or unprofessional image. A well-written, neat, and concise document—including correct spelling and grammar—will reflect good patient care. Consider using the old adage of "If you didn't write it, it didn't happen," or "If the report looks sloppy, the patient care was also sloppy."

These reports also provide valuable administrative information. For example, the report provides information for patient billing. It can also be used to evalu-

You are the Provider 2

You are able to ascertain from writing that his pain is a 4 on a 1 to 10 scale and he has a cardiac history. His pain was much worse, but he took his nitroglycerin and it is better. You place him on the stretcher in a position of comfort and apply oxygen via a nonrebreathing mask at 15 L/min. He is loaded in the ambulance and your partner obtains his baseline vital signs.

Once en route to the hospital you prepare your radio report. It is a busy day, and radio traffic should be kept to a minimum.

Vital Signs	Recording Time: 3 Minutes
Skin	Pale, diaphoretic
Pulse	96 beats/min, irregular
Blood pressure	152/98 mm Hg
Respirations	18 breaths/min, adequate

3. What should be included in your radio report?
4. Where should you sit in the ambulance?
5. What is not pertinent to the report?

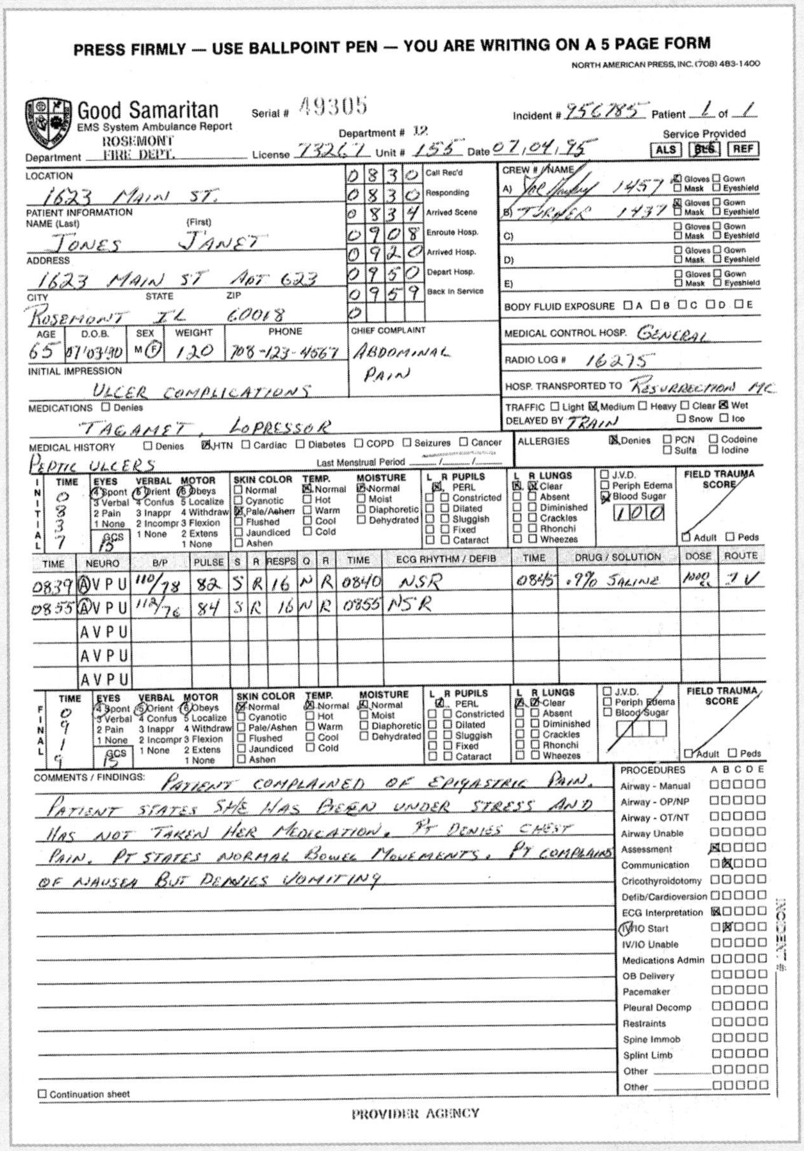
PRESS FIRMLY — USE BALLPOINT PEN — YOU ARE WRITING ON A 5 PAGE FORM

NORTH AMERICAN PRESS, INC. (708) 483-1400

Good Samaritan EMS System Ambulance Report

Serial # 49305

Incident # 956785 Patient 1 of 1

Department # 32 Service Provided ALS BLS REF

Department ROSEMONT FIRE DEPT. License 73267 Unit # 155 Date 07/04/95

0830	Call Rec'd	CREW # / NAME A) Joe Husky 1457
0830	Responding	B) Turner 1437
0834	Arrived Scene	C)
0908	Enroute Hosp.	D)
0920	Arrived Hosp.	E)
0950	Depart Hosp.	
0959	Back in Service	

LOCATION 1623 Main St.

PATIENT INFORMATION NAME (Last) Jones (First) Janet

ADDRESS 1623 Main St Apt 623

CITY Rosemont STATE IL ZIP 60018

AGE 65 D.O.B. 07/03/30 SEX F WEIGHT 120 PHONE 708-123-4567

CHIEF COMPLAINT Abdominal Pain

INITIAL IMPRESSION Ulcer complications

MEDICATIONS Tagamet, Lopressor

MEDICAL HISTORY HTN; Peptic ulcers

BODY FLUID EXPOSURE A B C D E

MEDICAL CONTROL HOSP. General

RADIO LOG # 16275

HOSP. TRANSPORTED TO Resurrection MC

TRAFFIC DELAYED BY Train

ALLERGIES Denies

TIME	NEURO	B/P	PULSE	R	ECG RHYTHM / DEFIB	TIME	DRUG / SOLUTION	DOSE	ROUTE
0839	A V P U	110/78	82	16	0840 NSR	0845	.9% Saline	1000	IV
0855	A V P U	112/76	84	16	0855 NSR				

COMMENTS / FINDINGS: Patient complained of epigastric pain. Patient states she has been under stress and has not taken her medication. Pt denies chest pain. Pt states normal bowel movements. Pt complains of nausea but denies vomiting.

PROVIDER AGENCY

Figure 7-8 The minimum data set includes both patient information and administrative information.

ate response times, equipment usage, and other areas of administrative responsibility.

Data may be obtained from the prehospital care forms to analyze causes, severity, and types of illness or injury requiring emergency medical care. These reports may also be used in an ongoing program for evaluation of the quality of patient care. All records are reviewed periodically by your system. The purpose of this review is to make sure that trauma triage and/or other prehospital care criteria have been met.

There are many requirements of a prehospital care report. Often, these requirements vary from jurisdiction to jurisdiction, mainly because so many agencies obtain information from them. While there is no universally accepted form, certain data points (uniform components of a prehospital care report) are common to many reports. The advantages of collecting such information are significant, as national trends can be detected.

Types of Forms

You most likely use one of two types of forms. The first type is the traditional written form with check boxes and a narrative section. The second type is a computerized version in which you fill in information using an electronic clipboard or similar device.

If your service uses written forms, be sure to fill in the boxes completely, and avoid making stray marks on the sheet. Make sure that you are familiar with the specific procedures for collecting, recording, and reporting the information in your area.

If you must complete a narrative section, be sure to describe what you see and what you do. Be sure to include significant negative findings and important observations about the scene. Do not record your conclusions about the incident. For example, you may write, "The patient admits to drinking today." This is a clear description that does not make any judgments about the patient's condition. However, a report that says, "The patient was drunk," makes a conclusion about the patient's condition. Also avoid radio codes, and use only standard abbreviations. When information is of a sensitive nature, note the source of the information. Be sure to spell words correctly, especially medical terms. If you do not know

Documentation Tips

REMEMBER:

If you didn't write it, it didn't happen.

If the report looks sloppy, the patient care was also sloppy.

how to spell a particular word, find out how to spell it, or use another word.

Remember that the report form itself and all the information on it are considered confidential documents. Be sure that you are familiar with state and local laws concerning confidentiality. All prehospital forms must be handled with care and stored in an appropriate manner once you have completed them. After you have completed a report, distribute the copies to the appropriate locations, according to state and local protocol. In most instances, a copy of the report will remain at the hospital and will become a part of the patient's record.

Reporting Errors

Everyone makes mistakes. If you leave something out of a report or record information incorrectly, do not try to cover it up. Rather, write down what did or did not happen and the steps that were taken to correct the situation. Falsifying information on the prehospital report may result in suspension and/or revocation of your certification/license. More important, falsifying information results in poor patient care, because other health care providers have a false impression of assessment findings or the treatment given. Document only the vital signs that were actually taken. If you did not give the patient oxygen, do not chart that the patient was given oxygen.

If you discover an error as you are writing your report, draw a single horizontal line through the error, initial it, and write the correct information next to it. Do not try to erase or cover the error with correction fluid. This may be interpreted as an attempt to cover up a mistake.

If an error is discovered after you submit your report, draw a single line through the error, preferably in a different color ink, initial it, and date it. Make sure to add a note with the correct information. If you left out information accidentally, add a note with the correct information, the date, and your initials.

Documenting Refusal of Care

Refusal of care is a common source of litigation in EMS. Thorough documentation is crucial. Competent adult patients have the right to refuse treatment and, in fact, must specifically provide permission for treatment to be provided by EMS or any other health care provider. Before you leave the scene, try to persuade the patient to go to the hospital and consult medical direction as directed by local protocol. Also make sure

Documentation Tips

When documenting a competent patient's refusal, be sure to include the following:

- All assessment findings
- Any care given
- Your explanation to the patient of potential risks associated with refusal of care
- Witness signatures
- That the patient was advised to call EMS back if needed

You are the Provider 3

Once you arrive at the hospital you should promptly give an oral report to the nurse in the emergency department. You obtain the appropriate signatures on your PCR and write the narrative.

Reassessment	Recording Time: 10 Minutes
Pulse	96 beats/min, irregular
Blood pressure	152/88 mm Hg
Respirations	16 breaths/min, good tidal volume
Breath sounds	Clear bilaterally
Pulse oximetry	97% on oxygen via nonrebreathing mask

6. What information should be given in the oral report?
7. What is the proper way to correct a mistake on a written report?
8. What six functions does the prehospital care report serve?

You are the Provider 4

You complete your written report and distribute the copies to the appropriate places. Your partner has cleaned and restocked the truck and once you turn in your paperwork, you are ready to head back to your substation in preparation for the next call.

that the patient is able to make a rational, informed decision and is not under the influence of alcohol or other drugs or the effects of an illness or injury. Explain to the patient why it is important to be examined by a physician at the hospital. Also explain what may happen if the patient is not examined by a physician. If the patient still refuses, suggest other means for the patient to obtain proper care. Explain that you are willing to return. If the patient still refuses, document any assessment findings and emergency medical care given, then have the patient sign a refusal form. You should also have a family member, police officer,

or bystander sign the form as a witness. If the patient refuses to sign the refusal form, have a family member, police officer, or bystander sign the form verifying that the patient refused to sign.

Be sure to complete the prehospital report, including the patient assessment findings. You'll need to document the advice you gave as to the risks associated with refusal of care. Note pertinent patient comments and any medical advice given to the patient by phone or radio by physician or medical control. Also include a description of the care that you wished to provide for the patient.

You are the Provider Summary

Patient care is your first priority. Take notes while attending the patient so that your report is accurate. Give a brief, thorough radio report to allow the emergency department time to prepare for your arrival. Once an oral report has been given and the patient is turned over at the ED, you should promptly write your trip report so as not to forget any pertinent details.

1. **What are your priorities for this patient?**

   ABCs; recognize that this is a load-and-go patient

2. **How will you try to communicate?**

   Try writing on a notepad, try a little universal sign language, position yourself so he can read your lips.

3. **What should be included in your radio report?**

   Include his age, chief complaint, vital signs, treatment, any response, any requested orders, ETA.

4. **Where should you sit in the ambulance?**

   You should be positioned in such a fashion that the patient can see you at all times.

5. **What is not pertinent to the report?**

   Medications, entire history, name, allergies not pertinent to present care, etc.

6. **What information should be given in the oral report?**

   You should give the same information included in the radio report, along with the patient's name, his medications and allergies, his physician's name, and any changes since your radio report.

7. **What is the proper way to correct a mistake on a written report?**

   Draw one line through it and initial the correction.

8. **What six functions does the prehospital care report serve?**

   - Continuity of care
   - Legal documentation
   - Education
   - Administrative
   - Essential research record
   - Evaluation and continuous quality improvement

Prep Kit

Ready for Review

- Excellent communication skills are crucial for relaying pertinent information to the hospital before arrival.
- Radio and telephone communications link you and your team to other members of the EMS, fire, and law enforcement communities.
- It is your job to know what your communication system can and cannot handle. You must be able to communicate effectively by sending precise, accurate reports about the scene, the patient's condition, and the treatment that you provide.
- Remember, the lines of communication are not always exclusive; therefore, you should speak in a professional manner at all times.
- In addition to radio and oral communications with hospital personnel, EMT-Bs must have excellent person-to-person communication skills. You should be able to interact with the patient and any family members, friends, or bystanders.
- It is important for you to remember that people who are sick or injured may not understand what you are doing or saying. Therefore, your body language and attitude are very important in gaining the trust of both the patient and family. You must also take special care of individuals such as children, geriatric patients, and hearing-impaired, visually impaired, and non-English-speaking patients.
- Along with your radio report and oral report, you must also complete a formal written report about the patient before you leave the hospital. This is a vital part of providing emergency medical care and ensuring the continuity of patient care. This information guarantees the proper transfer of responsibility, complies with the requirements of health departments and law enforcement agencies, and fulfills your administrative needs.
- Reporting and record-keeping duties are essential, but they should never come before the care of a patient.

Vital Vocabulary

Federal Communications Commission (FCC)   The federal agency that has jurisdiction over interstate and international telephone and telegraph services and satellite communications, all of which may involve EMS activity.

Refresher.EMSzone.com

Technology

Interactivities

Vocabulary Explorer

Anatomy Review

Web Links

Online Review Manual

Assessment in Action

Effective communication is an essential component of pre-hospital care. You must communicate via radio, telephone, and face-to-face with patients, family members, law enforcement, hospital personnel, firefighters, and others. This communication includes written documentation as well as verbal reports.

1. All radio operations in the United States are regulated by the _____.
   A. DHR
   B. FCC
   C. NHTSA
   D. FAA

2. What type of exchange helps to eliminate confusion and the possibility of poor patient care when communicating with medical control?
   A. medical control
   B. protocol
   C. direct
   D. echo

3. John Frances is a 52-year-old man with dyspnea. How should he be addressed?
   A. John
   B. John Frances
   C. Mr. Frances
   D. Hey, Buddy

4. A good prehospital care report documents _____.
   A. the patient's condition on arrival at the scene
   B. care that was provided
   C. changes in the patient's condition
   D. all of the above

5. What portion of the EMT's patient care interaction becomes part of the patient's permanent medical record?
   A. list of medications
   B. standing order
   C. written report
   D. verbal report

6. EMS-related responsibilities of the FCC include:
   A. establishing licensing standards and operating specifications for radio equipment.
   B. establishing limitations for transmitter power output.
   C. allocating specific radio frequencies.
   D. all of the above.

Challenging Questions

7. When treating an older patient who appears to have an altered mental status, do not assume that this is normal behavior. What should you do in this situation?

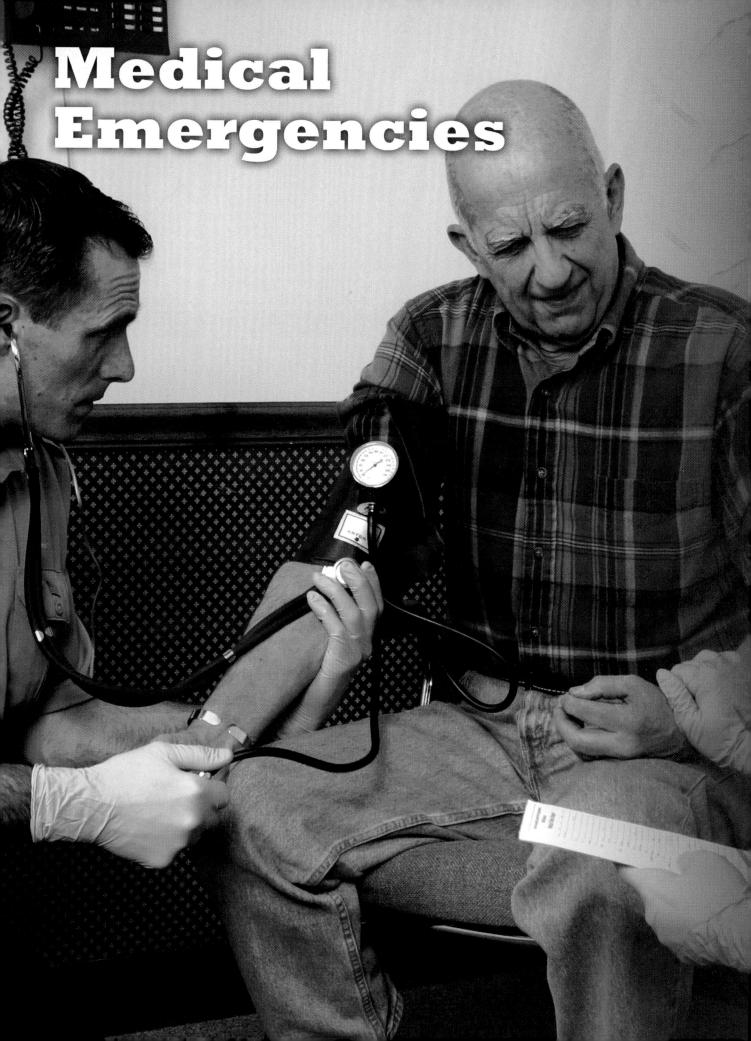

Medical Emergencies

Section 4

Cognitive Objectives

1. Provide treatment for a patient in respiratory distress. (Chapter 9, p 176)
   - List the signs and symptoms of difficulty breathing
   - Describe the emergency medical care of the patient with breathing difficulty.
   - Recognize the need for medical direction to assist in the emergency medical care of the patient with breathing difficulty.
   - State the generic name, medication forms, dose, administration, action, indications and contraindications for the prescribed inhaler.
2. Provide care to a patient experiencing chest pain/discomfort. (Chapter 10, p 190)
   - Describe the emergency medical care of the patient experiencing chest pain/discomfort.
   - Discuss the position of comfort for patients with various cardiac emergencies.
   - Recognize the need for medical direction of protocols to assist in the emergency medical care of the patient with chest pain.
   - List the indications for the use of nitroglycerin.
3. Attempt to resuscitate a patient in cardiac arrest. (Chapter 10, p 195)
   - Discuss the circumstances that may result in inappropriate shocks.
   - Explain the considerations for interruption of CPR when using the automated external defibrillator (AED).
   - List the steps in the operation of the AED.
   - Discuss the need to complete the Automated Defibrillator: Operator's Shift Checklist.
   - Explain the role medical direction plays in the use of automated external defibrillation.
4. Provide care to a patient with an altered mental status. (Chapter 12, p 233)
   - State the steps in the emergency medical care of the patient taking diabetic medicine with an altered mental status and a history of diabetes.
   - Evaluate the need for medical direction in the emergency medical care of the diabetic patient.
5. Provide care of the patient experiencing an allergic reaction. (Chapter 13, p 244)
   - Recognize the patient experiencing an allergic reaction.
   - Describe the emergency medical care of the patient with an allergic reaction.
   - State the generic and trade names, medication forms, dose, administration, action, and contraindications for the epinephrine auto-injector.
   - Evaluate the need for medical direction in the emergency medical care of the patient with an allergic reaction.
   - Differentiate between the general category of those patients having an allergic reaction and those patients having an allergic reaction and requiring immediate medical care, including immediate use of epinephrine auto-injector.
6. Provide care to a suspected poison/overdose patient. (Chapter 14, p 259)
   - Describe the steps in the emergency medical care for the patient with suspected poisoning.
   - Discuss the emergency medical care for the patient with possible overdose.

7. Provide care to a patient experiencing a behavioral problem. (Chapter 16, p 301)
  - Discuss the characteristics of an individual's behavior suggests that the patient is at risk for suicide.
  - Discuss the special considerations for assessing a patient with behavioral problems.
  - Discuss the general principles of an individual's behavior suggests that he is at risk for violence.
  - Discuss methods to calm behavioral emergency patients.

Affective Objectives

1. Defend the rationale for the EMT-Basic to carry and assist with medications. (Chapter 8, p 146)
2. Recognize and respond to the feelings of the patient who may require interventions to be performed. (Chapter 8, p 156)

Psychomotor Objectives

1. Given medical scenarios, demonstrate the ability to properly assess the patient and demonstrate the ability to properly utilize the intervention, to include inhaler, nitroglycerin, oral glucose, and activated charcoal. (Chapter 8)
2. Demonstrate the use of an epinephrine auto-injector. (Chapter 8, p 152)
3. Given a cardiac arrest scenario, demonstrate the use of the AED. (Chapter 10, p 195)

(The following objectives for Chapter 17 are from module VI of the DOT curriculum)

Cognitive Objectives

1. Assess and provide care to the obstetric patient. (Chapter 17, p 313)
2. Assist with the delivery of an infant. (Chapter 17, p 315)
3. Assess and provide care to the newborn. (Chapter 17, p 319)
4. Assess and provide care to the mother immediately following delivery of a newborn. (Chapter 17, p 320)
  - Identify predelivery emergencies.
  - State the steps to assist in the delivery.
  - Discuss the steps in the delivery of the placenta.
  - List the steps in the emergency medical care of the mother postdelivery.
  - Summarize neonatal resuscitation procedures.
  - Describe the procedures for abnormal deliveries.

Psychomotor Objectives

1. Demonstrate steps to assist in the normal cephalic delivery. (Chapter 17, p 315)
2. Demonstrate postdelivery care of the infant. (Chapter 17, p 319)
3. Demonstrate postdelivery care of the mother. (Chapter 17, p 320)

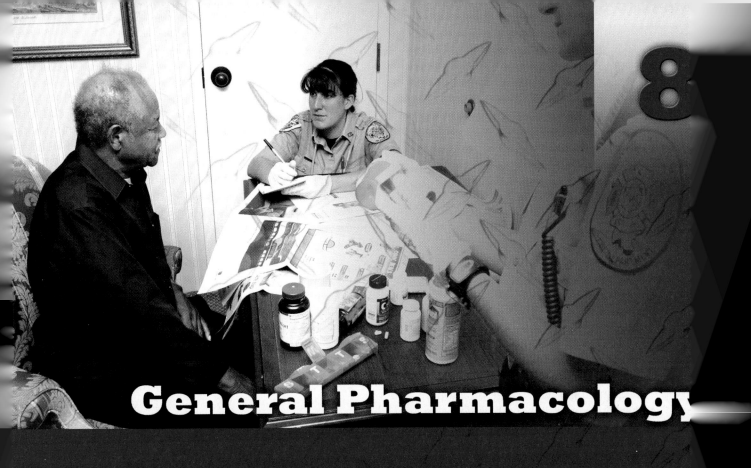

General Pharmacology

You are the Provider **1**

After a busy day, you and your EMT-B partner are relaxing at a substation when you hear a knock on the door. Your partner opens the door to find a lady asking for help with her husband. They were on their way home from a bowling tournament when he began experiencing chest pain. They saw the ambulance parked outside and stopped to ask for help. Her husband is waiting in the car.

Your partner locks up the station and calls the dispatcher while you go to assess the patient. You find a 56-year-old man who is diaphoretic, clutching his chest, and complaining of a "squeezing" pain.

Initial Assessment	Recording Time: 0 Minutes
Appearance	Pale, diaphoretic
Level of consciousness	Alert to person, place, and time
Airway	Open and clear
Breathing	A little fast and shallow
Circulation	Radials present, irregular

1. What are your priorities for this patient?
2. What questions should you ask about his pain?

Introduction

Medication administration is an intervention that can be lifesaving to your patients. It is also an EMT-B skill that should not be taken lightly. Used appropriately, a medication may alleviate pain or distress and improve a patient's well-being. However, used inappropriately, medication may cause harm and even death. As an EMT-B, you have been responsible for administering certain drugs to patients and helping them to self-administer others. You have experienced how these medications have helped patients and perhaps have also seen some of their side effects. By now, your experience has underscored the importance of knowing about those medications and the dangers associated with their administration. You are also aware that patients who require medication administration may also be experiencing a wide range of emotions. They are often anxious and afraid of what's going on around them. Your calm and reassuring approach helps to decrease the patient's anxiety and allows you to deal more effectively with the medical condition they are experiencing. The purpose of this chapter is to review the medications carried on the EMS unit and those that the EMT-B may assist patients in taking with approval by medical direction.

How Medications Work

Pharmacology is the science of drugs, including their ingredients, preparation, uses, and actions on the body. Although the terms "drugs" and "medications" are often used interchangeably, the term drugs may make some people think of narcotics or illegal

Technology

- Interactivities
- Vocabulary Explorer
- Anatomy Review
- Web Links
- Online Review Manual

Refresher.EMSzone.com

substances. For this reason, you should use the word "medications," especially when interviewing patients and families. In general terms, a medication is a chemical substance that is used to treat or prevent disease or relieve pain.

The dose is the amount of the medication that is given. The action is the therapeutic effect that a medication is expected to have on the body. For example, nitroglycerin relaxes the walls of the blood vessels and may dilate the arteries. This increases the blood flow and, thus, the supply of oxygen, to the heart muscle. By this action, nitroglycerin relieves chest pain. Nitroglycerin is indicated for cardiac chest pain. Indications are the reasons or conditions for which a particular medication is given.

As you recall, there are times when you should not give a patient medication, even if it usually is indicated for that person's condition. Contraindications are the reasons or conditions not to give a medication. Contraindications would harm the patient or have no positive effect on the patient's condition. For example, giving activated charcoal is indicated when a patient has swallowed a poison. Generally, activated charcoal, premixed with water, is used to prevent the body from absorbing a poison. However, activated charcoal is contraindicated if the patient is unconscious and cannot swallow.

Side effects are any actions of a medication other than the desired ones. Side effects may occur even when a medication is administered properly. For example, giving epinephrine to a patient who is having a severe allergic reaction should dilate the bronchioles and decrease wheezing. However, two side effects of epinephrine are cardiac stimulation and constriction of the arteries, which may elevate the patient's heart rate and blood pressure.

Medication Names

Medications usually have two types of names. The generic name of a medication (such as ibuprofen) is usually its original given name or the name which it is given by the original manufacturer. The generic name is not capitalized. Sometimes a medication is called by its generic name more often than by any of its trade names. For example, you may hear the term "nitroglycerin" used more often than the trade names Isordil and Nitrostat. All medications that are licensed for use in the United States are listed by their generic names in the United States Pharmacopoeia.

A trade name is the brand name that a manufacturer gives to a medication, such as Tylenol and Lasix.

As a proper noun, a trade name begins with a capital letter. Trade names are used in every aspect of our daily lives, not just in medications. Well-known examples include Jell-O gelatin, Band-Aid adhesive bandages, and Hershey chocolate candy. A medication may have many different trade names, depending on how many companies manufacture it. Advil, Nuprin, and Motrin all are trade names for the generic medication, ibuprofen. A trade name sometimes is also designated by a raised registered symbol, that is, Advil®.

Medications may be prescription medications or over-the-counter (OTC) medications. Prescription medications are distributed to patients only by pharmacists according to a physician's order. Medications that are OTC may be purchased directly, such as from a discount store or supermarket, without a prescription. In recent years, the number of prescription medications that have become available OTC has increased dramatically.

Routes of Administration

Absorption is the process by which medications travel through body tissues until they reach the bloodstream. Often the rate at which a medication is absorbed into the bloodstream depends on its route of administration.

Intravenous (IV) injection. Intravenous means into the vein. This is the fastest way to deliver a chemical substance, but the IV route cannot be used for all chemicals. For example, aspirin, oxygen, and charcoal cannot be given by the IV route.

Oral. Many medications are taken by mouth, or per os (PO), and enter the bloodstream through the digestive system. This process often takes as long as 1 hour.

Sublingual (SL). Sublingual means under the tongue. Medications given by the SL route, such as nitroglycerin tablets, enter through the oral mucosa under the tongue and are absorbed into the bloodstream within minutes. This route is faster than the oral route, and it protects medications from chemicals in the digestive system, such as acids, that can weaken or inactivate them.

Intramuscular (IM) injection. Intramuscular means into the muscle. Usually, medications that are administered by IM injection are absorbed quickly because muscles have a lot of blood vessels. However, not all medications can be administered by the IM route. Possible problems with IM injections are damage to muscle tissue and uneven, unreliable absorption, especially in people with decreased tissue perfusion or who are in shock.

Intraosseous (IO). Intraosseous means into the bone. Medications that are given by this route reach the bloodstream through the bone marrow. Giving a medication by the IO route requires drilling a needle into the outer layer of the bone. Because this is painful, the IO route is used most often in patients who are unconscious as a result of cardiac arrest or extreme shock. Most commonly, the IO route is used for children who have fewer available (or difficult to access) IV sites.

Subcutaneous (SC) injection. Subcutaneous means beneath the skin. An SC injection is given into the tissue between the skin and the muscle. Because there is less blood here than in the muscles, medications that are given by this route are generally absorbed more slowly, and their effects last longer. An SC injection is a useful way to give medications that cannot be taken by mouth, as long as they do not irritate or damage the tissue. Daily insulin injections for patients with diabetes are given by the SC route. Some forms of epinephrine can be given by the SC route. (Subcutaneous sometimes is abbreviated as SQ or sub-Q.)

Transcutaneous. Transcutaneous means through the skin. Some medications can be absorbed transcutaneously, such as the nicotine in patches used by people who are trying to quit smoking. On occasion, a medication that also comes in another form is administered transcutaneously to achieve a longer-lasting effect. An example is an adhesive patch containing nitroglycerin.

Inhalation. Some medications are inhaled into the lungs so that they can be absorbed into the bloodstream more quickly. Others are inhaled because they work directly in the lungs. Generally, inhalation helps minimize the effects of the medication in other body tissues. Such medications come in the form of aerosols, fine powders, and sprays.

Per rectum (PR). Per rectum means by rectum. This route of delivery is frequently used with children because of easier administration and more reliable absorption. For similar reasons, many medications that are used for nausea and vomiting come in a rectal suppository form. Some medications to control seizures are administered PR when it is impossible to administer them intravenously. The PR route also is used to give some medications when the patient cannot swallow or is unconscious.

■ Forms of Medication

The form of a medication usually dictates the route of administration. For example, a tablet or a spray cannot be given through a needle. The manufacturer chooses the form to ensure the proper route of administration, the timing of its release into the bloodstream, and its effects on the target organs or body systems. As an EMT-B, you should be familiar with the following seven medication forms.

Tablets and Capsules

Most medications that are given by mouth to adult patients are in tablet or capsule form. Capsules are gelatin shells filled with powdered or liquid medication. If the capsule contains liquid, the shell is sealed and usually soft. If the capsule contains powder, the shell can usually be pulled apart. In tablets, the medication is compressed under high pressure. Tablets often contain other materials that are mixed with the medication.

Some tablets are designed to dissolve very quickly in small amounts of liquid so that they can be given sublingually and absorbed rapidly. An example is the sublingual nitroglycerin tablet used to treat chest pain. These medications are especially useful in emergency situations. Generally, a medication that must be swallowed is less useful in an emergency because the digestive tract provides a slower route of delivery. For example, an oral pain medication is less useful than an IV pain medication when pain relief is needed within minutes.

Solutions and Suspensions

A solution is a liquid mixture of one or more substances that cannot be separated by filtering or allowing the mixture to stand. Solutions can be given by almost any route. When given by mouth, solutions may be absorbed from the stomach fairly quickly because the medication is already dissolved. For example, you may need to help in the sublingual delivery of a nitroglycerin spray **Figure 8-1 ▶**. Many solutions can be given as an IV, IM, or SC injection. If a patient has a severe allergic reaction, you may help to administer a solution of epinephrine using an auto-injector.

Many substances do not dissolve well in liquids. Some of these can be ground into fine particles and evenly distributed throughout a liquid by shaking or stirring. This type of mixture is called a suspension. An example is activated charcoal, which you may give

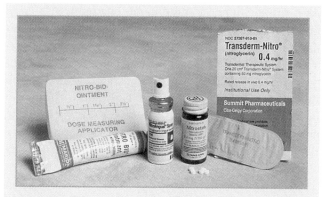

Figure 8-1 Nitroglycerin, which is prescribed for chest pain, is given in the prehospital setting sublingually (SL) as a spray or tablet.

to patients who have taken overdoses of certain medications or ingested certain poisons.

Suspensions separate if they stand or are filtered. It is very important that you shake or swirl a suspension before administering it to ensure that the patient receives the right amount of medication. For example, if you are a parent, you may have had to shake a suspension of oral antibiotic before giving it to your child.

Suspensions usually are administered by mouth but sometimes are given rectally. Injectable suspensions are given via IM or SC injection only. Certain hormone shots or vaccinations are given this way because of the suspended particles. They cannot be given by IV injection because the suspended particles do not remain dissolved.

Metered-Dose Inhalers

If liquids or solids are broken into small enough droplets or particles, they can be inhaled. A <u>metered-dose inhaler (MDI)</u> is a miniature spray canister used to direct such substances through the mouth and into the lungs **Figure 8-2 ▶**. An MDI delivers the same amount of medication each time it is used. Because an inhaled medication usually is suspended in a propellant, the MDI must be shaken vigorously before the medication is administered. An MDI is often used by a patient with respiratory conditions such as asthma or emphysema.

Topical Medications

Lotions, creams, and ointments are topical medications. These medications are applied to the surface of the skin and affect only that area. Lotions contain the

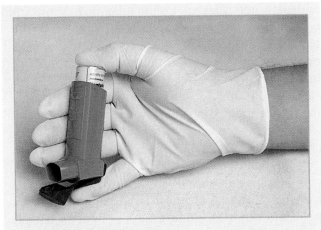

Figure 8-2 Metered-dose inhalers are used to give medications that are inhaled in the lungs so that they can be absorbed into the bloodstream quickly.

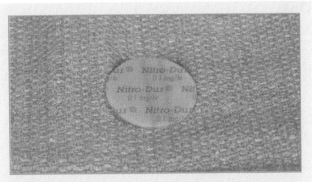

Figure 8-3 Transcutaneous medications, such as a nitroglycerin patch, deliver the medication through the skin.

most water and are absorbed the most rapidly. Ointments contain a lesser amount of water and are absorbed more slowly. Calamine lotion is an example of a medical lotion. Hydrocortisone cream, to diminish skin itching, is an example of a medical cream that can also be given in ointment form. Neosporin is an example of a first-aid ointment.

Transcutaneous Medications

Transdermal medications are designed to be absorbed through the skin, or by the transcutaneous route. Medications such as nitroglycerin paste usually have

properties or delivery systems that help to dilate the blood vessels in the skin and, thus, speed absorption into the bloodstream. In contrast with most topical medicines, which work directly on the application site, transdermal medications are usually intended for systemic (whole-body) effects. A note of caution: If you touch such a medication with your bare skin while administering it, you will absorb it just as readily as the patient will.

One of the newer delivery systems for transcutaneous medications is the adhesive patch. Patches attach to the skin and allow for an even absorption of a medication for many hours (Figure 8-3 ▲). Prescription and OTC medications come in this form. Common examples are nitroglycerin, nicotine, pain medications, and some oral contraceptives.

You are the Provider 2

After placing the patient on the stretcher in a position of comfort and loading him in the ambulance, you assess vital signs while your partner applies oxygen. The patient tells you that the pain is an 8 on a scale of 1 to 10 and it is moving down his left arm. He denies any nausea or vomiting.

Vital Signs	Recording Time: 2 Minutes
Skin	Pale, diaphoretic
Pulse	96 beats/min, irregular
Blood pressure	164/98 mm Hg
Respirations	22 breaths/min, slightly shallow

3. What type of oxygen does he need? Why?
4. What else do you need to know about this patient?
5. Name the pertinent negative in this scenario.

Gels

A gel is a semiliquid substance that is administered orally in capsule form or through plastic tubes. Gels usually have the consistency of pastes or creams but are transparent (clear). "Gelatinous" means thick and sticky, like gelatin. As an EMT-B, you may give oral glucose in gel form to patients with a low blood glucose level.

Gases for Inhalation

Gaseous medications are neither solid nor liquid and most often are given in an operating room. For EMS, oxygen is the best example of this medication form. Oxygen, in its concentrated form, is a potent medication that has systemic effects (throughout the body).

■ Medications Carried on the EMS Unit

By now, you are very familiar with the medications that may be carried on the EMS unit: oxygen, oral glucose, activated charcoal, aspirin, and epinephrine. Remember that you may administer these medications only according to standing orders in a protocol (off-line medical control) or a direct order (online medical control).

Oxygen

As you remember, all cells need oxygen to function properly. Because the heart and brain can only function for a few minutes without oxygen, oxygen should be your most commonly used on-board medication. Administration is usually by a nonrebreathing mask at 10 to 15 L/min, or a nasal cannula at 2 to 6 L/min. With a good seal, the nonrebreathing mask can provide up to 90% inspired oxygen. A nasal cannula can provide up to 24% to 44% inspired oxygen with the flow meter set at 1 to 6 L/min.

If the patient is not breathing, you should ventilate the patient with a bag-mask (BVM) device. Oxygen is usually delivered at 15 L/min with this technique.

Remember that, although oxygen itself does not burn, it allows other things to burn. If there is extra oxygen in the air, objects will burn more easily. So make sure there are no open flames, lit cigarettes, or sparks in the area in which you are administering oxygen.

Activated Charcoal

Many poisoning emergencies involve overdoses of medications taken by mouth. Many medications bind

with activated charcoal, keeping the medications from being absorbed by the body. Activated charcoal is often used for patients who have taken a drug overdose or swallowed a poison. Activated charcoal is ground into a very fine powder to provide the greatest possible surface area for binding. If your service carries this medication, you probably have a container with a premixed suspension of activated charcoal powder and water ◖ Figure 8-4 ▾ ◗.

The bond between the ingested substance (most commonly a medication) and the charcoal is not permanent. Activated charcoal is frequently suspended with another medication called sorbitol (a complex sugar). This suspension has a laxative effect that causes the entire mixture, including the ingested substance, to move quickly through the digestive system.

Common trade names are InstaChar, Actidose, and LiquiChar. The usual dose for an adult or child is 1 gram of activated charcoal per kilogram of body weight. The usual adult dose is 25 to 50 grams and the usual pediatric dose is 12.5 to 25 grams. Activated charcoal is given by mouth. Although sorbitol sweetens the suspension, the black charcoal makes it look unappealing. Remember that patients with an altered mental status and those who cannot swallow or

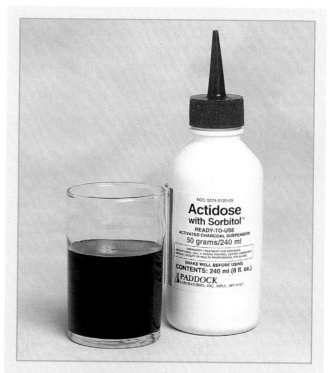

Figure 8-4 Activated charcoal is a suspension that is used for patients who have ingested a poison.

protect their own airway should not be given activated charcoal.

Oral Glucose

Glucose is a sugar that our cells use as fuel. Although some cells can use other sugars, brain cells must have glucose. If the level of glucose in the blood gets too low (hypoglycemia), a person can lose consciousness, have seizures, and ultimately die.

Diabetics self-administer insulin to control blood glucose levels. Hypoglycemia can be caused by an excess of insulin. Oral glucose that is carried in the EMS unit can counteract the effects of hypoglycemia in the same way as a candy bar or a drink that contains a lot of sugar, but much faster. Common table sugar (sucrose) and fruit sugars (fructose) are complex sugars that must be broken down before they can be absorbed. Oral glucose is a simple sugar that is readily absorbed by the bloodstream.

Hospital personnel and paramedics can give glucose ($D_{50}W$) through an IV line. As an EMT-B, you can give glucose only by mouth. Glucose is available as a gel designed to be spread on the mucous membranes between the cheek and gum; however, absorption through this route is not as quick as with injection. Because the patient may be conscious one moment and unconscious the next, you must be very careful when administering oral glucose. Never administer oral medications to an unconscious patient or to one who is unable to swallow or protect their own airway.

Aspirin

Aspirin (acetylsalicylic acid, or ASA) is an antipyretic (reduces fever), analgesic (reduces pain), and anti-inflammatory (reduces inflammation) and inhibits platelet aggregation (clumping). This last property makes it one of the most used medications today. Research has shown that platelets aggregating under certain conditions in the coronary arteries is one of the direct causes of heart attack. Patients at risk for coronary artery disease are often prescribed one or two "baby" (or children's) aspirins a day. During a potential heart attack, aspirin may be lifesaving. For these reasons, some states have added the administration of aspirin to the EMT-B scope of practice. Be sure to review your local protocol to see if it includes aspirin administration at the EMT-B level.

Contraindications for aspirin include documented hypersensitivity to aspirin, preexistent liver damage, bleeding disorders, and asthma. Because of the asso-

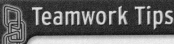

Teamwork Tips

When assisting with medications, one EMT-B should talk with and assess the patient while the second EMT-B readies the medication. Remember to check the medication for the expiration date, clarity, and prescription, and to obtain orders from medical control.

ciation of aspirin with Reye's syndrome, it should not be given to children during episodes of fever-causing illnesses.

Epinephrine

Epinephrine is the main hormone that controls the body's fight-or-flight response. It is released inside the body when there is sudden stress, such as during exercise or when the patient is suddenly scared. Because epinephrine is secreted by the adrenal glands, it is also known as adrenaline. Epinephrine has different effects on different body tissues and is used as a medication in several forms. Generally, epinephrine will increase heart rate and blood pressure and dilate passages in the lungs. Therefore, it can ease breathing problems caused by the bronchial spasms that are common in asthma and allergic reactions. Epinephrine also may help to maintain blood pressure when a patient is in anaphylactic shock.

Epinephrine has the following actions/characteristics:

- Secreted naturally by the adrenal glands
- Dilates passages in the lungs
- Constricts blood vessels, causing increased blood pressure
- Increases heart rate

Administering Epinephrine by Injection

Some states and EMS services now authorize the use of epinephrine by EMT-Bs for the treatment of life-threatening anaphylaxis. In certain individuals, insect venom or other allergens cause the body to release histamine, which lowers blood pressure by relaxing the small blood vessels and allowing them to leak. The release of histamine may also cause wheezing from bronchial spasms and swelling of the airway tissues (edema), which make it difficult for the patient to breathe. Epinephrine acts as a specific antidote to histamine, countering both of these harmful effects. It constricts the blood vessels, allowing blood pressure to rise and reducing the swelling. In the lungs, it has the opposite effect; it dilates the air passages, so the flow of air is less restricted. You can also expect the patient's heart rate to increase after administration of epinephrine.

You may be trained to administer SC and IM injections of epinephrine, depending on state and local protocol. Remember that an SC injection puts the epinephrine into the tissue between the skin and the muscle. Therefore, it is usually helpful to pinch the skin lightly to lift it away from the muscle. A syringe used for SC injections has a short, thin needle, typically between ½" and ⅝" long. The syringe for IM use has a longer, larger diameter needle that is between 1" and 1½" long so it can reach the muscle.

Follow these steps for an SC injection:

1. Prepare the skin with an appropriate antiseptic Figure 8-5A ▶ .
2. Pinch the skin and insert the needle into the pinched skin at a 45° angle. Aspirate by drawing the syringe's plunger back slightly before injecting the medication to verify you have not accidentally placed the needle in a small blood vessel Figure 8-5B ▶ . If blood returns, you will need to withdraw the needle and start again using the same syringe (assuming that the skin remains sterilized). If no blood returns, push the plunger on the syringe to inject the medication.
3. Place the needle and syringe in a biohazard sharps container.

Administering Epinephrine by Auto-injector

Epinephrine may also be dispensed from an auto-injector, which automatically delivers a preset amount of the medication. This is the method that you will most likely use to treat allergic reactions or anaphylaxis. Your medical director may authorize you to carry an epinephrine auto-injector (EpiPen) or to assist patients who have their own EpiPen. The adult system delivers 0.3 mg of epinephrine via an automatic needle and syringe system; the infant-child system delivers 0.15 mg Figure 8-6 ▶ .

If the patient is able to use the auto-injector on his or her own, your role is limited to helping them administer the medication. To use, or help the patient use, the auto-injector, you should first have permission from medical control (local protocol or

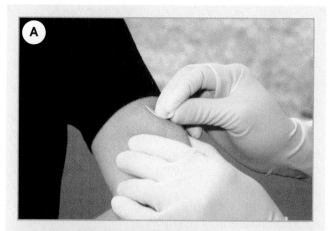
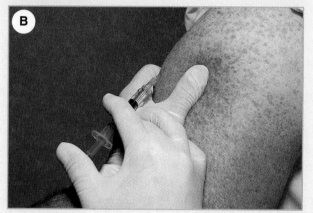

Figure 8-5 Administering epinephrine by SC injection. **A.** Cleanse the skin. **B.** Insert the needle into pinched skin, then draw the plunger back slightly.

standing order). Follow BSI precautions, and make sure the medication has been prescribed specifically for that patient. If it has not, do not give the medication: Inform medical control, and provide immediate transport. Finally, make sure the medication is not discolored and that the expiration date has not passed.

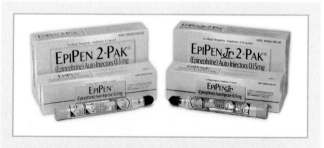

Figure 8-6 Patients who experience severe allergic reactions often carry their own epinephrine, which comes in a preset dose in an auto-injector (EpiPen and EpiPen Jr.).

To use the auto-injector, follow the steps in **Skill Drill 8-1 ▼**.

1. **Remove the safety cap** (hold the EpiPen in one hand without touching either end and remove the safety cap with the other hand to avoid accidentally activating the needle). If possible, wipe the patient's thigh with alcohol or some other antiseptic. However, do not delay administration of the drug (**Step ①**).

2. **Place the tip of the auto-injector** against the lateral part of the patient's thigh, midway between the waist and the knee (**Step ②**).

3. **Push the injector firmly** against the thigh until the injector activates. Provide steady pressure to prevent kickback from the spring in the syringe, and prevent the needle from being pushed out of the injection site too soon. Hold the injector in place until the medication has been injected (10 seconds) (**Step ③**).

4. **Remove the injector** from the patient's thigh and dispose of it in the proper biohazard container.

5. **Record the time and dose** of the injection on your patient care report (PCR).

6. **Reassess and record** the patient's vital signs after using the auto-injector.

■ Patient-Assisted Medications

The three medications that you may help patients self-administer are epinephrine, metered-dose inhalers (MDI) medications, and nitroglycerin. In your initial EMT-B training, you learned the risks and benefits of using these medications. As your experience with these medications has shown, it is important to understand how these medications work and when you should use them.

Epinephrine

You have already read the general information on epinephrine and its use by EMT-Bs for severe allergic reactions and anaphylaxis. Some services do not permit EMT-Bs to carry epinephrine but do allow them to assist patients in administering their own epinephrine by auto-injector in life-threatening anaphylactic reactions.

MDI Medications

Sometimes, a respiratory condition such as asthma is not severe enough to require the use of epinephrine. In such cases, patients may use one of the epinephrine "cousins" that are more narrowly focused on the lungs. These medications are delivered with an MDI. An MDI requires a great deal of coordination, something that may be in short supply when an individual is having trouble breathing. Patients must aim properly and spray just as they start to inhale; however, most of the medication tends to end up on the roof of the patient's mouth. An adapter, called a "spacer," which fits over the inhaler like a sleeve, can be used to

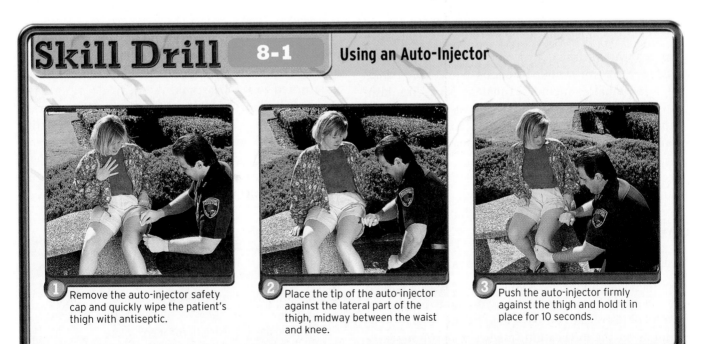

Skill Drill   8-1   Using an Auto-Injector

1. Remove the auto-injector safety cap and quickly wipe the patient's thigh with antiseptic.

2. Place the tip of the auto-injector against the lateral part of the thigh, midway between the waist and knee.

3. Push the auto-injector firmly against the thigh and hold it in place for 10 seconds.

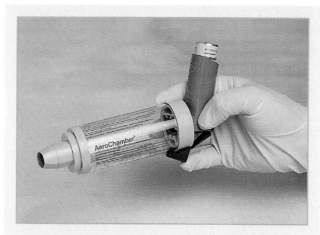

Figure 8-7 Some inhalers have spacer devices to better direct the medication spray.

avoid misdirecting the spray **Figure 8-7 ▲**. The inhaler fits into an opening on one end of the spacer's chamber, and the mouthpiece fits on the other end. The patient sprays the prescribed dose into the chamber and then breathes in and out of the mouthpiece until the mist is completely inhaled.

You can activate the spray by pressing the canister into the adapter just as the patient starts to inhale. If relief is not achieved, wait about 3 minutes and repeat this sequence according to the patient's prescription for the MDI. Above all, it is important to ensure that the patient inhales all the medication in a single-sprayed dose.

Administering Epinephrine by Metered-Dose Inhaler

Epinephrine is inhaled to relieve bronchial spasms due to asthma or allergic reactions. Some trade names of these inhalers include Primatene Mist, Bronkitin Mist, Bronkaid Mist, and Medihaler-Epi. Epinephrine tends to increase heart rate and blood pressure, so most patients with asthma use chemical cousins of epinephrine that produce fewer side effects. Metaproterenol (Alupent or Metaprel) and albuterol (Proventil or Ventolin) both work more on the bronchial spasms and less on the cardiovascular system.

Administration of a Metered-Dose Inhaler

Before you administer a medication or assist a patient to self-administer a medication, you must follow local protocol. Confirm you have medical authorization to administer the medication (medical control or standing orders), and check that you have the right medi-

cation, the right patient, and the right route. Review **Skill Drill 8-2 ▶** on assisting patients with an inhaler:

1. **Confirm that the patient is alert** enough to use the inhaler.
2. **Check to see whether the patient** has already taken any doses and make sure the inhaler is at room temperature or warmer.
3. **Check the expiration date** of the inhaler (**Step ①**).
4. **Shake the inhaler** vigorously several times.
5. **Stop administering supplemental oxygen** and remove any mask from the patient's face.
6. **Ask the patient to exhale deeply** and, before inhaling, to put his or her lips around the opening of the inhaler (**Step ②**).
7. **Have the patient depress** the inhaler as he or she begins to inhale deeply.
8. **Instruct the patient** to hold his or her breath for as long as is comfortable to help the body absorb the medication (**Step ③**).
9. **Continue to administer supplemental oxygen.** Repeat a second dose per direction from medical control or local protocol (**Step ④**).

Nitroglycerin

Many patients with cardiac conditions carry some form of fast-acting nitroglycerin to relieve the pain of angina pectoris. The cause of angina is lack of oxygen to the heart muscle, resulting from a blockage, narrowing, or even spasm of the blood vessels that supply the heart muscle.

Nitroglycerin increases blood flow by relaxing the muscular walls of the coronary arteries and veins. It also relaxes veins throughout the body, so less blood is returned to the heart and the heart does not have to work as hard each time it contracts. Blood pressure is decreased as a result. It is important to take the patient's blood pressure before and after administering nitroglycerin. If the systolic blood pressure is less than 100 mm Hg, the nitroglycerin may actually lower the blood flow to the heart's own blood vessels. Even a pa-

Documentation Tips

After assisting with a medication, document the type of medication, the route, the dose, the time, and any response to the medication.

Skill Drill 8-2 Assisting a Patient With a Metered-Dose Inhaler

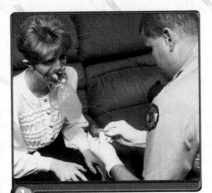

1 Check the expiration date on the inhaler and shake the container several times.

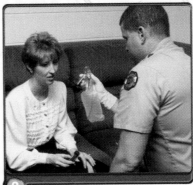

2 Remove the oxygen mask and instruct the patient to exhale deeply.

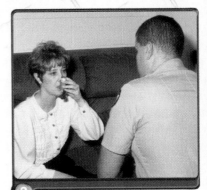

3 Instruct the patient to press the inhaler and inhale deeply. Have the patient hold the medication in as long as possible.

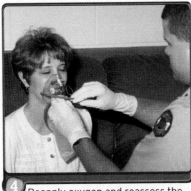

4 Reapply oxygen and reassess the patient. Repeat with a second dose if order/protocol allows.

tient who has adequate blood pressure should sit or lie down with the head elevated before taking this medication. A standing patient may faint when blood flow to the brain drops. If a significant drop in the patient's blood pressure (15 to 20 mm Hg) occurs and the patient suddenly feels dizzy or sick, lay the patient down and raise the legs.

During a heart attack (myocardial infarction, or MI), a blood clot in a narrowed coronary artery blocks blood flow to a section of heart muscle. If the blockage is not cleared in time, that section of muscle may die. If nitroglycerin no longer brings relief to a person in whom it has previously worked, the person may be experiencing an MI instead of an angina attack. Therefore, it is important to know—and report to medical control—how much nitroglycerin a patient has needed in the past to relieve chest pain, and how much has been taken during the current episode. Always report this information to medical control. Remember that you cannot administer this medication without approval from medical control or standing orders.

Nitroglycerin has the following effects:

- Relaxes the muscular walls of coronary arteries and veins
- Results in less blood returning to the heart (decreases preload)
- Decreases blood pressure
- Relaxes veins throughout the body
- Often causes a mild headache after administration

Administering Nitroglycerin

Nitroglycerin is administered by the sublingual route by tablet or spray. The tiny tablet is placed under the tongue where it dissolves. Patients who take nitroglycerin with a metered-dose spray must spray the medication on or under the tongue. Each spray is equivalent to one tablet.

Nitroglycerin should create a slight tingling or burning, unless it has lost its strength because of aging or improper storage. Be sure to check the expiration date on the bottle. Sublingual nitroglycerin tablets should be stored in their original glass container with the cap screwed on tightly. Exposure to light, heat, or air may degrade the strength of the medication.

To safely assist the patient with nitroglycerin, review the steps in Skill Drill 8-3 ▶:

1. **Obtain an order from medical direction**—either online or off-line protocol.
2. **Take the patient's blood pressure.** Nitroglycerin is contraindicated if the systolic blood pressure is less than 100 mm Hg (**Step 1**).
3. **Check that you have the right medication,** the right patient, and the right route. Check the expiration date.
4. **Question the patient** about the last dose he or she took and its effects. Be prepared to have the patient lie down to prevent fainting if the nitroglycerin substantially lowers the patient's blood pressure (the patient gets dizzy or feels faint) (**Step 2**).
5. **Place the tablet or spray the dose underneath the tongue** or have the patient do so. Have the patient keep his or her mouth closed with the tablet under the tongue until it is dissolved and absorbed. Caution the patient against chewing or swallowing the tablet (**Step 3**).
6. **Recheck blood pressure within 5 minutes.** Document the medication and the time of administration. Reevaluate the chest pain and note the response to the medication. If the chest pain persists and the patient still has a systolic blood pressure greater than 100 mm Hg, repeat the dose every 5 minutes as authorized by medical control. In general, a maximum of three doses of nitroglycerin are given for any one episode of chest pain (**Step 4**).

■ General Steps in Administering Medication

It is important to remember that the patient you are treating (especially a patient that requires a medica-

You are the Provider 3

Your partner applies a nonrebreathing mask at 15 L/min and moves up front to drive. You question the patient about his history and he tells you that he has had one myocardial infarction and takes warfarin, nitroglycerin, an aspirin, and some type of blood pressure medication. He has not taken any of his medications today, but he does have his nitroglycerin with him. You call medical control to request permission to assist him with a nitroglycerin tablet. Medical control tells you to go ahead.

Reassessment	Recording Time: 5 Minutes
Pulse	96 beats/min, irregular
Blood pressure	164/98 mm Hg
Respirations	20 breaths/min, not quite as shallow
Breath sounds	Clear bilaterally
Pulse oximetry	97% on oxygen via nonrebreathing mask

6. What do you need to know before assisting with nitroglycerin?
7. What should you verify before assisting with any medication?
8. How are nitroglycerin tablets administered?
9. What side effect do you expect?
10. What is the most common contraindication for any drug?

Skill Drill   8-3   Administration of Nitroglycerin

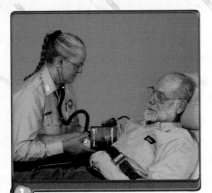

1 Verify medical direction authorization. Take the patient's blood pressure. Do not administer nitroglycerin if the systolic blood pressure is less than 100 mm Hg.

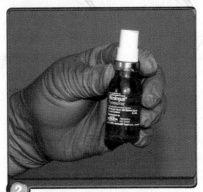

2 Check the medication and expiration date. Be prepared to lie the patient down if he or she gets dizzy or lightheaded.

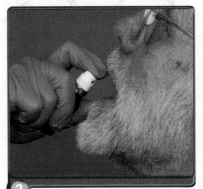

3 Place the tablet or spray underneath the tongue. Have the patient keep his or her mouth closed and tell the patient not to chew or swallow.

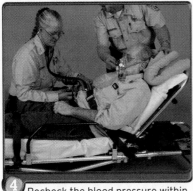

4 Recheck the blood pressure within 5 minutes. Reassess the patient's chest pain and repeat if indicated.

tion administration) is experiencing a medical emergency. Recognize that your patient may be scared and anxious. Your professionalism, care, and reassurance will help the patient through the incident. Remember to always use BSI precautions. Review the following general steps of administering any medication to a patient:

1. **Obtain an order from medical control.** This order may be online medical control (telephone or radio) or off-line medical control (through protocols that contain standing orders for the administration of certain medications).

2. **Verify the proper medication and prescription.** Once you have assessed the patient and determined that the patient is a candidate for the medication, you must make sure that the medication you are about to give is the correct medication. Carefully read the label. Make sure that the medication is the patient's own and does not belong to a friend or relative. You should never give a medication to a patient that has been prescribed for someone else.

3. **Verify the form, dose, and route of the medication.** You must make sure that the form of the medication, the dose, and the route all match the protocol you are following or the order you received.

4. **Check the expiration date** and condition of the medication. The last step before administering a medication is to make sure the expiration

date has not passed. Check the date. If no date can be found, you should examine the medication with suspicion. In addition, if you find discoloration, cloudiness, or particles in a liquid medication, you should not use it.

5. **Reassess the vital signs,** especially heart rate and blood pressure, at least every 5 minutes or sooner if the patient's condition changes.

6. **Document.** Remember the EMS rule: The work is not done until the paperwork is done. Once the medication has been given, you must document your actions and the patient's response. This includes the time you gave the medication and the name, dose, and route of administration. Did the patient's condition improve, worsen, or not change? Were there any side effects?

■ Patient Medications

Part of your patient assessment includes finding out what medications your patient is taking. This information may provide vital clues to your patient's condition that may help guide your treatment or be extremely useful to the emergency department physician. Often, knowing what medications a patient takes may be the only way you can determine what chronic or underlying conditions your patient may have. The patient may be unresponsive, confused, not knowledgeable of his or her medical history, uncooperative, or unable to communicate. Discovering what the patient takes and taking the medications or a list of them with you to the emergency department can be crucial in assessing your patient's needs.

In addition to prescription medications, patients often take nonprescription OTC medications and herbal medications. Many times, they do not consider these substances "medications" and will not report them to you unless you ask about them specifically. Herbal medications and OTC medications may be as potent as prescription medications and can have interactions and effects on the patient's health and condition that are just as important. Be sure to ask specifically about these also and relay that information to the hospital. ⬢ Table 8-1 ▶ ⬢ lists the top 100 prescribed medications and their uses.

Patients are naturally reluctant to tell you about any illegal drugs they may have taken or overdoses of medication. It is important to ask, and you can assure them that your only interest in asking is to be able to treat them appropriately.

You are the Provider   4

On arrival at the emergency department, the pain is now a 3 on a scale of 1 to 10. The patient's respirations are 16 breaths/min with good tidal volume, the pulse is 84 beats/minute and still irregular, and his blood pressure is 144/92 mm Hg. He is treated for stable angina and released to follow up with his cardiologist.

Table 8-1 Commonly Prescribed Medications

Category	Drug Name—generic (Trade)	Description
High blood pressure medications	■ atenolol ■ furosemide ■ hydrochlorothiazide ■ triamterene/hydrochlorothiazide (HCTZ) ■ quinapril (Accupril) ■ ramipril (Altace) ■ valsartan (Diovan) ■ amlodipine/benazepril (Lotrel) ■ losartan (Cozaar) ■ valsartan/HCTZ (Diovan HCT) ■ benazepril (Lotensin) ■ clonidine ■ losartan/HCTZ (Hyzaar)	Lower blood pressure by reducing blood volume, affecting the heart, or dilating blood vessels.
Other cardiac medications	■ atorvastatin (Lipitor) ■ amlodipine (Norvasc) ■ lisinopril ■ metoprolol (Lopressor and Toprol XL) ■ simvastatin (Zocor) ■ pravastatin (Pravachol) ■ clopidogrel (Plavix) ■ potassium chloride ■ warfarin (Coumadin) ■ verapamil ■ digoxin ■ diltiazem ■ fenofibrate (Tricor)	Lower blood pressure, decrease work on the heart, strengthen heartbeat, or lower cholesterol (fat) in the blood. Some of these drugs are also used in relieving chest pain.
Respiratory medications	■ albuterol ■ cetirizine (Zyrtec) ■ fexofenadine (Allegra) ■ montelukast (Singulair) ■ salmeterol/fluticasone (Advair Diskus) ■ fluticasone (Flonase) ■ mometasone (Nasonex) ■ fexofenadine/pseudoephedrine (Allegra D) ■ fluticasone propionate (Flovent) ■ ipratropium/albuterol (Combivent)	Improve airflow in and out of the lungs or decrease secretions in the respiratory tract. Some of these drugs are used to control allergy symptoms such as sneezing and watery eyes.

continued

Table 8-1 Commonly Prescribed Medications (continued)

Category	Drug Name—generic (Trade)	Description
Analgesics	■ hydrocodone/acetaminophen (APAP) ■ propoxyphene N/APAP ■ ibuprofen ■ celecoxib (Celebrex) ■ acetaminophen/codeine ■ valdecoxib (Bextra) ■ naproxen ■ oxycodone/APAP ■ oxycodone ■ rofecoxib (Vioxx; withdrawn from the market, but some patients might have this medication from previous prescriptions)	Decrease pain. A few are narcotics or controlled substances and have potential for abuse. Some also lower fever and fight inflammation.
Behavioral medications	■ alprazolam ■ sertraline (Zoloft) ■ zolpidem (Ambien) ■ fluoxetine ■ venlafaxine (Effexor and Effexor SR) ■ lorazepam ■ citalopram (Celexa) ■ bupropion (Wellbutrin, Wellbutrin SR, and Wellbutrin XL) ■ paroxetine (Paxil) ■ amitriptyline ■ escitalopram (Lexapro) ■ trazodone ■ risperidone (Risperdal) ■ olanzapine (Zyprexa) ■ methylphenidate XR (Concerta)	This group includes sedatives, sleeping medications, and drugs to fight depression or other mental conditions. The sustained release form of bupropion is also used to help people stop smoking tobacco.
Endocrine and hormone medications	■ levothyroxine ■ conjugated estrogens (Premarin) ■ norgestimate/ethinyl estradiol (Ortho Tri-Cyclen) ■ glipizide (Glucotrol and Glucotrol XL) ■ norelgestromin/ethinyl estradiol (Ortho Evra) ■ rosiglitazone (Avandia) ■ pioglitazone (Actos) ■ glyburide ■ metformin (Glucophage and Glucophage XR) ■ glimepiride (Amaryl) ■ glyburide/metformin (Glucovance)	Includes hormone replacement (thyroid or estrogen), birth control medications, and drugs used to control blood glucose levels in diabetes.

Table 8-1 Commonly Prescribed Medications (continued)

Category	Drug Name—generic (Trade)	Description
Antibiotic, antibacterial, and antifungal medications	■ azithromycin (Zithromax) ■ amoxicillin ■ cephalexin ■ amoxicillin/clavulanate ■ levofloxacin (Levaquin) ■ fluconazole ■ penicillin VK ■ ciprofloxacin (Cipro) ■ sulfamethoxazole/trimethoprim	Fight bacterial or fungal infections.
Stomach and intestinal tract medications	■ lansoprazole (Prevacid) ■ esomeprazole (Nexium) ■ pantoprazole (Protonix) ■ ranitidine ■ omeprazole ■ rabeprazole (Aciphex)	Decrease acid production in the stomach and intestinal tract and allow ulcers to heal. May also be used to stop heartburn (burning sensation in throat and upper part of the chest).
Other medications	■ alendronate (Fosamax) ■ prednisone ■ gabapentin (Neurontin) ■ clonazepam ■ sildenafil (Viagra) ■ cyclobenzaprine ■ tamsulosin (Flomax) ■ raloxifene (Evista) ■ risedronate (Actonel) ■ latanoprost (Xalatan)	Alendronate, raloxifene, and risedronate used to prevent osteoporosis (weakened bones) in postmenopausal women. Prednisone used in asthma, allergic reactions, severe arthritis, cancer, and other conditions. Gabapentin used to treat seizures or neurologic (nerve) pain. Clonazepam prevents seizures. Sildenafil aids in erectile dysfunction (lowered male sexual arousal). Cyclobenzaprine used to relax or decrease spasms in muscles. Tamsulosin used to help older men with enlarged prostate glands start and sustain urine flow. Latanoprost used in glaucoma (increased pressure within the eye).

Note: Within each group, the drugs are listed from the most common to the least common. *Data Source:* rx.list.com. Accessed November 29, 2004.

You are the Provider Summary

It is essential to recognize the need for early intervention as well as to remember the steps for proper drug administration. Oxygen and position of comfort are the first steps when dealing with a nontrauma patient complaining of chest pain. Obtaining a good history is also vital to proper assessment and treatment.

1. What are your priorities for this patient?

ABCs; recognize that this is a load-and-go patient.

2. What questions should you ask about his pain?

- Does the pain radiate?
- On a scale of 1 to 10, how does this rate?
- Have you had any nausea or vomiting?

3. What type of oxygen does he need? Why?

Nonrebreathing mask. Chest pain is generally the result of a hypoxic myocardium. The patient is alert and probably will not tolerate a bag-mask device. Also, since his respirations are only slightly shallow, he should receive more than adequate oxygenation with a nonrebreathing mask.

4. What else do you need to know about this patient?

- What is his pertinent medical history?
- Does he take any medications?
- SAMPLE

5. Name the pertinent negative in this scenario.

He denies any nausea or vomiting. It is common for patients with chest pain to experience one or both.

6. What do you need to know before assisting with nitroglycerin?

What is his blood pressure? Do not assist with nitroglycerin if the patient's blood pressure is below 100 mm Hg systolic. Nitroglycerin is a potent vasodilator and can rapidly decrease blood pressure.

7. What should you verify before assisting with any medication?

- The prescription belongs to the patient
- The expiration date
- Permission from medical control

8. How are nitroglycerin tablets administered?

Sublingual—under the tongue. If the patient's mouth is dry, have him swish a little water around and spit it out to moisten the mucous membranes. This will help the tablet to dissolve quicker.

9. What side effect do you expect?

A decrease in blood pressure due to the vasodilatory effects.

10. What is the most common contraindication for any drug?

Hypersensitivity to that drug.

Prep Kit

Ready for Review

- Patients having a medical emergency that requires medication administration are often anxious and scared. Recognize and respect your patient's feelings.
- Medications come in many forms: tablets and capsules, solutions and suspensions, metered-dose inhalers, topical medications, transdermal medications, gels, and gases.
- Medications may be administered through several routes: intravenous, intramuscular and subcutaneous injection, oral, sublingual, intraosseous, transcutaneous, by inhalation, and rectally.
- In all but the intravenous injection route, the medication is absorbed into the bloodstream through various body tissues. These routes of administration often determine the speed with which the medication takes effect.
- Three medications are typically carried on the EMS unit: oxygen, oral glucose, and activated charcoal. Two medicines have recently been added to the EMT-B list by some states and services: aspirin and epinephrine.
- There are three additional medications that you may help the patient self-administer: metered-dose inhaler medications, nitroglycerin, and epinephrine. Remember, though, that the administration of the medications may differ depending on local protocol.
- The administration of any medication requires approval by medical control, through direct orders given online or standing orders that are part of the local protocols.
- The steps to follow in administering medications are:
  - Obtain an order from medical control
  - Verify the proper medication
  - Verify the dose and route
  - Check the expiration date of the medication
  - Reassess vital signs and the patient's response to the medication
  - Accurately document the care you provided

Vital Vocabulary

absorption The process by which medications travel through body tissues until they reach the bloodstream.

action The therapeutic effect of a medication on the body.

contraindications Conditions that make a particular medication or treatment inappropriate, for example, a condition in which a medication should not be given because it would not help or may actually harm a patient.

dose The amount of medication given on the basis of the patient's size and age.

generic name The original chemical name of a medication (in contrast with one of its "trade names"); the name is not capitalized.

indications The therapeutic uses for a specific medication.

inhalation Breathing into the lungs; a medication delivery route.

intramuscular (IM) injection An injection into a muscle; a medication delivery route.

intraosseous (IO) Into the bone; a medication delivery route.

intravenous (IV) injection An injection directly into a vein; a medication delivery route.

metered-dose inhaler (MDI) A miniature spray canister through which droplets or particles of medication may be inhaled.

oral By mouth; a medication delivery route.

per os (PO) Through the mouth; a medication delivery route; same as oral.

per rectum (PR) Through the rectum; a medication delivery route.

pharmacology The study of the properties and effects of medications.

side effects Any effects of a medication other than the desired ones.

subcutaneous (SC) injection Injection into the tissue between the skin and muscle; a medication delivery route.

sublingual (SL) Under the tongue; a medication delivery route.

trade name The brand name that a manufacturer gives a medication; the name is capitalized.

transcutaneous Through the skin; a medication delivery route.

transdermal medications Medications that are designed to be absorbed through the skin (transcutaneously).

Technology

- Interactivities
- Vocabulary Explorer
- Anatomy Review
- Web Links
- Online Review Manual

Refresher.EMSzone.com

Assessment in Action

You are called to the scene of a person with "difficulty breathing." On arrival you find a 17-year-old girl who presents with wheezing and peripheral cyanosis. She has an albuterol metered-dose inhaler but has not used it.

1. An EMT-B can assist with all of the following medications EXCEPT:
   - **A.** albuterol in a metered-dose inhaler.
   - **B.** insulin.
   - **C.** nitroglycerin.
   - **D.** an EpiPen.

2. Before assisting with any medication, you should:
   - **A.** obtain permission from medical control to assist with the medication.
   - **B.** ensure that the prescription is for the patient.
   - **C.** check the expiration date.
   - **D.** all of the above.

3. What side effects do you expect after assisting with the metered-dose inhaler?
   - **A.** bradycardia
   - **B.** diaphoresis
   - **C.** tachycardia
   - **D.** hemoptysis

4. What is the next step after assisting with any medication?
   - **A.** Ask the patient about any allergies.
   - **B.** Call medical control.
   - **C.** Recheck the expiration date of the medication.
   - **D.** Monitor the patient.

5. What is the therapeutic effect of a medication?
   - **A.** any side effect
   - **B.** a contraindication
   - **C.** the action of the medication
   - **D.** the dose

6. What is the desired effect of albuterol?
   - **A.** tachycardia
   - **B.** bronchodilation
   - **C.** bronchoconstriction
   - **D.** tachypnea

Challenging Questions

7. Albuterol is a beta-2 selective sympathomimetic drug. What does this mean?

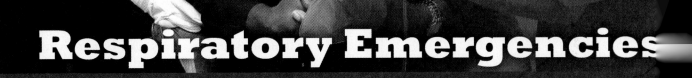

Respiratory Emergencies

9

You are the Provider 1

It is early on a Sunday morning in January when you and your partner are called for a patient who is having difficulty breathing. On arrival you find an 87-year-old woman lying in bed looking very ill. Her husband tells you that she refused to go to the doctor and she is much worse than she was last night.

Initial Assessment	Recording Time: 0 Minutes
Appearance	Flushed, diaphoretic
Level of consciousness	Alert and oriented, but sluggish to respond
Airway	Open and clear
Breathing	A little fast and shallow
Circulation	Radials present, irregular

1. What are your priorities for this patient?
2. What questions should you ask about this episode?

Introduction

Dyspnea, the feeling of being short of breath, is one of the most common complaints encountered in the field. As you know, the origin of the problem may range from asthma to pneumonia to a heart attack. Even though you may not be able to determine the exact cause of the dyspnea, you have the tools to identify a potential threat to life and, in some cases, even to save a life.

This chapter begins with a basic review of respiratory anatomy and physiology. It then looks at common medical problems that cause dyspnea, including acute pulmonary edema, chronic obstructive pulmonary disease, and asthma. We will review the signs and symptoms of each condition. You should keep these possible medical conditions in mind as you take the patient's history and perform a physical assessment, a process that the chapter describes in detail. Remember, the sensation of not getting enough air can be terrifying to the patient, regardless of its cause. As an EMT-B, you should be prepared to provide emergency medical care to the patient and to address the emotional needs of your patient with a calm and reassuring approach.

Anatomy and Physiology

The respiratory system consists of all the structures of the body that contribute to the breathing process. Important anatomic features include the upper and lower airways, the lungs, and the diaphragm `Figure 9-1 ▶`. Air enters the upper airway through the nose and mouth and moves past the epiglottis into the trachea.

Technology

Interactivities

Vocabulary Explorer

Anatomy Review

Web Links

Online Review Manual

Refresher.EMSzone.com

It then moves along the bronchial tubes to the alveoli where oxygen and carbon dioxide are exchanged.

The principal function of the lungs is respiration, which is the exchange of oxygen and carbon dioxide. The two processes that occur during respiration are inspiration, the act of breathing in or inhaling, and expiration, the act of breathing out or exhaling. During respiration, oxygen is provided to the blood and carbon dioxide is removed from it. This exchange of gases takes place rapidly in normal lungs in the alveoli. Alveoli are microscopic, thin-walled air sacs that lie against the pulmonary capillary vessels. Oxygen and carbon dioxide must be able to pass freely between the alveoli and the capillaries. Oxygen enters the alveoli through tiny passages in the alveolar wall into the capillaries, which carry the oxygen to the heart. The heart pumps the oxygen around the body. Carbon dioxide produced by the body's cells returns to the lungs in the blood that circulates through and around the alveolar air spaces. The carbon dioxide diffuses back into the alveoli and travels back up the bronchial tree and out the upper airways during exhalation `Figure 9-2 ▶`. Again, carbon dioxide is "exchanged" for oxygen, which travels in exactly the opposite direction (during inhalation). The brain stem senses the level of carbon dioxide in the arterial blood. The level of carbon dioxide bathing the brain stem stimulates a healthy person to breathe. If the level drops too low, the person automatically breathes at a slower rate and less deeply. As a result, less carbon dioxide is expired, allowing the carbon dioxide level in the blood to return to normal. If the level of carbon dioxide in the arterial blood rises above normal, the patient breathes more rapidly and more deeply. When more fresh air (containing no carbon dioxide) is brought into the alveoli, more carbon dioxide diffuses out of the bloodstream, thereby lowering the level.

The following are the characteristics of adequate breathing:

- Normal rate and depth
- Regular pattern of inhalation and exhalation
- Good audible breath sounds on both sides of the chest
- Regular rise and fall movement on both sides of the chest
- Pink, warm, dry skin

Pathophysiology

Respiratory emergencies can be the result of several causes. One common cause is an increased level of

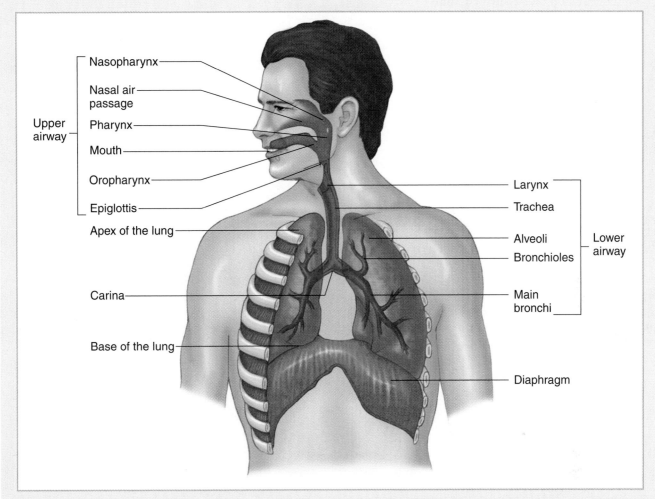

Figure 9-1 The upper airway includes the mouth, nose, pharynx, and oropharynx. The lower airway includes the larynx, trachea, mainstem bronchi, bronchioles, and alveoli.

carbon dioxide in the arterial blood to a level above normal. Frequently, this is caused by an impaired exhalation process that is from various types of lung disease. The body may also produce too much carbon dioxide, temporarily or chronically, depending on the disease or abnormality.

If, for a period of years, the arterial carbon dioxide level rises slowly to an abnormally high level and remains there, the respiratory center in the brain, which senses the carbon dioxide level and controls breathing, may work less efficiently. The failure of this center to respond normally to a rise in the arterial level of carbon dioxide is called chronic carbon dioxide retention. If the condition is severe, respiration will stop, unless there is a secondary drive, called <u>hypoxic drive</u>, to stimulate the respiratory center. Hypoxic drive works by sensing the low blood oxy-

gen level. When detected, the respiratory center responds and stimulates the person to breathe. If the arterial level of oxygen is then raised, which happens when the patient is given additional oxygen, there is no longer any stimulus to breathe; the high carbon dioxide and low oxygen drives are lost. Patients with chronic lung diseases frequently have a chronically high level of carbon dioxide in the blood. Therefore, giving too much oxygen to them (for a long period) may actually depress, or completely stop, the respirations.

In most disorders of the respiratory system, one or more of the following situations exists:

- The pulmonary veins and arteries are actually obstructed from absorbing oxygen or releasing carbon dioxide by fluid, infection, or collapsed air spaces.

- The alveoli are damaged and cannot transport gases properly across their own walls.
- The air passages are obstructed by muscle spasm, mucus, or weakened, floppy airway walls.
- Blood flow to the lungs is obstructed by blood clots.
- The pleural space is filled with air or excess fluid, so the lungs cannot properly expand.

All of these conditions prevent the proper exchange of oxygen and carbon dioxide. In addition, the pulmonary blood vessels themselves may have abnormalities that interfere with blood flow and, thus, with the transfer of gases.

The following are signs of inadequate breathing:

- A rate slower than 12 breaths/min or faster than 20 breaths/min in an adult
- Unequal chest expansion
- Decreased breath sounds on one or both sides of the chest
- Muscle retractions above the clavicles, between the ribs, and below the rib cage, especially in children
- Pale or cyanotic skin
- Cool, damp (clammy) skin
- Shallow or irregular respirations
- Pursed lips and nasal flaring

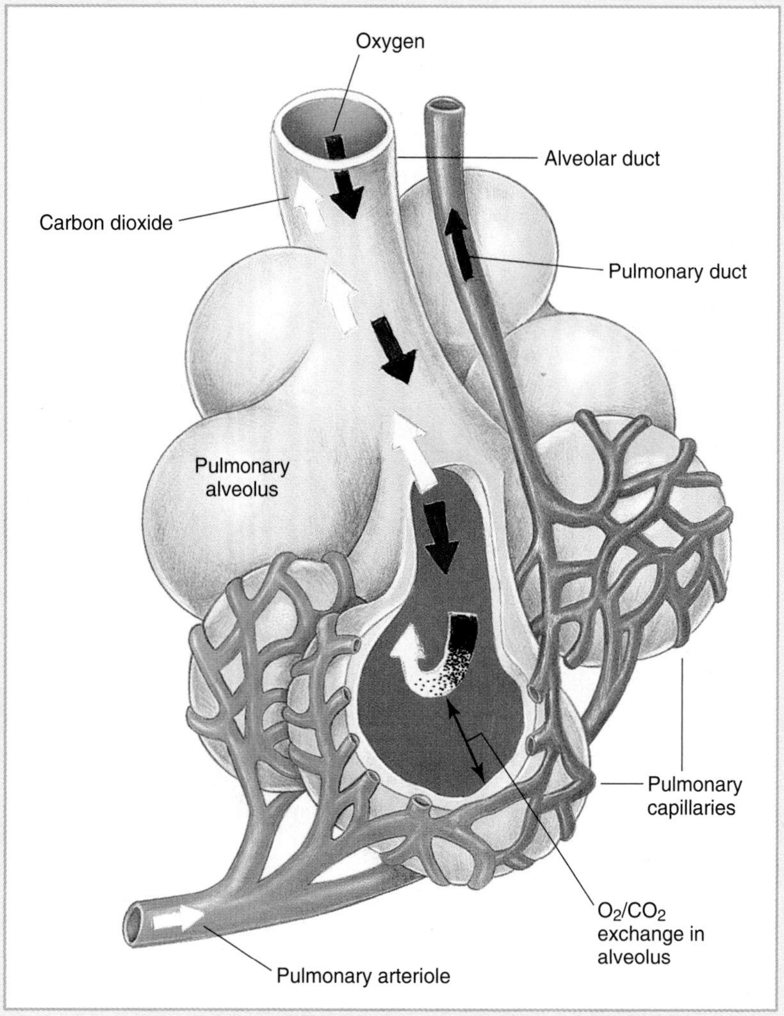

Figure 9-2 An enlarged view of a single alveolus that shows oxygen and carbon dioxide exchange between the air in the sac and blood in the pulmonary capillaries.

Causes of Dyspnea

Dyspnea is shortness of breath or difficulty breathing. Remember that if the problem is severe and the brain is deprived of oxygen, the patient may not be alert enough to complain of shortness of breath. Altered mental status is a sign of hypoxia of the brain.

Common respiratory emergencies include the following:

- Upper or lower airway infection
- Acute pulmonary edema
- Chronic obstructive pulmonary disease (COPD)
- Asthma or allergic reactions
- Spontaneous pneumothorax
- Anaphylactic reactions
- Prolonged seizures
- Airway obstruction
- Pulmonary embolism
- Hyperventilation
- Severe pain, particularly chest pain

Upper or Lower Airway Infection

Infectious diseases causing dyspnea may affect all parts of the airway. Some cause mild discomfort. Others obstruct the airway to the point that patients require a full range of respiratory support. In general, the problem is always some form of obstruction to the flow of air in the major passages (colds, diphtheria, epiglottitis, and croup) or to the exchange of gases between the alveoli and the capillaries (pneumonia).

Acute Pulmonary Edema

Sometimes, the heart muscle is so injured after a heart attack or other illness that it cannot pump blood efficiently. In these cases, the left side of the heart cannot remove blood from the lung as fast as the right side delivers it. As a result, fluid builds up within the alveoli and in the lung tissue between the alveoli and the pulmonary capillaries. This accumulation of fluid in the space between the alveoli and the pulmonary capillaries, called pulmonary edema, can develop quickly after a major heart attack. By physically separating alveoli from pulmonary capillary vessels, the edema interferes with the exchange of carbon dioxide and oxygen. The patient usually experiences dyspnea with rapid, shallow respirations. In severe cases, you will see frothy, pink sputum coming from the mouth and nose.

In most cases, patients have a medical history of congestive heart failure (CHF) that is usually controlled by medication. However, an acute onset may occur if the patient stops taking the medication, eats food that is too salty, or has a stressful illness, a new heart attack, or an abnormal heart rhythm. Pulmonary edema is one of the most common causes of hospital admission in the United States. It is common for patients to have recurring episodes of pulmonary edema.

Some patients who have pulmonary edema do not have heart disease. Poisonings from inhaling large amounts of smoke or toxic chemical fumes can produce pulmonary edema, as can traumatic injuries of the chest. In these cases, fluid collects in the alveoli and lung tissue in response to damage to the tissues of the lungs or the bronchi.

Chronic Obstructive Pulmonary Disease

Chronic obstructive pulmonary disease (COPD) is a common lung condition, affecting 10% to 20% of the entire adult population in the United States. It is the end of a slow process, which during several years results in disruption of the airways, the alveoli, and the pulmonary blood vessels. The process itself may be a result of direct lung and airway damage from repeated infections or inhalation of toxic agents such as industrial gases and particles, but most often, it results from cigarette smoking. Although it is well known that cigarettes are a direct cause of lung cancer, their role in the development of COPD is far more significant and less well publicized.

Tobacco smoke is itself a bronchial irritant and can create chronic bronchitis, an ongoing irritation of the trachea and bronchi. With bronchitis, excess mucus is constantly produced, obstructing small airways and alveoli. Protective cells and lung mechanisms that remove foreign particles are destroyed, further weakening the patient's respiratory system. Chronic oxygenation problems can also lead to right-sided heart failure and fluid retention, such as peripheral edema in the legs. Pneumonia develops easily when the passages are persistently obstructed. Ultimately, repeated episodes of irritation and pneumonia cause scarring in the lung and some dilation of the obstructed alveoli, leading to COPD.

Another type of COPD is called emphysema. Emphysema is a loss of the elastic material around the air spaces as a result of chronic stretching of the alveoli when inflamed airways obstruct the expulsion of gases. Smoking can also directly destroy the elasticity of the lung tissue. Normally, lungs act like a spongy balloon that is inflated; once they are inflated, they will naturally recoil because of their elastic nature, expelling gas rapidly. However, when they are constantly obstructed or when the balloon's elasticity is diminished, air is no longer expelled rapidly, and the walls of the alveoli eventually fall apart, leaving large "holes" in the lung that resemble large air pockets or cavities. This condition is called emphysema.

Most patients with COPD have elements of chronic bronchitis and emphysema. Some patients will have more elements of one condition than the other; few patients will have only emphysema or bronchitis. Most patients with COPD chronically produce sputum, have a chronic cough, and have difficulty expelling air from their lungs, with long expiration phases and wheezing. These patients present with abnormal breath sounds such as rales, crackles, rhonchi, and wheezes, which are discussed in the section on patient assessment later in this chapter.

Asthma

Asthma is an acute spasm of the smaller air passages called bronchioles, associated with excessive mucus production and with swelling of the mucous lining of the respiratory passages. It is a common but serious disease, affecting about 6 million Americans and killing 4,000 to 5,000 Americans each year. Asthma produces characteristic wheezing as patients attempt to exhale through partially obstructed air passages. These same air passages open easily during inspiration. In other words, when patients inhale, breathing appears relatively normal; the wheezing is most often heard when they exhale. This wheezing may be so loud that you can hear it without a stethoscope. In other cases, the airways are so blocked that no air movement is heard. In severe cases, the actual work of exhaling is very tiring. Respiratory arrest may develop quickly.

Asthma affects patients of all ages and is usually the result of an allergic reaction to an inhaled, ingested, or injected substance. Note that the substance itself is not the cause of the allergic reaction; rather, it is an exaggerated response of the body's immune system to that substance that causes the reaction. In some cases, however, there is no identifiable substance, or allergen, that triggers the body's immune system. An allergic response to certain foods or some other allergen may produce an acute asthma attack. Between attacks, patients may breathe normally. In its most severe form, an allergic reaction can produce anaphylaxis and even anaphylactic shock. This, in turn, may cause respiratory distress severe enough to result in coma and death. Asthma attacks may also be caused by severe emotional stress, exercise, and respiratory infections.

Most patients with asthma are familiar with their symptoms and know when an attack is imminent. Typically, they will have appropriate medication with them or at home. You should listen carefully to what these patients tell you; they often know exactly what they need.

Spontaneous Pneumothorax

When the surface of the lung is disrupted (from a weakened area or trauma), air escapes into the pleural cavity, and the negative vacuum pressure in the lung is lost. The natural elasticity of the lung tissue causes the lung to collapse. The accumulation of air in the pleural space, which may be mild or severe, is called a pneumothorax. A pneumothorax is most often caused by trauma, but it can also be caused by medical conditions. In these patients, the condition is called a "spontaneous" pneumothorax.

Spontaneous pneumothorax may occur in patients with certain chronic lung infections or in young people born with weak areas of the lung. Patients with emphysema and asthma are at high risk for spontaneous pneumothorax when a weakened portion of lung ruptures, often during a coughing episode. A patient with a spontaneous pneumothorax becomes short of breath and might complain of pleuritic chest pain, a sharp, stabbing pain on one side that is worse during inspiration and expiration or with certain movement of the chest wall. By listening to the chest with the stethoscope, you can sometimes tell that breath sounds are absent or decreased on the affected side. Spontaneous pneumothorax may be the cause of sudden dyspnea in a patient with underlying emphysema.

Anaphylactic Reactions

Patients who do not have asthma may still have severe allergic reactions. An allergen, a substance that a person is sensitive to, may cause an allergic reaction or may cause anaphylaxis, a reaction characterized by airway swelling and dilation of blood vessels all over the body (which lowers the blood pressure significantly). Anaphylaxis may be associated with widespread itching and the same signs and symptoms as asthma. The airway may swell so much that breathing problems can progress from extreme difficulty breathing to total airway obstruction in a matter of a few minutes. Most anaphylactic reactions occur within 30 minutes of exposure to the allergen, which can be anything from eating certain nuts to receiving a penicillin injection. In severe cases, epinephrine is the treatment of choice.

Mechanical Obstruction of the Airway

You should always be aware of the possibility that a patient with dyspnea may have a mechanical obstruction of the airway and be prepared to treat it quickly. In semiconscious and unconscious people, the obstruction may be the result of aspiration of vomitus or a foreign object or of a position of the head that causes obstruction by the tongue. Opening the airway with the head tilt–chin lift maneuver may solve the problem. If simply opening the airway does not correct the breathing problem, you will have to assess for an airway obstruction.

Always consider upper airway obstruction from a foreign body first in patients who were eating just before becoming short of breath. The same is true of young children, especially crawling babies, who might have swallowed and choked on a small object.

Pulmonary Embolism

An embolus is anything in the circulatory system that moves from its point of origin to a distant site and lodges there, obstructing blood flow in that area. Beyond the point of the obstruction, circulation can be completely cut off or at least markedly decreased, which can result in a serious, life-threatening condition. Emboli can be fragments of blood clots in an artery or vein that break off and travel through the bloodstream. They also can be foreign bodies that enter the circulation, such as a bullet or a bubble of air.

A pulmonary embolism is a blood clot formed in a vein, usually in the legs or pelvis, that breaks off and circulates through the venous system. The large clot moves through the right side of the heart and into the pulmonary artery, where it becomes lodged, significantly decreasing or blocking blood flow. Even though the lung is actively involved in inhalation and exhalation of air, no exchange of oxygen or carbon dioxide takes place in the areas of blocked blood flow because there is no effective circulation. In this circumstance, the level of arterial carbon dioxide usually rises, and the oxygen level may drop enough to cause cyanosis and significant dyspnea.

Pulmonary emboli may occur as a result of damage to the lining of vessels, a tendency for blood to clot unusually fast, or, most often, slow blood flow in a lower extremity. Slow blood flow in the legs is usually caused by long-term bed rest, which can lead to the collapse of veins. Patients whose legs are immobilized following a fracture or recent surgery are at risk for pulmonary emboli for days or weeks after the incident. A pulmonary embolism is rare in active, healthy people. Although they are fairly common, pulmonary emboli are difficult to diagnose. They occur about 650,000 times a year in the United States, some of them immediately fatal.

Hyperventilation Syndrome

Hyperventilation is defined as overbreathing to the point that the level of arterial carbon dioxide falls below normal. This may be an indicator of a major life-threatening illness. For example, a patient with diabetes who has a very high blood glucose level, a patient who has taken an overdose of aspirin, or a patient with a severe infection is likely to hyperventilate. In these patients, rapid, deep breathing is the body's attempt to stay alive. The body is trying to compensate for acidosis, the buildup of excess acid in the blood or body tissues that results from the primary illness. Because carbon dioxide mixed with water in the bloodstream can add to the blood's acidity, lowering the level of carbon dioxide helps compensate for the other acids.

Similarly, in an otherwise healthy person, blood acidity can be diminished by excessive breathing, because it "blows off" too much carbon dioxide. The result is a relative lack of acids. The resulting condition, alkalosis, is the buildup of excess base (lack of acids) in the body fluids.

Alkalosis is the cause of many of the symptoms associated with hyperventilation syndrome, including anxiety, dizziness, numbness, tingling of the hands and feet, and even a sense of dyspnea despite the rapid breathing. Although hyperventilation can be the response to illness and a buildup of acids, hyperventilation syndrome occurs in the absence of other physical problems. It is common during psychological stress,

You are the Provider 2

As you are performing your assessment and taking baseline vital signs you note that the patient is very warm to the touch. Her husband tells you that she has been coughing a lot and has just started complaining of a sore throat. She does not have a history of respiratory problems and only takes medication for her heart condition. She started feeling bad on Thursday and it has been progressively worsening.

Vital Signs	Recording Time: 2 Minutes
Skin	Flushed, diaphoretic
Pulse	96 beats/min, irregular
Blood pressure	110/76 mm Hg
Respirations	22 breaths/min, slightly shallow

3. What type of oxygen does she need? Why?
4. What should you ask about the fever?
5. What should you ask about the cough?

Teamwork Tips

While you are assessing the patient and coaching his or her breathing, your partner should set up the oxygen and talk to any family members or bystanders to obtain a history.

affecting some 10% of the population at one time or another. The respirations of a person who is experiencing hyperventilation syndrome may be as high as more than 40 shallow breaths/min or as low as only 20 very deep breaths/min. The decision whether hyperventilation is being caused by a life-threatening illness or a panic attack should not be made outside the hospital. All patients who are hyperventilating should be given supplemental oxygen and transported to the hospital.

■ Assessment of the Patient in Respiratory Distress

Patients in respiratory distress are usually quite anxious. A calm and systematic assessment will help to decrease their anxiety level.

Scene Size-up

Body substance isolation precautions include gloves and, if you suspect a respiratory infection, a mask and protective eyewear. Scene safety may be as simple as ensuring safe access to the patient and considering safe lifting and moving of the patient. Or you may need to consider that the respiratory emergency may have been caused by a toxic substance that was inhaled, absorbed, or ingested.

Once you have determined that the scene is safe, you need to consider the nature of illness or mechanism of injury and whether there is a need to consider taking spinal immobilization precautions. Then determine how many patients there are and whether you need additional resources. In situations with multiple people with dyspnea, you should consider the possibility of an airborne hazardous material release.

Initial Assessment

General Impression

As you approach and begin interacting with the patient, you need to form a general or initial impression of the patient. Does the patient appear calm? Is he or she anxious, restless? Does the patient appear listless and tired? This initial impression will help you decide whether the patient's condition is stable or unstable.

At the same time, you should determine the patient's level of consciousness using the AVPU scale. If the patient is alert or responding to verbal stimuli, the brain is still receiving oxygen. If the patient is responsive to painful stimuli or unresponsive, the brain may not be oxygenated well and the potential for an airway or breathing problem is more likely. If the patient is alert or responding to verbal stimuli, what is the patient's chief complaint? Within seconds, you will be able to determine whether there are any immediate threats to life.

Airway and Breathing

Assess the airway. Is it patent? Is it adequate? Air must flow in and out of the chest easily for the airway to be considered patent and adequate. If snoring sounds are heard in an unresponsive patient, reposition the airway and insert an oral or nasal airway if necessary to maintain the airway. If you hear <u>stridor</u>, position the patient so he or she can breathe easily. If gurgling sounds are heard, suction as necessary.

If the airway is open and clear, you should next evaluate your patient's breathing. Is the patient breathing? Is the patient breathing adequately? If the patient is not breathing, give two ventilations immediately. As you ventilate, you need to evaluate if your ventilations are adequate.

1. Is the air going in?
2. Does the chest expand with each breath?
3. Does the chest fall after each breath?
4. Is the rate adequate for the patient's age?

Refer to Chapter 5 for a review of ventilation techniques. Remember, you will need to continue to monitor the airway for fluid, secretions, or other problems as you move on to assess the adequacy of your patient's breathing. If the patient is breathing, ensure that the breathing is adequate. Listen to breath sounds to determine whether they are equal and clear. Is there adequate rise and fall of the chest? Are the patient's respirations labored? If the patient can only speak one or two words at a time before gasping for a breath, ventilations are considered labored. Is the patient using accessory muscles to assist the respiratory effort? If the respiratory effort is inadequate, you must provide the necessary intervention. If the patient is in respiratory distress, place him or her in a position that facilitates easier breathing and begin administering oxygen at 15 L/min via a nonrebreathing mask. If the patient has inadequate depth in breathing or the rate is too slow, the patient's ventilations may need to be assisted with bag-valve ventilation.

Circulation

Evaluating the adequacy of the pulse and the patient's skin can give you an indication of the patient's breathing status. If the pulse rate is normal, the patient is most likely receiving enough oxygen. If the pulse rate is too fast or too slow, the patient may not be getting enough oxygen. Assessing a patient's circulation includes an evaluation of shock and bleeding. Respiratory distress in a patient could be from a lack of red blood cells to transport the oxygen. This loss of perfusion may be from chronic anemia, a wound, internal bleeding, or simply from shock overwhelming the body's ability to compensate for the illness. Recheck everything. Is the oxygen bottle hooked up to the mask? Is the oxygen turned on? Is the flow rate adequate (10 to 15 L/min)? Is there a good face-mask seal? Is the chest rising and falling with each breath? Is the airway blocked with vomitus or the tongue? Control any bleeding no matter how mild and treat your patient for shock.

Transport Decision

The last step in the initial assessment is to make a transport decision. If the patient's condition is stable and there are no life threats, you may decide to perform a focused history and physical exam on scene. If the patient's condition is unstable and there is a possible life threat, proceed with rapid transport. Perform a focused history and physical exam en route to the hospital.

Focused History and Physical Exam

After you have completed your initial assessment and addressed any potential or real life threats, you can now focus your assessment on the patient's respiratory emergency. Begin the focused history and physical exam by asking questions about the present illness. Use SAMPLE and OPQRST to guide you in your questioning.

SAMPLE History

With patients in respiratory distress, many of the SAMPLE questions can be answered by the family or bystanders. Limit the number of questions to pertinent ones—a patient who is in respiratory distress doesn't need to be using any additional air to answer questions. To help determine the cause of your patient's condition, look for medications, medical alert bracelets, environmental conditions, and other clues to what may be causing the problem. Each part of the SAMPLE history may give you clues.

Ask the patient to describe the problem. Begin by asking an open-ended question, "What can you tell me about your breathing?" Pay close attention to OPQRST: when the problem began (onset), what makes the breathing difficulty worse (provocation), how the breathing feels (quality), and whether the discomfort moves (radiation). How much of a problem is the patient having (severity)? Is the problem continuous or intermittent (time)?

Find out what the patient has already done for the breathing problem. Does the patient use a prescribed inhaler? If so, when was it used last? How many doses have been taken? Does the patient use more than one inhaler? Be sure to record the name of each inhaler and when it was used.

Different respiratory complaints offer different clues and different challenges. Patients with chronic conditions may have long periods when they are able to live relatively normal lives, but they sometimes experience acute worsening of their conditions. That's when you are called, and it is important to be able to determine your patient's baseline status, in other words, the patient's usual condition, and what is different at this time that resulted in a call to you. For example, patients with COPD (emphysema and chronic bronchitis) cannot handle pulmonary infections well because the existing airway damage makes them unable to cough up the mucus or sputum produced by the infection. The chronic lower airway obstruction makes it difficult to breathe deeply enough to clear the lungs. Gradually, the arterial oxygen level falls, and the carbon dioxide level rises. If a new infection of the lung occurs in a patient with COPD, the arterial oxygen level may fall rapidly. In a few patients, the carbon dioxide level may rise high enough to cause sleepiness. These patients require respiratory support and careful administration of oxygen.

A patient with COPD usually presents with a long history of dyspnea with a sudden increase in shortness of breath. There is rarely a history of chest pain. More often, the patient will remember having had a recent "chest cold" with fever and an inability to cough up mucus or a sudden increase in sputum. If the patient is able to cough up sputum, it will be thick and is often green or yellow. The blood pressure of patients with COPD is normal; however, the pulse is rapid and occasionally irregular. Pay particular attention to the respirations. They may be rapid, or they may be very slow.

Patients with asthma may have different "triggers," different causes of acute attacks. These include allergens, cold, exercise, stress, infection, and not taking medications as prescribed. It is important to try to determine what may have triggered the attack so that it can be treated appropriately.

Patients with CHF often walk a fine line between compensating for their diminished cardiac capacity and decompensating. Many take several medications, most often including diuretics ("water pills") and blood pressure medications. Your history taking should include obtaining a list of all their medications and paying special attention to the events leading up to the present problem.

Focused Physical Exam

Patients with COPD usually are older than 50 years. They usually will have a history of recurring respiratory problems and are almost always long-term cigarette smokers. Patients with COPD may complain of tightness in the chest and constant fatigue. Because air has been gradually and continuously trapped in their lungs in increasing amounts, their chests often have a barrel-like appearance. If you listen to the chest with a stethoscope, you will hear abnormal breath sounds. These sounds may include crackles, which are crackling, rattling sounds that are usually associated with fluid in the lungs, but in COPD are related to chronic scarring of small airways; rhonchi, which are coarse, gravelly sounds caused by mucus in the upper airways; and <u>wheezing</u>, a high-pitched whistling or crackling sound, most often heard on exhalation. Because of diminished airflow, breath sounds can be difficult to hear and may be detected only high up on the posterior part of the chest. Patients with COPD will often exhale through pursed lips in an attempt to maintain airway pressures.

Documentation Tips

Patients with dyspnea due to chronic obstructive pulmonary disease (COPD) or congestive heart failure (CHF) may feel claustrophobic with an oxygen mask and may only tolerate a nasal cannula or blow-by oxygen. Be sure and document why your oxygen delivery device is inappropriate.

Patient would not tolerate NRB, applied O_2 via NC at 4 L/M.

In addition to the signs of air hunger present in all patients with respiratory distress, such as tripod positioning, rapid breathing, and use of accessory muscles, restriction of the small lower airways in patients with asthma often causes wheezing. Patients may have a prolonged expiratory phase of breathing as they attempt to exhale trapped air from their lungs. In severe cases, you may not actually hear wheezing because of insufficient airflow. As your patient tires from the effort of breathing and the oxygen level drops, respiratory and heart rates may actually decrease, and your patient may seem to relax or go to sleep. These signs indicate impending respiratory arrest, and you must act immediately.

You are the Provider   3

Your partner applies a nonrebreathing mask at 15 L/min and listens to her breath sounds. She has rales bilaterally. Her husband tells you that she has been coughing up a thick phlegm that has changed from a light yellow on Friday to a greenish-brown today.

You and your partner place her on the stretcher and wrap her with blankets. She is having chills with the fever. Her cough is getting worse and it is harder for her to cough anything up. She is getting very tired and more dyspneic from the effort.

Reassessment	Recording Time: 5 Minutes
Pulse	98 beats/min, irregular
Blood pressure	110/76 mm Hg
Respirations	20 breaths/min, not quite as shallow
Breath sounds	Rales bilaterally
Pulse oximetry	95% on oxygen via a nonrebreathing mask

  6. What does the phlegm tell you?
  7. Is there any medication with which you might assist her?
  8. What might help with the cough?
  9. In what position should she be transported?
10. What do you think is wrong with the patient?

When patients with CHF decompensate, they will often experience pulmonary edema as fluid backs up in their circulatory system and into the lungs. High blood pressure and low cardiac output often trigger this "flash" (sudden) pulmonary edema. These patients are among the most sick, afraid, and anxious patients you encounter. They are literally drowning in their own fluid. In addition to the classic signs of respiratory distress, they may have pink, frothy sputum coming from their mouths. Their lung sounds are not clear. You will often hear breath sounds that are wet (rales, rhonchi, crackles) but sometimes dry sounding (wheezes). Their legs and feet may be swollen (pedal edema) from the backup of fluid in their system.

Sometimes it is not possible to determine quickly and definitively what is causing your patient's respiratory distress. The 20-year-old at a picnic in whom difficulty breathing and hives rapidly develop after a bee sting offers a clear-cut diagnostic picture. The older woman receiving 12 medications in a nursing home who has a cough and increasing shortness of breath that developed during a week's time is more challenging. Keep an open mind, obtain as complete a history as possible, and perform a focused physical exam.

Baseline Vital Signs

In addition to pulse, respirations, and blood pressure, other signs such as skin color, level of consciousness, and pain measurement are key in evaluating the patient in respiratory distress. It is essential to look at the whole clinical picture when evaluating the patient in respiratory distress and not fixate on any one vital sign or symptom. This baseline evaluation of vital signs may be used later to determine trends. For example, your patient may present with a rapid respiratory rate to compensate for a failing heart. After you administer oxygen, a decrease in the breathing rate toward normal may indicate that your patient is getting better. On the other hand, it may indicate that your patient is decompensating, no longer able to maintain the effort of rapid breathing, and the patient's condition may quickly deteriorate. Patients initially compensate for respiratory distress by increased respiratory and heart rates. If they are able to maintain adequate oxygenation, they will be able to maintain their level of consciousness and skin color, temperature, and dryness. Blood pressure will vary with the patient's baseline status and condition. It is often elevated in pulmonary edema due to CHF.

The brain needs a constant, adequate supply of oxygen to function normally. When the oxygen level drops, you will notice an altered level of consciousness. This may manifest as confusion, lack of coordination, bizarre behavior, or even combativeness. Change in affect or level of consciousness is one of the early warning signs of respiratory inadequacy.

When there is inadequate oxygen in the blood, the body will attempt to divert blood from the extremities to the core in an attempt to keep the vital organs, including the brain, functioning. This will result in pale skin and delayed capillary refill in the hands and feet. Feel the skin temperature, and look for color changes. Cyanosis is a late sign and can be seen first in the lips and mucous membranes.

Pulse oximetry is an effective diagnostic tool when used in conjunction with experience, good assessment skills, and clinical judgment. Pulse oximeters measure the percentage of hemoglobin that is saturated by oxygen. In patients with normal levels of hemoglobin, pulse oximetry can be an important tool for evaluating oxygenation. To use pulse oximetry properly, it is important for you to be able to evaluate the quality of the reading and correlate it to the patient's condition.

Interventions

Now that you have completed the focused history and physical exam, it is time to provide interventions for any problems you have identified. Interventions for respiratory emergencies may include the following:

- Oxygen via a nonrebreathing mask at 15 L/min
- Positive-pressure ventilations using bag-valve ventilation, a pocket mask, or a flow-restricted, oxygen-powered ventilation device
- Airway management techniques such as use of an oropharyngeal airway, a nasopharyngeal airway, suctioning, or airway positioning

◆ Geriatric Needs

Most geriatric patients take medications to treat various ailments that are part of the aging process. Some of these medications will blunt the body's normal reaction to stress and the mechanisms the body uses to compensate for respiratory compromise and hypoxia. For example, beta blockers, used for a variety of conditions, prevent the heart from speeding up and the veins from constricting to compensate for a loss of blood pressure or oxygenation. Keep this in mind when evaluating vital signs in geriatric patients.

- Positioning the patient in the high Fowler's position or a position of choice to facilitate breathing
- Assisting the patient with using his or her prescribed inhaler
- Documentation of your assessment, including all medications given

Detailed Physical Exam

In respiratory emergencies as in all other emergencies, you should only proceed to the detailed physical exam once all life threats have been identified and treated. If you are busy treating airway or breathing problems, you may not have the opportunity to proceed to a detailed physical exam before arriving at the emergency department. Never compromise the assessment and treatment of airway and breathing problems to conduct the detailed physical exam.

Keep in mind that there may be additional pieces to the assessment that you may find in the detailed physical exam. For example, in treating a patient in acute respiratory distress who is breathing 40 times a minute with audible wheezing, you may not know whether the patient has CHF or is having an asthma attack. The detailed physical exam may provide you with some clues, such as a consistently elevated blood pressure and pedal edema, which would lead you in the direction of CHF.

Ongoing Assessment

You need to monitor patients with shortness of breath carefully. Repeat your initial assessment. Have there been any changes in the patient's condition? Obtain vital signs at least every 5 minutes for a patient in unstable condition and/or after the patient uses an inhaler. If the patient's condition is stable and no life threat exists, vital signs should be obtained at least every 15 minutes. Perform a focused reassessment of the respiratory system. Ask the patient whether the treatment made any difference. Look at the patient's chest to see whether accessory muscles are still being used to breathe. Listen to the patient's speech pattern. Keep in mind that the patient may get worse instead of better. Be prepared to assist with bag-valve ventilation.

Communications and Documentation

Contact medical control with any change in the level of consciousness or difficulty breathing. Depending on local protocol, contact medical control before assisting with any prescribed medications. Be sure to document any changes (and the time) and any orders given by medical control.

■ Emergency Care of Respiratory Emergencies

When taking the initial vital signs of a person with dyspnea, you should give particular attention to respirations. Always speak with assurance and assume a concerned, professional approach to reassure the patient. You will usually administer oxygen. Reevaluate the respirations and the patient's response to oxygen repeatedly, at least every 5 minutes, until you reach the emergency department. Patients with COPD should be closely monitored. There is a small chance that supplemental oxygen, given for a long period, could take away the secondary respiratory oxygen drive and cause respiratory arrest. These patients will not stop breathing instantly but will start to show changes in their breathing status. Do not withhold oxygen for fear of depressing or stopping breathing in a patient with COPD who needs oxygen. A decreased respiratory rate after the administration of oxygen does not necessarily mean that the patient no longer needs the oxygen; he or she may need it even more. If respirations are slow and the patient becomes unconscious, you should assist breathing with bag-mask ventilation.

Supplemental Oxygen

If a patient complains of breathing difficulty, you should administer supplemental oxygen during the focused history and physical exam if it was not done during the initial assessment. Put a nonrebreathing face mask on the patient, and supply oxygen at a rate of 10 to 15 L/min (enough to maintain the reservoir bag) in a patient with difficulty breathing.

You are the Provider 4

You call medical control and alert the emergency department that you are transporting an elderly woman with possible pneumonia and that her distress is getting worse. When you arrive a respiratory therapist is standing by to administer a breathing treatment and collect a sputum culture.

She is admitted and pneumonia is the confirmed diagnosis. She is treated with antibiotics and antipyretics and is released from the hospital the following week.

Prescribed Inhalers (MDI)

Frequently, patients who call for help because of breathing difficulty are likely to have had the same trouble before. Some of them have prescribed medications to use that are delivered by inhaler. If so, you may be able to help them use it. Consult medical control or go by standing orders if they allow for this. Remember to report what the medication is, when the patient last took a puff, how many puffs were used at that time, and what the label states regarding dosage. If medical control or standing orders permit, you may assist the patient to self-administer the medication. Be certain that the inhaler belongs to the patient and contains the correct medication, the expiration date has not passed, and the correct dose is being administered. Administer repeated doses of the medication if the maximum dosage has not been exceeded and the patient is still experiencing shortness of breath.

Some of the most common medications used for shortness of breath are called inhaled beta-agonists, which dilate breathing passages. Typical trade names are Proventil, Ventolin, Alupent, Metaprel, and Brethine. The generic name for Proventil and Ventolin is albuterol; for Alupent and Metaprel, it is metaproterenol; and for Brethine, it is terbutaline. Most of these medications relax the muscles that surround the bronchioles in the lungs, leading to enlargement (dilation) of the airways and easier passage of air. Common side effects of inhalers include increased pulse rate, nervousness, and muscle tremors. To assist a patient with his or her prescribed inhaler, see Skill Drill 8-2 in Chapter 8.

You are the Provider Summary

The very old and the very young do not respond well to illness and injury. It is imperative to recognize distress early on and treat them aggressively. A patient who is breathing well enough prior to transport may rapidly tire and require ventilation. Monitor the patient closely and be prepared to ventilate if needed.

1. **What are your priorities for this patient?**

   ABCs; recognize that this is a load-and-go patient.

2. **What questions should you ask about this episode?**
   - Does she have a history of respiratory problems?
   - Has this happened before? If so, what did the doctor tell her?
   - Does she take any medication for respiratory problems?
   - How long has this been going on?
   - Has she taken any medication to treat this particular episode?

3. **What type of oxygen does she need? Why?**

   She should be placed on a nonrebreathing mask at 15L/min. She is alert enough not to tolerate a bag-mask device.

4. **What should you ask about the fever?**
   - How long has she felt this warm?
   - Has she taken any medication to reduce the fever?

5. **What should you ask about the cough?**
   - Does she have a productive cough? (Is she coughing up anything?)
   - If so, what is the color and consistency?

6. **What does the phlegm tell you?**

   She may have pneumonia.

7. **Is there any medication with which you might assist her?**

   Possibly aspirin or acetaminophen for the fever. Medical control should be consulted prior to administering any medication.

8. **What might help with the cough?**

   Humidified oxygen may help soothe the throat as well as thin mucous making it easier to cough up. Pour saline or sterile water in the bowl of a nebulizer and administer it through a mask.

9. **In what position should she be transported?**

   Position of comfort.

10. **What do you think is wrong with the patient?**

    Pneumonia

Respiratory Distress

Scene Size-up	Body substance isolation should include a minimum of gloves and eye protection. Ensure scene safety and determine nature of illness or mechanism of injury. Consider the number of patients, the need for additional help, and c-spine stabilization.
Initial Assessment	
■ General impression	Determine priority of care based on environment and patient's chief complaint. Determine level of consciousness and find and treat any immediate threats to life.
■ Airway	Ensure patent airway.
■ Breathing	Evaluate depth and rate of respirations and provide ventilations as needed. Auscultate and note breath sounds, providing high-flow oxygen.
■ Circulation	Evaluate pulse rate and quality; observe skin color, temperature, and condition. If stable condition and no life threats, proceed with focused history and physical exam. If unstable condition or possible life threat, proceed with rapid transportation.
■ Transport decision	If stable condition and no life threats, proceed with focused history and physical exam. If unstable condition or possible life threat, proceed with rapid transportation.
Focused History and Physical Exam	*NOTE: The order of the steps in the focused history and physical exam differs depending on whether the patient is conscious or unconscious. The following order is for a conscious patient. For an unconscious patient, perform a rapid physical exam, obtain vital signs, and obtain the history.*
■ SAMPLE history	Ask for pertinent SAMPLE and OPQRST information. Be sure to ask if and what interventions were taken before your arrival, how many times the interventions were used, and at what time.
■ Focused physical exam	Perform a focused physical exam, keying in on patient's physical appearance, cyanosis, work of breathing, tripod positioning, pursed lips, use of accessory muscles, adventitious lung sounds, wheezing, and pedal edema.
■ Baseline vital signs	Take vital signs, noting skin color and temperature and patient's level of consciousness. Use pulse oximetry if available.
■ Interventions	Support patient with oxygen, positive-pressure ventilation, adjuncts, proper positioning, and assisting with medication(s) per local protocol. Many of these interventions may need to be performed earlier, in the initial assessment.
Detailed Physical Exam	Consider a detailed physical exam if time and the situation permit.
Ongoing Assessment	Repeat the initial assessment and focused assessment, and reassess interventions performed. Reassess vital signs every 5 minutes for patient in unstable condition or when an inhaler is used. For the patient in stable condition or not using inhalers, reassess vital signs every 15 minutes. Reassure and calm the patient.
■ Communications and documentation	Contact medical control with any change in level of consciousness or difficulty breathing. Depending on local protocol, contact medical control before assisting with any prescribed medications. Document any changes, the time, and any orders from medical control.

NOTE: While the steps below are widely accepted, be sure to consult and follow your local protocol.

Respiratory Distress

Administer oxygen by placing a nonrebreathing mask on the patient and supplying oxygen at a rate of 10 to 15 L/min. For any patient in respiratory distress, use positioning, airway adjuncts (oropharyngeal or nasopharyngeal airway), or positive-pressure ventilation as indicated.

Asthma

Administer oxygen. Allow patient to sit in an upright position.

Suction large amounts of mucus.

Help patient self-administer a metered-dose inhaler:

1. Obtain order from medical control.
2. Check expiration date and whether patient has taken other doses.
3. Ensure inhaler is at room temperature or warmer.
4. Shake inhaler vigorously several times.
5. Remove oxygen mask. Instruct patient to exhale deeply.
6. Instruct patient to press inhaler and inhale. Instruct patient to hold breath as long as is comfortable.
7. Reapply oxygen.

Acute Pulmonary Edema

Administer 100% oxygen, and suction any secretions from the airway as necessary.

Place in position of comfort, and provide ventilatory support as needed.

Transport promptly.

Chronic Obstructive Pulmonary Disease

Provide full-flow oxygen via nonrebreathing mask at 15 L/min.

If patient is prescribed an inhaler, administer it according to local protocol. Document time and effect on patient with each use.

Place in the position of comfort, and provide prompt transport.

Spontaneous Pneumothorax

Provide supplemental oxygen, and place in position of comfort.

Transport promptly.

Support airway, breathing, and circulation as necessary.

Obstruction of the Upper Airway

For partial or complete foreign body airway obstructions, clear by following BLS guidelines, apply full-flow oxygen at 15 L/min as necessary, and transport promptly.

Pulmonary Embolism

Clear airway, and provide full-flow oxygen at 15 L/min.

Place in position of comfort, and provide prompt transport.

Provide ventilatory support as necessary, and be prepared for cardiac arrest.

Hyperventilation

Provide full-flow oxygen at 15 L/min, and coach respirations slower in a calm manner.

Complete an initial assessment and focused history and physical exam.

Transport promptly for evaluation.

Assessment and Emergency Care

Prep Kit

Ready for Review

- Dyspnea is a common EMS dispatch that has several causes, including infections of the upper or lower airways, acute pulmonary edema, chronic obstructive pulmonary disease, spontaneous pneumothorax, asthma or allergic reactions, mechanical obstruction of the airway, pulmonary embolism, and hyperventilation.
- Each of these lung disorders interferes in one way or another with the exchange of oxygen and carbon dioxide that takes place during respiration. This interference may be in the form of damage to the alveoli, separation of the alveoli from the pulmonary vessels by fluid or infection, obstruction of the air passages, or air or excess fluid in the pleural space.
- Patients with longstanding lung diseases often have chronically high levels of blood carbon dioxide; in some cases, giving too much oxygen to these patients may depress or stop respirations. However, oxygen administration is always an important priority in patients with dyspnea.
- Signs and symptoms of breathing difficulty include unusual breath sounds, including wheezing, stridor, rales, and rhonchi; nasal flaring; pursed-lip breathing; cyanosis; inability to talk; use of accessory muscles to breathe; and sitting in the tripod position, which allows the diaphragm the most room to function.
- In treating dyspnea, it is important to reassure the patient and provide supplemental oxygen. Remember to maintain the patient in a position that is comfortable for breathing, usually sitting upright.
- If the patient is not breathing, use bag-mask ventilation to assist breathing. If the patient is breathing inadequately, apply oxygen by nonrebreathing face mask with the oxygen flow set at 10 to 15 L/min.
- Perform a focused history and physical exam, including vital signs. If the patient has a prescribed inhaler or an epinephrine auto-injector, consult medical control to assist with its use, or follow standing orders.
- Remember, a patient who is breathing rapidly may not be getting enough oxygen as a result of respiratory distress from a variety of problems, including pneumonia or a pulmonary embolism; trying to "blow off" more carbon dioxide to compensate for acidosis caused by a poison, a severe infection, or a high level of blood glucose; or may be having a stress reaction.
- In every case, prompt recognition of the problem, administration of oxygen, and prompt transport are essential.

Vital Vocabulary

asthma A disease of the lungs in which muscle spasm in the small air passageways and the production of large amounts of mucus with swelling of the mucous lining of the respiratory passages result in airway obstruction.

chronic bronchitis Inflammation of the major lung passageways from infectious disease or irritants such as smoke.

chronic obstructive pulmonary disease (COPD) A slow process of dilation and disruption of the airways and alveoli caused by chronic bronchial obstruction.

dyspnea Shortness of breath or difficulty breathing.

emphysema A disease of the lungs in which there is extreme dilation and eventual destruction of pulmonary alveoli with poor exchange of oxygen and carbon dioxide; it is one form of chronic obstructive pulmonary disease (COPD).

hyperventilation Rapid or deep breathing that lowers the blood carbon dioxide level below normal.

hypoxia A condition in which the body's cells and tissues do not have enough oxygen.

hypoxic drive Backup system to control respirations when the oxygen level falls.

pneumothorax A partial or complete accumulation of air in the pleural space.

pulmonary edema A buildup of fluid in the lungs, usually as a result of congestive heart failure.

stridor A harsh, high-pitched, barking inspiratory sound often heard in acute laryngeal (upper airway) obstruction.

wheezing A high-pitched, whistling breath sound, characteristically heard on expiration in patients with asthma or COPD.

Technology

- Interactivities
- Vocabulary Explorer
- Anatomy Review
- Web Links
- Online Review Manual

Assessment in Action

Patients with dyspnea need aggressive treatment including oxygen and possible assistance with their medications. You should recognize the signs and symptoms of distress and prepare for rapid transport. You should also have a good understanding of respiratory medications that the patient may need assistance to use.

1. A focused assessment of the respiratory system includes:
   A. looking for use of the accessory muscles.
   B. listening to the patient's speech.
   C. inquiring about any treatment administered.
   D. all of the above.

2. Signs of inadequate breathing include:
   A. pale or cyanotic skin.
   B. cool, damp skin.
   C. shallow or irregular respirations.
   D. all of the above.

3. All of the following are signs of adequate breathing EXCEPT:
   A. pink, warm, dry skin.
   B. a normal rate and depth.
   C. inspiratory stridor.
   D. a regular pattern of inhalation and exhalation.

4. _____ is heard as a patient tries to exhale through partially obstructed air passages.
   A. Rales
   B. Stridor
   C. Rhonchi
   D. Wheezing

5. Which of the following is considered a sign of hypoxia of the brain?
   A. bradycardia
   B. decreased blood pressure
   C. altered mental status
   D. dyspnea

6. Inhaled beta-agonists work by:
   A. increasing blood flow through the lungs.
   B. dilating breathing passages.
   C. stimulating the hypoxic drive.
   D. decreasing gas exchange.

Challenging Questions

7. Explain what is meant by chronic carbon dioxide retention.

8. Explain how the hypoxic drive works.

10

Cardiovascular Emergencies

You are the Provider   1

You are called to the supermarket for a 48-year-old woman complaining of chest pain. On arrival you find the patient seated on a sofa in the employee lounge. She is pale and diaphoretic.

Initial Assessment	Recording Time: 0 Minutes
Appearance	Pale, diaphoretic
Level of consciousness	Alert and oriented
Airway	Open and clear
Breathing	Within normal limits
Circulation	Radials present, irregular

1. What are your first priorities in caring for this patient?
2. What might you learn from your general impression?
3. What should you ask about this episode?

Introduction

Experienced EMTs quickly learn that patient complaints involving the heart and that heart-related problems account for many of their calls. Indeed, heart disease is the leading cause of death in the United States, with nearly 1 million persons dying of cardiovascular disease annually. About one third of Americans will eventually die as a result of heart disease.

It is important for EMS providers to understand that many of these deaths may have been avoided by people living healthier lifestyles and by better access to improved medical technology. EMS can help reduce these deaths with better public awareness, early access, increased numbers of laypersons trained in CPR, support of public access to defibrillation, and the recognition of the need for advanced life support services.

This chapter begins with a brief review of the heart and how it works. It then reviews the conditions of cardiac compromise (chest pain and acute myocardial infarction [classic heart attack]), the complications of sudden death, cardiogenic shock, and congestive heart failure. Treatment issues will also be discussed, including assisting with nitroglycerin and aspirin administration. The last part of the chapter is devoted to the use and maintenance of the automated external defibrillator (AED), including a review of pediatric AED guidelines.

Anatomy and Physiology (Cardiac Structure and Function)

The heart is a relatively simple organ with a simple job. It has to pump blood to supply oxygen-enriched

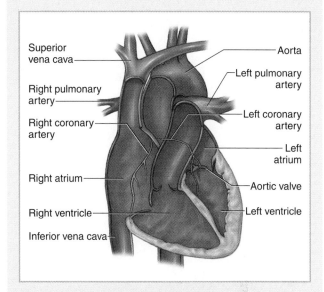

Figure 10-1 The heart is a four-chambered muscle that pumps blood to all parts of the body.

red blood cells to the tissues of the body. The heart is divided down the middle into two sides (left and right) by a wall called the septum. Each side of the heart has an <u>atrium</u>, or upper chamber, to receive incoming blood and a <u>ventricle</u>, or lower chamber, to pump outgoing blood Figure 10-1▲. Blood leaves each of the four chambers of the heart through a one-way valve. These valves keep the blood moving through the circulatory system in the proper direction and help to prevent backflow. The <u>aorta</u>, the body's main artery, receives the blood ejected from the left ventricle and delivers it to the tissues of the body.

The right side of the heart receives oxygen-poor (deoxygenated) blood from the veins of the body Figure 10-2A ▶. Blood enters the right atrium from the vena cava and then fills the right ventricle. After contraction of the right ventricle, blood flows into the pulmonary artery and the pulmonary circulation, where the blood is oxygenated. The left side of the heart receives oxygen-rich (oxygenated) blood from the lungs through the pulmonary veins Figure 10-2B ▶. Blood enters the left atrium and then passes into the left ventricle. The left side of the heart is more muscular than the right side because it must pump blood into the aorta and all the other arteries of the body.

The heart contains more than muscle tissue. The heart's electrical system, which is distributed throughout the entire heart, controls the heart rate and enables the atria and ventricles to work together.

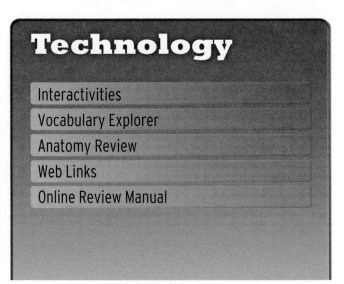

Technology

Interactivities

Vocabulary Explorer

Anatomy Review

Web Links

Online Review Manual

Refresher.EMSzone.com

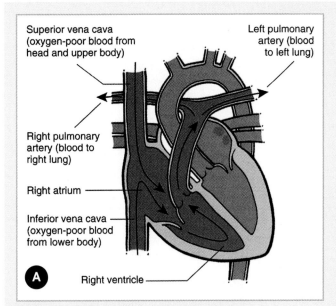

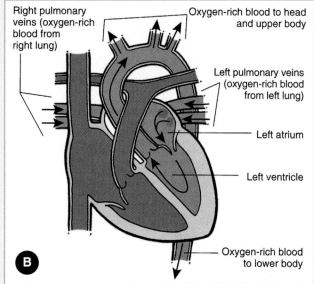

Figure 10-2 **A.** The right side of the heart receives oxygen-poor blood from the veins. **B.** The left side of the heart receives oxygen-rich blood from the lungs through the pulmonary veins.

Normal electrical impulses begin in the sinus node, just above the atria. The impulses travel across both atria, causing them to contract. Between the atria and the ventricles, the impulses cross over a bridge of special electrical tissue called the atrioventricular (AV) node. Here, the signal is slowed for about one tenth to two tenths of a second to allow blood time to pass from the atria to the ventricles. Then the impulses exit the AV node and spread throughout both ventricles, causing the ventricular muscle cells to contract.

Circulation

To carry out its function of pumping blood, the myocardium, or heart muscle, must have a continuous supply of oxygen and nutrients. During periods of physical exertion or stress, the myocardium requires more oxygen, so the heart must increase its output of blood flow. In the normal heart, the increased need for blood is easily supplied by dilation, or widening, of the coronary arteries, which increases blood flow. The <u>coronary arteries</u> are the blood vessels that supply blood to the heart muscle **Figure 10-3 ▶**. They start at the first part of the aorta, just above the <u>aortic valve</u>. The right coro-

nary artery supplies blood to the right ventricle and, in most people, the bottom part, or inferior wall, of the left ventricle. The left coronary artery divides into

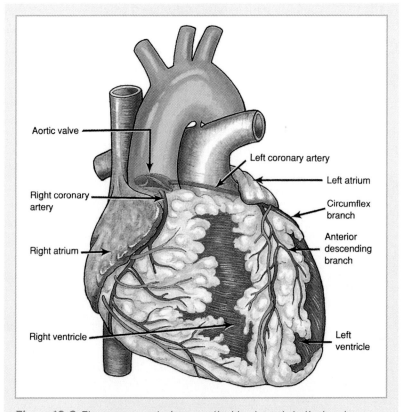

Figure 10-3 The coronary arteries carry the blood supply to the heart.

two major branches, both of which supply the left ventricle.

Blood exits the heart to the body via the aorta. Major arteries branching from the aorta supply blood to the extremities and body organs. After blood travels through the arteries, it enters smaller vessels called arterioles and capillaries. The capillaries are tiny blood vessels about one cell thick that connect arterioles to venules. Capillaries, which are found in all parts of the body, allow the exchange of nutrients and waste at the cellular level.

Venules are the smallest branches of veins. After traveling through the capillaries, blood enters the system of veins, starting with the venules, on its way back to the heart. The veins become larger and eventually form the two large venae cavae: the upper vena cava and the lower vena cava. The superior vena cava (upper) carries blood from the head and arms back to the right atrium. The inferior vena cava (lower) carries blood from the abdomen, kidneys, and legs back to the right atrium. The superior and inferior venae cavae join at the right atrium of the heart, where blood is eventually returned into the pulmonary circulation for oxygenation.

Blood consists of several types of cells and fluid. Red blood cells are the most numerous and give blood its color. Red blood cells carry oxygen to the body's tissues and then remove carbon dioxide. Larger white blood cells help fight infection. Platelets, which help the blood clot, are much smaller than the red and white blood cells. Plasma, the fluid that the cells float in, is a mixture of water, salts, nutrients, and proteins.

■ Pathophysiology (Cardiac Compromise)

Chest pain or discomfort that is related to the heart usually stems from a condition called <u>ischemia</u>, or insufficient blood supply, which results in insufficient oxygen. Because of a partial or complete blockage of blood flow through the coronary arteries, heart tissue fails to get enough oxygen and nutrients. The tissue soon begins to starve and, if blood flow is not restored, eventually dies.

Atherosclerosis

Most often, the low blood flow to heart tissue is caused by coronary artery atherosclerosis. <u>Atherosclerosis</u> is a disorder in which calcium and a fatty material (cholesterol) build up and form a plaque inside the walls of blood vessels, obstructing flow and inter-

fering with their ability to dilate or contract. Eventually, atherosclerosis can cause complete blockage of a coronary artery. Atherosclerosis typically involves other arteries of the body as well.

For reasons that are not completely understood, an area of this plaque buildup becomes brittle and will sometimes develop a crack that exposes the inside of the atherosclerotic wall. Acting like a torn blood vessel, the ragged edge of the crack activates the blood-clotting system, just as it does when an injury has caused bleeding. In this situation, however, the resulting blood clot will partially or completely block the opening (lumen) of the artery. Tissues downstream from the blood clot will not have sufficient oxygen (ischemia). If blood flow is resumed in a short time, the ischemic tissues will recover. However, if too much time goes by before blood flow is resumed, the tissues will die. In the heart, this sequence of events leads to an <u>acute myocardial infarction (AMI)</u>, a classic heart attack Figure 10-4 ▾ . Infarction means the death of tissue. The same sequence may also cause the death of cells in other organs, such as the brain. The death of heart muscle can significantly reduce the heart's ability to pump and, in extreme cases, can result in cardiac arrest.

In the United States, coronary artery disease is the number one cause of death for men and women. The peak incidence of heart disease occurs between ages

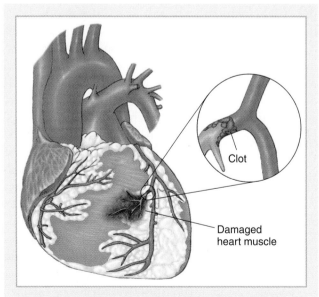

Figure 10-4 An acute myocardial infarction (heart attack) occurs when a blood clot prevents blood flow to an area of the heart muscle. If left untreated, this can result in death of heart tissue.

40 and 70 years, but it can also strike teens or people in their 90s. You must be alert to the possibility that, although less likely, a 26-year-old person with chest pain could actually be having a heart attack, especially if he or she has a higher than usual risk.

The major controllable risk factors for cardiovascular disease and heart attacks are cigarette smoking, high blood pressure, elevated cholesterol levels, elevated blood glucose level (diabetes), lack of exercise, and stress. The major risk factors that cannot be controlled are older age, family history of atherosclerotic coronary artery disease, and male gender.

Angina Pectoris

Chest pain does not always mean that a person is having an AMI. When, for a brief period, heart tissues are not getting enough oxygen, the pain is called angina pectoris, or angina. Although angina can result from a spasm of the artery, it is most often a symptom of atherosclerotic coronary artery disease. Angina occurs when the heart's need for oxygen exceeds its supply, usually during periods of physical or emotional stress (when the heart is working hard). When the increased oxygen demand goes away (for example, the person stops exercising), the pain typically goes away.

Angina pain is typically described as crushing, squeezing, or "like somebody is standing on my chest." It is usually felt in the middle of the chest, under the sternum. Chest pain can radiate to the jaw, the arms (frequently the left arm), the midback, or the epigastrium (the upper-middle region of the abdomen). The pain usually lasts from 3 to 8 minutes, rarely longer than 15 minutes. It may be associated with shortness of breath, nausea, or sweating. It disappears promptly with rest, supplemental oxygen, or nitroglycerin, all of which increase the supply of oxygen to the heart. Although angina pectoris is frightening, it does not mean that heart cells are dying, nor does it usually lead to death or permanent heart damage. It is, however, a warning that you and the patient should take seriously. Even with angina, because oxygen supply to the heart is diminished, the electrical system can be compromised and the person is at risk for significant cardiac rhythm problems.

Angina can be further differentiated into "stable" and "unstable" angina. Unstable angina is characterized by pain of coronary origin in the chest that occurs in response to progressively less exercise or fewer other stimuli than those ordinarily required to produce angina. If untreated, it can often lead to myocardial infarction. Stable angina is characterized by chest pain of cardiac origin that is relieved by simple steps, such as resting or taking nitroglycerin. Emergency medical services personnel usually become involved when stable angina become unstable, such as when a patient whose pain is normally relieved by sitting down and taking one nitroglycerin tablet has taken three tablets with no relief. Keep in mind that it can be very difficult even for physicians in hospitals to distinguish between the pain of angina and the pain of an AMI. Patients experiencing chest pain, therefore, should always be treated as if they are having an AMI.

Heart Attack

The pain of AMI signals the actual death of cells in the area of the heart where blood flow is obstructed. Once dead, the cells cannot be revived. Eventually these areas turn into scar tissue and become a burden to the beating heart. This is why fast action is so critical in treating a heart attack. The sooner the blockage can be cleared, the fewer the cells that may die. About 30 minutes after blood flow is cut off, some heart muscle cells begin to die. After about 2 hours, as many as half of the cells in the area can be dead; in most cases, after 4 to 6 hours, more than 90% will be dead. In many cases, however, opening the coronary artery with "clot-busting" (thrombolytic) medications or angioplasty (mechanical clearing of the artery) can prevent damage to the heart muscle if done within the first hour after the onset of symptoms. Immediate treatment and transport to the emergency department are essential.

Signs and Symptoms of Heart Attack

A patient with a heart attack may show any of the following signs and symptoms:

- Sudden onset of weakness, nausea, and sweating without an obvious cause
- Chest pain or discomfort that is often crushing or squeezing and that does not change with each breath
- Pain in the lower jaw, arms, back, abdomen, or neck
- Sudden arrhythmia with syncope (fainting)
- Shortness of breath or dyspnea
- Pulmonary edema
- Sudden death

The pain of an AMI differs from the pain of angina in three ways:

- It may or may not be caused by exertion but can occur at any time, sometimes when a person is sitting quietly or even sleeping.
- It does not resolve in a few minutes; rather, it can last between 30 minutes and several hours.
- It may or may not be relieved by rest or nitroglycerin.

As you know, not all patients who are having an AMI experience chest pain or recognize it when it does occur. In fact, about a third of patients never seek medical attention. This can be attributed, in part, to fear of dying and not wanting to face the possibility that symptoms may be serious (cardiac denial). Middle-aged men, in particular, are likely to minimize their symptoms. However, a few patients, particularly older people, women, and people with diabetes do not experience any pain during an AMI but will have other common complaints associated with ischemia discussed earlier. Others may feel only mild discomfort and call it "indigestion." It is common for the only complaint, especially in older women, to be fatigue.

Physical Findings of AMI and Cardiac Compromise

The physical findings of AMI vary, depending on the extent and severity of heart muscle damage. The following are common:

- **Pulse.** Generally, the pulse rate increases as a normal response to pain, stress, fear, or actual injury to the myocardium. Because arrhythmias are common in AMI, you may feel an irregularity of the pulse.
- **Blood pressure.** Blood pressure may fall as a result of diminished cardiac output and diminished capability of the left ventricle to pump. However, most patients with AMI will have a normal or, most likely, elevated blood pressure.
- **Respiration.** Respirations are usually normal unless the patient has congestive heart failure. In that case, respirations may become rapid and labored.
- **General appearance** and skin color, temperature, and dryness. The patient often appears frightened. There may be nausea, vomiting, and a cold sweat. The skin is often ashen gray because of inadequate cardiac output and the loss of perfusion. Occasionally, the skin is cyanotic as a result of inadequate oxygenation of the circulating blood.

- **Mental status.** Patients with AMI sometimes experience an almost overwhelming feeling of impending doom. If a patient tells you, "I think I am going to die," pay attention.

Sudden Death

Approximately 40% of all patients with AMI never reach the hospital. Sudden death is usually the result of cardiac arrest, in which the heart fails to generate effective blood flow.

A variety of lethal and nonlethal abnormal heart rhythms (arrhythmias) may follow AMI, usually within the first hour. Common rhythms following a heart attack that are life threatening or potentially life threatening include the following:

- Tachycardia. Rapid beating of the heart, 100 beats/min or more.
- Bradycardia. Unusually slow beating of the heart, 60 beats/min or less.
- Ventricular tachycardia (VT). Rapid heart rhythm, usually at a rate of 150 to 200 beats/min. The electrical activity starts in the ventricle instead of the atrium. This rhythm usually does not allow adequate time between beats for the left ventricle to fill with blood. The blood pressure may fall, and the patient may lose a pulse altogether. The patient may complain of weakness or lightheadedness or may become unresponsive. Most cases of VT will be sustained and may deteriorate into ventricular fibrillation.
- Ventricular fibrillation. Disorganized, ineffective quivering of the ventricles. No blood is pumped through the body, and the patient becomes unconscious within seconds. The only way to treat this arrhythmia is to defibrillate the heart. To defibrillate means to shock the heart with a specialized electrical current in an attempt to stop the chaotic, disorganized contraction of the myocardial cells and allow them to start again in a synchronized manner to restore a normal rhythmic beat. Defibrillation is highly successful in terms of saving lives if delivered within the first few minutes of sudden death (ie, witnessed cardiac arrest). However, studies have shown that survival rates from sudden death of greater than 4 to 5 minutes duration (ie, unwitnessed cardiac arrest) are higher if CPR is performed for 2 minutes prior to defibrillation.

If uncorrected, unstable ventricular tachycardia or ventricular fibrillation will eventually lead to <u>asystole</u>, the absence of all heart electrical activity. Without CPR, this may occur within minutes. Because it reflects a long period of ischemia, nearly all patients you find in asystole will die.

Cardiogenic Shock

Shock is present when body tissues do not get enough oxygen, causing body organs to malfunction. In <u>cardiogenic shock</u> (most often caused by a heart attack), the heart lacks enough power to force the proper volume of blood through the circulatory system. Cardiogenic shock can occur immediately or as late as 24 hours after the onset of the AMI. The signs and symptoms of cardiogenic shock are produced by the improper functioning of the body's organs. The challenge for you is to recognize shock in its early stages, when treatment is much more successful.

Congestive Heart Failure

Failure of the heart occurs when the ventricular heart muscle is so damaged that it can no longer keep up with the return flow of blood from the atria. <u>Congestive heart failure (CHF)</u> can occur any time after a myocardial infarction, heart valve damage, or long-standing high blood pressure, but it usually happens between the first few hours and the first few days after a heart attack.

Just as the pumping function of the left ventricle can be damaged by coronary artery disease, it can also be damaged by diseased heart valves or chronic hypertension. In any of these cases, when the muscle can no longer contract effectively, the heart tries other ways to maintain adequate cardiac output. Two specific changes in heart function occur: The heart rate increases, and the left ventricle enlarges in an effort to increase the amount of blood pumped each minute. When these adaptations can no longer make up for the decreased heart function, CHF eventually develops. It is called "congestive" heart failure because the lungs become congested with fluid once the heart fails to pump the blood effectively. Blood tends to back up in the pulmonary veins, increasing the pressure in the capillaries of the lungs. When the pressure in the capillaries exceeds a certain level, fluid (mostly water) passes through the walls of the capillary vessels and into the alveoli. This condition is called pulmonary edema. It may occur suddenly, as in AMI, or slowly over months, as in chronic CHF. Sometimes, patients with an acute onset of CHF will develop severe pulmonary edema, in which the patient has pink, frothy sputum and severe dyspnea.

If the right side of the heart is damaged, fluid collects in the body, often showing in the feet and legs. The collection of fluid in the part of the body that is closest to the ground is called dependent edema. The swelling causes relatively few symptoms other than discomfort. However, chronic dependent edema may

You are the Provider 2

Your partner learns from a friend of the patient that she has a cardiac history. She had an acute myocardial infarction (AMI) last year and has angina and congestive heart failure. She has a prescription for nitroglycerin and a "water pill."

After placing the patient on the stretcher in a position of comfort, you apply oxygen via a nonrebreathing mask at 15 L/min. She says that she is nauseated but has not vomited.

Vital Signs	Recording Time: 2 Minutes
Skin	Pale, diaphoretic
Pulse	112 beats/min, irregular
Blood pressure	198/106 mm Hg
Respirations	22 breaths/min, slightly shallow

4. Should you apply the AED? Why or why not?
5. What should you check before assisting the patient with her nitroglycerin?
6. What other signs and symptoms do you expect the patient to present with?

indicate underlying heart disease, even in the absence of pain or other symptoms.

Assessment of the Patient With Chest Pain

While en route, consider body substance isolation (BSI) precautions that will be needed. These precautions can be as simple as gloves when caring for a patient with chest pain or full BSI precautions for a patient in cardiac arrest. Remember, the patient's condition can change rapidly from the time you are dispatched.

Scene Size-up

Always ensure that the scene is safe for you, your partner, your patient, and bystanders. As you approach the scene, determine the nature of illness (NOI) and how many patients there are. From the nature of the call and first glance at your patient, determine whether you will need additional resources to assist in moving the patient. If you are in a tiered-response system, request that paramedics be dispatched to your location. You will need to assess the scene quickly to determine whether spinal stabilization is needed.

Initial Assessment
General Impression

All patient assessments begin by determining whether the patient is responsive. If the patient is not responsive, evaluate the ABCs (airway, breathing, and circulation) and be ready to use the AED.

If the patient is responsive, begin by asking the chief complaint. Remember that many patients present differently when experiencing an AMI. A chief complaint of chest pain or discomfort, shortness of breath, or dizziness should be taken seriously. Many patients who suspect that something is wrong appear anxious. Act professionally, and be calm. Remember, some patients may act carefree, while others may be demanding. Most patients, however, are frightened. Your professional attitude may be the single most important factor in winning the patient's cooperation and helping the patient through this event. Patients often have a good idea about what is happening, so do not lie or offer false reassurance.

Airway and Breathing

Unless the patient is unresponsive, the airway will most likely be open. Responsive patients should be able to maintain their own airway. Some episodes of

Documentation Tips

Document all findings including **pertinent negatives.** *Patient is complaining of substernal chest pain; denies any nausea or vomiting.* Also remember to use the patient's own words. *Patient states, "It feels like an elephant sitting on my chest."*

cardiac compromise may result in syncope (fainting) or dizziness. If either of these have occurred, be suspicious of spinal injuries from a fall. Assess and treat the patient as appropriate.

Assess the patient's breathing to determine whether the rate, depth, and effort are adequate. You should also listen to breath sounds. Some patients feel short of breath even though there are no obvious signs of respiratory distress. Apply oxygen with a nonrebreathing mask at 10 to 15 L/min. If the patient is not breathing or has inadequate breathing, ensure adequate breathing with bag-mask ventilation and 100% oxygen.

Circulation

Assess the patient's circulation. Determine the rate and quality of the patient's pulse. Is the pulse rhythm regular or irregular? Is it too fast or too slow? Pulses that are too fast, too slow, or irregular indicate abnormal heart rhythms. Assess the patient's skin condition, color, and temperature. Patients who are complaining of chest pain and are diaphoretic (sweaty) are usually having a significant cardiac event. Place the patient in a comfortable position, usually sitting up and well supported. Provide reassurance to reduce the patient's anxiety.

Transport Decision

Make a transport decision. Does the patient need to be transported rapidly? Is the patient's condition life threatening, or is it stable enough to allow for performing a focused history and physical exam on scene? Generally speaking, most patients with chest pain should be transported immediately. As a general rule, responsive cardiac patients should be transported in the most gentle, stress-relieving manner possible. Try not to allow the patient to exert himself or herself or to walk.

Your decision of where to transport the patient will depend on your local protocol. Patients are generally transported to the closest appropriate facility. Some EMS systems have written protocols requiring patients with suspected cardiac emergencies to be transported to medical centers with certain capabilities, such as emergency angioplasty. Others require the patient to be transported to the nearest facility for stabilization before transporting to a specialty hospital.

Focused History and Physical Exam

SAMPLE History

For a conscious patient, begin with taking a brief history. Friends or family members often have helpful information. Ask the following questions:

- Has the patient ever had a heart attack before?
- Has anyone ever told the patient that he or she has heart problems?
- Are there any risk factors for coronary artery disease, such as smoking, high blood pressure, or high-stress lifestyle?

The SAMPLE history provides basic information on the patient's overall medical history. The more signs and symptoms a patient has, the easier it is to identify a particular problem. In addition, ask whether the patient has had the same pain before. If so, ask "Do you take any medications for the pain?" and "Do you have any of the medication with you?" If the patient has had a heart attack or angina before, ask whether the pain is similar.

Be sure to also include the OPQRST questions. Using OPQRST helps you to understand the details of the patient's specific complaints (such as chest pain) Table 10-1 ▶ . Even when a patient may not be able to articulate his or her exact medical condition, knowing the patient's medications may give you important clues.

Focused Physical Exam

Give particular attention to the cardiovascular system, but also check the respiratory system. How well is the heart working? Assess skin color, temperature, and condition. Is it cool, moist? How do the mucous membranes look? Are they pink, ashen, or cyanotic? Are the lung sounds clear? Are the neck veins distended?

Baseline Vital Signs

Measure and record the patient's vital signs. As you obtain the SAMPLE history, have your partner take the patient's baseline vital signs, including pulse, blood pressure, and respirations. You must obtain readings for systolic and diastolic blood pressures. If available, use pulse oximetry. Note the time that vital signs are taken.

Table 10-1 OPQRST Mnemonic for Assessing Pain

- **Onset.** Determine what time the discomfort that motivated the call for help began.
- **Provocation.** Ask what makes the pain or discomfort worse. Is it positional? Does a deep breath or palpation of the chest make it worse?
- **Quality.** Ask what type of pain it is. Let the patient use his or her own words to describe what is happening. Try to avoid supplying the patient with only one option. Do not ask "Does it feel like an elephant is sitting on your chest?" Instead, say "Tell me what the pain feels like." If the patient cannot answer an open-ended question, then provide a list of alternatives. "There are lots of different kinds of pain. Is your pain more like heaviness, pressure, burning, tearing, dull ache, stabbing, or needlelike?"
- **Radiation.** Ask whether the pain travels to another part of the body.
- **Severity.** Ask the patient to rate the pain on a simple scale. Often, a scale ranging from 0 to 10 is used, in which 0 represents no pain at all and 10 represents the worst pain imaginable. Do not use the patient's answer to determine whether the pain has a serious cause. Instead, use it to check whether the pain is getting better or worse. After a few minutes of oxygen or administration of a nitroglycerin pill, ask the patient to rate the pain again.
- **Time.** Find out how long the pain lasts when it is present and whether it has been intermittent or continuous.

Interventions

Depending on local protocol, you may administer "baby" aspirin (also called children's aspirin) and/or assist with prescribed nitroglycerin. Check the condition of the medication and its expiration date. Administer aspirin according to local protocol, and ensure that the patient is not allergic to aspirin. Baby aspirin comes in 81-mg chewable tablets. The recommended dose is 162 mg (two tablets) to 324 mg (four tablets). Aspirin (acetylsalicylic acid [ASA]) prevents clots from forming or getting bigger. To achieve a rapid blood level of aspirin, instruct the patient to chew the tablets prior to swallowing them.

After obtaining permission from medical control, help the patient administer prescribed nitroglycerin. Nitroglycerin works in most patients within 5 minutes to relieve the pain of angina. Most patients who have been prescribed nitroglycerin carry a supply with them. Patients take one dose of nitroglycerin whenever they have an episode of angina that does not immediately go away with rest. If the pain is still present after 5 minutes, patients are typically instructed by their physicians to take a second dose. If the second dose does not work, most patients are told to take a third dose and then call for EMS. If the patient has not taken all three doses, you can help to administer the medication, if you are allowed to do so by local protocol.

Nitroglycerin comes in several forms—as a small white pill, as a spray, or as a skin patch applied to the chest. In any form, the effect is the same. Nitroglycerin relaxes the muscle of blood vessel walls, dilates coronary arteries, increases blood flow and the supply of oxygen to the heart muscle, and decreases the workload of the heart. Nitroglycerin also dilates blood vessels in other parts of the body and can sometimes cause low blood pressure and/or a severe headache. Other side effects include changes in the patient's pulse rate, including tachycardia and bradycardia. For this reason, you should take the patient's blood pressure within 5 minutes after each dose. If the systolic blood pressure is less than 100 mm Hg, do not give more medication. Other contraindications include the presence of a head injury and the maximum prescribed dose has already been given. To safely assist the patient with nitroglycerin, review the steps in Skill Drill 8-4 .

Reevaluate your transport decision. Early, prompt transport to the emergency department is critical so that treatments such as clot-busting medications or angioplasty can be initiated. To be most effective, these treatments must be started as soon as possible after the onset of the attack. If the patient does not have prescribed nitroglycerin, move ahead with your focused assessment and prepare to transport. Do not delay transport to assist with administration of nitroglycerin. The drug can be given en route.

Detailed Physical Exam

If necessary, perform a detailed physical exam to elicit further information about the patient's condition. If you have time, you can talk with the patient about risk factors for heart disease such as cholesterol level, smoking, activity levels, and family history of heart disease. Do not obtain this information unless your patient's condition is stable and everything else is done.

Ongoing Assessment

Repeat your initial assessment by checking to see if the patient's condition has improved or is deteriorating. Vital signs should be reassessed at least every 5 minutes or as significant changes in the patient's condition occur. It is essential to monitor the patient with

You are the Provider 3

The patient is loaded into the ambulance and your partner goes up front to drive. Her blood pressure is sufficient to support administration of nitroglycerin. You call medical control to obtain orders and report that the patient is a 48-year-old woman with a cardiac history who is complaining of midsternal chest pain radiating into her jaw and left arm. She is pale, diaphoretic, nauseous, and a little dyspneic. On auscultation of her breath sounds you hear rales bilaterally. Medical control authorizes assisting the patient with her nitroglycerin, so you give her one tablet sublingually.

Reassessment	Recording Time: 7 Minutes
Pulse	96 beats/min, irregular
Blood pressure	164/98 mm Hg
Respirations	20 breaths/min, not quite as shallow
Breath sounds	Rales bilaterally
Pulse oximetry	94% on oxygen via nonrebreathing mask

7. Why should this patient be transported immediately?
8. What might help with her dyspnea?
9. How does the pain of an AMI differ from that of angina?
10. If the pulmonary edema worsens, how would you expect the signs and symptoms to change?

a suspected AMI closely because sudden cardiac arrest is always a risk. If cardiac arrest occurs, you must be ready to start CPR and use the AED. Reassess your interventions. It is important to continue reassessing to see whether the interventions are helping and whether the patient's condition is improving. Reassess vital signs after administering medications.

Communication and Documentation

It is important to document your assessment and care of the patient. You must record the interventions performed. It must be clear in your documentation that the patient was reassessed appropriately following any intervention. The patient's response to the intervention must also be recorded.

■ Heart Surgeries and Pacemakers

During the last 20 years, hundreds of thousands of open heart surgeries were performed to bypass damaged segments of coronary arteries in the heart. In a coronary artery bypass graft, a blood vessel from the chest or leg is sewn directly from the aorta to a coronary artery beyond the point of the obstruction. Other patients may have had a procedure called percutaneous transluminal coronary angioplasty, which aims to dilate, rather than bypass, the coronary artery. In this procedure, usually called an angioplasty or balloon angioplasty, a tiny balloon is attached to the end of a long, thin tube. The tube is introduced through the skin into a large artery, usually in the groin, and then threaded into the narrowed coronary artery. Once the balloon is in position inside the coronary artery, it is inflated. The balloon is then deflated, and the tube is removed from the body. Sometimes, a metal mesh called a stent is placed inside the artery instead of or after the balloon. The stent is left in place permanently to help keep the artery from narrowing again.

A patient who has had an AMI or angina will almost certainly have had one of these procedures. Patients who have had a bypass graft will have a long surgical scar on their chest from the operation.

Patients who have had an angioplasty or coronary artery stent usually will not. However, newer "keyhole" surgical techniques may not produce a large scar. You should not assume that a patient who has a small scar has not had bypass surgery. Chest pain in a patient who has had any of these procedures should be treated the same as chest pain in patients who have not had any heart surgery. Carry out all the described tasks, and transport the patient promptly to the emergency department of the hospital. If CPR is required, perform it in the usual way, regardless of the scar on the patient's chest. Likewise, if indicated, an AED should be used.

Many people with heart disease in the United States have cardiac pacemakers to maintain a regular cardiac rhythm and rate. Pacemakers are inserted when the electrical control system of the heart is so damaged that it cannot function properly. These battery-powered devices deliver an electrical impulse through wires that are in direct contact with the heart (myocardium). The generating unit is generally placed under a heavy muscle or a fold of skin; it typically resembles a small silver dollar under the skin in the left upper part of the chest Figure 10-5 ▼ .

Normally, you do not need to be concerned about problems with pacemakers. Thanks to modern technology, an implanted unit will not require replacement or a battery charge for years. Wires are well protected and rarely broken. In the past, pacemakers sometimes malfunctioned when a patient got too close to

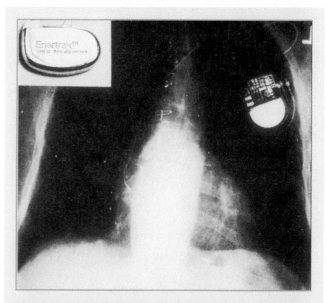

Figure 10-5 A pacemaker, which is typically inserted under the skin in the left upper chest, delivers an electrical impulse to regulate heartbeat.

an electrical radiation source, such as a microwave oven, but this is no longer the case. Every patient with a pacemaker should be aware of the precautions, if any, that must be taken to maintain its proper functioning.

If a pacemaker does not function properly, as when the battery wears out, the patient may experience syncope, dizziness, or weakness because of an excessively slow heart rate. The pulse ordinarily will be less than 60 beats/min because the heart is beating without the stimulus of the pacemaker and without the regulation of its own electrical system, which may be damaged. In these circumstances, the heart tends to assume a fixed slow rate that is not fast enough to allow the patient to function normally. A patient with a malfunctioning pacemaker should be promptly transported to the emergency department; repair of the problem may require surgery. When an AED is used, the pads should not be placed directly over the pacemaker, if possible. This will ensure a better flow of electricity through the patient's body.

Automatic Implantable Cardiac Defibrillators

More and more patients who survive ventricular fibrillation cardiac arrests have a small automatic implantable cardiac defibrillator (AICD) implanted Figure 10-6 ▶. Some patients who are at particularly high risk for a cardiac arrest have them as well. These devices are attached directly to the heart and can prolong the lives of certain patients. They continuously monitor the heart rhythm, delivering shocks as needed. Regardless of whether a patient having an AMI has an AICD, he or she should be treated like all other patients. Treatment should include performing CPR and using an AED if the patient goes into cardiac arrest. Generally, the electricity from an AICD is so low that it will have no effect on rescuers. You should not be concerned about getting shocked if the AICD fires and you are touching the patient. If you are using the AED on a patient with an AICD, do not place the AED pad directly over the device if possible.

■ Cardiac Arrest

Cardiac arrest is the complete cessation of cardiac activity—electrical, mechanical, or both. It is indicated in the field by the absence of a carotid pulse. Until the advent of CPR and external defibrillation in the 1960s, cardiac arrest was virtually always a terminal event. Now, although it is still infrequent for a patient to survive a cardiac arrest without neurologic

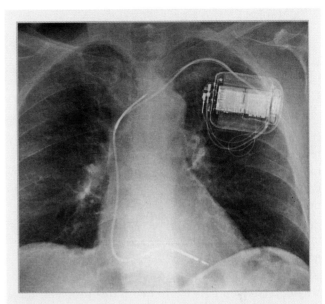

Figure 10-6 An AICD is attached directly to the heart and continuously monitors heart rhythm, delivering shocks as needed. The electricity from the AICD is so low that is has no effect on rescuers.

damage, great strides have been made in resuscitation science during the last 40 years.

Automated External Defibrillation

The AED machines come in different models with different features. All of them require a certain degree of operator interaction (applying the pads, turning the machine on, and pushing the shock button). Most AEDs have voice and screen message prompts that direct the user through the procedure. Some have an analyze button; other models start analyzing automatically when the pads are applied and the unit is powered on. In the United States, the majority of the AEDs are semiautomated. Even though most defibrillators are now semiautomated, we are using the term automated external defibrillator (AED) as a general term to describe all of these machines.

AEDs are manufactured to deliver a monophasic shock or a biphasic shock. Monophasic means to send the energy in one direction, from negative to positive, and biphasic means to send the energy in two directions simultaneously. The advantage of biphasic shock is that it produces more efficient defibrillation and may require a lower energy setting. Recommended energy settings for AED units are now based on whether the AED unit delivers a monophasic or a biphasic shock:

- Monophasic: First shock and all other shocks, 360 joules

- Biphasic (two types)
    - First shock, 150 to 200 joules or
    - First shock, 120 joules
    - With both biphasic types, the second and all other shocks are delivered at the same or a higher energy setting.

In general, AED manufacturers will have the dose (energy settings) printed on the AED unit. You should review the AED unit that your service uses to become familiar with these settings. Remember that your AED unit is automatic and will be programmed to deliver the defibrillations at the manufacturer-set recommended doses.

As you know, AED units are safe and effective when used appropriately. Statistically, we know that if there has been a complication with the use of an AED unit, it is usually the operator's fault. The most common is not having a charged battery. To avoid this problem, most AED companies have manufactured the AED units to warn the user that the battery charge is low. However, some of the older models do not have this feature. You should check the AED daily and exercise the battery as often as the manufacturer recommends. It is your responsibility to maintain your equipment.

The AED should only be used on patients who are assessed to be pulseless, apneic, and unresponsive. Remember that the unit is designed to analyze the heart rhythm of a motionless victim; it will not analyze if patient movement is detected. No one should be touching the patient when the AED is analyzing or shocking. You should not use the AED to analyze or shock a patient in a moving ambulance. Stop the ambulance to perform these procedures.

Most AED units will analyze and identify a particular heart rhythm that is faster than 150 or 180 beats/min (ventricular tachycardia) as a rhythm that should be shocked. Remember that you must determine whether the patient has a pulse; the AED unit cannot. Again, you should apply the AED only to unresponsive patients with no pulse.

Not all patients in cardiac arrest require an electrical shock. Although all patients in cardiac arrest should have analysis with an AED, some do not have shockable rhythms (for example, pulseless electrical activity and asystole). Asystole (flatline) indicates that no electrical activity remains. Pulseless electrical activity usually refers to a state of cardiac arrest despite an organized electrical complex. In both cases, CPR should be initiated as soon as possible.

AED Maintenance

One of your primary missions as an EMT-B is to deliver an electrical shock to a patient in ventricular

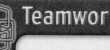

Teamwork Tips

One EMT-B should assess the patient and initiate CPR while the second EMT-B readies the AED.

fibrillation. To accomplish this mission, you need to have a functioning AED. You must become familiar with the maintenance procedures required for the brand of AED your service uses. Read the operator's manual. If your defibrillator does not work on the scene, someone will want to know what went wrong. That person may be your system's administrator, your medical director, the local newspaper reporter, or the family's attorney. You will be asked to show proof that you maintained the defibrillator properly and attended any mandatory in-service classes.

The main legal risk in using the AED is failing to deliver a shock when one was needed. The most common reason for this failure is that the battery did not work, usually because it was not properly maintained. Another problem is operator error. This means not pushing the analyze or shock buttons when the machine advises you to do so or failing to apply the AED to a patient in cardiac arrest. Of course, the AED is like any other manufactured item. It can fail, although this is rare. Ideally, you will encounter any such failure while doing routine maintenance, not while caring for a patient in cardiac arrest. Check your equipment, including your AED, at the beginning of each shift.

Medical Direction

Defibrillation of the heart is a medical procedure. Although AEDs have made this process much simpler, there is still a benefit in having a physician's involvement. Your medical director grants the authority for you to use the AED by developing and approving the protocols that you follow for caring for patients in cardiac arrest. He or she may also specify any training or refresher classes for you to attend to maintain your AED skills.

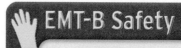

EMT-B Safety

Do not defibrillate any patient who is lying in pooled water or who is touching metal that others are touching. Carefully remove any medication patches with a gloved hand and wipe the area clean to prevent ignition of the patch.

There should be a review of each incident in which the AED is used. After returning from the hospital or the scene, sit down with the rest of the team and go over what happened. This discussion will help all members of the team learn from the incident. Review the patient care report and the events of the call with any documentation or reports that your particular AED unit provides. There is usually a review of the call with your medical director or quality improvement officer. All EMS systems continuously work on improving patient care. Mandatory continuing education with skill competency review is generally required for EMS providers, with a continuing competency skill review on the AED every 3 to 6 months for EMT-Bs.

Emergency Care for Cardiac Arrest

Preparation

Remember to follow BSI precautions. On arrival at the scene, make sure that the scene is safe for you and your partner to enter. If dispatch reports an unresponsive patient with CPR being performed, the AED is probably one of the first pieces of equipment you will gather from the ambulance. As the operator of the AED, you are responsible for making sure that the electricity injures no one, including yourself. Remote defibrillation using pads allows you to distance yourself safely from the patient. As long as you place the pads in the correct position and make sure no one is touching the patient, you should be safe. Do not defibrillate a patient who is in pooled (puddle) water. Although there is some danger to you if you are also in the water, there is another problem. Electricity follows the path of least resistance; instead of traveling between the pads and through the patient's heart, it will diffuse into the water. Therefore, the heart will not receive enough electricity to cause defibrillation. You can defibrillate a soaking wet patient, but first try to dry the patient's chest. Do not defibrillate someone who is touching metal that others are touching, and carefully remove any medication patches from the pa-

tient's chest and wipe the area with a dry towel before defibrillation to prevent ignition of the patch. Remember that you might have to shave any chest hair that prevents the AED pads from making good contact. Be sure to consult local protocols for issues such as pad placement and preparation of the pad site.

Determine the nature of illness and/or mechanism of injury. If the incident involves trauma, perform spinal stabilization as you begin the initial assessment. Is there only one patient? If you are in a tiered system and the patient is in cardiac arrest, call for ALS assistance.

Performing Defibrillation (Adult Patients)

It is important to review the general principles of using the AED:

- Minimize the amount of time chest compressions are *not* being performed (no more than 10 seconds except to insert an advanced airway or to use the AED).
- Use the AED immediately on any adult patient that you witness collapsing into cardiac arrest.
- For unwitnessed adult cardiac arrest, perform CPR for 2 minutes (5 cycles of 30 compressions to 2 breaths) before using the AED.
- Administer 1 shock and then provide CPR (starting with compressions) for 2 minutes before analyzing and shocking a second time.
- Do not stop compressions to check circulation in between shocks.

Review the steps in **Skill Drill 10-1 ▶** to use an AED on adult patients (cardiac arrest not witnessed by EMS personnel):

1. Arrive on scene and perform your initial assessment. Verify patient is unresponsive, apneic, and pulseless. If the patient is responsive, do not apply the AED.

2. If the patient is unresponsive and not breathing or has agonal respirations (slow, gasping breaths), give two breaths using a bag-mask or pocket mask device and then check pulse. If there is no pulse, perform CPR for 2 minutes (5 cycles of 30 compressions to 2 ventilations) (**Step 1**).

You are the Provider 4

You assist the patient in sitting more upright to alleviate some of her respiratory distress. The nitroglycerin has helped slightly with her pain, but it is still a 7 on a scale of 1 to 10.

On arrival at the hospital she is evaluated and sent for a cardiac catheterization. She has two arteries that are almost entirely blocked. Two stents are placed, and after 24 hours of observation in the hospital she is able to go home.

Skill Drill 10-1 AED and CPR

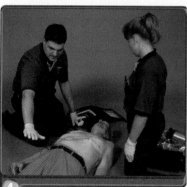

1 Perform your initial assessment. Verify patient is unresponsive, apneic, and pulseless. If not breathing, give two breaths and check for a pulse. If no pulse, perform CPR for 2 minutes (5 cycles of 30 compressions to 2 breaths).

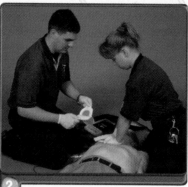

2 Prepare the AED pads and power on the AED unit.

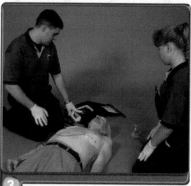

3 Stop CPR and prepare to analyze the cardiac rhythm.

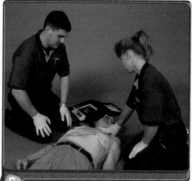

4 Call "clear" and make sure no one is touching the patient. Push the analyze button, if there is one, and wait for the AED to analyze the rhythm. If no shock advised, perform CPR for 2 minutes and then reanalyze. If shock advised, recheck that everyone is clear of patient, push the shock button, and immediately resume CPR.

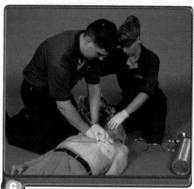

5 After 2 minutes of CPR, check for a pulse and analyze the cardiac rhythm. If the patient has a pulse, check the patient's breathing. If the patient is breathing adequately, give oxygen via nonrebreathing mask and transport. If the patient is not breathing adequately, perform artificial ventilation with high-flow oxygen and transport.

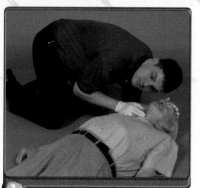

6 If no pulse, perform CPR for 2 minutes. Clear the patient and analyze again. If necessary, repeat the cycle of one shock and 2 minutes of CPR as indicated by the AED. Prepare to package and transport the patient. Continue CPR as needed.

3. Prepare to use the AED. Power on the AED unit (**Step 2**).

4. Remove any clothing from the patient's chest if not already done. Apply the pads to the chest; one to the right of the upper sternum just below the clavicle, the other on the lower left chest wall (top of pad 2" to 3" below the armpit). Ensure that the pads are attached to the patient cables (and that they are attached to the AED in some models).

5. Stop CPR and prepare to analyze the cardiac rhythm (**Step 3**).

6. Make sure that no one is touching the patient, and loudly call "clear."

7. Push the analyze button, if there is one. (Some AED units will automatically analyze once the AED pads are properly placed.)

8. If a shock is not indicated, perform CPR for 2 minutes and then reassess pulse and analyze cardiac rhythm. If a shock is advised, make

sure that no one is touching the patient. When the patient and the area around the patient are clear, push the shock button. Resume CPR for 2 minutes, starting with compressions, after the shock has been delivered (**Step ④**).

9. After 2 minutes of CPR, check for a pulse and reanalyze the cardiac rhythm. If the patient has a pulse, check the patient's breathing. If the patient is breathing adequately, give oxygen via nonrebreathing mask and transport. If the patient is not breathing adequately, perform artificial ventilation with high-flow oxygen and transport (**Step ⑤**).

10. If the patient has no pulse, perform 2 minutes of CPR, starting with compressions.

11. After 2 minutes of CPR, check the pulse and analyze the cardiac rhythm (as applicable).

12. If necessary, repeat the cycle of administering one shock and performing 2 minutes of CPR.

13. Prepare to package and transport the patient according to local protocol (**Step ⑥**).

You are the Provider Summary

The pain of AMI signals the actual death of cells in the area of the heart where blood flow is obstructed. Once dead, the cells cannot be revived. Early recognition and treatment are key when assessing a patient complaining of chest pain. It is also important to remember that not all patients present with the same set of symptoms. When unsure, err on the side of caution and treat as if the patient is having an AMI.

1. **What are your first priorities in caring for this patient?**

   Position of comfort and ABCs

2. **What might you learn from your general impression?**

   The patient is pale and diaphoretic. You can see evidence of some respiratory distress. Patients who are complaining of chest pain and are diaphoretic are usually having a significant cardiac event.

3. **What should you ask about this episode?**

   OPQRST

4. **Should you apply the AED? Why or why not?**

   No. An AED should only be applied to a pulseless apneic patient.

5. **What should you check before assisting the patient with her nitroglycerin?**

   Blood pressure, the medication, obtain orders from medical control.

6. **What other signs and symptoms do you expect the patient to present with?**
   - Weakness
   - Nausea/vomiting
   - Chest pain/discomfort that does not change
   - Pain in the lower jaw, arms, back, abdomen, or neck
   - Syncope
   - Dyspnea
   - Pulmonary edema
   - Sudden death

7. **Why should this patient be transported immediately?**

   Thrombolytic medications or angioplasty can prevent damage to the heart muscle if done within the first hour after the onset of symptoms.

8. **What might help with her dyspnea?**

   Sitting upright to allow the pulmonary edema to pool in the lower lobes of the lungs

9. **How does the pain of an AMI differ from that of angina?**
   - It may or may not be caused by exertion but can occur at any time, sometimes when a person is sitting quietly or even sleeping.
   - It does not resolve in a few minutes; rather, it can last between 30 minutes and several hours.
   - It may or may not be relieved by rest or nitroglycerin.

10. **If the pulmonary edema worsens, how would you expect the signs and symptoms to change?**

    You may see pink, frothy sputum and severe dyspnea that can lead to sudden death.

Assessment and Emergency Care

	Chest Pain	Cardiac Arrest
Scene Size-up	Use BSI precautions. Ensure scene safety. Determine NOI from patient and/or bystanders. Request additional resources if needed. Determine if spinal stabilization is needed.	Use BSI precautions. Ensure scene safety. Bring AED. Determine NOI/MOI. Determine if spinal stabilization is needed.
Initial Assessment		
■ General impression	Determine if patient is responsive. If so, ask about chief complaint. If not, evaluate ABCs. If patient has lost consciousness and possibly fallen, consider spinal stabilization.	Determine patient's LOC and chief complaint. If patient is unresponsive and pulseless, prepare to defibrillate.
■ Airway	Ensure that the airway is patent.	
■ Breathing	If patient is short of breath or in respiratory distress, provide oxygen via nonrebreathing mask at 10-15 L/min. If patient is not breathing, provide bag-mask ventilation and 100% oxygen.	Check scene safety—do not defibrillate a patient in pooled water.
■ Circulation	Assess the pulse and skin. Place patient in position of comfort. Provide reassurance.	
■ Transport decision	Transport patients with chest pain immediately in gentle, stress-relieving manner.	
Focused History and Physical Exam	*NOTE: The order of the steps in the focused history and physical exam differs depending on whether the patient is conscious or unconscious. The order below is for a conscious patient. For an unconscious patient, perform a rapid physical exam, obtain vital signs, and obtain the history.*	
■ SAMPLE history	If patient is conscious, take brief SAMPLE history and ask OPQRST questions. Specifically, ask if the patient has had: ■ a previous heart attack? ■ heart problems? ■ risk factors: smoking, high blood pressure, high stress? ■ medications?	Not applicable to a cardiac arrest patient. See emergency care table on opposite page for summary of AED procedure.
■ Focused physical exam	Perform a focused physical exam, focusing on the cardiovascular and respiratory systems. Assess skin color, temperature, and condition. Is cyanosis present? Are neck veins distended? Check mucous membranes.	
■ Baseline vital signs	Take vital signs, including systolic and diastolic blood pressures. Use pulse oximetry if available.	
■ Communication	Report to medical control and the hospital; follow instructions from medical control.	
■ Interventions	Depending on local protocol, administer baby aspirin and assist with prescribed nitroglycerin. Obtain permission from medical control before assisting with prescribed nitroglycerin.	
Detailed Physical Exam	If time permits and patient is stable, perform detailed physical exam and ask patient about risk factors for heart disease.	Not applicable to a cardiac arrest patient. See emergency care table on opposite page for summary of AED procedure.
Ongoing Assessment	Monitor patient very closely. Reassess vital signs every 5 minutes or as patient's condition changes. Reassess interventions.	
■ Communication and documentation	If cardiac arrest occurs, begin defibrillation or CPR immediately. Record all interventions. Obtain medical control physician's signature if required.	

NOTE: While the steps below are widely accepted, be sure to consult and follow your local protocol.

Chest Pain

Depending on local protocol, prepare to administer baby aspirin and assist with prescribed nitroglycerin. Check condition of medication(s) and expiration date(s).

Aspirin

Administer according to protocols.

Nitroglycerin

1. Obtain permission from medical control.

2. Take patient's blood pressure. Continue only if systolic pressure greater than 100 mm Hg.

3. Check that you have the right medication, right patient, and right delivery route.

4. Question patient about last dose and effects. Ensure patient understands route of administration. Prepare to have the patient lie down to prevent fainting.

5. Ask patient to lift his or her tongue. Place tablet underneath tongue or spray under tongue if medication is in spray form. Have patient keep mouth closed until dissolved or absorbed.

6. Recheck blood pressure within 5 minutes. Record medication and time of administration. If chest pain persists and systolic blood pressure is greater than 100 mm Hg, repeat the dose every 5 minutes as authorized by medical control.

Reevaluate transport decision. Do not delay transport to assist with nitroglycerin.

Cardiac Arrest

Defibrillation

For witnessed, confirmed adult cardiac arrest, immediately apply and use the AED.

For unwitnessed adult cardiac arrest:

1. Arrive on scene and perform your initial assessment. Verify patient is unresponsive, apneic, and pulseless. If the patient is responsive, do not apply the AED.

2. If there is no pulse, perform CPR for 2 minutes (5 cycles of 30 compressions to 2 breaths).

3. Prepare to use the AED. Power on the AED unit.

4. Remove any clothing from the patient's chest area if not already done. Apply the pads to the chest: one to the right of the sternum just below the clavicle, the other on the lower left chest wall (top of pad 2" to 3" below the armpit).

5. Stop CPR. Make sure that no one is touching the patient and loudly call "clear."

6. Push the analyze button, if there is one, and wait for the AED unit to analyze.

7. If a shock is not indicated, perform CPR for 2 minutes and then reassess pulse and analyze cardiac rhythm. If a shock is advised, make sure that no one is touching the patient. When the patient and the area around the patient are clear, push the shock button. Resume CPR, starting with compressions, immediately after the shock has been delivered.

8. After 2 minutes of CPR, check for a pulse and analyze the cardiac rhythm. If the patient has a pulse, check the patient's breathing. If the patient is breathing adequately, give oxygen via nonrebreathing mask and transport. If the patient is not breathing adequately, perform artificial ventilation with high-flow oxygen and transport.

9. If the patient has no pulse, perform 2 minutes of CPR, starting with compressions.

10. After 2 minutes of CPR, check for a pulse and analyze the cardiac rhythm (as applicable).

11. If necessary, repeat the cycle of administering one shock and performing 2 minutes of CPR.

12. Prepare to package and transport the patient according to local protocol.

Assessment and Emergency Care

Prep Kit

Ready for Review

- The heart is divided down the middle into two sides, right and left, each with an upper chamber called the atrium and a lower chamber called the ventricle.
- The largest of the four heart valves that keep blood moving through the circulatory system in the proper direction is the aortic valve, which lies between the left ventricle and the aorta, the body's main artery.
- The heart's electrical system controls heart rate and helps the atria and ventricles work together.
- During periods of exertion or stress, the myocardium requires more oxygen. This oxygen is supplied by dilation of the coronary arteries, which increases blood flow.
- Low blood flow to the heart is usually caused by coronary artery atherosclerosis, a disease in which cholesterol plaques build up inside blood vessels, eventually occluding them.
- Occasionally, a brittle plaque will crack, causing a blood clot to form. Heart tissue downstream receives insufficient oxygen and, within 30 minutes, will begin to die. In the heart, this is called an acute myocardial infarction (AMI), or heart attack.
- Heart tissues that are not getting enough oxygen but are not yet dying can cause pain called angina. The pain of AMI is different from the pain of angina in that it can come at any time, not just with exertion; it lasts up to several hours, rather than just a few moments; and it is not relieved by rest or nitroglycerin.
- In addition to crushing chest pain, signs of AMI include sudden onset of weakness, nausea, and sweating; sudden arrhythmia; pulmonary edema; and even sudden death.
- Heart attacks can have three serious consequences. One is sudden death, usually the result of cardiac arrest caused by abnormal heart rhythms called arrhythmias. These include tachycardia, bradycardia, ventricular tachycardia, and, most commonly, ventricular fibrillation.
- The second consequence is cardiogenic shock. Symptoms include restlessness; anxiety; pale, clammy skin; pulse rate higher than normal; and blood pressure lower than normal. Patients with these symptoms should receive oxygen, assisted ventilations as needed, and immediate transport.
- The third consequence of AMI is congestive heart failure (CHF), in which damaged heart muscle can no longer contract effectively enough to pump blood through the body. The lungs become congested with fluid, breathing becomes difficult, the heart rate increases, and the left ventricle enlarges.
- Signs include swollen ankles from dependent edema, high blood pressure, rapid heart rate and respirations, rales (crackles), and sometimes the pink sputum and dyspnea of pulmonary edema.
- Treat a patient with CHF as you would a patient with chest pain. Monitor the patient's vital signs. Give the patient oxygen via nonrebreathing face mask. Allow the patient to remain sitting up.
- In treating patients with chest pain, obtain a SAMPLE history, following the OPQRST mnemonic to assess the pain; measure and record vital signs; ensure the patient is in a comfortable position, usually semireclining or half sitting up; administer prescribed nitroglycerin and oxygen; and transport the patient.
- The AED requires the operator to apply the pads, power on the unit, follow the AED prompts, and press the shock button as indicated. The computer inside the AED recognizes rhythms that require shocking and will advise you to shock or not shock.
- The most common errors in using certain AEDs are failure to keep a charged battery in the machine and applying the AED to a patient who is moving or being transported.
- Do not touch the patient while the AED is analyzing the heart rhythm or delivering shocks.
- Application of an AED, analysis of heart rhythm, and defibrillation are a higher priority than CPR when you witness an adult patient's cardiac arrest. Stop CPR as soon as an AED is available, and treat the patient following the prompts from the AED.
- For unwitnessed adult cardiac arrest, perform CPR for 2 minutes before using the AED.
- Do not stop CPR for longer than 10 seconds unless needed for advanced airway management or to use the AED.
- If ALS service is responding to the scene, stay where you are and continue the sequence of shocks and CPR.
- If an unconscious patient has a pulse but loses it during transport, you must stop the vehicle, reanalyze the rhythm, and defibrillate again or begin CPR as appropriate.

Technology

- Interactivities
- Vocabulary Explorer
- Anatomy Review
- Web Links
- Online Review Manual

Vital Vocabulary

acute myocardial infarction (AMI) Heart attack; death of heart muscle following obstruction of blood flow to it. Acute in this context means "new" or "happening right now."

angina pectoris Transient (short-lived) chest discomfort caused by partial or temporary blockage of blood flow to the heart muscle.

aorta The main artery, which receives blood from the left ventricle and delivers it to all the other arteries that carry blood to the tissues of the body.

aortic valve The one-way valve that lies between the left ventricle and the aorta. It keeps blood from flowing back into the left ventricle after the left ventricle ejects blood into the aorta; one of four heart valves.

asystole Complete absence of heart electrical activity.

atherosclerosis A disorder in which cholesterol and calcium build up inside the walls of blood vessels, eventually leading to partial or complete blockage of blood flow.

atrium One of two (right and left) upper chambers of the heart. The right atrium receives blood from the vena cava and delivers it to the right ventricle. The left atrium receives blood from pulmonary veins and delivers it to the left ventricle.

bradycardia Slow heart rate, less than 60 beats/min.

cardiogenic shock A state in which not enough oxygen is delivered to the tissues of the body, caused by low output of blood from the heart. It can be a severe complication of a large acute myocardial infarction and of other conditions.

congestive heart failure (CHF) A disorder in which the heart loses part of its ability to effectively pump blood, usually as a result of damage to the heart muscle and usually resulting in a backup of fluid into the lungs.

coronary arteries Blood vessels that carry blood and nutrients to the heart muscle.

defibrillate To shock a fibrillating (chaotically beating) heart with specialized electrical current in an attempt to restore a normal, rhythmic beat.

ischemia A lack of oxygen that deprives tissues of necessary nutrients, resulting from partial or complete blockage of blood flow; potentially reversible because permanent injury has not yet occurred.

syncope Fainting spell or transient loss of consciousness.

tachycardia Rapid heart rhythm, more than 100 beats/min.

ventricle One of two (right and left) lower chambers of the heart. The left ventricle receives blood from the left atrium (upper chamber) and delivers blood to the aorta. The right ventricle receives blood from the right atrium and pumps it into the pulmonary artery.

ventricular fibrillation Disorganized, ineffective twitching of the ventricles, resulting in no blood flow and a state of cardiac arrest.

ventricular tachycardia (VT) Rapid heart rhythm in which the electrical impulse begins in the ventricle (instead of the atrium), which may result in inadequate blood flow and eventually deteriorate into cardiac arrest.

Assessment in Action

As part of your annual recertification you must take a refresher course in CPR. This also includes the use of an AED. You and your partner decide to brush up before your evaluation next week.

1. What is the main legal risk in using the AED?
   A. shocking a pediatric patient
   B. failing to deliver a shock when needed
   C. operator error
   D. manual defibrillation

2. What is the first step for an unwitnessed cardiac arrest?
   A. Perform a precordial thump.
   B. Use the AED.
   C. Administer one shock, then provide CPR.
   D. Perform CPR for 2 minutes, then use the AED.

3. What is the next step after determining a patient is apneic or has agonal respirations?
   A. Apply the AED.
   B. Assess for a carotid pulse.
   C. Give two ventilations.
   D. Assess for a radial pulse.

4. Once a patient has been defibrillated, when should the next analyze/shock be performed?
   A. immediately following the first shock
   B. after contacting medical control
   C. after reassessing ABCs
   D. after 2 minutes of CPR

5. When applying an AED, what should you do about medication patches on the patient's chest?
   A. Leave the patch where it is and do not place the AED pads over it.
   B. Shave the chest around the medication patch.
   C. Remove the patch and wipe the area with a towel.
   D. Place the AED pads over the medication patch.

6. What is the advantage of using a biphasic AED?
   A. Energy travels in only one direction, reducing the risk to the patient.
   B. It produces a more efficient defibrillation.
   C. The first shock is at 360 joules.
   D. It is the only type of AED that can detect a pulse.

Challenging Questions

7. What is the proper procedure for using an AED in a moving ambulance?

8. Why should you not use an AED on a patient who has a pulse?

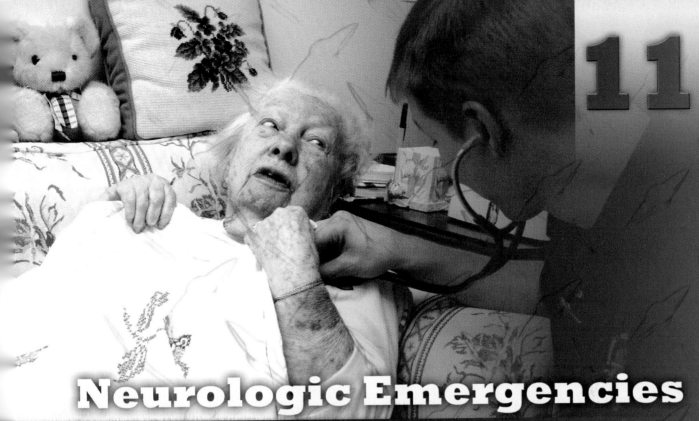

11

Neurologic Emergencies

You are the Provider 1

A call goes out for a residence several streets over from where you happen to be en route back to the station. You recognize that you are closer than the unit dispatched and advise dispatch that you will handle the call.

You arrive on scene to find a 72-year-old man who is "not acting right." Family members tell you that he was taking a nap and when he woke up he was "acting funny." He is sitting in a recliner in the family room.

Initial Assessment	Recording Time: 0 Minutes
Appearance	Pale, diaphoretic
Level of consciousness	Alert, but sluggish
Airway	Open and clear
Breathing	A little fast and shallow
Circulation	Radials present, a little slow

1. What are your priorities for this patient?
2. What questions should you ask about this episode?

Introduction

Stroke is the third leading cause of death in the United States, after heart disease and cancer. In the past few years, we have seen significant advances in the treatment of stroke. Emergency physicians, neurologists, and neurosurgeons can help some patients with acute stroke to avoid the most devastating consequences of this disease, assuming that the patients get to the hospital in time for treatments to be effective.

Seizures and altered mental status may also occur when there is a disorder in the brain. Seizures may occur as a result of a recent or old head injury, a brain tumor, a metabolic problem, or simply a genetic disposition. Your ability to recognize when a seizure has occurred or is occurring is critical for the patient.

Altered mental status (AMS) is a common presentation in patients with a wide variety of medical problems. There are many possible causes for AMS—intoxication, head injury, hypoxia, stroke, metabolic disturbances, and many more. As you may have already experienced, patients with AMS present a particular challenge because they may be difficult to handle and frustrating to treat. Your professionalism is paramount in these situations. This chapter reviews the structure and function of the brain and the most common causes of brain disorders, including stroke, seizure, and AMS. The chapter then reviews the signs, symptoms, and management of each condition.

Anatomy and Physiology (Brain Structure and Function)

The brain is the body's computer. It controls breathing, speech, and all other body functions. All your

thoughts, memories, wants, needs, and desires reside in the brain. Different parts of the brain perform different functions. For example, some receive input from the senses, including sight, hearing, taste, smell, and touch; others control the muscles and movement, while others control the formation of speech.

The brain is divided into three major parts: the brain stem, the cerebellum, and the largest part, the cerebrum Figure 11-1 ▶. The brain stem controls the most basic functions of the body, such as breathing, blood pressure, swallowing, and pupil constriction. Just behind the brain stem, the cerebellum controls muscle and body coordination. It is responsible for coordinating complex tasks that involve many muscles, such as standing on one foot without falling, walking, writing, picking up a coin, and playing the piano.

The cerebrum, located above the cerebellum, is divided down the middle into the right and left cerebral hemispheres. Each hemisphere controls activities on the opposite side of the body. The front part of the cerebrum controls emotion and thought, and the middle part controls touch and movement. The back part of the cerebrum processes sight. In most people, speech is controlled on the left side of the brain near the middle of the cerebrum.

All the messages traveling to and from the brain travel along nerves. Twelve cranial nerves run directly from the brain to various parts of the head, such as the eyes, ears, nose, and face. The other major nerves exit the brain through a large hole in the base of the skull called the foramen magnum. At each vertebra in the neck and back, two nerves, called spinal nerves, branch out from the spinal cord and carry signals to and from the body.

Common Causes of Brain Disorders

Many disorders can cause brain dysfunction or other neurologic symptoms and can affect the level of consciousness, speech, or voluntary muscle control. As a general rule, if the brain problem is caused primarily by disorders in the heart and lungs, the entire brain will be affected. For example, without any blood flow (cardiac arrest), the patient will go into a coma and can have permanent brain damage within minutes, even if CPR is performed immediately. However, if the primary problem is in the brain, such as an inadequate blood supply to the middle part of the left cerebral hemisphere, the patient may not be able to move some parts of the right side of the body. This might

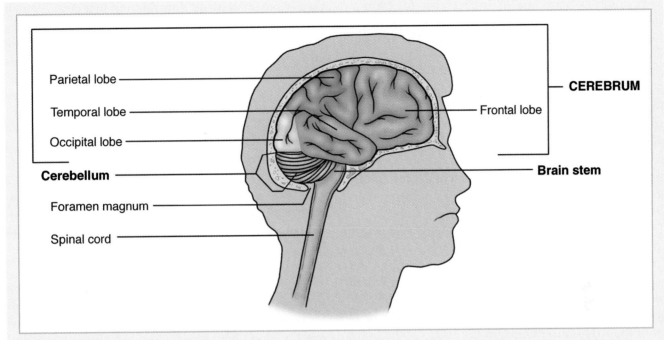

Figure 11-1 The brain lies well protected within the skull. Its major parts are the cerebrum, the cerebellum, and the brain stem.

be the right arm, the right leg, or the facial muscles. Low oxygen levels in the bloodstream will affect the entire brain, often causing anxiety, restlessness, and confusion.

Stroke is a common cause of brain disorder that is potentially treatable. Other brain disorders include infection and tumor. Although these specific problems are not reviewed in this chapter, the seizures or AMS that often accompany them are. The information in this chapter will help you better understand, communicate with, and care for patients who have experienced some type of neurologic emergency.

■ Stroke

A <u>cerebrovascular accident (CVA)</u> is an interruption of blood flow to the brain that results in the loss of brain function. <u>Stroke</u> is another term for CVA. Without sufficient oxygen, brain cells stop working and begin to die. Medical science currently has little to offer these cells once they are dead. However, it may take several hours or more for cell death to occur, even when it appears that severe disability will occur. Also, in some cases, a trickle of blood may still be getting through to the affected area of the brain. This blood may supply enough oxygen to keep cells alive, but not enough to let them work properly. For example, if cells that are responsible for controlling the left

arm are oxygen-starved, the patient will not be able to move that arm. If normal blood flow is restored to that area of the brain in time, the patient may regain use of the arm.

Interruption of cerebral blood flow may result from the following:

- <u>Thrombosis</u>: formation or presence of a blood clot in an artery
- <u>Arterial rupture</u>: rupture of an artery
- <u>Cerebral embolism</u>: obstruction of a cerebral artery caused by a clot that was formed elsewhere in the body and traveled to the brain

There are two main types of stroke: hemorrhagic (usually from arterial rupture) and ischemic (from embolism or thrombosis). Their symptoms are similar, although the events taking place inside the brain are different.

Types of Stroke
Hemorrhagic Stroke

A <u>hemorrhagic stroke</u> accounts for approximately 10% of all strokes and occurs as a result of bleeding inside the brain. The free blood then forms a clot, which squeezes the brain tissue next to it. When that tissue is compressed, oxygenated blood cannot get into the area, and the surrounding cells begin to die.

Certain patients are at higher risk for hemorrhagic stroke, which occurs more commonly in patients experiencing stress or exertion. The patients with highest risk are those who have very high blood pressure or chronically elevated blood pressure that is not treated. After many years of high pressure, the blood vessels in the brain weaken. Eventually, one of the vessels may rupture, and blood will spurt into the brain, increasing the pressure inside the cranium. Cerebral hemorrhages are often fatal, although proper treatment of high blood pressure can help prevent this long-term damage to the blood vessels, reducing morbidity and mortality.

Some people may have been born with weaknesses in the walls of the arteries. An <u>aneurysm</u> is a swelling or enlargement of part of an artery, resulting from weakening of the arterial wall. Many people in whom an aneurysm ruptures have a sudden onset of "the worst headache I've had in my life." The headache is from the irritation of blood on the tissue of the brain after the vessel swells and ruptures. When a hemorrhagic stroke occurs in an otherwise healthy young person, the likely cause is often a weakness in a blood vessel called a berry aneurysm. This type of aneurysm resembles a tiny balloon (or berry) that juts out from the artery. When the aneurysm is overstretched and ruptures, blood spurts into an area around the coverings of the brain called the subarachnoid space. Therefore, these types of strokes are called subarachnoid hemorrhages. Again, patients with this type of stroke experience a sudden severe headache. If the patient seeks medical attention immediately, surgeons may be able to repair the aneurysm; yet like other bleeding in the brain, subarachnoid hemorrhages are often fatal.

Ischemic Stroke

When blood flow to a particular part of the brain is cut off by a blockage inside a blood vessel, the result is an <u>ischemic stroke</u>. This can be from a thrombosis or an embolism that blocks blood flow. As with coronary artery disease, atherosclerosis in the blood vessels is often the cause. <u>Atherosclerosis</u> is a disorder in which calcium and cholesterol build up, forming a plaque inside the walls of blood vessels. This plaque may obstruct blood flow and interfere with the vessel's ability to dilate. Eventually, atherosclerosis may cause complete blockage of an artery. In other cases, an atherosclerotic plaque in the carotid artery in the neck will rupture. A blood clot will form over the crack in the plaque, sometimes growing big enough to com-

pletely block all blood flow through that artery. When deprived of oxygen, the parts of the brain supplied by the artery will stop working. Patients with ischemic strokes will have dramatic symptoms, including loss of movement (paralysis) on the opposite side of the body.

Even if the blockage in the carotid artery is not complete, smaller pieces of the clot may embolize (break off and be carried by the blood flow) deep into the brain, heart, or lungs. If a piece ends up in the brain, it will lodge in a branch blood vessel. This cerebral embolism then blocks blood flow **Figure 11-2 ▾** . Depending on the location of the clot, the patient may experience a range of symptoms from none to complete paralysis.

Transient Ischemic Attack

In some patients, normal processes in the body will break up a blood clot in the brain. When that happens quickly, blood flow is restored to the affected area, and the patient will regain use of the affected body

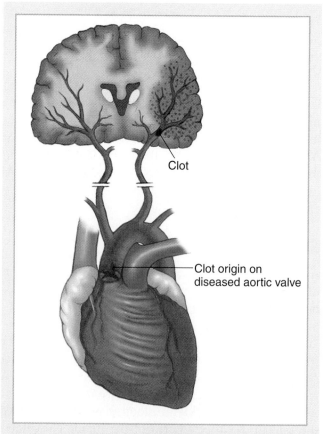

Figure 11-2 An embolus, a blood clot usually formed on a diseased heart valve, can travel through the body's vascular system, lodge in a cerebral artery, and cause a stroke.

Clot

Clot origin on diseased aortic valve

part. This often indicates that the patient has a serious medical condition that may eventually prove fatal. When stroke symptoms resolve without treatment in less than 24 hours, the event is called a <u>transient ischemic attack (TIA)</u>. Some patients call these mini-strokes.

Although most patients with TIAs do well, every TIA is an emergency. It may be a warning sign that a larger, permanent stroke is about to occur. For this reason, all patients with a new TIA should be evaluated by a physician to determine whether preventive action can be taken.

Signs and Symptoms of Stroke

Left Hemisphere Problems

If the left side of the brain has been affected, the patient may not be able to speak or to understand speech. Speech problems can vary widely. Some patients will have trouble understanding speech but still be able speak clearly. You can detect this problem by asking the patient a question such as "What day is today?" In response, the patient may say "Green." The speech is clear, but the answer does not make sense. Other patients will be able to understand the question but cannot produce the right sounds in order to answer. They may only be able to grunt or make incomprehensible sounds. Strokes that affect the left side of the brain can also cause paralysis of the right side of the body.

Right Hemisphere Problems

If the right side of the brain is not getting enough blood, patients will have trouble moving the muscles on the left side of the body. Usually, they will understand language and be able to speak, but their words may be slurred and hard to understand.

Patients with right hemisphere strokes may be completely oblivious to their problem. If you ask these patients to lift their left arm and they cannot, they will lift their right arm instead. They seem to have forgotten that the left arm even exists (called neglect). Patients with a problem affecting the back part of the cerebrum may neglect certain parts of their vision. Generally, this is hard to detect in the field owing to the patient's ability to compensate without conscious effort. Nevertheless, you should be aware of the possibility. Try to sit or stand on the patient's "good" side because he or she may be unable to see things on the "bad" side.

The problem of neglect causes many patients who have had large strokes to delay seeking help. Strokes may not be painful. Therefore, a patient may be unaware that there is a problem until a family member or friend points out that some part of the patient's body is not working correctly.

Bleeding in the Brain

Patients who have bleeding in their brain (a cerebral hemorrhage) may have very high blood pressure or cerebral aneurysms. Oftentimes, high blood pressure is the cause of the bleeding, but many times it is a response to the bleeding: The brain is raising the blood pressure in an attempt to force more oxygen into its injured parts. Quite often, blood pressure will return to normal or may drop significantly on its own.

Other Conditions

Because oxygen and glucose are needed for brain metabolism, a patient with hypoglycemia may look like a patient who is having a stroke. With good patient assessment, you should find out whether the patient has diabetes and takes insulin or another glucose-lowering medication.

A patient who has experienced a seizure may look like a patient who is having a stroke. This is often referred to as the postictal state. However, in most cases, a patient having a seizure will recover rapidly, within several minutes.

Subdural and epidural bleeding usually occur as a result of trauma. The dura is a leathery covering over the brain, next to the skull. A fracture near the temples may cause an artery to bleed on top of the dura, resulting in pressure on the brain. Onset of this epidural bleeding is usually very rapid after injury. In other cases, the veins just below the dura may be torn and bleed; this condition is referred to as subdural bleeding. Onset occurs more slowly, sometimes over several days. The onset of strokelike signs and symptoms may be subtle, and the patient may not even remember the original injury.

Scene Size-up

Strokes present in different ways. Dispatchers are not trained to diagnose particular problems but to recognize a set of specific conditions. Because a stroke can present in many different ways, the signs and symptoms may be easily confused with other conditions, particularly when signs and symptoms are described over the phone. Be aware of the information that dispatch provides you, but also consider other possibilities such as trauma and other illnesses that might mimic a stroke. For example, hypoglycemia associated with diabetes and seizures from other causes can present with symptoms similar to those of a stroke.

Do not be distracted by the seriousness of the situation or by frightened family members who want you to rush. Look first for threats to your safety and follow body substance isolation precautions. Most calls involving AMS require ALS backup or intercept, if available.

Initial Assessment

General Impression

Check the patient's ABCs (airway, breathing, and circulation) and care for immediate problems. Problems with the ABCs are initially found by asking the patient, "What is wrong?" or "How may we help you?" The chief complaint will guide you to what the patient is most concerned about. For patients having a stroke, the chief complaint may be highly variable and may include confusion, slurred speech, or unresponsiveness. Determining the patient's level of consciousness should be first in the list of assessment actions for anyone with AMS.

Airway and Breathing

Strokes affect how the body functions in many ways. Patients may have difficulty swallowing and are at risk for choking on their own saliva. Evaluate the airway of an unresponsive patient to make sure it is patent and will remain that way   Figure 11-3 ▶ . If the patient

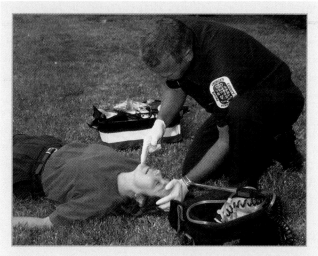

Figure 11-3 Securing and maintaining the airway in a patient who is unconscious is critical; also be sure to have suction readily available in the event that the patient vomits.

requires assistance maintaining an airway, consider an oropharyngeal or nasopharyngeal airway based on the level of consciousness and the presence of a gag reflex. Provide suction, and position the patient to prevent aspiration. If you determine that the patient cannot protect his or her own airway, place the patient in the recovery position to help prevent secretions from entering the airway. Suction as necessary. Evaluate the patient's breathing. Is the rate within normal parameters? Is the depth adequate? Is the patient using accessory muscles? As you perform the initial assessment,

You are the Provider 2

The family tells you that he has a history of "mini-strokes," but this is the first time this has happened and has not cleared up almost immediately. The patient's speech is slurred and he is unable to move his left side. When asked to raise his left arm, he raises his right arm.

Vital Signs	Recording Time: 2 Minutes
Skin	Pale, diaphoretic
Pulse	66 beats/min, irregular
Blood pressure	224/162 mm Hg
Respirations	22 breaths/min, slightly shallow

3. What type of oxygen does he need?
4. What do you think is wrong?
5. What is neglect?
6. Name another test that could be performed to detect facial drooping.

administer supplemental oxygen. If necessary, provide assisted ventilation.

Circulation

Your assessment of the patient's circulation should begin with checking a pulse if the patient is unresponsive. If there is no pulse, follow your protocol for CPR and AED. If the patient is responsive, determine whether the pulse is fast or slow, weak or strong. Is the patient in shock? Oxygen administration is helpful for limiting the effects of hypoperfusion to the brain. Quickly assess for external bleeding based on the chief complaint. It is unlikely your stroke patient has experienced trauma, but you should consider the possibility and assess appropriately.

Transport Decision

Controversial evidence exists that new therapies, such as thrombolytics (clot dissolvers), may reverse stroke symptoms and even stop the stroke if given within 2 to 3 hours of the onset of symptoms. These therapies may not work for all patients, and they cannot be given to patients with bleeding-type (hemorrhagic) strokes. Because hospital personnel will ultimately make these ongoing treatment decisions, you should proceed under the assumption that an area of the brain can still be saved. The sooner the treatment is begun, the better the prognosis for the patient.

Spend as little time at the scene as possible. Remember, stroke is an emergency. There may be treatment available for the patient at the hospital, and rapid transport is essential to maximize the possibility of recovery. Place the patient on one side, with the paralyzed side down and well protected with padding. This will help prevent aspiration of secretions in patients who cannot swallow well, and protect their airway. If a recovery position or left supine position is used, the patient's head should be elevated about 6" to maximize drainage of secretions. A patient's paralyzed extremities will require protection from harm. Remember that the patient cannot move if an arm gets pinched or a hand gets caught in a doorway while being transported. Calm and reassure the patient throughout transport.

Focused History and Physical Exam

Once you have concluded your initial assessment and addressed all life threats, begin the next step in the patient assessment process—the focused history and physical exam. If the patient is unresponsive, begin

EMT-B Safety

Regardless of the way the call is dispatched, you must always be alert for scene safety. Frightened family members, pets, and other seemingly innocuous situations can quickly become dangerous for rescuers.

with a rapid physical exam and then obtain baseline vital signs and a SAMPLE history. A situation in which patients are unresponsive after AMS was noted is much more serious than when patients are awake but confused. Quickly looking for explanations (trauma, medical tags, track marks) for the AMS may help identify the cause of the unresponsiveness and, therefore, guide you to appropriate treatment more quickly. When your rapid physical exam is complete, continue with obtaining the patient's vital signs and history. In a responsive medical patient, begin with a SAMPLE history, giving special attention to any information that may explain the patient's AMS. Perform a focused physical exam, and obtain the patient's baseline vital signs.

SAMPLE History

If the patient is responsive and breathing, obtain a SAMPLE history. Also try to speak with relatives or friends who may be able to explain the events before the AMS; remember that time is critical, and make a special effort to determine the exact time that the patient last seemed to be "normal." This information will help physicians in the emergency department understand whether it is safe to begin certain treatments that must be given within the first hours after onset of symptoms. You may be the only person on the emergency medical team with the opportunity to speak with bystanders to obtain this critical information. Collect or list all medications the patient has taken. When possible, determine allergies and the patient's last oral intake. This information may be helpful if the patient requires surgery.

Although a patient who has had a stroke may appear to be unconscious and unable to speak, the patient may still be able to hear and understand what is taking place. Therefore, as in any situation, avoid all unnecessary or inappropriate remarks. Try to communicate with the patient by looking for indications that the patient can understand you, such as a glance, gaze, motion or pressure of the hand, effort to speak, or head nod. Establishing effective communication can help you calm the patient and lessen the fear that accompanies the inability to communicate. Try to keep in mind that the patient has just experienced a potentially life-threatening event and that anxiety, frustration, and embarrassment may inhibit communication with you.

You should perform at least three key physical tests on patients you suspect of having had a stroke: tests of speech, facial movement, and arm movement. If any one of the three is abnormal, the patient may be having a stroke. Many EMS services use the Cincinnati Stroke Scale, which tests speech, facial droop, and arm drift (Table 11-1 ▼). To test speech, simply ask the patient to repeat a simple phrase such as "The sky is blue in Cincinnati." If the patient does this correctly, you know that he or she understands and can produce speech. If the patient cannot repeat the phrase, the problem may be with either function: understanding speech or producing it.

To test facial movement, ask the patient to show his or her teeth. Watch to see that both sides of the face around the mouth move equally. If only one side is moving well, you know that something is wrong with the control of the muscles on the other side.

To test arm movement, ask the patient to hold both arms in front of his or her body, palms up toward the sky, with eyes closed and without moving. For the next 10 seconds, watch the patient's hands. If you see one side drift down toward the ground, you know that side is weak. If both arms stay up and do not move, you know that both sides of the brain are working.

If both arms fall to the ground, you have not really learned anything. Perhaps the patient did not understand your instructions. Try the arm test again, but this time move the patient's arms into position your-self. Another possibility to consider is that the patient is having a problem other than a stroke.

Baseline Vital Signs

The last step of the focused history and physical exam is to obtain a baseline set of vital signs. These will be important to compare with vital signs obtained in the ongoing assessment. During severe situations, a great deal of pressure from bleeding in the brain may slow the pulse and cause respirations to be irregular. Blood pressure is usually high to compensate for poor perfusion in the brain.

Interventions

The cause of AMS may be unknown, even after arrival at the hospital. This makes it difficult to provide definitive care in the prehospital environment. Most of your interventions will be based on your assessment findings. For example, if the blood glucose level is low, you may give oral glucose according to protocol, or if a patient is unresponsive, you may need to position him or her in the recovery position to protect the airway. Your best treatment in these situations is to perform a thorough assessment and maintain the ABCs.

Detailed Physical Exam

A thorough detailed exam should be performed when time and conditions permit. A detailed physical exam includes inspection, palpation, and auscultation to identify DCAP-BTLS in all areas of the body. Because this exam is thorough and time-intensive, it is not often performed when attention is required to continuously treat the ABCs. Every effort should be made to complete this exam, especially when patients are unresponsive and unable to tell you about symptoms. Because of the time sensitivity of treatment options, this

Table 11-1 Cincinnati Stroke Scale

Test	Normal	Abnormal
Facial Droop (Ask patient to show teeth or smile.)	Both sides of face move equally well.	One side of face does not move as well as other.
Arm Drift (Ask patient to close eyes and hold both arms out with palms up.)	Both arms move the same, or both arms do not move.	One arm does not move, or one arm drifts down compared with the other side.
Speech (Ask patient to say, "The sky is blue in Cincinnati.")	Patient uses correct words with no slurring.	Patient slurs words, uses inappropriate words, or is unable to speak.

is generally performed during transport to the hospital. Do not delay transport to perform this on scene.

Ongoing Assessment

The ongoing assessment should focus on three main goals: reassessing the ABCs, interventions, and vital signs. In patients who have had a stroke, a previously patent airway can become obstructed or patients can stop breathing without warning. Multiple interventions may be necessary. The effectiveness of airway adjuncts, positive-pressure ventilation, and other treatments can only be determined with immediate and continuous observation after providing the intervention.

Communication and Documentation

After you begin transport, you should relay the information you have learned as soon as possible. Notify the receiving facility personnel that it is possible your patient had a stroke so that staff there can prepare to test and treat the patient without delay. Be sure to include the time that the patient was last seen to be normal, the findings of your neurologic exam, and the time you anticipate arriving at the hospital.

One of the key pieces of information to document is the time of onset of the patient's signs and symptoms. If the physician's diagnosis is an ischemic stroke, time of onset of the signs and symptoms is critical in determining whether the patient is a candidate for treatment with clot-dissolving drugs.

Definitive Care for Patients Who Have Had a Stroke

In most patients with suspected stroke, physicians need to determine whether there is bleeding in the brain. If there is no bleeding, the patient may be a candidate for medication to help break up the blood clot

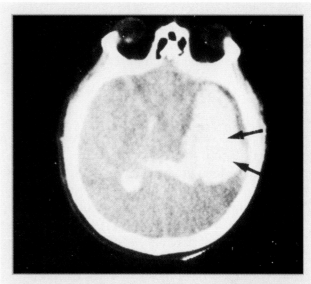

Figure 11-4 A computed tomographic scan of a ruptured cerebral aneurysm. The light area represents hemorrhage into the brain tissue (arrows).

or to help brain cells survive the reduced amount of oxygen. The only reliable way to tell whether there is bleeding is with a special type of x-ray test called computed tomography (CT) of the head. Blood is usually easy to see on the CT scan (**Figure 11-4 ▲**).

Keep in mind that most treatments for stroke must be started as soon as possible after the onset of the event. Few, if any, current treatments do any good if they are started more than 3 to 6 hours after the stroke begins. Even if 3 hours have passed, prompt action on your part is essential. Some EMS systems designate specific hospitals for stroke patients. These institutions have CT scanner technicians, radiologists, and neurosurgeons on duty 24 hours a day.

■ Seizures

Types of Seizures

A <u>seizure</u>, or convulsion, is a temporary alteration in behavior or consciousness and is typically characterized by unconsciousness and a generalized severe twitching of all of the body's muscles that lasts several minutes or longer. This type of seizure is often called a generalized tonic-clonic seizure (formerly called grand mal seizure). In other cases, the seizure may simply be characterized by a brief lapse of consciousness without loss of composure in which the patient seems to stare and not to respond to anyone. Other characteristics may be lip smacking, eye blinking, or

---

Documentation Tips

For potential stroke patients, be sure to include the following in your documentation:

- Time of onset of the patient's signs and symptoms
- Findings of your neurologic exam
- Any pertinent history and medications
- Any medication allergies

isolated convulsions or jerking of the body. This type of seizure, called an absence (sometimes pronounced ob-sáhnz) seizure (formerly called petit mal seizure), typically occurs in children from 4 to 12 years old.

Signs and Symptoms

Some seizures occur on only one side of the body. Others begin on one side and gradually progress to a generalized seizure that affects the entire body. Most people with lifelong or chronic seizures tolerate these events reasonably well without complications, but in some situations, seizures may signal life-threatening conditions.

Often, a patient may have experienced a warning before the event, which is referred to as an aura. The seizure is characterized by sudden loss of consciousness, chaotic muscle movement and tone, and apnea. The patient may also experience a tonic phase, usually lasting only seconds, in which the there will be a period of extensor muscle tone activity, tongue biting, or bladder or bowel incontinence. During the tonic-clonic phase, the patient may exhibit bilateral movement characterized by muscle rigidity and relaxation usually lasting 1 to 3 minutes. Throughout the tonic-clonic phase, the patient experiences tachycardia, hyperventilation, and intense salivation. Most seizures last 3 to 5 minutes and are followed by a lengthy period (5 to 30 minutes or more) called a <u>postictal state</u>, in which the patient is unresponsive at first and gradually regains consciousness. The postictal state is over when the patient regains a complete level of consciousness. Gradually, in most cases, the patient will begin to recover and awaken but appear dazed, confused, and fatigued. In contrast, an absence seizure can last for just a fraction of a minute, after which the patient fully recovers immediately with only a brief lapse of memory of the event.

Seizures that continue every few minutes without the patient regaining consciousness or last longer than 30 minutes are referred to as <u>status epilepticus</u>. For obvious reasons, recurring seizures should be considered potentially life-threatening situations in which patients need emergency medical care.

Causes of Seizures

Some seizure disorders, such as epilepsy, are congenital, which means that the patient was born with the condition. Other types of seizures may be due to high fevers, structural problems in the brain, or metabolic or chemical problems in the body. Epileptic seizures

can usually be controlled with medications such as phenytoin (Dilantin), phenobarbital, or carbamazepine (Tegretol). Patients with epilepsy will often have seizures if they stop taking their medications or if they do not take the prescribed dose on a regular basis.

Seizures may also be caused by tumors, an infection (brain abscess), or scar tissue from some type of injury. Seizures from a metabolic cause can result from abnormal levels of certain blood chemicals (for example, extremely low sodium levels), hypoglycemia, poisons, drug overdoses, or sudden withdrawal from routine heavy alcohol or drug use. Phenytoin, a drug that is used to control seizures, can cause seizures itself if the person takes too much.

Seizures can also result from sudden high fevers, particularly in children. <u>Febrile seizures</u> are usually very unnerving for parents to observe but are generally well tolerated by the child. You must transport a child who has had a febrile seizure because this condition needs to be evaluated in the hospital.

The Importance of Recognizing Seizures

Regardless of the type of seizure, it is important for you to recognize when a seizure is occurring or whether one has already occurred. You must also determine whether this episode differs from any previous ones. For example, if the previous seizure occurred on only one side of the body and this seizure occurred over the entire body, some additional or new problem may be involved. In addition to recognizing that seizure activity has occurred and/or that something different may now be occurring, you must also recognize the postictal state and the complications of seizures.

Because most seizures involve a vigorous twitching of the muscles, the muscles use a lot of oxygen. This excessive demand consumes oxygen being delivered by the circulation for the vital functions of the body. As a result, there is a buildup of acids in the bloodstream, and the patient may be cyanotic from the lack of oxygen. Often, the seizures themselves prevent the patient from breathing normally, making the problem worse. In patients with diabetes, blood glucose values may drop because of the excessive muscular contraction of a seizure. Monitor blood glucose levels closely after a patient with diabetes has a seizure.

Recognizing seizure activity also means looking at other problems associated with the seizure. For example, the patient may have fallen during the seizure episode and injured some part of the body. Patients having a generalized seizure may experience inconti-

Teamwork Tips

For those patients in *status epilepticus*, time is of the essence. Early recognition and rendezvous with an ALS unit may save the patient from morbidity due to hypoxia.

nence, meaning that they may lose bowel and bladder control. Although incontinence is possible with other medical conditions, sudden incontinence is very likely a sign that a seizure has occurred. When such patients regain their faculties, they are naturally embarrassed by this temporary loss of control. Do what you can to minimize this discomfort by covering the patient and giving assurance that incontinence is part of the loss of control that accompanies a seizure.

The Postictal State

Once a seizure has stopped, the patient's muscles relax and breathing becomes labored (fast and deep) in an attempt to compensate for the buildup of acids in the bloodstream. By breathing faster and more deeply, the body can balance the acidity in the bloodstream. With normal circulation and liver function, the acids clear away within minutes, and the patient will begin to breathe more normally. The longer and harder the seizure, the longer it will take for this imbalance to cor-

rect itself. Likewise, longer and more severe seizures will result in longer postictal unresponsiveness and confusion. Once the patient regains a normal level of consciousness, typically oriented to person, place, and time, the postictal state is over.

In some situations, the postictal state may be characterized by weakness on one side of the body, resembling a stroke. Unlike the typical stroke, this soon goes away. Most commonly, the postictal state is characterized by lethargy and confusion to the point that the patient may be combative and appear angry. You must be prepared for these circumstances in your approach to scene control and in your treatment of the patient's symptoms. If the patient's condition does not improve, you should consider other possible underlying problems, including hypoglycemia and infection.

Assessing the Seizure Patient

You are typically called to care for a patient who has had a seizure because someone witnessed the seizure. However, you may also be called to see an unresponsive patient when the patient is found in a postictal state. In other situations, you may be called to care for a patient who is having seizures and find that the patient has some other medical problem, such as cardiac arrest or a psychological problem.

In most cases, you will arrive sometime after the seizure has occurred because it only lasts a few minutes. By the time someone recognizes the problem, calls for help, and receives a response, the patient

You are the Provider 3

Your partner applies a nonrebreathing mask at 15 L/min, and the two of you lift the patient onto the stretcher. You note that he is incontinent of bladder. You ask him about any pain and he shakes his head "no."

Reassessment	Recording Time: 5 Minutes
Pulse	72 beats/min, irregular
Blood pressure	228/160 mm Hg
Respirations	20 breaths/min, not quite as shallow
Breath sounds	Clear bilaterally
Pulse oximetry	96% on oxygen via nonrebreathing mask

7. How should he be positioned on the stretcher?
8. What is the optimal time frame for treatment of a cerebrovascular accident (CVA)?
9. What else should you rule out while assessing the patient?
10. What conditions can mimic a CVA?

Geriatric Needs

When you are called to care for a geriatric patient with an AMS, consider the possibility of a stroke or transient ischemic attack (TIA). At the scene of a motor vehicle crash involving an older driver, consider a stroke or TIA as the precipitating factor in the crash. Be alert of altered mental status or unusual pupil responses (ie, constricted pupils in dim light, unequal pupils).

is usually in a postictal state. You must obtain as much information as possible from family or bystanders to verify that a seizure occurred and to obtain a description of the way the seizure developed.

Scene Size-up

Dispatchers are frequently given information about a seizure from the caller. Even if the caller has never seen a seizure before, the description often indicates a seizure is taking place. Although this may be an obvious nature-of-illness (NOI) problem as reported by bystanders, a mechanism of injury (MOI) may still be present. Consider the need for spinal precautions based on dispatch information and your assessment of the scene as you approach the patient. Ensure the scene is safe, and use appropriate BSI precautions. Gloves and eye protection, at a minimum, should be worn. ALS is not typically needed for a simple seizure; however, when complications such as severe trauma or prolonged seizures are present, you should call for ALS.

Initial Assessment

General Impression

Most seizures last only a few minutes at most. As you approach your patient and observe the level of consciousness, you should be able to tell whether the patient is still having a seizure. If the patient is still having a seizure when you arrive, the potentially life-threatening condition of status epilepticus may be present. If the patient is in the postictal stage of the seizure, he or she may be unresponsive or starting to regain awareness of the surroundings.

Airway, Breathing, and Circulation

As with any other situation, you should focus on the patient's ABCs on arrival. Bystanders may have tried to put objects in the patient's mouth to prevent the patient from swallowing his or her tongue. Assess the patient for adequate ventilation. Even if ventilation is adequate, administer high-flow oxygen at 15 L/min via nonrebreathing mask. Seizures will use up oxygen quickly and cause patients to be hypoxic. Breathing and circulation should be confirmed as normal or treated as necessary. Again, in the immediate postictal state following a major seizure, you should anticipate rapid, deep respirations and an accompanying fast heart rate due to the stress of the seizure. However, respirations and heart rate should begin to slow to normal rates after several minutes.

Transport Decision

Make sure that before packaging you have assessed the patient for trauma and have taken appropriate spinal precautions, if indicated. Never attempt to restrain a patient during a seizure because injury could result. Use soft materials for padding, and move any objects out of the way that may harm your patient.

Not every patient who has had a seizure wants to be transported. It is usually in the best interest of the patient to be evaluated by a physician in the emergency department after a seizure. Your goal is to encourage the patient to be seen in the emergency department. Follow your local protocols on releasing patients who refuse care.

Focused History and Physical Exam

As with other unresponsive medical patients, perform a rapid physical exam, quickly checking the patient from head to toe, looking for any obvious trauma or explanations as to why the seizure occurred. Vital

You are the Provider 4

The patient is transported promptly to the emergency department where he receives treatment for a right hemisphere stroke. He is released from the hospital a week later but still has a small deficit on his left side. The doctor assures you that without the prompt treatment, his residual damage would have been much worse.

signs and history can then be obtained as the patient regains consciousness. If the patient is responding to questions, begin with a SAMPLE history and baseline vital signs. Perform a focused physical exam to look for any injuries.

SAMPLE History

You should obtain a SAMPLE history, including whether the patient has a history of seizures. If so, it is important to find out how the patient's seizures typically occur and whether this episode differs in some way from previous episodes. You should also ask what medications the patient has been taking. You might find that the patient ran out of seizure medication or stopped taking the medication.

Baseline Vital Signs

Vital signs are generally normal in patients in the postictal period. Obtain pulse rate, rhythm, and quality; respiratory rate, rhythm, and quality; blood pressure; skin color, temperature, and condition; and pupil size and reactivity. If the patient has a history of diabetes and you have the ability to check a finger-stick blood glucose level, the result should be included in your vital signs. Compare these baseline vital signs with vital signs obtained in the ongoing assessment.

Interventions

Seizures are usually limited in duration. Most will not require a lot of intervention because they will be over by the time you arrive. For patients having a seizure, protect them from harm, maintain a clear airway by suctioning as necessary, and provide oxygen as quickly as possible. Treat any trauma you find as you would for any other patient.

For patients who continue to have seizures, as in status epilepticus, suction the airway according to protocol, provide positive pressure ventilations, and transport quickly to the hospital. If you have the option to rendezvous with ALS, you should do so. ALS providers can administer medications that can stop a prolonged seizure.

Detailed Physical Exam

Once the initial assessment and focused history and physical exam are completed, you can consider performing a detailed physical exam. The patient should be checked for injuries, including head lacerations, shoulder dislocations, tongue lacerations, and extremity fractures. Also assess the patient for weakness or loss of sensation on one side of the body.

Ongoing Assessment

If another seizure occurs, note whether the seizure starts at a focal part of the body (for example, one arm or one leg) and then progresses to the rest of the body. Most important, evaluate the patient's ABCs, vital signs, and mental status. Monitor the patient's mental status every several minutes to verify progressive improvement. Check to see whether interventions are providing the benefits you want.

Communication and Documentation

Report and record your findings of the initial assessment and interventions performed. Give a description of the episode and include bystanders' comments, especially if they witnessed the seizure. Document the onset and duration of the seizure. Record any evidence of trauma and interventions performed. Document whether this is the patient's first seizure or whether the patient has a history of seizures. If the patient has a history of seizure activity, how often does he or she have them? When you are documenting your interventions, record the time the intervention was performed and the patient's response to the intervention.

Definitive Care for the Patient Who Has Had a Seizure

In most situations, patients who have had a seizure require definitive evaluation and treatment in the hospital. Even a patient who has a history of chronic epilepsy that is controlled with medications may have an occasional seizure. At the hospital, blood levels of seizure medications are checked to ensure that patients are receiving the correct dose. Clearly, patients who have just had their first seizure or those with chronic seizures who have had an episode that is "different" require immediate examination to rule out life-threatening conditions. Unless the patient has a well-established history of seizures and is completely alert and oriented, supplemental oxygen is strongly advised, not only to provide extra oxygen, but also to help prevent another seizure.

Depending on local protocols, you should assess and treat the patient for possible hypoglycemia (for example, a person with diabetes with AMS who takes insulin or oral agents that lower blood glucose levels). If trauma is suspected, provide spinal immobilization. With recurrent seizures, protect the patient from further injury and manage the airway once the seizure ceases.

If you are treating a child who you suspect is having a febrile seizure, you should attempt to lower the child's temperature by removing his or her clothing and cooling the child with tepid water, particularly about the head and neck, and then fanning the moistened areas. Be careful not to make the patient shiver, which will increase temperature.

If the patient has been exposed to a toxin or poison, you should safely remove the source if possible. Suction should be readily available in case a patient with a decreased level of consciousness begins to vomit. In all cases, you should show patience and tolerance because many patients are likely to be confused and possibly frightened. Many patients who experience seizures are frustrated with their condition and may refuse transport. Kindness and professional behavior are required to help convince the patient that transport is necessary for definitive care.

■ Altered Mental Status

Aside from stroke and seizures, the most common type of neurologic emergency that you encounter is AMS, which means that the patient is not thinking clearly or is incapable of being aroused. Patients with AMS can be alert but confused or may be unconscious. There are many causes of AMS, including hypoglycemia, hypoxemia, intoxication, drug overdose, unrecognized head injury, brain infection, and brain tumors.

Causes of AMS
Hypoglycemia

Patients with a low blood glucose level can have signs and symptoms that mimic stroke, and they can have seizures. Patients with hypoglycemia commonly, but not always, take medications that lower the blood glucose level. Check for and report medications, but remember that not all patients who have diabetes take insulin or other medications to lower the blood glucose level. Remember also that patients with a decreased level of consciousness should not be given anything by mouth.

Patients with hypoglycemia can also experience seizures, and you may arrive at the scene to find the patient in a postictal state. The mental status of a patient who has had a typical seizure is likely to improve; however, in a patient with hypoglycemia, the mental status is not likely to improve, even after several minutes. You should also consider hypoglycemia in a patient who has AMS after an injury such as a motor vehicle crash, even when there is the possi-

bility of an accompanying head injury. As with any other patient, you should look for medical identification bracelets or medications that might confirm your suspicions.

Other Causes of AMS

Altered mental status can occur as a result of hypoglycemia, but there are many other possibilities as well, including unrecognized head injury or severe alcohol intoxication. In most cases, a patient who appears intoxicated most likely is just that; however, you must consider other problems as well; electrolyte imbalance and hypoglycemia also can cause behavior that mimics that of intoxication. People with chronic alcoholism can have abnormalities in liver function and in their blood-clotting and immune systems, which can predispose them to intracranial bleeding, brain and bloodstream infections, and hypoglycemia.

Psychological problems and complications from medications are also possible causes of AMS. A person who appears to have a psychological problem may also have an underlying medical condition. Infections are another possible cause of AMS, particularly those involving the brain or bloodstream. Infections in these areas are life threatening and need immediate attention. Patients may not demonstrate typical signs of infection, such as fever, particularly if they are very young or very old or have impaired immune systems.

▲ Pediatric Needs

Children can have AMS caused by strokes, seizures, high or low blood glucose levels, infections (meningitis), poisoning, or tumors. Hemorrhagic strokes are usually caused by congenital defects in blood vessels; these defects are called berry aneurysms. Ischemic strokes can be due to disorders such as sickle cell anemia. However, children who have subarachnoid hemorrhages may not have a berry aneurysm; instead, they may have a congenital problem with the blood vessels in the brain. Children who have sickle cell anemia are at particularly high risk for ischemic stroke. Treat stroke and AMS in children the same way that you do in adults.

Altered mental status can also be caused by drug overdose or poisonings; therefore, you should monitor patients closely for accompanying cardiac and breathing problems. The presentation of AMS varies widely from simple confusion to coma. No matter what the cause, you should consider AMS to be an emergency that requires immediate attention.

Assessment of the Patient With AMS

The patient assessment process for patients with AMS is the same as for patients with potential stroke and seizure, with a few differences. The most significant difference between AMS and other emergencies is that your patient cannot tell you reliably what is wrong, and there may be more than one cause. Therefore, being vigilant in your ongoing assessment is essential to find possible causes of your patient's condition and to monitor your patient's condition for changes and deterioration. Prompt transport is necessary, with close monitoring of vital signs en route and careful attention to the airway, positioning the patient to avoid aspiration and maintain comfort.

You are the Provider Summary

It is essential to recognize the need for early intervention. Remember to monitor the airway for secretions that should be suctioned. Spend as little time on scene as possible and always place the patient in the recovery position with the weak side down for transport. Also remember that a stroke can be a terrifying event for the patient, so constantly reassure him en route to the hospital.

1. **What are your priorities for this patient?**

   ABCs, gather a SAMPLE history

2. **What questions should you ask about this episode?**
   - Does he have any medical history?
   - Does he take any medications?
   - Is he allergic to anything?
   - Has this happened before?
   - If so, what did the doctor say then?
   - When did this start?
   - Signs and symptoms?
   - Last oral intake?

3. **What type of oxygen does he need?**

   Since his breathing is shallow, he needs to be ventilated with a bag-mask device. However, since he is alert he probably will not tolerate the bag-mask and should be placed on a nonrebreathing mask at 15 L/min.

4. **What do you think is wrong?**

   He is presenting with the signs of a right hemisphere CVA.

5. **What is neglect?**

   When asked to raise his left arm, he raises his right. He seems to have forgotten the left arm even exists.

6. **Name another test that could be performed to detect facial drooping.**

   Ask the patient to smile.

7. **How should he be positioned on the stretcher?**

   The weak side should be down with the arm strapped in.

8. **What is the optimal time frame for treatment of a CVA?**

   Within 3 hours of the onset of symptoms

9. **What else should you rule out while assessing the patient?**

   Hypoglycemia

10. **What conditions can mimic a CVA?**

    Seizures, hypoglycemia

Assessment and Emergency Care

	Stroke	Seizure	Altered Mental Status
Scene Size-up	Body substance isolation precautions should include a minimum of gloves and eye protection. Ensure scene safety and determine NOI/MOI. Consider the number of patients, the need for additional help/ALS, and c-spine stabilization.	Body substance isolation precautions should include a minimum of gloves and eye protection. Ensure scene safety and determine NOI/MOI. Consider the number of patients, the need for additional help, and c-spine stabilization.	Body substance isolation precautions should include a minimum of gloves and eye protection. Ensure scene safety and determine NOI/MOI. Consider the number of patients, the need for additional help, and c-spine stabilization.
Initial Assessment ■ General impression	Determine level of consciousness, and find and treat any immediate threats to life. Determine priority of care based on environment and patient's chief complaint.	Determine level of consciousness, and find and treat any immediate threats to life. If the seizure is still taking place on your arrival, life-threatening status epilepticus may be taking place. Call for ALS.	Determine priority of care based on environment and patient's chief complaint. Determine level of consciousness, and find and treat any immediate threats to life.
■ Airway	Ensure patent airway, place in the recovery position, and suction as necessary.	Clear mouth, and ensure patent airway. Use airway adjuncts according to local protocol.	Ensure patent airway, and place in the recovery position as necessary.
■ Breathing	Provide high-flow oxygen at 15 L/min. Evaluate depth and rate of the respiratory cycle, and provide ventilatory support as needed.	Evaluate depth and rate of the respiratory cycle, and provide ventilatory support as needed. Provide high-flow oxygen at 15 L/min.	Evaluate depth and rate of the respiratory cycle, and provide ventilatory support as needed. Auscultate and note breath sounds, providing high-flow oxygen at 15 L/min.
■ Circulation	Evaluate pulse rate and quality; observe skin color, temperature, and condition, and treat accordingly.	Evaluate pulse rate and quality; observe skin color, temperature, and condition.	Evaluate pulse rate and quality; observe skin color, temperature, and condition.
■ Transport decision	Rapid transport to stroke center if available	Transport based on assessment and local guidelines	Rapid transport based on initial assessment
Focused History and Physical Exam	*NOTE: The order of the steps in the focused history and physical exam differs depending on whether the patient is conscious or unconscious. The order below is for a conscious patient. For an unconscious patient, perform a rapid physical exam, obtain vital signs, and obtain the history.*		
■ SAMPLE history	Ask pertinent SAMPLE and OPQRST. Be sure to ask if and what interventions were taken before your arrival, how many interventions, and at what time. Ascertain when the patient last appeared normal.	Ask pertinent SAMPLE and OPQRST. How do seizures typically occur, and did this one differ from the norm? Has patient been compliant with medications?	Ask pertinent SAMPLE and OPQRST. Be sure to ask if and what interventions were taken before your arrival, how many interventions, and at what time.
■ Focused physical exam	Perform a focused neurologic exam using the Cincinnati Stroke Scale, and/or the Glasgow Coma Scale.	Perform focused physical exam for AMS, speech, and thinking ability. Determine blood glucose level and Glasgow Coma Scale score.	Perform a focused neurologic exam for AMS. Determine blood glucose level and Glasgow Coma Scale score.
■ Baseline vital signs	Take vital signs, noting skin color and temperature and patient's level of consciousness. Use pulse oximetry if available.	Take vital signs, noting skin color and temperature, patient's level of consciousness, and pupil size and reactivity. Use pulse oximetry if available.	Take vital signs, noting skin color and temperature and patient's level of consciousness. Use pulse oximetry if available.

	Stroke	Seizure	Altered Mental Status
■ Interventions	Support patient as needed. Consider the use of oxygen, positive-pressure ventilation, airway adjuncts, and proper positioning of the patient.	Protect patient from harm, maintain a clear airway by suctioning as necessary, and provide oxygen as quickly as possible. Treat any trauma injury you find. For patients who continue to seize, suction airway according to protocol, provide positive-pressure ventilation, and transport quickly to the hospital.	Support patient as needed. Consider the use of oxygen, positive pressure ventilation, airway adjuncts, and proper positioning. Treat low glucose levels according to local protocols.
Detailed Physical Exam	Complete a detailed physical exam.	Complete a detailed physical exam.	Complete a detailed physical exam.
Ongoing Assessment	Repeat the initial assessment, focused assessment, and reassess interventions performed. Reassess vital signs and the Glasgow Coma Scale score every 5 minutes for the unstable patient, every 15 minutes for the stable patient. Reassure and calm the patient.	Repeat the initial assessment, focused assessment, and reassess interventions performed. Reassess vital signs every 5 minutes for the unstable patient, every 15 minutes for the stable patient.	Repeat the initial assessment, focused assessment, and reassess interventions performed. Reassess vital signs every 5 minutes for the unstable patient, every 15 minutes for the stable patient. Reassure and calm the patient.
■ Communication and documentation	Contact medical control with a radio report that gives information on patient's condition and the last time patient appeared normal. Relay any change in level of consciousness or difficulty breathing. Be sure to document any changes, at what time, and any Cincinnati Stroke Scale or Glasgow Coma Scale results.	Report and record your findings. Document the onset and duration of the seizure, recording the time of each intervention performed, the patient's response, and continued reassessments.	Report and record your findings. Document each intervention performed, the patient's response, and the continued reassessments.

NOTE: While the steps below are widely accepted, be sure to consult and follow your local protocol.

Stroke	Seizure		Altered Mental Status
Cincinnati Stroke Scale	**Glasgow Coma Scale**		Use the Cincinnati Stroke Scale and/or the Glasgow Coma Scale to aid in your assessment.
1. Ask patient to show teeth or smile to determine facial droop.	*Eye Opening* Spontaneous 4 Responsive to speech 3 Responsive to pain 2 None 1	*Best Motor Response* Obeys commands 6 Localizes pain 5 Withdraws to pain 4 Abnormal flexion 3 Abnormal extension 2 None 1	
2. Ask patient to close eyes and hold both arms out with palms up to measure arm drift.	*Best Verbal Response* Oriented conversation 5 Confused conversation 4 Inappropriate words 3 Incomprehensible sounds 2 None 1	Add the total points selected from all three categories to determine the patient's Glasgow Coma Scale score.	
3. Ask patient to say, "The sky is blue in Cincinnati," to monitor speech.			

Prep Kit

Ready for Review

- Strokes occur when part of the blood flow to the brain is suddenly cut off; within minutes, brain cells begin to die.
- Seizures and altered mental status (AMS) are also common, and you must learn to recognize the signs and symptoms of each.
- Other causes of neurologic emergencies include coma, infections, and tumors.
- Signs and symptoms of stroke include the inability to speak or understand what people are saying, inappropriate responses to questions, muscle weakness or numbness on one side, and facial droop.
- There are three neurologic tests (Cincinnati Stroke Scale) to use to assess patients you suspect of having a stroke: testing speech, facial movement, and arm movement.
- In a transient ischemic attack (TIA), normal body processes break up the blood clot, restoring blood flow and ending symptoms in less than 24 hours. Patients with TIA are at risk for a stroke.
- Because current treatments must be administered within 3 to 6 hours (and preferably within 2 hours) of the onset of symptoms to be most effective, you should provide prompt transport for patients you suspect are having a stroke.
- Always notify the hospital as soon as possible that you are bringing in a possible stroke patient so that staff there can prepare to test and treat the patient without delay.
- Seizures are characterized by unconsciousness and generalized twitching of all or part of the body.
- Most seizures last between 3 and 5 minutes and are followed by a postictal state in which the patient may be unresponsive and have labored breathing. Many seizure patients will be incontinent and may have bit their tongue or lip.
- AMS is a common EMS call. Signs and symptoms vary widely, as do the causes. Common causes are hypoglycemia, intoxication, drug overdose, and poisoning.

- As you assess a patient with AMS, do not always assume intoxication; hypoglycemia is just as likely a cause. Prompt transport with close monitoring of vital signs en route is indicated.

Vital Vocabulary

altered mental status (AMS) A condition in which a person is disoriented or does not respond normally to selected stimuli (for example, is confused or stares rather than speaking).

aneurysm A bulging, weakened area in an artery that might burst. Rupture of an aneurysm in the brain might result in stroke or death.

arterial rupture Sudden breakage of an artery. When arterial rupture occurs in the brain, a stroke or death might result.

atherosclerosis A condition in which cholesterol and calcium build up on the walls of blood vessels, forming plaque, which leads to partial or complete blockage of blood flow or formation of emboli.

cerebral embolism Obstruction of a cerebral artery caused by a clot formed elsewhere in the body or other object or air that travels to the brain and obstructs blood flow.

cerebrovascular accident (CVA) An interruption of blood flow to the brain that results in the loss of brain function.

coma A state of profound unconsciousness from which one cannot be roused.

febrile seizures Convulsions that result from sudden high fevers, particularly in children.

hemorrhagic stroke One of the two main types of stroke; occurs as a result of bleeding inside the brain.

ischemic stroke One of the two main types of stroke; occurs when blood flow to a particular part of the brain is cut off by a blockage (for example, a clot) inside a blood vessel.

postictal state Period following a seizure that lasts between 5 and 30 minutes, characterized by labored respirations and some degree of altered mental status.

seizure Generalized, uncoordinated muscular activity associated with loss of consciousness; a convulsion.

status epilepticus A condition in which seizures recur every few minutes or last more than 30 minutes.

stroke A synonym for cerebrovascular accident (CVA). Usually caused by obstruction of the blood vessels in the brain that feed oxygen to the brain cells.

thrombosis The formation or presence of a blood clot.

transient ischemic attack (TIA) A disorder of the brain in which brain cells temporarily stop working because of insufficient oxygen, causing strokelike symptoms that resolve completely within 24 hours of onset.

Technology

Interactivities

Vocabulary Explorer

Anatomy Review

Web Links

Online Review Manual

Assessment in Action

You are called for a patient exhibiting "seizure-like" activity. On arrival you find a 15-month-old girl who is lethargic and has vomited. She is extremely warm to touch, and the mother tells you she has had an ear infection for almost a week and the medication is not working.

1. What type of seizures result from sudden high fevers?
   - A. focal motor
   - B. febrile
   - C. petite mal
   - D. grand mal

2. Seizures may be the result of _____.
   - A. tumors
   - B. infection
   - C. scar tissue
   - D. all of the above

3. Due to the buildup of acids in the bloodstream, what type of respirations are typically seen after a seizure?
   - A. slow and steady
   - B. slow and shallow
   - C. rapid and deep
   - D. rapid and shallow

4. What type of seizures are recurrent without an intervening period of consciousness?
   - A. grand mal seizures
   - B. epilepsy
   - C. the postictal phase
   - D. status epilepticus

5. What is the treatment of choice for a child who has experienced a febrile seizure?
   - A. cooling with tepid water
   - B. removing the clothing
   - C. fanning moistened areas
   - D. all of the above

Challenging Questions

6. Why should you monitor glucose levels closely after a patient with diabetes mellitus has a seizure?

7. What causes the buildup of acids in the bloodstream during seizure activity?

12

Diabetic Emergencies

You are the Provider 1

You are called to the scene of a 17-year-old boy playing basketball at the local high school who is "not acting right." On arrival, the coach tells you that he got confused and shot at the wrong basket and then became very combative with his best friend. He is pacing on the sideline and rips his shirt off as you approach.

Initial Assessment	Recording Time: 0 Minutes
Appearance	Flushed, extremely diaphoretic
Level of consciousness	Confused
Airway	Open and clear
Breathing	A little fast and shallow
Circulation	Radials present, rapid

1. What is your first consideration?
2. What questions should you ask his friend and the coach?
3. What else might you look for while surveying the scene?

Diabetic Emergencies

Diabetes is a common disease that affects about 6% of the population. It is a disorder of glucose metabolism or difficulty in breaking down carbohydrates, fats, and proteins. Without treatment, the blood glucose level becomes too high and can cause coma and death. If properly treated, most people with diabetes can live a relatively normal life. However, diabetes can have many severe complications that affect the length and quality of life, including blindness, cardiovascular disease, and kidney failure. Also, treatment to lower a high blood glucose level can sometimes cause a life-threatening state of hypoglycemia (low blood glucose level). As an EMS provider, you need to know the signs and symptoms of a blood glucose level that is too high or too low so that you can administer the proper treatment.

This chapter explains two types of diabetes and how they are controlled, including the role of glucose and insulin. We will also review how to distinguish between hyperglycemia and hypoglycemia. The chapter discusses how to identify and treat diabetic emergencies in the prehospital setting. Complications, such as seizures, altered mental status, and heart attack, are also briefly discussed.

Diabetes

Defining Diabetes

Literally, "diabetes" means "a passer through; a siphon." Medically, the term refers to a metabolic disorder in which the body's ability to metabolize simple carbohydrates (glucose) is impaired. It is characterized by the passage of large quantities of urine con-

taining glucose, significant thirst, and deterioration of body functions. Glucose, or dextrose, is one of the basic sugars in the body and, along with oxygen, is the primary fuel for cellular metabolism.

The primary problem in diabetes is the lack or ineffective action of insulin, a hormone that is normally produced by the pancreas. Insulin is needed to enable glucose to enter the cells. A hormone is a chemical substance produced by a gland that has special regulatory effects on other body organs and tissues. Without insulin, cells begin to "starve" because the glucose cannot get into the cells. Insulin acts like a key to allow the glucose to enter the cells.

Diabetes mellitus means "sweet diabetes." This refers to the presence of glucose (sugar) in the urine. Diabetes mellitus is considered a metabolic disorder in which the body cannot metabolize glucose, usually because of the lack of insulin. The body wastes the glucose that it is unable to use by excreting it in the urine. *Diabetes insipidus,* a rare condition, also involves excessive urination, but it is caused by inadequate amounts of the hormone that regulates fluid reabsorption (antidiuretic hormone) or failure of the kidney tubules to respond to the hormone. In this text, the term "diabetes" always refers to diabetes mellitus.

Left untreated, diabetes leads to wasting of body tissues and death. Even with medical care, some patients with particularly aggressive forms of diabetes will die relatively young of one or more complications of the disease. Most patients with diabetes live a normal life span, but they must be willing to adjust their lives to the demands of the disease, especially their eating habits and activities.

Types of Diabetes

Diabetes is a disease with two distinct onset patterns. It may become evident when the patient is a child, or it may develop in later life, usually when the patient is middle-aged.

In type 1 diabetes, most patients do not produce insulin at all; they are insulin-dependent. (This type of diabetes formerly was called insulin-dependent diabetes mellitus, or IDDM.) Patients with type 1 diabetes need daily injections of supplemental, synthetic insulin throughout their lives to control their blood glucose levels. This type generally strikes children as opposed to adults (previously called juvenile diabetes) but, in many cases, can develop later in life as well. Patients with type 1 diabetes are more likely to have

Technology

- Interactivities
- Vocabulary Explorer
- Anatomy Review
- Web Links
- Online Review Manual

problems such as blindness, heart disease, kidney failure, and nerve disorders.

In type 2 diabetes, which usually appears later in life, patients produce inadequate amounts of insulin or they may produce a normal amount but the insulin does not function effectively. Although some patients with type 2 diabetes (formerly called non–insulin-dependent diabetes mellitus, or NIDDM) may require some supplemental insulin, most can be treated with diet, exercise, and non–insulin-type oral medications (hypoglycemic agents), such as chlorpropamide (Diabinese), tolbutamide (Orinase), glyburide (Micronase), glipizide (Glucotrol), metformin (Glucophage), and rosiglitazone (Avandia). These medications stimulate the pancreas to produce more insulin, which results in a lower blood glucose level. In some cases, these medications can lead to hypoglycemia, particularly when patient activity and exercise levels are too vigorous or excessive. Type 2 diabetes used to be called adult (maturity)-onset diabetes.

The two types of diabetes are equally serious, although type 2 diabetes is easier to regulate. Both can affect many tissues and functions other than the glucose-regulating mechanism, and both require lifelong medical management. Type 1 diabetes is considered an autoimmune problem, in which the body becomes allergic to the insulin-producing cells of the endocrine parts of the pancreas and literally destroys them. The severity of diabetic complications is related to how high the average blood glucose level is and how early in life the diabetes begins.

The Role of Glucose and Insulin

Glucose is the major source of energy for the body, and all cells need it to function properly. Some cells will not function at all without glucose. A constant supply of glucose is as important as oxygen to the brain. Without glucose, or with a very low level, brain cells rapidly suffer permanent damage. With the exception of the brain, insulin is needed to allow glucose to enter individual body cells Figure 12-1 ▶ .

Without insulin, glucose from food remains in the blood and gradually rises to an extremely high level (hyperglycemia). Once the blood glucose levels reach 200 mg/dL or more, or twice the usual amount (normal is 80 to 120 mg/dL), excess glucose is excreted by the kidney. This process requires a large amount of water. The loss of water in such large amounts causes the classic symptoms of uncontrolled diabetes, the "3 Ps":

- Polyuria: frequent and plentiful urination
- Polydipsia: frequent drinking of liquid to satisfy continuous thirst (secondary to the loss of so much body water)
- Polyphagia: excessive eating as a result of cellular "hunger"; seen only occasionally

Without glucose to supply energy for cells, the body must turn to other fuel sources. The most abun-

You are the Provider 2

His best friend tells your partner that the patient has been a diabetic since before they started school and has always taken shots. They were playing basketball like they do every afternoon in the gym and the patient suddenly started acting funny. They tried to give him a soda and he knocked it to the ground.

When you try to place a nonrebreathing mask on him, he will not tolerate it. You switch to a nasal cannula and he also refuses to allow you to place it on him.

Vital Signs	Recording Time: 2 Minutes
Skin	Becoming slightly pale, very diaphoretic
Pulse	108 beats/min, regular
Blood pressure	110/70 mm Hg
Respirations	26 breaths/min, slightly shallow

4. What other questions might you ask?
5. Do you think his blood glucose may be high or low? Why?
6. What should you do next?

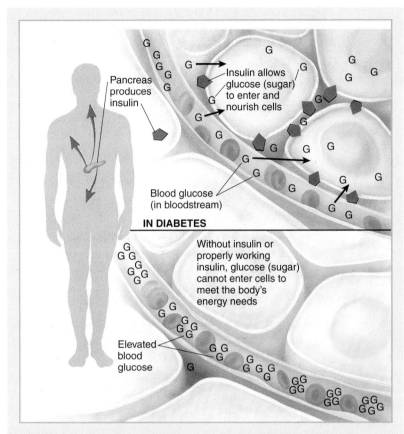

Figure 12-1 Diabetes is defined as a lack of or ineffective action of insulin. Without insulin, cells begin to "starve" because insulin is needed to allow glucose to enter and nourish the cells.

dant fuel source is fat. Unfortunately, when fat is used as an immediate energy source, chemicals called *ketones* and *fatty acids* are formed as waste products and are difficult for the body to excrete. As they accumulate in blood and tissue, certain ketones can produce a dangerous condition called <u>acidosis</u>. The form of acidosis seen in uncontrolled diabetes is called <u>diabetic ketoacidosis (DKA)</u>, in which an accumulation of certain acids occurs when insulin is not available in the body. Signs and symptoms of DKA include vomiting, abdominal pain, and a type of deep, rapid breathing called <u>Kussmaul respirations</u>. When the acid levels in the body become too high, individual cells will cease to function. If the patient is not given proper fluid and insulin to reverse fat metabolism and restore use of glucose as a source of energy, ketoacidosis will progress to unconsciousness, diabetic coma, and, eventually, death.

Diabetes is a treatable condition, but treatment must be tailored for the individual patient. The patient's need for glucose must be balanced with the available supply of insulin by testing the blood or the

urine. Most patients with type 1 diabetes monitor their blood glucose level several times a day with a glucometer. A drop of blood, usually from the fingertip, is touched to a disposable sensor and read by the machine. The readings are in milligrams per deciliter of blood; remember that the normal blood glucose level is between 80 and 120 mg/dL. In some EMS systems, EMT-Bs are allowed to use glucometers (Figure 12-2 ▼) as part of their patient assessment. You should review your own protocol on this issue.

Hyperglycemia and Hypoglycemia

Two conditions can lead to a diabetic emergency: hyperglycemia and hypoglycemia. <u>Hyperglycemia</u> is a state in which the blood glucose level is above normal. <u>Hypoglycemia</u> is a state in which the blood glucose level is below normal. Extremes of both hyperglycemia and hypoglycemia can lead to diabetic emergencies (Figure 12-3 ▶). Ketoacidosis results from prolonged and exceptionally high hyperglycemia. Diabetic coma results when ketoacidosis is not treated adequately. Hypoglycemia, on the other hand, will progress into unresponsiveness and eventually insulin shock. As you recall, the signs and symptoms of hypoglycemia and hyperglycemia can be quite similar (Table 12-1 ▶).

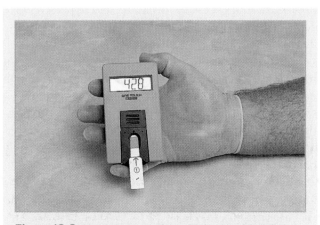

Figure 12-2 Blood glucose self-monitoring kit with digital meter is a device used by patients at home or by EMT-Bs in some areas.

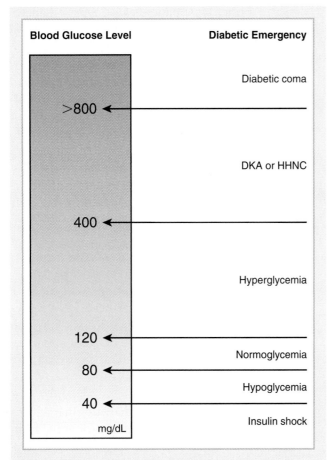

Blood Glucose Level | Diabetic Emergency

Diabetic coma

>800

DKA or HHNC

400

Hyperglycemia

120

Normoglycemia

80

Hypoglycemia

40

mg/dL

Insulin shock

Figure 12-3 The two most common diabetic emergencies, ketoacidosis and insulin shock, develop when the patient has too much or too little glucose in the blood, respectively.

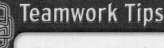

Teamwork Tips

While you are assessing a patient with an altered mental status, your partner should look for signs that may indicate that he or she is a diabetic. Look in the refrigerator (usually in the butter dish on the door) for insulin. A dish of candy on a nightstand may also be a clue.

- A rapid, weak ("thready") pulse
- A normal or slightly low blood pressure
- Varying degrees of unresponsiveness

Insulin Shock

In insulin shock, the problem is hypoglycemia (low blood glucose level). When the insulin level remains high, glucose is rapidly taken out of the blood to fuel the cells. If the glucose level gets too low, there may be an insufficient amount to supply the brain. If the blood glucose level remains low, unconsciousness and permanent brain damage can quickly follow.

Insulin shock occurs when the patient has done one of the following:
- Taken too much insulin
- Taken a regular dose of insulin, but has not eaten enough food
- Had an unusual amount of activity or vigorous exercise and used up all available glucose

Insulin shock may also occur with no identifiable predisposing factor.

Children who have diabetes may pose a particular management problem. First, their high levels of activity mean that they can use up circulating glucose more quickly than adults do, even after a normal insulin injection. Second, they do not always eat correctly and on schedule. As a result, insulin shock can develop more often and more severely in children than in adults.

Insulin shock develops much more quickly than diabetic coma. In some cases, it can occur in a matter of minutes. Signs and symptoms of hypoglycemia include the following:
- Normal or rapid respirations
- Pale, moist (clammy) skin
- Diaphoresis (sweating)
- Dizziness, headache

Diabetic Coma

Diabetic coma is a state of unconsciousness resulting from several problems, including ketoacidosis, dehydration because of excessive urination, and hyperglycemia. Too much blood glucose by itself does not always cause diabetic coma, but on some occasions, it can lead to it.

Diabetic coma may occur in a patient who is not receiving medical treatment, who does not take enough insulin, who markedly overeats, or who is undergoing some sort of stress (infection, illness, overexertion, fatigue, or drinking alcohol). Usually, ketoacidosis develops during hours to days. The patient may ultimately be found comatose with the following physical signs:
- Kussmaul respirations
- Dehydration, as indicated by dry, warm skin and sunken eyes
- A sweet or fruity (acetone) odor on the breath, caused by the unusual waste products in the blood (ketones)

Table 12-1 Characteristics of Diabetic Emergencies

	Diabetic Coma	Insulin Shock
History		
Food intake	Excessive	Insufficient
Insulin dosage	Insufficient	Excessive
Onset	Gradual	Rapid, within minutes
Skin	Warm and dry	Pale and moist
Infection	Common	Uncommon
Gastrointestinal tract		
Thirst	Intense	Absent
Hunger	Absent	Intense
Vomiting	Common	Uncommon
Respiratory system		
Breathing	Air hunger	Normal or rapid
Odor of breath	Sweet, fruity	Normal
Cardiovascular system		
Blood pressure	Low	Normal to low
Pulse	Rapid, weak	Normal or rapid and full
Nervous system		
Headache	Absent	Present
Consciousness	Restlessness progressing to coma	Irritability, confusion, seizure, or coma
Urine		
Sugar	Present	Absent
Acetone	Present	Absent
Treatment		
Response	Gradual, within 6 to 12 hours following medication and fluid	Immediately after glucose administration

- Rapid pulse
- Normal to low blood pressure
- Altered mental status (aggressive, confused, lethargic, or unusual behavior)
- Hunger

✋ EMT-B Safety

A patient in insulin shock may exhibit all types of bizarre behavior. Personal safety is still the first step. If necessary, call for law enforcement to restrain the patient so that you can continue your assessment and care.

- Seizure, fainting, or coma
- Weakness on one side of the body (may mimic stroke)

Diabetic coma and insulin shock produce unconsciousness and, in some cases, death. Diabetic coma is a complex metabolic condition that usually develops over time and involves all the tissues of the body. Correcting this condition may take many hours in a well-controlled hospital setting. Insulin shock, however, is an acute condition that can develop rapidly. A patient with diabetes who has taken his or her standard insulin dose and missed lunch may be in insulin shock before dinner. The condition is just as quickly reversed by giving the patient glucose. Without glucose, however, the patient will have permanent brain damage. Minutes count.

Most people with diabetes understand and manage their disease well. Still, emergencies occur. In addition to diabetic coma and insulin shock, patients with diabetes may have "silent," or painless, heart attacks, a possibility that you should always consider. Their only symptom may be "not feeling so well."

■ Assessment of Diabetic Patients

Scene Size-up

Although your report from dispatch may be for a patient with altered mental status, remember that trauma may also have occurred because of a medical incident. Body substance isolation precautions should consist of gloves and an eye shield at a minimum.

Do not let your guard down, even on what appears to be a routine call. Evaluate scene safety as you arrive on scene and as you approach the patient. Remember that diabetic patients often use syringes to administer insulin. It is possible you may be stuck by a used needle that was not disposed of properly. Insulin syringes on the bed stand, insulin bottles in the refrigerator, a plate of food, or glass of orange juice are important clues that may help you decide what is possibly wrong with your patient. Question bystanders on events of the situation as you approach. Determine whether this is your only patient, the nature of the illness, and whether trauma was involved. Decide whether you will need any additional resources. Perform cervical spine stabilization if necessary.

Initial Assessment

General Impression

Form a general impression of the patient. Does the patient appear anxious, restless, or listless? Is the patient interacting with his or her environment appropriately? These initial observations may help you to suspect a high or low blood glucose value. Determine the patient's level of consciousness. If the patient is conscious, what is the chief complaint? If a suspected diabetic patient is unresponsive, call for ALS immediately.

Airway and Breathing

As you are forming your general impression, assess the patient's airway and breathing. Patients showing signs of inadequate breathing or altered mental status should receive high-flow oxygen at 10 to 15 L/min via nonrebreathing mask. A patient in a diabetic coma who is hyperglycemic may have rapid, deep respirations (Kussmaul respirations) and sweet, fruity breath. A patient in insulin shock who is hypoglycemic will have normal to rapid respirations. If the patient is not breathing or is having difficulty breathing, open the airway, give oxygen, and assist ventilation. Continue to monitor the airway as you provide care.

You are the Provider 3

You are unable to obtain a glucose level reading. Your partner has brought candy from the coach's office and you are able to get the patient to eat a few pieces of chocolate. He refuses to take any more, but his friend gets him to drink some of the soda to wash down the candy.

Reassessment	Recording Time: 5 Minutes
Level of consciousness	Alert, less combative
Pulse	96 beats/min, irregular
Blood pressure	112/70 mm Hg
Respirations	20 breaths/min
Pulse oximetry	97% on room air

7. What is the next step?
8. What should you verify before giving anything by mouth?
9. Should you call for an ALS unit?
10. What type of consent is used to treat this patient initially?

Documentation Tips

Document the patient's history and medications. Many diabetics keep a log of glucose levels each day and how much insulin they are taking. If possible, take this with you to the hospital.

Circulation

Once you have assessed airway and breathing and have performed the necessary interventions, check the patient's circulatory status. A patient with dry and warm skin indicates diabetic coma, whereas a patient with moist and pale skin indicates insulin shock. The patient in insulin shock will have a rapid, weak pulse.

Transport Decision

Whether you decide to transport will depend on the patient's level of consciousness and ability to swallow. Patients with altered mental status and impaired ability to swallow should be transported promptly. Patients who have the ability to swallow and are conscious enough to maintain their own airway may be further evaluated on scene and interventions performed.

Focused History and Physical Exam

Assess unresponsive medical patients first from head to toe with a rapid physical exam, looking for clues to their condition. The patient may have experienced trauma resulting from changes in the level of consciousness or dizziness. Next, obtain the patient's vital signs and assess history. Remember that the environment, bystanders, and a medical identification symbol may provide important clues about your patient's condition.

Responsive medical patients are able to provide their own medical history to help you identify a cause for their altered mental status. Next, perform a focused physical exam and obtain your patient's baseline vital signs.

SAMPLE History

Ask the following questions of a known diabetic patient in addition to obtaining a SAMPLE history:

- Do you take insulin or any pills that lower your blood sugar?
- Have you taken your usual dose of insulin (or pills) today?
- Have you eaten normally today?
- Have you had any illness, unusual amount of activity, or stress today?

If the patient has eaten but has not taken insulin, it is more likely that DKA is developing. If the patient has taken insulin but has not eaten, the problem is more likely to be insulin shock. A patient with diabetes will often know what is wrong. If the patient is not thinking or speaking clearly (or is unconscious), ask a family member or bystander the same questions.

When you are assessing a patient who might have diabetes, check to see whether he or she has an emergency medical identification symbol—a wallet card, necklace, or bracelet—or ask the patient or a family member. Remember that even though a person has diabetes, the diabetes may not be causing the current problem. A heart attack, stroke, or other medical emergency may be the cause. For this reason, you must always do a thorough, careful assessment, paying attention to the ABCs.

Focused Physical Exam

When you suspect a diabetes-related problem, the focused physical exam should focus on the patient's mental status and ability to swallow and protect the airway. Obtain a Glasgow Coma Scale score to track the patient's mental ability. Otherwise, physical signs such as tremors, abdominal cramps, vomiting, a fruity breath odor, or a dry mouth may guide you in determining whether the patient is hypoglycemic or hyperglycemic.

Baseline Vital Signs

Obtain a complete set of vital signs, including checking the patient's blood glucose level using a glucometer if available. In hypoglycemia, respirations are normal to rapid, pulse is weak and rapid, skin is typically pale and clammy, and the blood pressure is normal to low. In hyperglycemia, respirations are deep and rapid, pulse is full and bounding at a normal or fast rate, the skin is warm and dry, and the blood pressure is normal. At times, the blood pressure may be low. Remember, the patient may have abnormal vital signs and a normal blood glucose value. When this is the case, something else may be causing the patient's altered mental status.

Interventions

If your patient is conscious and able to swallow without the risk of aspiration, you should encourage him or her to drink juice or milk or other drinks that contain sugar. If allowed by protocol, you may also administer oral glucose. The patient will usually become more alert within minutes.

If your patient is unconscious, or if there is any risk of aspiration, the patient will need intravenous (IV) glucose, which EMT-Bs are not authorized to give. Your responsibility is to provide prompt transport to the hospital, where the proper care can be given. If you are working in a tiered system, EMT-Is and paramedics are able to administer IV glucose.

If no one else is present and you know that the unconscious patient has diabetes, you must use your knowledge of the signs and symptoms to decide whether the problem is diabetic coma or insulin shock. This distinction should not prevent you from providing prompt treatment and transport. The primary visible difference will be the patient's breathing—deep, sighing respirations in diabetic coma and normal or rapid respirations in insulin shock. The patient with diabetes who is unconscious and having seizures is more likely to be in insulin shock.

Keep in mind that any unconscious patient may have undiagnosed diabetes. In patients with altered mental status, you may be able to determine this in the field, if you have the proper equipment to test the blood glucose level. Provide emergency medical care, particularly airway management, and provide prompt transport.

A patient in insulin shock (rapid onset of altered mental status, hypoglycemia) needs sugar immediately, and a patient in diabetic coma (acidosis, dehydration, hyperglycemia) needs insulin and IV fluid therapy. These patients need prompt transport to the hospital for appropriate medical care.

For a conscious patient who is hypoglycemic, protocols usually recommend oral glucose. Glucose will usually reverse the reaction within several minutes. Do not give sugar-free drinks that are sweetened with saccharin or other synthetic sweetening compounds because they will have little or no effect. Remember that even if the patient responds after receiving glucose, he or she may still need additional treatment and transport to the hospital.

When there is any doubt about whether a conscious patient with diabetes is going into insulin shock or diabetic coma, most protocols will err on the side of giving glucose, even though the patient may be hyperglycemic. Untreated insulin shock will result in loss of consciousness and can quickly cause

significant brain damage or death. Hypoglycemia is far more critical and far more likely to cause permanent damage than a high blood glucose level. Furthermore, the amount of sugar that is typically given to a patient in insulin shock is very unlikely to significantly worsen the condition of a patient with DKA.

Detailed Physical Exam

As in every call, you should perform a detailed physical exam when time permits. With unconscious patients or patients with altered mental status, you must play detective and look for problems or injuries that are not obvious because the patient is unable to communicate these to you. Although altered mental status may be caused by a blood glucose level that is too high or too low, the patient may have sustained trauma or be having another medical emergency. The altered mental status may also be caused by something else, such as intoxication, poisoning, or a head injury. A careful physical exam may provide you with information essential to proper patient care.

Ongoing Assessment

It is important to reevaluate diabetic patients frequently to assess changes. Is there an improvement in the patient's mental status? Are the ABCs still intact? How is the patient responding to the interventions performed? How must you adjust or change the interventions? In many patients with diabetes, you will note marked improvement with appropriate treatment. Base your glucose administration on serial readings if you have access to a glucometer. If a glucometer is unavailable, a deteriorating level of consciousness indicates that you need to provide more glucose. Again, the use of glucometers and the administration of glucose will be based on your service's protocols and standing orders.

Communication and Documentation

Your run report is the only legal document you have to say that appropriate care was provided. Document clearly your assessment findings as the basis for your treatment. Patients who refuse transport because you "cured" them with oral glucose should only be allowed to refuse based on your local protocol. Refusals require complete and accurate documentation.

■ Emergency Care of Diabetic Emergencies

Oral Glucose Administration

Oral glucose is a commercially available gel that dissolves when placed in the mouth. Trade names for oral glucose include Glutose and Insta-Glucose. Glucose gel acts to increase a patient's blood glucose level. If authorized by your system, you should administer glucose gel to any patient with altered mental status who has a history of diabetes. The only contraindications to glucose are an inability to swallow or unconsciousness, because aspiration (inhalation of the substance) can occur. Oral glucose itself has no side effects if it is administered properly; however, the risk of aspiration in a patient who does not have a gag reflex can be dangerous.

As always, be sure to wear gloves before placing anything into a patient's mouth. After you have confirmed that the patient is conscious and able to swallow and have obtained an online or off-line order, follow these steps to administer oral glucose **Skill Drill 12-1** :

1. **Examine the tube** to ensure that it is not open or broken. Check the expiration date (**Step 1**).
2. **Squeeze a generous amount** onto the bottom third of a bite stick or tongue depressor (**Step 2**).
3. Open the patient's mouth.
4. **Place the tongue depressor** on the mucous membranes between the cheek and gum, with the gel side next to the cheek (**Step 3**). Once the gel is dissolved, or if the patient loses consciousness or has a seizure, remove the tongue depressor. Repeat until the entire tube has been used. Instruct the patient to not swallow the gel, it acts more quickly when dissolved in the mouth.

Reassess the patient's condition regularly after giving glucose, even if you see rapid improvement.

Watch for airway problems, sudden loss of consciousness, and seizures.

■ Complications of Diabetes

Diabetes is a systemic disease affecting all tissues of the body, especially the kidneys, eyes, small arteries, and peripheral nerves. You are likely to be called to treat patients with a variety of complications of diabetes, such as heart disease, visual disturbances, renal failure, stroke, and ulcers or infections of the feet or toes. With the exception of heart attack and stroke, most of these will not be acute emergencies. Considering that diabetes is a major risk factor for cardiovascular disease, people with diabetes should always be suspected of having a potential for heart attack, particularly older patients, even when they do not present with classic symptoms, such as chest pain.

■ Associated Problems

Conditions associated with diabetes include seizures, altered mental status, and airway problems. You should consider that patients may also be having a diabetic emergency when they present with these conditions.

Seizures

Seizures, which may be brief or prolonged, are caused by fever, infections, poisoning, hypoglycemia, trauma, and decreased levels of oxygen. They can also be idiopathic (of unknown cause) in children. Although brief seizures are not harmful, they may indicate a more dangerous and potentially life-threatening underlying condition. Because seizures can be caused by a head injury, consider trauma as a cause. In patients with diabetes, you should also consider hypoglycemia.

Emergency medical care of seizures includes ensuring that the airway is clear and placing the patient on his or her side if there is no possibility of cervical

You are the Provider 4

After all of the candy and the soda, his mental status is back to normal. His mother has arrived on scene and does not wish to have him transported. She tells you that he has recently changed to a different type of insulin and has not been eating properly. After you explain why you feel he should be transported, she still refuses and he says he just wants to go home. His mother signs the refusal, witnessed by the coach.

Several days later you and your partner are called into the supervisor's office and are shown a thank-you note from the mother praising the exemplary conduct of your team.

Skill Drill   12-1   Administering Oral Glucose

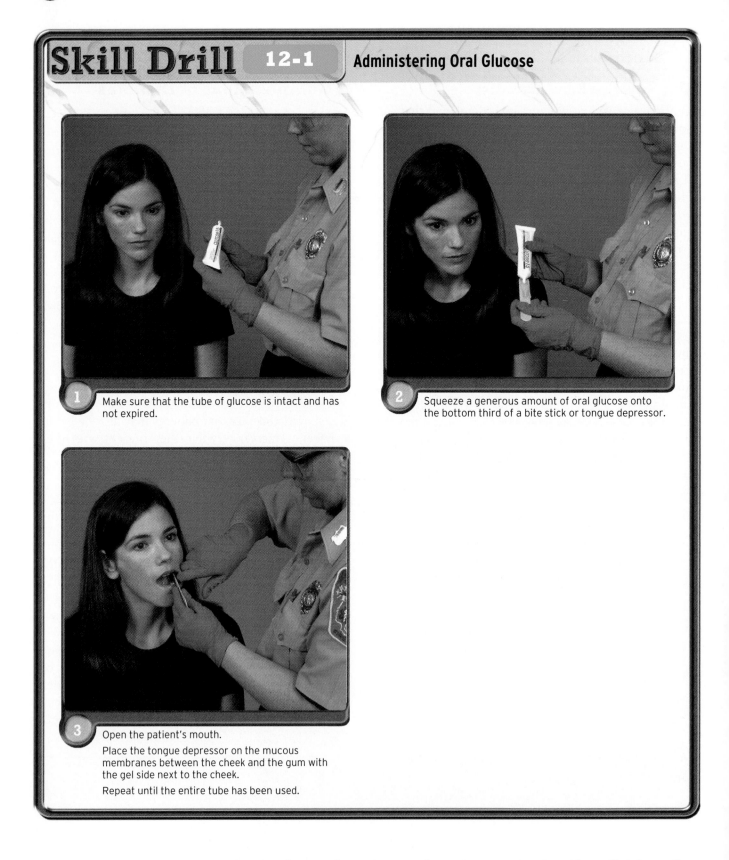

1   Make sure that the tube of glucose is intact and has not expired.

2   Squeeze a generous amount of oral glucose onto the bottom third of a bite stick or tongue depressor.

3   Open the patient's mouth.

Place the tongue depressor on the mucous membranes between the cheek and the gum with the gel side next to the cheek.

Repeat until the entire tube has been used.

spine trauma. Do not attempt to place anything in the patient's mouth (for example, a bite stick or an oral airway). Be sure to have suctioning equipment ready in case the patient vomits. Provide artificial ventilation if the patient is cyanotic or seems to be breathing inadequately, and provide prompt transport.

Altered Mental Status

Although altered mental status is often caused by a diabetic emergency, it may also be caused by other conditions, including poisoning, seizure, infection, head injury, and a decreased level of oxygen. In diabetes, altered mental status can be caused by a low or high blood glucose level.

Begin emergency medical care of altered mental status by ensuring that the airway is clear. Be prepared to provide artificial ventilation and suctioning in case the patient vomits, and provide prompt transport.

Alcoholism

Occasionally, patients in insulin shock or a diabetic coma are thought to be intoxicated, especially if their condition has caused a motor vehicle crash or other incident. Often, only a blood glucose test performed at the scene or in the emergency department will identify the real problem. In some EMS systems, you will be trained and allowed to use a glucometer. If not, you should always suspect hypoglycemia in any patient with altered mental status.

■ Relationship to Airway Management

Patients with altered mental status, particularly those who are difficult to awaken, are at risk for losing their gag reflex. When the gag reflex is not working, patients cannot protect their airway from foreign materials in their mouth (including vomit), and their tongues will often relax and obstruct the airway. You should carefully monitor the airway in patients with hypoglycemia, diabetic coma, or a diabetic complication such as stroke or seizure. Place the patient in a lateral recumbent position, and make sure suction is readily available.

You are the Provider Summary

Diabetic emergencies are a common call for EMS. Remember that it is essential to give glucose any time you are unable to check blood glucose levels. The brain must have glucose to function. If the patient's blood glucose is high, giving glucose will not raise it enough to create a problem; however, if the blood glucose is low, it may save the patient's life.

1. **What is your first consideration?**

   Personal safety. The patient is already agitated and combative.

2. **What questions should you ask his friend and the coach?**

   Try to obtain a SAMPLE history. Pay close attention to the events leading up to this episode and any patient history.

3. **What else might you look for while surveying the scene?**

   Do you see any medic alert tags or anything else that may lead you in the appropriate direction?

4. **What other questions might you ask?**

   What has the patient been doing today? Did he take any insulin/medication? Has he eaten?

5. **Do you think his blood glucose may be high or low? Why?**

   Low, based on the presenting signs/symptoms. Sudden onset, tachycardic, diaphoretic, altered mental status.

6. **What should you do next?**

   Check his blood glucose if possible. If not, try to give oral glucose.

7. **What is the next step?**

   Assess his glucose level.

8. **What should you verify before giving anything by mouth?**

   That the patient is alert enough to swallow without aspirating.

9. **Should you call for an ALS unit?**

   It is not necessary if the patient is alert and willing to take more glucose by mouth. However, if he becomes combative again it may be necessary.

10. **What type of consent is used to treat this patient initially?**

    The patient is a minor and also has an altered mental status, so he is treated under implied consent.

Assessment and Emergency Care

Diabetic Emergencies

Scene Size-up	Body substance isolation precautions should include a minimum of gloves and eye protection. Ensure scene safety and determine NOI/MOI. Consider the number of patients, the need for additional help/ALS, and c-spine stabilization.
Initial Assessment	
■ General impression	Determine level of consciousness and find and treat any immediate threats to life. Determine priority of care based on environment and patient's chief complaint.
■ Airway	Ensure patent airway.
■ Breathing	Provide high-flow oxygen at 15 L/min. Evaluate depth and rate of the respirations and provide ventilations as needed.
■ Circulation	Evaluate pulse rate and quality; observe skin color, temperature, and condition and treat accordingly. Determine if bleeding is present and control if life threatening.
■ Transport decision	Rapid transport
Focused History and Physical Exam	*NOTE: The order of the steps in the focused history and physical exam differs depending on whether the patient is conscious or unconscious. The order below is for a conscious patient. For an unconscious patient, perform a rapid physical exam, obtain vital signs, and obtain the history.*
■ SAMPLE history	Ask pertinent SAMPLE and OPQRST questions. Be sure to ask if and what interventions were taken before your arrival, how many interventions, and at what time.
■ Focused physical exam	Perform focused physical exam and ascertain if patient has taken any insulin or pills for diabetes. Has the patient been compliant with his or her diet and medications? Learn of any recent illness, physical activity, or stress. Determine the blood glucose level and Glasgow Coma Scale score.
■ Baseline vital signs	Take vital signs, noting skin color and temperature as well as patient's level of consciousness. Use pulse oximetry if available.
■ Interventions	A conscious patient who is able to swallow can be given fluids with a high sugar content, or a highly concentrated sugar gel as protocols allow.
Detailed Physical Exam	Complete a detailed physical exam.
Ongoing Assessment	Repeat the initial assessment and focused assessment, and reassess interventions performed. Reassess vital signs and blood glucose levels every 5 minutes for the unstable patient, every 15 minutes for the stable patient. Reassure and calm the patient.
■ Communication and documentation	Contact medical control with a radio report, informing patient's condition and blood glucose level(s). Relay any change in level of consciousness or difficulty breathing. Be sure to document any changes, at what time, and blood glucose readings.

NOTE: While the steps below are widely accepted, be sure to consult and follow your local protocol.

Diabetic Emergencies

Administering Glucose
1. Examine the tube to ensure that it is not open or broken. Check the expiration date.
2. Squeeze a generous amount onto the bottom third of a bite stick or tongue depressor.
3. Open the patient's mouth. Place the tongue depressor on the mucous membranes between the cheek and gum, with the gel side next to the cheek.

Prep Kit

Ready for Review

- Diabetes is a disorder of glucose metabolism or difficulty metabolizing carbohydrates, fats, and proteins.
- There are two types of diabetes. Type 1 diabetes, or insulin-dependent diabetes, usually starts in childhood and requires daily insulin to control blood glucose. Type 2 diabetes, or non-insulin-dependent diabetes, usually develops in middle age and often can be controlled with diet and oral medications.
- Both types of diabetes are significant diseases and can affect the kidneys, eyes, small arteries, and peripheral nerves.
- Patients with diabetes have chronic complications that place them at risk for other diseases such as heart attack, stroke, and infections. Most often, however, you will be called on to treat the acute complications of blood glucose imbalance. These include hyperglycemia (high blood glucose level) and hypoglycemia (low blood glucose level).
- Symptoms of hypoglycemia classically include confusion; rapid respirations; pale, moist skin; diaphoresis; dizziness; fainting; and even coma and seizures. This condition, called insulin shock, is rapidly reversible with the administration of glucose or sugar. Without treatment, however, permanent brain damage and death can occur.
- Hyperglycemia is usually associated with dehydration and ketoacidosis. It can result in diabetic coma, marked by rapid (often deep) respirations; warm, dry skin; a weak pulse; and a fruity breath odor. Hyperglycemia must be treated in the hospital with insulin and IV fluids.
- Because a blood glucose level that is too high or too low can result in altered mental status, you must perform a thorough history and patient assessment. When you cannot determine the nature of the problem, treat the patient for hypoglycemia.
- Administer oral glucose to a conscious patient who is confused or has slightly altered mental status. Do not give oral glucose to a patient who is unconscious or otherwise unable to swallow properly or protect his or her own airway.
- Remember that providing emergency medical care and prompt transport is your primary responsibility.

Vital Vocabulary

acidosis A pathologic condition resulting from the accumulation of acids in the body.

diabetes mellitus A metabolic disorder in which the ability to metabolize carbohydrates (sugars) is impaired, usually because of a lack of insulin.

diabetic coma Unconsciousness caused by dehydration, a very high blood glucose level, and acidosis in diabetes.

diabetic ketoacidosis (DKA) A form of acidosis in uncontrolled diabetes in which certain acids accumulate when insulin is not available.

glucose One of the basic sugars; it is the primary fuel, along with oxygen, for cellular metabolism.

hormone A chemical substance that regulates the activity of body organs and tissues; produced by a gland.

hyperglycemia Abnormally high glucose level in the blood.

hypoglycemia Abnormally low glucose level in the blood.

insulin A hormone produced by the islets of Langerhans (one of the endocrine parts of the pancreas) that enables glucose in the blood to enter the cells of the body; used in synthetic form to treat and control diabetes mellitus.

insulin shock Unconsciousness or altered mental status in a patient with diabetes, caused by significant hypoglycemia; usually the result of excessive exercise and activity or failure to eat after a routine dose of insulin.

Kussmaul respirations Deep, rapid breathing; usually the result of an accumulation of certain acids when insulin is not available in the body.

polydipsia Excessive thirst persisting for long periods despite reasonable fluid intake; often the result of excessive urination.

polyphagia Excessive eating; in diabetes, the inability to use glucose properly can cause a sense of hunger.

polyuria The passage of an unusually large volume of urine in a given period; in diabetes, this can result from wasting of glucose in the urine.

type 1 diabetes The type of diabetic disease that usually starts in childhood and requires insulin for proper treatment and control.

type 2 diabetes The type of diabetic disease that usually starts in later life and often can be controlled through diet and oral medications.

Technology

Interactivities

Vocabulary Explorer

Anatomy Review

Web Links

Online Review Manual

Refresher.EMSzone.com

Assessment in Action

A large number of calls at your EMS service are for diabetic emergencies. You and your partner decide to review so that you can provide the best possible care for your patients.

1. In diabetes mellitus, the body cannot metabolize glucose usually because of a lack of _____.
   - **A.** epinephrine
   - **B.** insulin
   - **C.** bile
   - **D.** oxygen

2. Diabetic coma may present with which of the following signs and symptoms?
   - **A.** rapid, weak pulse
   - **B.** normal or slightly low blood pressure
   - **C.** dehydration
   - **D.** all of the above

3. What is the problem in insulin shock?
   - **A.** hyperglycemia
   - **B.** increased glucose levels
   - **C.** hypoglycemia
   - **D.** too little insulin

4. Diabetes mellitus is considered what type of disease?
   - **A.** renal
   - **B.** optic
   - **C.** neuropathic
   - **D.** systemic

5. Seizures may be caused by _____.
   - **A.** increased oxygen levels
   - **B.** increased blood glucose levels
   - **C.** hypoglycemia
   - **D.** hyperglycemia

6. Which of the following organs is the only one that does not require insulin to use glucose?
   - **A.** heart
   - **B.** brain
   - **C.** liver
   - **D.** pancreas

Challenging Questions

7. Explain the cause of the "3 Ps" associated with diabetic ketoacidosis.

8. List the possible causes of insulin shock.

13

Allergic Reactions and Envenomations

You are the Provider 1

A call comes in for an individual with dyspnea at a restaurant very near your substation. You arrive on scene to find a 32-year-old woman who is flushed and complaining of some shortness of breath. She was eating lunch with her family when her chest began to feel tight and her husband noticed that her face was flushed.

Initial Assessment	Recording Time: 0 Minutes
Appearance	Flushed
Level of consciousness	Alert to person, place, and time
Airway	Open and clear
Breathing	Normal, a little rapid
Circulation	Radials present

1. What is your first concern?
2. What questions should you ask?
3. In what direction do the symptoms lead you?

■ Introduction

Every year, at least 1,000 Americans die of acute allergic reactions. In dealing with allergy-related emergencies, you must be aware of the possibility of acute airway obstruction and cardiovascular collapse and be prepared to treat these life-threatening complications. Your ability to recognize and manage the many signs and symptoms of allergic reactions may be the only thing standing between a patient's life and imminent death.

This chapter reviews the five most common substances that cause allergic reactions. You will learn what to look for in assessing patients who may be having an allergic reaction and how to care for them, including administration of epinephrine.

■ Allergic Reactions

An allergic reaction is an exaggerated immune response to any substance. The body's immune system releases chemicals (histamines and leukotrienes) to combat the stimulus. An allergic reaction may be mild and local, including hives, itching, or tenderness, or it may be severe and systemic, resulting in shock and respiratory failure.

Anaphylaxis is an extreme allergic reaction that is usually life threatening and typically involves multiple organ systems. In severe cases, anaphylaxis can rapidly result in death. Two of the most common signs of anaphylaxis are wheezing, a high-pitched, whistling breath sound usually resulting from bronchospasm and typically heard on expiration, and widespread hives (urticaria). Urticaria consists of small areas of generalized itching or burning that appear as multiple, small, raised areas on the skin.

Technology

Interactivities

Vocabulary Explorer

Anatomy Review

Web Links

Online Review Manual

Refresher.EMSzone.com

Almost any substance can trigger the body's immune system and cause an allergic reaction: animal bites, food, latex gloves, and many other substances can be allergens. The following five general categories are the most common allergens:

- **Insect bites and stings.** When an insect bites and injects the venom with its bite, the act is called envenomation or, more commonly, a sting. The sting of a honeybee, a wasp, an ant, a yellow jacket, or a hornet may cause a severe reaction. The reaction may be local, causing swelling and itchiness in the surrounding tissue, or it may be systemic, involving the entire body. Such a total body reaction would be considered an anaphylactic reaction.
- **Medications.** Injection of medications, such as penicillin, may cause an immediate (within 30 minutes) and severe allergic reaction Figure 13-1 ▶. Reactions to oral medications, such as oral penicillin, may be slower in onset (more than 30 minutes), but just as severe. The fact that a person has taken a medication once without experiencing an allergic reaction is no guarantee that he or she will not have an allergic reaction to it the next time around.
- **Plants.** People who inhale dusts, pollens, or other plant materials to which they are sensitive may experience a rapid and severe allergic reaction.
- **Food.** Eating certain foods, such as shellfish or nuts, may result in a relatively slow (more than 30 minutes) reaction that still can be quite severe. The person may be unaware of the exposure or what food caused the reaction.
- **Chemicals.** Certain chemicals, makeup, soap, latex, and various other substances can cause severe allergic reactions.

Insect Stings

There are more than 100,000 species of bees, wasps, and hornets. Deaths due to anaphylactic reactions to stinging insects far outnumber deaths due to snake bites. The stinging organ of most bees, wasps, yellow jackets, and hornets is a small hollow spine projecting from the abdomen. Venom can be injected through this spine directly into the skin. The stinger of the honeybee is barbed, so the bee cannot withdraw it. Therefore, the bee leaves a part of its abdomen embedded with the stinger and dies shortly after flying away. Wasps and hornets have no such handicap; they can sting repeatedly. Because these insects usually fly

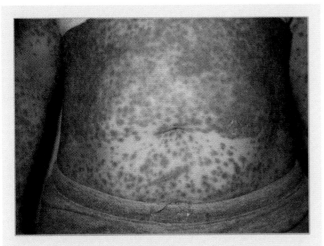

Figure 13-1 A severe allergic reaction to medication.

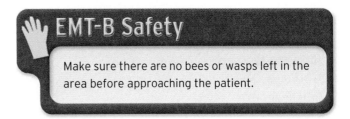

EMT-B Safety

Make sure there are no bees or wasps left in the area before approaching the patient.

away after stinging, it is often impossible to identify which species was responsible for the injury.

Some ants, especially the fire ant (*Formicoidea*), also strike repeatedly, often injecting a particularly irritating toxin, or poison, at the bite sites. It is common for a patient to sustain multiple ant bites, usually on the feet and legs Figure 13-2 ▾.

Signs and symptoms of insect stings or bites include sudden pain, swelling, localized heat, and redness in light-skinned people, usually at the site of

injury. There may be itching and sometimes a wheal, which is a raised, swollen, well-defined area on the skin Figure 13-3 ▶. There is no specific treatment for these injuries, although applying ice sometimes makes them less irritating. The swelling associated with an insect bite may be dramatic and sometimes frightening to patients, but it usually is not serious.

Because the stinger of the honeybee remains in the wound, it can continue to inject venom for up to 20 minutes after the bee has flown away. In caring for a patient who has been stung by a honeybee, you should gently attempt to remove the stinger by scraping the skin with the edge of a sharp, stiff object, such as a credit card Figure 13-4 ▶. Generally, you should not use tweezers or forceps because squeezing may cause the stinger to inject more venom into the wound. Gently wash the area with soap and water or a mild antiseptic. You should remove any jewelry from the area before swelling begins. Position the injection site slightly

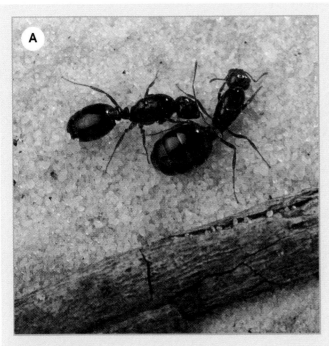

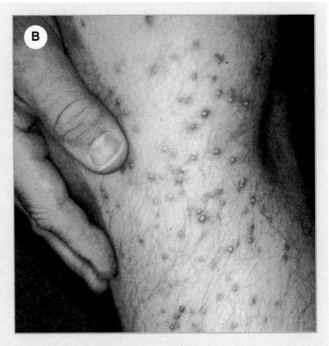

Figure 13-2 **A.** The fire ant. **B.** Fire ants inject an irritating toxin at multiple sites, usually on the feet and legs.

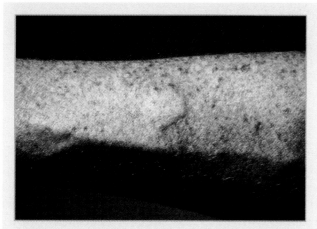

Figure 13-3 A wheal is a whitish, firm elevation of the skin that occurs after an insect sting or bite.

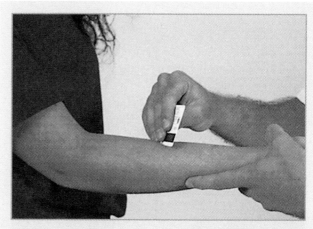

Figure 13-4 To remove the stinger of a honeybee, gently scrape the skin with the edge of a sharp, stiff object such as a credit card.

below the level of the heart, and apply ice or cold packs to the area, but not directly on the skin, to help relieve pain and slow the absorption of the toxin. Be alert for vomiting or any signs of shock or allergic reaction, and do not give the patient anything by mouth. Place the patient in the shock position, and give oxygen if needed. Monitor the patient's vital signs, and be prepared to provide further support as needed.

Anaphylactic Reaction to Stings

Approximately 5% of all people are allergic to the venom of the bee, hornet, yellow jacket, or wasp. This type of allergy, which accounts for about 200 deaths per year, can cause very severe reactions, including anaphylaxis. Patients may experience generalized itching and burning, widespread hives, swelling of the lips and tongue, bronchospasm and wheezing, chest tightness and coughing, dyspnea, anxiety, abdominal cramps, and hypotension. Occasionally, respiratory failure occurs. If untreated, such an anaphylactic reaction can proceed rapidly to death. In fact, more than two thirds of patients who die of anaphylaxis do so within the first half hour.

You are the Provider 2

While your partner is applying oxygen via a nonrebreathing mask at 15 L/m, her husband tells you that she is allergic to shellfish but is very careful not to eat any. She is not allergic to sulfites. They have been at the restaurant for about 35 minutes and she has eaten half of her dinner. The symptoms started shortly after they started the main course.

As you are assisting her onto the stretcher you note that she is scratching her arms and there appears to be some urticaria.

Vital Signs	Recording Time: 3 Minutes
Skin	Flushed, urticaria on the arms
Pulse	98 beats/min, regular
Blood pressure	122/74 mm Hg
Respirations	20 breaths/min, very slight distress

4. What else do you need to know?
5. Does she need pharmacologic intervention at this point?

Assessment of a Patient With an Allergic Reaction

Scene Size-up

The environment the patient is in or the activity he or she was performing may indicate the source of the reaction, such as a sting or bite from an insect, a food allergy at a restaurant, or a new medication. A respiratory problem reported by dispatch may be an allergic reaction. If many people are affected, it could be an inhaled poison or terrorist event. As you proceed to the patient, observe for safety threats to yourself and your partner and determine the number of patients at the scene. Gloves and eye protection should be the minimum BSI precautions. Call for additional resources as needed.

Initial Assessment

General Impression

Allergic reactions may present as respiratory distress or as cardiovascular distress in the form of shock. Patients experiencing a severe allergic reaction will often be very anxious and feel like they are going to die. If your first impression finds the person anxious and in distress, call for ALS backup if available. Some patients who are known to be severely allergic to bee stings, certain medications, or other substances wear a medical identification tag. If conscious, they will provide this information to you. Some may have even already taken their own medications. If they are unresponsive, immediately assess and treat airway, breathing, and circulation (ABCs).

Airway and Breathing

The most severe form of allergic reaction, anaphylaxis, can cause rapid swelling of the upper airway. You may have only a few minutes to assess the airway and provide lifesaving treatment. Remember that not all allergic reactions are anaphylactic reactions. Work quickly to assess the patient to determine the severity of the symptoms. Position the conscious patient in a sitting position, leaning forward. This position will help facilitate air entry into the lungs and may help the patient relax. Quickly listen to the lungs on each side of the chest. If wheezing is heard, the lower airways are also closing, preventing oxygen from entering the circulatory system. Do not hesitate to initiate high-flow oxygen therapy. You may have to assist with ventilation for a patient with a severe allergic reaction. This can be done in a semiresponsive or unresponsive patient. The positive-pressure ventilation you provide will force air through the swelling in the throat and into the lungs while you are waiting for more

You are the Provider 3

Your partner asks about an EpiPen and the patient tells him that she has one in her purse. He asks her husband to get it for him.

After checking with the restaurant manager you find out that the pasta salad she was eating has crab in it. You note that her breathing is becoming a little more distressed and you hear stridor. She is also becoming confused and lethargic and she is pale and diaphoretic.

Reassessment	Recording Time: 6 Minutes
Pulse	116 beats/min, thready
Blood pressure	106/54 mm Hg
Respirations	24 breaths/min, shallow
Breath sounds	Bilateral wheezing
Pulse oximetry	95% on oxygen via nonrebreathing mask

6. What must you do before assisting with the EpiPen?
7. What should you verify before assisting with any medication?
8. How is an EpiPen administered?
9. What side effects do you expect?
10. What are the indications for administering the EpiPen?

definitive treatment. In severe situations, the definitive care needed is an injection of epinephrine.

Circulation

While respiratory complaints are most common, some patients in anaphylaxis may not present with severe respiratory symptoms, but primarily with signs and symptoms of a cardiovascular emergency. Palpating a radial pulse will help identify how the circulatory system is responding to the reaction. If the patient is unresponsive and does not have a pulse, follow your protocol for CPR and AED. Hypoperfusion may be present if you assess and find a rapid heart rate and skin that is pale, cool, and moist. Your initial treatment for shock should include oxygen, the shock position, and maintaining normal body temperature. The definitive treatment for anaphylactic shock is epinephrine.

Transport Decision

Always provide prompt transport for any patient who may be having an allergic reaction. Take with you all medications and auto-injectors the patient has. Make your transport decision based on findings in the initial assessment. If the patient has signs of respiratory distress or shock, treat those conditions and transport. If the patient is calm and has no signs of respiratory distress or shock after contact with a substance that causes an allergic reaction, continue with the focused history and physical exam.

Focused History and Physical Exam

If the allergic reaction has left the patient unresponsive, perform a rapid physical exam to determine hidden trauma or other problems and then obtain the vital signs and history. If the patient is responsive, begin with obtaining the SAMPLE history and asking questions specific to an allergic reaction. Find out what interventions have been completed. Find out whether the patient has any prescribed medications for allergic reactions (such as an EpiPen or an inhaler). After obtaining the necessary history, perform a focused physical exam to look for bee stingers or contact with chemicals and other indications of a reaction. Finish by obtaining a complete set of vital signs.

SAMPLE History

Obtain a SAMPLE history. Areas to focus on with a possible allergic reaction may include the following:

- **Symptoms:** Any respiratory involvement is significant because a patient's condition can

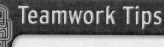

Teamwork Tips

While one EMT-B is assessing the patient and applying oxygen, the second EMT-B should obtain the patient's EpiPen and check that it is prescribed for the patient, in date, and obtain permission from medical control to assist with the medication.

rapidly deteriorate. Other signs and symptoms may include itching, rash, hives, bite or sting marks, or altered mental status.

- **Allergies:** Patients may have a history of the specific allergy involved in this case or of other allergies.
- **Medications:** Patients who have had severe allergic reactions in the past may carry an epinephrine auto-injector or antihistamines (diphenhydramine [Benadryl]) or chlorpheniramine (found in an AnaKit) or an inhaler such as albuterol.
- **Past medical history:** Ask about previous allergic reactions, asthma, and hospitalizations.
- **Last oral intake:** Find out what and when your patient ate last. This information may help you determine the cause of the reaction. Peanuts, chocolate, and shellfish can be potent allergens.
- **Events:** Determine what the patient was doing and what he or she was exposed to before the onset of symptoms.

Focused Physical Exam

Your assessment of the patient experiencing an allergic reaction should include the respiratory system, circulatory system, mental status, and the skin. Assess for altered mental status, which may be the result of hypoxia or systemic shock. Thoroughly assess breathing, including any increased work of breathing or accessory muscle use. Listen to lung sounds.

Wheezing occurs because of narrowing of the air passages, which is mainly due to contraction of muscles around the bronchioles in reaction to the allergen. Exhalation, normally the passive, relaxed part of breathing, becomes more difficult as the patient tries to cough up the secretions or move air past the constricted airways. The fluid in the air passages and the constricted bronchi together produce the wheezing sound. Prolonged respiratory distress can cause a rapid heartbeat (tachycardia), shock, and even death. Stridor, a harsh, high-pitched inspiratory sound, occurs when swelling in the upper airway (near the vocal cords and throat) closes off the airway; the swelling can eventually lead to total obstruction.

Remember, the presence of hypoperfusion (shock) or respiratory distress indicates that the patient is having a severe life-threatening allergic reaction. Common signs and symptoms of an allergic reaction are listed in Table 13-1 ▾. Carefully assess the skin for swelling, rash, hives, or signs of the source of the reaction: bite, sting, or contact marks. A rapidly spreading rash may indicate a systemic reaction. Red, hot skin may also indicate a systemic reaction as the blood ves-

sels lose their ability to constrict and blood moves to the extremities.

Baseline Vital Signs

Vital signs help determine how the body is compensating. Assess baseline vital signs. Rapid, labored breathing indicates airway obstruction. Rapid respiratory and heart rates may indicate respiratory distress or systemic shock. Fast pulse and hypotension are ominous signs, indicating systemic vascular collapse and shock. Changes in skin color, temperature, and condition (moist or dry) may be an unreliable indicator of hypoperfusion because of rashes and swelling.

Interventions

Some allergic reactions will produce severe signs and symptoms in a matter of minutes and threaten the patient's life. Others will have a slower onset and cause less severe distress. Epinephrine and ventilatory support are required for severe reactions. Milder reactions, without respiratory or cardiovascular distress, may only require supportive care, such as oxygen.

Detailed Physical Exam

Consider performing a detailed physical exam if the patient presents with a confusing history or complaint, if there is an extended transport time, or if there is a need to clarify findings from earlier in the assessment. In severe reactions, a detailed physical exam may be omitted when time must be spent managing ABCs or when transport distances are short.

Ongoing Assessment

The patient experiencing a suspected allergic reaction should be closely monitored because deterioration of the patient's condition can be rapid and fatal. Special attention should be given to any signs of airway compromise, including increasing work of breathing, stridor, and wheezing. Also, watch the skin for signs of shock, including pallor and diaphoresis, and for flushing due to vascular collapse. Serial vital signs are important in monitoring your patient's status. Any increase in the respiratory or heart rate or decrease in blood pressure should be noted.

If you administered epinephrine, what was the effect? Is the patient's condition improving? Do you need to consider giving a second dose? You may need to give more than one injection of epinephrine if you note that the patient has decreasing mental status, increased breathing difficulty, or decreasing blood

Table 13-1 Common Signs and Symptoms of Allergic Reaction

Respiratory System
- Sneezing or an itchy, runny nose (initially)
- Tightness in the chest or throat
- Irritating, persistent dry cough
- Hoarseness
- Respirations that become rapid, labored, or noisy
- Wheezing and/or stridor

Circulatory System
- Decrease in blood pressure as the blood vessels dilate
- Increase in pulse rate (initially)
- Pale skin and dizziness as the vascular system fails
- Loss of consciousness and coma

Skin
- Flushing, itching, or burning skin; especially common over the face and upper part of the chest
- Urticaria over large areas of the body, both internally and externally
- Swelling, especially of the face, neck, hands, feet, and/or tongue
- Swelling and cyanosis or pallor around the lips
- Warm, tingling feeling in the face, mouth, chest, feet, and hands

Other Findings
- Anxiety; a sense of impending doom
- Abdominal cramps
- Headache
- Itchy, watery eyes
- Decreasing mental status

Documentation Tips

Document the medication given, the route, the time, the dosage, the site, and any response whether positive or negative.

pressure. Be sure to consult medical control first. Current auto-injectors give only one dose, and a patient who needs more than one dose will need to have more than one injector. Any patient in critical condition should have his or her vital signs taken at least every 5 minutes.

Communication and Documentation

When to contact medical control depends on your assessment findings and the urgency of care required. In some allergic reactions, you may use standing orders to administer epinephrine before calling medical control. At other times, the reaction may be less severe and you may question whether the patient needs an injection of epinephrine. Follow your local protocols, which may guide you in providing lifesaving care without needing to contact medical control.

Your documentation not only should include the signs and symptoms found during your assessment, but also should clearly show why you chose to provide the care you did. Be complete in your documentation, including not only assessment findings and treatment, but also the patient's response to your treatment.

◼ Emergency Medical Care

If the patient appears to be having a severe allergic (or anaphylactic) reaction, you should provide immediate emergency medical care and prompt transport.

You may want to request ALS backup if you work in a tiered response system. In addition to providing oxygen, you should be prepared to manage the patient's airway. Placing ice over the injury site has been thought to slow absorption of the toxin and diminish swelling, but ice packs placed directly on the skin may freeze it and cause more damage. Like any other attempt to reduce swelling with ice, you should be careful not to overdo the icing. In some EMS systems, you may be allowed to administer epinephrine or assist the patient with epinephrine administration.

Epinephrine works rapidly to raise the pulse rate and blood pressure by constricting the blood vessels. Epinephrine also inhibits the allergic reaction and dilates the bronchioles. All bee-sting kits should contain a prepared syringe of epinephrine, ready for intramuscular injection, along with instructions for its use. Your EMS service may or may not allow you to help patients self-administer epinephrine. In some places, the medical director may authorize you to carry an epinephrine auto-injector (EpiPen) or to assist patients who have their own EpiPen. The adult system delivers 0.3 mg of epinephrine via an automatic needle and syringe system; the infant–child system delivers 0.15 mg Figure 13-5 ▶ .

If the patient is able to use the auto-injector on his or her own, your role is limited to helping. To use, or help the patient use, the auto-injector, you should first receive a direct order from medical control or follow local protocols or standing orders. Follow BSI precautions, and make sure the medication has been prescribed specifically for that patient. If it has not, do not give the medication: inform medical control, support the ABCs, and provide immediate transport. Finally, make sure the medication is not discolored and that the expiration date has not passed. See **Skill Drill 8-1** to review the steps in using the EpiPen auto-injector.

You are the Provider 4

You receive orders from medical control to assist her with her EpiPen. After administration you reassess vital signs every 5 minutes. You call medical control to update the patient's condition and your estimated time of arrival.

On arrival at the emergency department, the patient is breathing fine and the urticaria is better. Her mental status is normal.

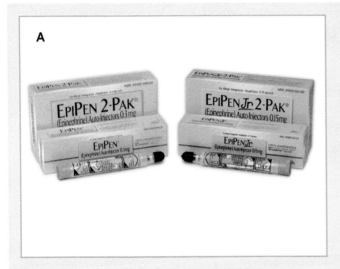
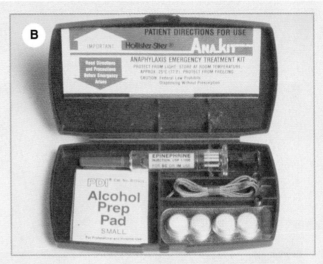

Figure 13-5 Patients who experience severe allergic reactions often carry their own epinephrine, which comes predosed in an auto-injector or a standard syringe. **A.** EpiPen auto-injectors. **B.** AnaKit with epinephrine syringe.

If the patient has a medical history of severe allergic reactions, he or she might carry a commercial bee-sting kit (AnaKit) that contains a standard syringe of epinephrine for intramuscular injection. Be sure to review your local protocol, some EMS systems only allow EMT-Bs to administer epinephrine with an auto-injector. If you are authorized to administer an AnaKit, take the same general precautions as for an auto-injector: Confirm medical control authorization, take BSI precautions. Make sure the medicine belongs to your patient, that it is not discolored, and the expiration date has not passed. Follow the steps in ▶ **Skill Drill 13-1** ▶ to administer epinephrine from an AnaKit.

1. **Prepare the injection site** with an alcohol wipe or other antiseptic, if there is time. Remove the needle cover (**Step ①**).
2. **Hold the syringe upright** so any air inside rises to the base of the needle. Remove the air by depressing the syringe plunger until it stops (**Step ②**).
3. **Turn the plunger** one-quarter turn (**Step ③**).
4. **Insert the needle quickly,** straight into the injection site, deep enough to place the tip into the muscle beneath the skin and subcutaneous fat (**Step ④**).
5. **Holding the syringe steady,** push the plunger until it stops, to ensure that all medication is injected (**Step ⑤**).

6. **Have the patient chew and swallow the Chlo-Amine antihistamine tablets** in the kit (**Step ⑥**).
7. If you have or can **make a cold pack,** apply it to the site of the sting to reduce swelling and minimize the amount of venom that enters the circulation (**Step ⑦**). The syringe from the AnaKit holds a second injection if needed.

Other bee-sting kits contain some oral or intramuscular antihistamines. These work relatively slowly, within several minutes to 1 hour. Because epinephrine can have an effect within 1 minute, it is the primary way to save the life of someone having a severe anaphylactic reaction.

In some areas of the country, EMT-B squads can administer epinephrine for anaphylaxis. Follow your local protocols or medical direction. Be aware that epinephrine may cause significant tachycardia and increased anxiety or nervousness and palpitations.

Epinephrine constricts blood vessels and may cause the patient's blood pressure to rise significantly. Other side effects include tachycardia, pallor, dizziness, chest pain, headache, nausea, and vomiting. All these effects may cause the patient to feel anxious or excited. In life-threatening situations, the risk of these side effects is acceptable. Patients who are not wheezing or who have no signs of respiratory compromise or hypotension should not be given epinephrine.

Skill Drill 13-1   Using an AnaKit

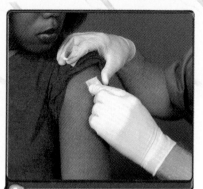

1 Prepare the injection site with antiseptic, and remove the needle cover.

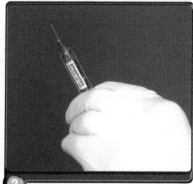

2 Hold the syringe upright, and carefully use the plunger to remove air.

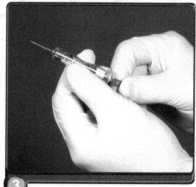

3 Turn the plunger one-quarter turn.

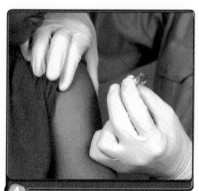

4 Quickly insert the needle into the muscle.

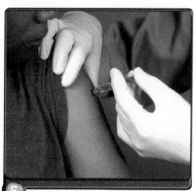

5 Hold the syringe steady, and push the plunger until it stops.

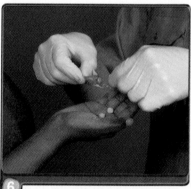

6 Have the patient chew and swallow the Chlo-Amine antihistamine tablets provided in the kit.

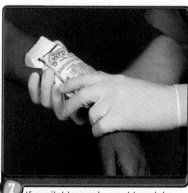

7 If available, apply a cold pack to the sting site.

You are the Provider Summary

Early recognition and pharmacologic intervention are essential when treating a patient having an allergic reaction. You must treat aggressively to prevent the airway from closing and cardiovascular collapse.

1. **What is your first concern?**

   Airway. The airway may close quickly in a patient experiencing an allergic reaction.

2. **What questions should you ask?**

   What was she doing when this started? Does she have any medical problems? Is she allergic to anything? What was she doing before coming to the restaurant? What has she eaten?

3. **In what direction do the symptoms lead you?**

   Possible allergic reaction. A sudden onset of dyspnea and facial flushing should lead you to think she has been exposed to something to which she is allergic.

4. **What else do you need to know?**

   Does she have an EpiPen?

5. **Does she need pharmacologic intervention at this point?**

   Yes. She is experiencing dyspnea, facial flushing, hives, and her pulse is a little elevated.

6. **What must you do before assisting with the EpiPen?**

   Obtain permission from medical control.

7. **What should you verify before assisting with any medication?**

   That it is the proper medication, it is prescribed for the patient, it is not expired, and that you have permission to assist with the medication.

8. **How is an EpiPen administered?**

   It is an intramuscular injection given at a 90° angle in the lateral aspect of the upper arm or the lateral thigh.

9. **What side effects do you expect?**

   Tachycardia, pallor, dizziness, chest pain, headache, nausea, and vomiting

Assessment and Emergency Care

Allergic Reactions

Scene Size-up	Body substance isolation precautions should include a minimum of gloves and eye protection. Ensure scene safety, and determine NOI/MOI. Consider the number of patients, the need for additional help/ALS, and cervical spine stabilization.
Initial Assessment	
■ General impression	Determine level of consciousness, and find and treat any immediate threats to life. Determine priority of care based on environment and patient's chief complaint. If the patient appears anxious or fears death, call for ALS assistance.
■ Airway	Ensure patent airway.
■ Breathing	Provide high-flow oxygen at 15 L/min. If possible, place patient in a tripod position and evaluate depth and rate of the respiratory cycle, and provide ventilatory support as needed.
■ Circulation	Evaluate pulse rate and quality; observe skin color, temperature, and condition, and treat accordingly.
■ Transport decision	Rapid transport
Focused History and Physical Exam	*NOTE: The order of the steps in the focused history and physical exam differs depending on whether the patient is conscious or unconscious. The order below is for a conscious patient. For an unconscious patient, perform a rapid physical exam, obtain vital signs, and obtain the history.*
■ SAMPLE history	Ask SAMPLE questions and determine if patient has prescribed auto-injector(s)/inhaler. Be sure to ask if and what interventions were taken before your arrival, how many interventions were performed, and at what time.
■ Focused physical exam	Perform focused physical exam, keying in on the respiratory drive, adequate ventilation, the adequacy and effectiveness of the circulatory system, and the patient's mental status.
■ Baseline vital signs	Take vital signs, noting skin color and temperature and the patient's level of consciousness. Use pulse oximetry if available.
■ Interventions	Support patient as needed. Consider the use of oxygen, positive pressure ventilation, adjuncts, and proper positioning of the patient. Assist with the use of auto-injector(s) or inhaler as defined by local protocol.
Detailed Physical Exam	Consider a detailed physical exam.
Ongoing Assessment	Repeat the initial assessment and focused assessment, and reassess interventions performed. Reassess vital signs every 5 minutes for a patient in unstable condition and every 15 minutes for a patient in stable condition. Note and treat the patient as necessary.
■ Communication and documentation	Contact medical control with a radio report, providing information on the patient's condition. Relay any significant changes, including level of consciousness or difficulty in breathing. Be sure to document any changes, at what time, and any interventions performed.

NOTE: While the steps below are widely accepted, be sure to consult and follow your local protocol.

Allergic Reations

Using an AnaKit

1. Prepare the injection site with antiseptic, and remove the needle cover.
2. Hold the syringe upright, and carefully use the plunger to remove air.
3. Turn the plunger one-quarter turn.
4. Quickly insert the needle into the muscle.
5. Hold the syringe steady, and push the plunger until it stops.
6. Have the patient chew and swallow the Chlo-Amine antihistamine tablets provided in the kit.
7. If available, apply a cold pack to the sting site.

Prep Kit

Ready for Review

- An allergic reaction is a response to chemicals the body releases to combat allergens.
- Allergic reactions occur most often in response to insect bites and stings, medications, food, plants, and chemicals.
- The reaction may be mild and local, involving itching, redness, and tenderness, or it may be severe and systemic, including shock and respiratory failure.
- Anaphylaxis is a life-threatening allergic reaction mounted by multiple organ systems, which must be treated with epinephrine.
- Wheezing and skin wheals can be signs of anaphylaxis.
- People who know that they are allergic to bee, hornet, yellow jacket, or wasp venom often carry a bee-sting kit that contains epinephrine in an auto-injector. You may help administer this medication in this form with authorization from medical control.
- All patients with suspected anaphylaxis require oxygen.
- In assessing a person who may be having an allergic reaction, you should check for flushing, itching and swelling skin, hives, wheezing and stridor, cough, a decrease in blood pressure, a weak pulse, dizziness, abdominal cramps, and headache.
- Always provide prompt transport to the hospital for any patient who is having an allergic reaction. Remember that signs and symptoms can rapidly become more severe. Carefully monitor the patient's vital signs en route, especially for airway compromise.

Vital Vocabulary

allergens Substances that cause allergic reactions.

allergic reaction The body's exaggerated immune response to an internal or surface agent.

anaphylaxis An extreme, possibly life-threatening systemic allergic reaction that may include shock and respiratory failure.

stridor A harsh, high-pitched respiratory sound, generally heard during inspiration, that is caused by partial blockage or narrowing of the upper airway.

toxin A poison or harmful substance.

wheezing A high-pitched, whistling breath sound, usually caused by a constriction of the smaller tubes of the lungs and typically heard on expiration.

Technology

- Interactivities
- Vocabulary Explorer
- Anatomy Review
- Web Links
- Online Review Manual

Refresher.EMSzone.com

Assessment in Action

As an EMT-B you may be called on to help administer medications for allergic reactions. You must be familiar with the indications, contraindications, side effects, adverse reactions, and possible antidotes. You must also recognize the signs and symptoms associated with allergic reactions and treat patients properly and at times, aggressively.

1. Two of the most common signs of anaphylaxis are wheezing and _____.
   A. hypotension
   B. urticaria
   C. abdominal pain
   D. bradycardia

2. Wheezing is the result of:
   A. swelling in the upper airway.
   B. pulmonary hypoperfusion.
   C. tachypnea and tachycardia.
   D. narrowing of the air passages.

3. Assess the skin for signs of shock, including _____.
   A. pallor
   B. diaphoresis
   C. flushing
   D. all of the above

4. The dose of epinephrine in an adult EpiPen is how many milligrams?
   A. 0.15 mg
   B. 0.3 mg
   C. 1.5 mg
   D. 3.0 mg

5. Common allergens include _____.
   A. insect bites and stings
   B. plants
   C. chemicals
   D. all of the above

6. When treating a sting from a honeybee, you should:
   A. remove the stinger with a credit card.
   B. wash the area with soap and water.
   C. apply cold packs to the area.
   D. all of the above.

Challenging Questions

7. Describe the procedure for using an AnaKit.

14

Substance Abuse and Poisoning

You are called to a residence for a possible accidental ingestion of iron by a 2-year-old girl. The hysterical mother meets you at the door with an empty prescription bottle and tells you that she found the girl in the kitchen with a bottle of her 5-year-old child's chocolate-flavored iron pills. The top was off the bottle and some were scattered on the floor. She took one out of the child's mouth.

Initial Assessment	Recording Time: 0 Minutes
Appearance	Flushed, crying
Level of consciousness	Alert and oriented
Airway	Open and clear
Breathing	Rapid, good tidal volume
Circulation	Strong radials

1. What questions should you ask the mother?
2. What is the primary treatment goal for this patient?
3. How is this accomplished?

■ Introduction

Acute poisoning affects some 5 million children and adults each year. Chronic poisoning, often caused by abuse of medications and other substances, including tobacco and alcohol, is much more common. Fortunately, deaths due to poisoning are fairly rare. Rates of death due to poisoning in children have decreased steadily since the 1960s, when safety caps were introduced for drug bottles and containers. Deaths due to poisoning in adults, though, have been rising, the majority the result of drug abuse.

This chapter reviews how to identify a patient who has been poisoned and how to obtain information about the poison. It describes the different ways in which poison is introduced into the body. It then discusses the signs, symptoms, and treatment of specific poisonings and overdoses, including some drugs that are abused (sedatives and opioids—medicines with actions similar to morphine).

■ Identifying the Patient and the Poison

A poison is any substance with a chemical action that can damage body structures or impair body function. Poisons act by changing the normal metabolism of cells or by actually destroying them. Poisons may act acutely, as in an overdose of heroin, or chronically, as in years of alcohol or other substance abuse. Substance abuse is the misuse of any substance to produce a desired effect (for example, methamphetamine use).

Remember that very small amounts of some poisons can cause considerable damage or death. Signs

and symptoms of poisoning vary according to the specific agent, as shown in Table 14-1 ▼. Some poisons cause the pulse to speed up, while others cause it to slow down; some cause the pupils to dilate, while others cause the pupils to constrict. Some chemical compounds will irritate or burn the skin or mucous membranes. The presence of such injuries at the mouth strongly suggests the ingestion (swallowing) of a poison.

Consider asking the suspected poisoning patient the following questions:

- What substance did you take?
- When did you take it (or become exposed to it)?

Refresher.EMSzone.com

Technology

Interactivities
Vocabulary Explorer
Anatomy Review
Web Links
Online Review Manual

Table 14-1 Toxidromes: Typical Signs and Symptoms of Specific Drug Overdoses

Drug	Signs and Symptoms
Opioid (Examples: heroin, oxycodone)	■ Hypoventilation or respiratory arrest ■ Pinpoint pupils ■ Sedation or coma ■ Hypotension
Sympathomimetics (Examples: epinephrine, albuterol, cocaine, methamphetamine)	■ Hypertension ■ Tachycardia ■ Dilated pupils ■ Agitation or seizures ■ Hyperthermia
Sedative-hypnotics (Examples: diazepam [Valium], secobarbital [Seconal], flunitrazepam [Rohypnol])	■ Slurred speech ■ Sedation or coma ■ Hypoventilation ■ Hypotension
Anticholinergics (Examples: atropine, Jimson weed)	■ Tachycardia ■ Hyperthermia ■ Hypertension ■ Dilated pupils ■ Dry skin and mucous membranes ■ Sedation, agitation, seizures, coma, or delirium ■ Decreased bowel sounds
Cholinergics (Examples: cimetidine, pilocarpine, nerve gas)	■ Excess defecation or urination ■ Muscle fasciculations ■ Pinpoint pupils ■ Excess lacrimation (tearing) or salivation ■ Airway compromise ■ Nausea or vomiting

- How much did you ingest?
- What actions have been taken?

Try to determine what substance is involved. Objects at the scene may provide clues: an overturned bottle, a needle or syringe, scattered pills, chemicals, even an overturned or damaged plant. The remains of any nearby food or drink may also be important. Place any suspicious material in a plastic bag and take it to the hospital.

Containers can provide critical information. In addition to the name and concentration of the drug, a pill bottle label may list specific ingredients, the number of pills that were originally in the bottle, the name of the manufacturer, and the dose that was prescribed. This information can help emergency department physicians determine how much has been ingested and what specific treatment may be required. For certain food poisonings, a food container that lists the name and location of the maker or the vendor may be of equal importance in saving

the life of the patient. If the patient vomits, examine the contents for pill fragments. Note anything unusual that you see. You may collect the vomitus in a separate plastic bag so that it can be analyzed at the hospital.

■ How Poisons Enter the Body

Emergency care for a patient who has been poisoned or overdosed usually does not include administering a specific antidote. Most substances do not have one. In general, the most important treatment for poisoning is diluting and/or physically removing the poisonous agent. How this is accomplished depends on how the poison entered the patient's body. The four routes to consider are:

- Inhalation Figure 14-1A ▾
- Absorption (surface contact) Figure 14-1B ▾
- Ingestion Figure 14-1C ▾
- Injection Figure 14-1D ▾

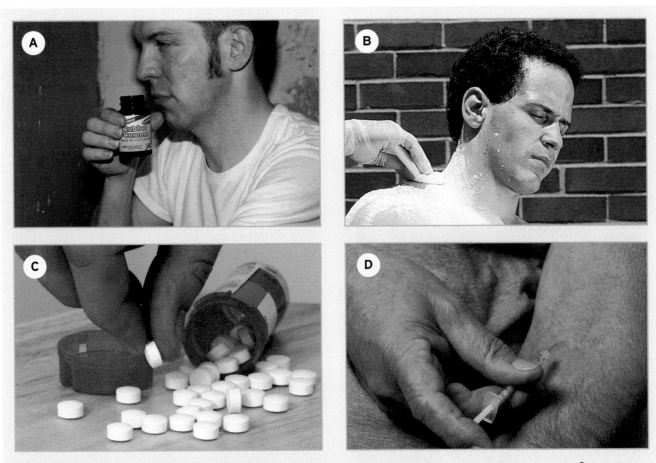

Figure 14-1 There are four routes by which a poison can enter the body. **A.** Inhalation. **B.** Absorption (surface contact). **C.** Ingestion. **D.** Injection.

Injection may be the most significant route of poisoning because it is difficult to remove or dilute injected poisons. You can administer oxygen to a patient who has inhaled a poison. You can give activated charcoal to a patient who has ingested a poison, and you can flood the skin with water and wash out the eyes of one who has contacted a poison. However, all routes of poisoning are potentially fatal.

Inhaled Poisons

Patients who have any type of toxic inhalation should be moved to fresh air immediately **Figure 14-2 ▼**. Most patients will require supplemental oxygen. If you are not specifically trained in the use of an SCBA (self-contained breathing apparatus) or do not have appropriately fit-tested equipment available, do not enter the scene. Patients may need to be decontaminated

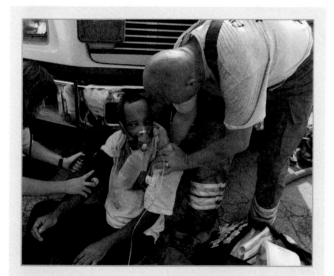

Figure 14-2 Patients who have inhaled poisons need supplemental oxygen and prompt transport to the emergency department.

by HazMat personnel before you can assess and treat them.

Some inhaled poisons, such as carbon monoxide, are odorless and produce severe hypoxia without damaging or even irritating the lungs. Others, such as chlorine, are very irritating and cause airway obstruction and pulmonary edema. The patient may have the following signs and symptoms: burning eyes, sore throat, cough, chest pain, hoarseness, wheezing, respiratory distress, dizziness, confusion, headache, or, in severe cases, stridor. The patient may also have seizures or altered mental status. Some inhaled agents cause progressive lung damage, even after the patient has been removed from direct exposure (the damage may not be evident for a few hours). All patients who have inhaled poison require treatment and immediate transport to an emergency department. Be prepared to use supplemental oxygen via nonrebreathing mask and/or provide bag-mask ventilation. Make sure a suctioning unit is available in case the patient vomits. As with other poisonings, it is helpful to take the containers, bottles, and labels when you transport the patient to the hospital.

Absorbed and Surface Contact Poisons

Poisons that come in contact with the surface of the body can affect the patient in many ways. Many corrosive substances will damage the skin, mucous membranes, or eyes, causing chemical burns, telltale rashes, or lesions. Acids, alkalis, and some petroleum (hydrocarbon) products are very destructive. Other substances are absorbed into the bloodstream through the skin and have systemic effects, just like medications or drugs that are swallowed or injected. Poison ivy or poison oak may just cause an itchy rash without being dangerous to health. It is important to distinguish between contact burns and contact absorption.

Signs and symptoms of absorbed poisoning include a history of exposure, liquid or powder on a patient's skin, burns, itching, irritation, redness of the skin, and typical odors of the substance.

The two general guidelines in providing treatment for a contact poisoning are:

1. Avoid contaminating yourself or others.
2. Remove the irritating or corrosive substance from the patient as rapidly as possible.

Remove all clothing that has been contaminated, thoroughly brush off any dry chemicals, flush the skin with running water, and then wash the skin with soap and water. When a large amount of material has been spilled on a patient, flooding the affected part for at

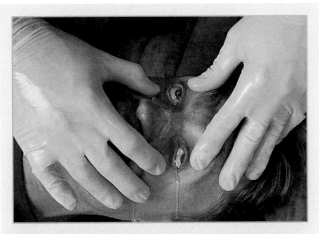

Figure 14-3 If chemical agents are in the patient's eyes, irrigate the eyes quickly and thoroughly, ensuring that the irrigation fluid runs from the bridge of the nose outward. (Use of a nasal cannula is pictured.)

least 20 minutes may be the fastest and most effective treatment. If the patient has a chemical agent in the eyes, you should irrigate them quickly and thoroughly, at least 5 to 10 minutes for acid substances and 15 to 20 minutes for alkaline substances. To avoid contaminating the other eye, make sure that the fluid runs from the bridge of the nose outward Figure 14-3 ▲ .

Many chemical burns occur in industrial settings, where showers and specific protocols for handling surface burns are available. There are usually trained people there to assist you. Do not spend time trying to neutralize substances on the skin with additional chemicals because this may actually be more harmful. Instead, wash the substance off immediately with plenty of water. Obtain material safety data sheets from industrial sites and, if available, transport them with the patient.

The only time you should not irrigate the contact area with water is when a poison reacts violently with water, such as contamination with phosphorus or elemental sodium. These substances ignite when they come into contact with water. Instead, brush the chemical off the patient, remove contaminated clothing, and apply a dry dressing to the burn area. Be sure to wear appropriate protective gloves and clothing. Provide prompt transport to the emergency department for definitive care. En route, continue irrigation and provide oxygen if needed.

Ingested Poisons

Approximately 80% of all poisoning is by mouth (ingestion). Ingested poisons include liquids, household cleaners, contaminated food, plants, and, in the majority of cases, drugs. Ingested poisoning is usually accidental in children and, except for contaminated food, intentional in adults. Plant poisonings are common among children, who like to explore and often bite the leaves of the plants.

Your goal as an EMT-B is to rapidly remove as much of the poison as possible from the gastrointestinal tract. Many EMS systems carry activated charcoal to treat patients who have ingested a poison. Activated charcoal comes as a suspension that binds to the poison in the stomach and carries it out of the system. Because activated charcoal is a black, thick fluid, you may have to do some coaxing to get the patient to drink it. Try to give it to the patient in a covered cup with a straw. Remember, you should never force this (or any other) liquid into a patient's mouth.

Although every poison will result in a specific set of signs and symptoms, you should always assess the airway, breathing, and circulation (ABCs) of every patient who has been poisoned. Many patients have died as a result of problems with the ABCs that might have been managed easily. Be prepared to provide aggressive ventilatory support and CPR to a patient who has ingested an opiate, sedative, or barbiturate, each of which can cause depression of the central nervous system (CNS) and slow breathing. Whenever poisoning is involved, you should provide prompt transport to the emergency department. If you work in a tiered system, ALS backup also may be appropriate.

Injected Poisons

Poisoning by injection is usually the result of drug abuse, such as heroin, cocaine, or methamphetamine Figure 14-4 ▶ . Signs and symptoms of poisoning by injection include weakness, dizziness, fever, chills, diaphoresis, increased body temperature, unresponsiveness, and respiratory depression.

In general, injected poisons are impossible to dilute or remove because they are usually absorbed quickly into the body or cause intense local tissue destruction. If you suspect poisoning by injection, monitor the patient's airway, provide high-flow oxygen, and be alert for nausea and vomiting. Remove rings, watches, and bracelets from areas around the injection site if swelling occurs. Prompt transport to the emergency department is essential. Take all containers, bottles, and labels with the patient to the hospital.

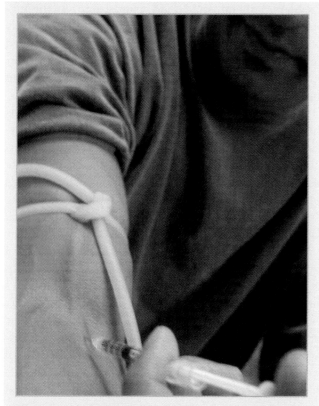

Figure 14-4 Injected poisons are impossible to dilute or remove from the body in the field; therefore, prompt transport to the emergency department is critical.

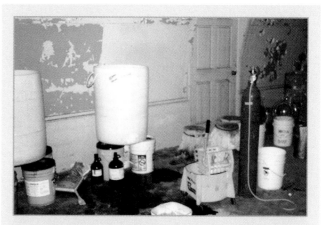

Figure 14-5 A laboratory capable of producing large quantities of methamphetamine.

■ Assessment for Poisonings and Overdoses

Because of the risk of possible cross-contamination by poisons that can be inhaled, ingested, and injected, you must take appropriate BSI precautions. Use the appropriate personal protective equipment necessary to avoid being contaminated.

Scene Size-up

This is a situation in which a well-trained dispatcher is of great value. Dispatchers with an appropriate set of protocols and excellent interrogation skills can obtain important information pertaining to a poisoning call that will help anticipate the proper protection needed to ensure safety. The dispatcher may be able to obtain information pertaining to the number of patients involved, whether additional resources are needed, and whether trauma is involved. You must take the time to assess the scene thoroughly to ensure safety and to determine the nature of the illness, the number of patients involved, the need for additional resources, and whether spinal stabilization is required.

As you approach the scene, you should look for clues that might indicate the substance and/or poison involved.

- Are there medicine bottles lying around the patient and scene? If so, is there medication missing that might indicate an overdose?
- Are there alcoholic beverage containers present?
- Are there syringes or other drug paraphernalia on the scene?
- Is there an unpleasant or odd odor in the room? If so, is the scene safe?

A suspicious odor and/or drug paraphernalia may indicate the presence of a drug laboratory. Drug laboratories can be very volatile, so ensure scene safety Figure 14-5 ▲ . Conducting a scene size-up will help ensure safety, help determine the appropriate actions you need to take, and ensure that patient care begins successfully.

Initial Assessment
General Impression

By obtaining a general impression of the patient, chief complaint, apparent life threats, and level of consciousness, you are trying to determine the severity of the patient's condition. With substance abuse and poisonings, do not be complacent about a conscious, alert, and oriented patient who seems to be in stable condition and has no apparent life threats. The patient may have a harmful or even lethal amount of poison in his or her system that has not had time to produce systemic reactions. An initial assessment that reveals a patient with signs of distress and/or altered mental status gives you early confirmation that the substance involved is causing systemic reactions.

Airway and Breathing

Quickly ensure that the patient has an open airway and adequate ventilation. Do not hesitate to begin oxygen therapy for the patient. If the patient is unresponsive to painful stimuli, you need to consider inserting an airway adjunct to ensure an open airway. Have suction available because these patients frequently vomit. You may also have to assist a patient's breathing with bag-mask ventilation. As you assess and manage the patient's airway and breathing, you must consider the potential for spinal injury. Spinal precautions in an unresponsive patient must begin when the airway is first opened and continued when positive pressure ventilation is needed.

Circulation

Once the airway and breathing have been assessed and appropriate interventions performed, assess the patient's circulatory status. You will find variations in a patient's circulatory status depending on the substance involved. Assess the pulse and skin condition. Some poisons are stimulants, and others are depressants. Some poisons will cause vasoconstriction, and others may cause vasodilation; either condition may cause a change in perfusion status and skin color, temperature, and condition (dry or moist).

Transport Decision

Patients with unstable ABCs or those for whom you have a poor general impression should be considered for immediate transport. A delay on the scene to further assess and treat patients is rarely indicated. Some industrial settings may have specific decontamination stations and antidotes available at the site. Most of the time, decontamination and antidote administration will have been initiated by the industrial response team before your arrival and should not delay rapid transport. For your safety, patients should be decontaminated before being treated or placed in the ambulance.

Focused History and Physical Exam

Once initial life threats have been addressed, you may begin the next step of your assessment, the focused history and physical exam. In most situations, this can be performed in the ambulance en route to the hospital. If no trauma is involved and the patient remains unresponsive after your initial assessment, begin with a rapid physical exam to assess for hidden problems or indications of a poisoning or an exposure. Obtain baseline vital signs and obtain as much of a SAMPLE history as you can.

If your patient is responsive and can answer questions, begin with an evaluation of the exposure and the SAMPLE history. This will guide you in a focused physical exam of the area exposed or the

You are the Provider 2

You take the child and try to calm her down while your partner talks to the mother. He is able to find out that she can account for all but about five pills. She is not positive of how many were in the bottle but is guessing based on when the prescription was filled.

The girl is no longer crying and is eyeing you warily. You allow her to play with the stethoscope and she laughs and tries to listen to her chest.

Vital Signs	Recording Time: 2 Minutes
Skin	Flushed
Pulse	132 beats/min, regular
Respirations	26 breaths/min
Oxygen saturation	99% on room air

4. The patient is alert and in no apparent distress. How should she be treated?

5. What is the dose of activated charcoal for this patient?

6. What do her vital signs suggest?

most concerning problems. The history will guide your focus as you continue to assess the patient's condition.

SAMPLE History

As part of the SAMPLE history, you should ask the following questions:

- What is the substance involved? If you know the substance involved, you will be better able to access the appropriate resource, such as the poison center to determine appropriate interventions.
- When did the patient ingest or become exposed to the substance?
- How much did the patient ingest or what was the level of exposure?
- Over what period did the patient take the substance? Did the patient take the substance all at once or during minutes or hours?
- Has the patient or a bystander provided any treatments? Interventions by the patient or a bystander may cause more complications. The emergency physician will also need to know this information.

Focused Physical Exam

Your focused physical exam should focus on the area of the body or the route of exposure. For example, if a person has ingested a poison, inspect the mouth for indications of poisoning. Are there burns from caustic chemicals? Are there plant or pill fragments? If the person's skin came in contact with a poison, is there a rash or burns? How large an area was involved? If a respiratory exposure occurred, listen to the lungs. Is there good air movement in and out of the lungs? Do you hear any wheezing or crackles? Much of what you would focus on in your physical exam is based on the route of exposure and the particular drug or chemical to which the patient was exposed. Take the time to become familiar with the effects of general classes of drugs and chemicals.

Baseline Vital Signs

A complete set of baseline vital signs is important to determine how your patient is doing. Many poisons have no outward indications of the seriousness of the exposure. Changes in mental status, pulse, respirations, blood pressure, and skin are more sensitive indicators that something serious is wrong.

Interventions

The treatment you provide for patients with a poisoning or an overdose depends a great deal on what they were exposed to, how they were exposed, and other signs and symptoms found in your assessment. Supporting the ABCs is most important. Some poisons can be easily diluted or decontaminated before transport or en route to the hospital. Dilute airborne exposures with oxygen, remove contact exposures with copious amounts of water unless contraindicated, and consider activated charcoal for ingested poisons. Contact your medical control or a poison center to discuss treatment options for particular poisonings.

Detailed Physical Exam

Often a detailed exam will provide additional information on the exposure the patient experienced. A general review of all body systems may help identify systemic problems. This review should be performed, at a minimum, on patients with extensive chemical burns or other significant trauma and on patients who are unresponsive. Management of the ABCs should be the priority assessment and treatment goal. These interventions would take precedence over a detailed physical exam.

Ongoing Assessment

The condition of patients exposed to poisons may change suddenly and without warning. You should continually reassess the adequacy of the patient's ABCs. Repeat assessment of the vital signs, and compare them with the baseline set obtained earlier. Evaluate the effectiveness of interventions you have provided. If the patient is in unstable condition, check the vital signs every 5 minutes. If the patient

Documentation Tips

Document the type of chemical exposure, the duration of the exposure, the route of exposure, and any interventions prior to EMS arrival. Also document if the patient has vomited since exposure.

If an MSDS (Material Safety Data Sheet) is immediately available, take that with you to the emergency department.

is in stable condition and there are no life threats, reassess every 15 minutes. If the poison or the level of exposure (for example, the number and type of pills taken) is unknown, careful and frequent reassessment is mandatory.

Communication and Documentation

Once you have completed your focused history and physical exam, including baseline vital signs, report to the hospital as much information as you have about the poison or chemical to which the patient was exposed. If a material safety data sheet is immediately available in a work setting, take it with you. If it is not immediately available, ask the company to fax it to the receiving hospital while you are en route.

■ Emergency Medical Care

Decontamination of the patient is a priority for your safety and for the patient's safety. Remove tablets or fragments from the patient's mouth, and wash or brush poison from the patient's skin. Assess and maintain the ABCs, and monitor the patient's breathing closely. Activated charcoal may be indicted for patients who have ingested a poison, if approved by medical control or local protocol. Charcoal is not indicated for patients who have ingested an acid, an alkali, or a petroleum product; who have a decreased level of consciousness and cannot protect their airway; or who are unable to swallow.

Remember that activated charcoal adsorbs, or sticks to, many commonly ingested poisons, preventing the toxin (poison) from being absorbed into the body by the stomach or intestines. If local protocol permits, you will likely carry activated charcoal. Some common trade names for the suspension form are InstaChar, Actidose, and LiquiChar. The usual dose for an adult or child is 1 g of activated charcoal per kilogram of body weight. The usual adult dose is 25 to 50 g, and the usual pediatric dose is 12.5 to 25 g. Review **Skill Drill 8-1** for the steps in administering activated charcoal. If the patient has ingested a poison that causes nausea, he or she may vomit after drinking the activated charcoal. If the patient vomits, you may have to repeat the dose. As you reassess the patient, be prepared for vomiting, nausea, and possible airway problems.

■ Specific Poisons

A person with an addiction has an overwhelming desire or need to continue using the agent, at whatever cost, with a tendency to increase the dose. Almost any substance can be abused, including street drugs, alcohol, prescription medications, laxatives, nasal decongestants, vitamins, and food.

The importance of safety awareness and BSI precautions in caring for victims of drug abuse cannot be discussed enough. Known drug abusers have a fairly high incidence of serious and undiagnosed infections,

You are the Provider 3

The patient is loaded into the ambulance and you prepare for rapid transport. Medical control advised not to administer the activated charcoal because the child is so small and the dose was unsure. The hospital is only a few minutes away.

Reassessment	Recording Time: 5 Minutes
Pulse	130 beats/min, irregular
Skin	Warm and dry
Respirations	24 breaths/min
Breath sounds	Clear bilaterally
Pulse oximetry	99% on room air

7. What else might you consider if the transport time was longer?
8. What should you take along to the hospital?
9. What physical response may occur as a result of ingestion and how should you prepare?

including human immunodeficiency virus (HIV) and hepatitis. These patients, when under the influence, may bite, spit, hit, or otherwise injure you, causing you to come into contact with their blood and other body fluids. Always be sure to wear appropriate protective equipment. A calm, professional approach can defuse frightening situations, but keep your safety and that of your team uppermost in mind. Expect the unexpected, and remember: the drug user, not the drug, can pose the greatest threat.

Alcohol

The most commonly abused drug in the United States is alcohol. It affects people from all walks of life and kills more than 200,000 people each year. More than 40% of all traffic deaths and injuries, 67% of murders, and 33% of suicides are related to alcohol. Alcoholism is one of the greatest national health problems, along with heart disease, cancer, and stroke.

Alcohol is a powerful CNS depressant. It is a sedative, a substance that decreases activity and excitement, and a hypnotic, meaning that it induces sleep. In general, alcohol dulls the sense of awareness, slows reflexes, and reduces reaction time. It may also cause aggressive and inappropriate behavior and lack of coordination. However, a person who appears intoxicated may have other medical problems as well. Look for signs of head trauma, toxic reactions, or uncontrolled diabetes. Severe acute alcohol ingestion may cause hypoglycemia. At the very least, you should assume that all intoxicated patients are experiencing a drug overdose and require thorough examination by a physician. In most states, intoxicated patients cannot legally refuse transport.

If a patient exhibits signs of serious CNS depression, you must provide respiratory support. Respiratory depression can also cause vomiting. The vomiting may be forceful or even bloody (hematemesis) because large amounts of alcohol irritate the stomach. Internal bleeding should also be considered if the patient appears to be in shock (hypoperfusion) because blood might not clot effectively in a patient who has a prolonged history of alcohol abuse.

A patient in alcohol withdrawal may experience frightening hallucinations, or delirium tremens (DTs), a syndrome characterized by restlessness, fever, sweating, disorientation, agitation, and even seizures. These conditions may develop if patients no longer have their daily source of alcohol. Alcoholic hallucinations come and go. A patient with an otherwise fairly clear

mental state may see fantastic shapes or figures or hear odd voices. Such auditory and visual hallucinations often precede DTs, which are a much more severe complication.

Provide prompt transport for these patients after you have completed your assessment and given necessary care. A person who is experiencing hallucinations or DTs is extremely ill. Be prepared for seizures. The patient should not be restrained, although you must protect him or her from injury. Give the patient oxygen, and monitor for vomiting. Hypovolemia may develop due to sweating, fluid loss, insufficient fluid intake, or vomiting associated with DTs. If you see signs of shock, elevate the patient's feet slightly, clear the airway, and turn the head to one side to minimize the chance of aspiration during transport.

Narcotics (Opioids)

The pain relievers called opioid analgesics are named for the opium in poppy seeds, the origin of heroin, codeine, and morphine. On the list of frequently abused drugs, they have been joined by a number of synthetic narcotics (manufactured in a laboratory). Commonly abused narcotics include meperidine (Demerol), hydromorphone (Dilaudid), propoxyphene (Darvon), oxycodone (Percocet), oxycodone hydrochloride (OxyContin), hydrocodone (Vicodin), and methadone. Most of these drugs have legitimate medical uses. With the exception of heroin, which is illegal in the United States, many addicts may have started using the drug with an appropriate medical prescription.

Narcotics are CNS depressants and can cause severe respiratory depression. In general, emergency medical problems related to narcotic abuse are caused by respiratory depression. Patients typically appear sedated and have pinpoint pupils. Treatment includes supporting the airway and breathing. Always open the airway, give supplemental oxygen, and be prepared for vomiting. The only effective antidote to reverse the symptoms and signs of opioid overdose are certain narcotic antagonists such as naloxone (Narcan). Patients will respond within 2 minutes to naloxone when it is given intravenously. Naloxone can be administered by paramedics or physicians.

Sedative-Hypnotic Drugs

Barbiturates and benzodiazepines have been a part of legitimate medicine for a long time. They are easy to obtain and relatively cheap. People sometimes solicit prescriptions from several physicians for the same hypnotics or a variety of sedative-hypnotics. These drugs are CNS depressants and alter the level of consciousness, with effects similar to those of alcohol, so that the patient may appear drowsy, peaceful, or intoxicated `Table 14-2 ▾`. By themselves, these drugs do not relieve pain nor do they produce a specific high, although users often take alcohol or a narcotic at the same time to boost the effect.

You may be called to a scene of an attempted suicide in which the patient has taken large quantities of these drugs. In these situations, patients will have significant respiratory depression and may be in a coma. Sedative-hypnotic drugs may also be given to unsuspecting people as a "knock-out" drink, or "Mickey Finn." More recently, drugs such as flunitrazepam (Rohypnol) have been abused as a "date rape drug," causing an unwary person to become sedated and even unconscious. The person later awakens, confused and unable to remember what happened.

In general, your treatment of patients who have overdosed with sedative-hypnotics and have respiratory depression is to provide airway clearance, ventilatory assistance, and prompt transport. Give supplemental oxygen, and be ready to assist ventilation. A specific antidote (flumazenil) is available for acute benzodiazepine overdose. As multidrug use becomes more common, you may find it increasingly difficult to determine what agents patients have taken. Your best approach is to treat any obvious injuries or illnesses. Focus on the ABCs, especially the possibility of airway problems (relaxation of the tongue, causing obstruction), vomiting, respiratory depression, and, in severe cases, cardiac arrest.

Abused Inhalants

Many abused inhalants depress the CNS. Some of the more common agents include acetone, toluene, xylene, and hexane, which are found in glues, cleaning compounds, paint thinners, and lacquers. Similarly, gasoline and various halogenated hydrocarbons, such as Freon, used as propellants in aerosol sprays, are also abused as inhalants. Because these are products that can be bought in hardware stores, they are commonly abused by teenagers seeking an alcohollike high. The effective dose and the lethal dose are very close, making these extremely dangerous drugs. The low cost and relative availability make them favorites of children and curious experimenters.

Always use special care in dealing with a patient who may have used inhalants. Their effects range from mild drowsiness to coma, but unlike most other sedative-hypnotics, these agents can cause seizures. Also, halogenated hydrocarbon solvents can make the heart supersensitive to the patient's own adrenaline, putting the patient at high risk for sudden cardiac death due to ventricular fibrillation; even the action of walking may release enough adrenaline to cause a fatal ventricular arrhythmia. You must try to keep such patients from struggling with you or exerting themselves. Give supplemental oxygen, and use a stretcher to move the patient. Prompt transport to the hospital is essential; monitor vital signs en route.

Sympathomimetics (Stimulants)

Sympathomimetics are CNS stimulants that frequently cause hypertension, tachycardia, and dilated pupils. A <u>stimulant</u> is an agent that produces an ex-

---

Table 14-2 Examples of Sedative-Hypnotic Drugs

Barbiturates	Benzodiazepines	Others
Amobarbital (Amytal)	Alprazolam (Xanax)	Carisoprodol (Soma)
Butabarbital (Butisol)	Chlordiazepoxide (Librium)	Chloral hydrate ("Mickey Finn")
Pentobarbital (Nembutal)	Diazepam (Valium)	Cyclobenzaprine (Flexeril)
Phenobarbital (Luminal)	Flunitrazepam (Rohypnol)	Ethchlorvynol (Placidyl)
Secobarbital (Seconal)	Lorazepam (Ativan)	Ethyl alcohol (drinking alcohol)
	Oxazepam (Serax)	Glutethimide (Doriden)
	Temazepam (Restoril)	Hydrocarbon inhalants
		Isopropyl alcohol (rubbing alcohol)
		Meprobamate (Equagesic)

cited state. Amphetamine and methamphetamine ("ice") are commonly taken by mouth, but are also injected by abusers. They typically are taken to make the user "feel good," improve task performance, suppress appetite, or prevent sleepiness. They may just as easily produce irritability, anxiety, lack of concentration, or seizures. Other common examples include phentermine and amphetamine sulfate (Benzedrine). Caffeine, theophylline, and phenylpropanolamine (a nasal decongestant) are all mild sympathomimetics. So-called designer drugs, such as Ecstasy and Eve, are also frequently abused in certain areas of the United States.

These drugs are frequently called "uppers" Table 14-3 ▾ . Someone using one of these agents may display disorganized behavior, restlessness, and sometimes anxiety or great fear. Paranoia and delusions are common.

Cocaine may be taken in a number of different ways. Classically, it is inhaled into the nose and absorbed through the nasal mucosa, damaging tissue, causing nosebleeds, and ultimately destroying the nasal septum. It can also be injected intravenously or subcutaneously (skin-popping). Cocaine can be absorbed through all mucous membranes and even

across the skin. In any form, the immediate effects of a given dose last less than an hour.

Another method of abusing cocaine is by smoking it. Crack is pure cocaine. It melts at 93°F (34°C) and vaporizes at a slightly higher temperature. Therefore, crack is easily smoked. In this form, it reaches the capillary network of the lungs and is absorbed by the body in seconds. The immediate outflow of blood from the heart speeds the drug to the brain, so its effect is felt at once. Smoked crack produces the most rapid means of absorption and the most potent effect.

Cocaine is one of the most addicting substances known. Its immediate effects include excitement and euphoria. Acute cocaine overdose is a true emergency because patients are at high risk for seizures and cardiac arrhythmias. Long-term cocaine abuse may cause hallucinations; patients with "cocaine bugs" think that bugs are crawling out of their skin.

You should be aware that these patients can be severely agitated and become tachycardic and hypertensive. Patients may also be paranoid, putting you and others in danger. Law enforcement officers should be at the scene to restrain the patient, if necessary.

These patients need prompt transport to the emergency department because of their risk of seizures, cardiac arrhythmias, and stroke. You may see blood pressures as high as 250/150 mm Hg. Give supplemental oxygen, and be ready to provide suctioning. If the patient is having a seizure, protect him or her from further injury.

Marijuana

The flowering hemp plant, *Cannabis sativa*, called marijuana, is abused throughout the world. It has been estimated that as many as 20 million people use marijuana daily in the United States. Inhaling marijuana smoke from a cigarette or pipe produces euphoria, relaxation, and drowsiness. An altered perception of time is common, and anxiety and panic can occur. With very high doses, patients experience hallucinations.

A person who has been using marijuana rarely needs transport to the hospital. Exceptions may include someone who is hallucinating, very anxious, or paranoid. However, you should be aware that marijuana is often used as a vehicle to get other drugs into the body. For example, it may be covered with crack or PCP (phencyclidine hydrochloride), also known as "angel dust."

Table 14-3 Street Names for Amphetamines

Street Name	Drug Name
Adam	3,4-Methylenedioxymethamphetamine (MDMA)
Bennies	Amphetamines
Crank	Crack cocaine, heroin, amphetamine, methamphetamine, methcathinone
DOM	4-Methyl-2,5-dimethoxyamphetamine
Ecstasy	MDMA
Eve	MDMA
Fen-phen	Phentermine
Golden eagle	4-Methylthioamphetamine
Ice	Cocaine, crack cocaine, smokable methamphetamine, methamphetamine, MDMA, phencyclidine (PCP)
MDA	Methaqualone
Meth	Methamphetamine
Speed	Crack cocaine, amphetamine, methamphetamine
STP	PCP
Uppers	Amphetamines

EMT-B Safety

Be very careful when dealing with patients who have taken hallucinogens or other mind-altering drugs. The associated behavioral changes may cause patients to inflict harm on themselves or others.

Hallucinogens

Hallucinogens alter a person's sensory perceptions (Table 14-4 ▼). The classic hallucinogen is lysergic acid diethylamide (LSD). Abuse of another hallucinogen, PCP, or angel dust, is no longer common with young adults. Phencyclidine is a dissociative anesthetic that is easily synthesized and highly potent. Its effectiveness by oral, nasal, pulmonary, and intravenous routes makes it easy to add to other street drugs. It is dangerous because it causes severe behavioral changes in which people who use it often inflict injury on themselves.

All of these agents cause visual hallucinations, intensify vision and hearing, and generally separate the user from reality. At some point, you are bound to encounter patients who are having a "bad trip." They will usually be hypertensive, tachycardic, anxious, and probably paranoid.

Use a calm, professional manner, and provide emotional support. Do not use restraints unless you or the patient is in danger of injury, and then always use them within the guidelines specified by local authorities. These patients may suddenly experience hallucinations or odd perceptions, so you must watch them carefully throughout transport.

Anticholinergic Agents

The classic picture of a person who has taken too much of an anticholinergic medication is "hot as a hare, blind as a bat, dry as a bone, red as a beet, and mad as a hatter." These are medications that have properties that, among other effects, block the parasympathetic nerves. These drugs include atropine, diphenhydramine (Benadryl), Jimson weed, and certain tricyclic antidepressants. With the exception of Jimson weed, these medications usually are not abused drugs but may be taken as an intentional overdose. These patients may be agitated and tachycardic and have dilated pupils.

Because newer, safer antidepressants such as fluoxetine (Prozac) and sertraline (Zoloft) are now being prescribed, you can expect to see fewer overdoses of tricyclic antidepressants such as amitriptyline (Elavil) and imipramine (Tofranil). In addition to its anticholinergic effects, a tricyclic antidepressant overdose may cause life-threatening cardiac arrhythmias. Patients with acute tricyclic antidepressant overdose must be transported immediately to the emergency department; they may go from appearing "normal" to having a seizure and dying within 30 minutes. The seizures and cardiac arrhythmias caused by a severe tricyclic antidepressant overdose are best treated in the hospital with intravenous sodium bicarbonate. If you work in a tiered system, you should consider calling for ALS backup when you are en route to the scene.

Table 14-4 Commonly Abused Hallucinogens

Bufotenine (toad skin)	Mescaline
Dimethyltryptamine (DMT)	Morning glory
Hashish	Mushrooms
Jimson weed	Nutmeg
LSD	PCP
Marijuana	Psilocybin (mushroom)

You are the Provider 4

The patient remains stable on the way to the hospital. You keep suction and an emesis bag available, but she remains stable with no vomiting. On arrival at the hospital, a pediatric specialist is standing by with the information from poison control. She is treated with a gastric lavage and admitted overnight for observation. She is released the following day with no ill effects.

Cholinergic Agents

The "nerve gases" designed for chemical warfare are cholinergic agents. These agents overstimulate normal body functions that are controlled by parasympathetic nerves, resulting in salivation, mucus secretion, urination, crying, and abnormal heart rate. You are unlikely to encounter nerve agents. However, you may be called to care for patients who have been exposed to an organophosphate insecticide or certain wild mushrooms, which are also cholinergic agents. The signs and symptoms of cholinergic drug poisoning are easy to remember with the mnemonic DUMBELS:

- Defecation
- Urination
- Miosis (constriction of the pupils)
- Bronchorrhea (discharge of mucus from the lungs)
- Emesis
- Lacrimation (tearing)
- Salivation

Alternatively, you can use the mnemonic SLUDGE:

- Salivation
- Lacrimation
- Urination
- Defecation
- GI (gastrointestinal) irritation
- Eye constriction and emesis

In this situation, patients will have excessive amounts of body secretions. In addition, patients may have bradycardia or tachycardia. The most important consideration in caring for a patient who has been exposed to an organophosphate insecticide or some other cholinergic agent is to avoid exposure yourself. Because such agents may cling to a patient's clothing and skin, decontamination may take priority over immediate transport to the emergency department. Hospital staff or paramedics can use the anticholinergic drug atropine to dry up the patient's secretions. In the meantime, your priorities after decontamination are to decrease the secretions in the mouth and trachea that threaten to suffocate the patient and provide airway support. Depending on your local EMS protocol, this may be treated as a HazMat (hazardous materials) situation.

Miscellaneous Drugs

Although not as common as it was 30 years ago, aspirin poisoning remains a potentially lethal condition. Ingesting too many aspirin tablets, in the short- or long-term, may result in nausea, vomiting, hyperventilation, and ringing in the ears. Patients with this problem are frequently anxious, confused, tachypneic (rapid respirations), hyperthermic, and in danger of having seizures. They should be transported quickly to the hospital.

Overdosing with acetaminophen is common, probably because acetaminophen is available in so many different preparations, such as Tylenol. Acetaminophen is generally not very toxic. A healthy patient could ingest 140 mg of acetaminophen for every kilogram of body weight without serious adverse effects. The bad news is that the symptoms of an overdose generally do not appear until it is too late. For example, massive liver failure may not be apparent for a full week. Obtaining information at the scene is very important. By finding an empty acetaminophen bottle, you may save a patient's life. If given early enough (before liver failure occurs), a specific antidote may prevent liver damage.

Be extremely careful in dealing with a child who has unintentionally ingested a poisonous substance. Although such incidents usually do not lead to death, family members may be distraught, and your professional attitude will help ease the tension. Remember, however, that a single swallow of some substances can kill a child Table 14-5 ▼.

Some alcohols, including methyl alcohol and ethylene glycol, are even more toxic than ethyl alcohol (drinking alcohol). Although they may be used as a substitute by a person with chronic alcoholism who is unable to obtain ethyl alcohol, they are more often taken by someone attempting suicide. In either case, immediate transport to the emergency department is essential. Methyl alcohol is found in dry gas products and Sterno; ethylene gly-

Table 14-5 Fatal Ingested Poisons

Benzocaine	Methylsalicylate (oil of wintergreen)
Calcium channel blockers (verapamil, nifedipine, diltiazem)	Phenothiazines (Thorazine)
	Quinine
Camphor	Theophylline
Chloroquine	Tricyclic antidepressants (amitriptyline [Elavil], imipramine [Tofranil], nortriptyline [Pamelor])
Hydrocarbon solvents	
Lomotil	
Methanol and ethylene glycol	Visine

col is found in some antifreeze products. Left untreated, they will cause severe tachypnea, blindness (methyl alcohol), renal failure (ethylene glycol), and eventually death. Even ethyl alcohol (typical drinking alcohol) can stop a patient's breathing if taken in too high a dose or too fast, particularly by children.

Food Poisoning

Food poisoning is almost always caused by eating food that is contaminated by bacteria. The food may appear perfectly good, with little or no decay or odor to suggest danger. There are two main types of food poisoning. In one, the organism itself causes disease. In the other, the organism produces toxins that cause disease. A toxin is a poison or harmful substance produced by bacteria, animals, and plants.

One organism that produces direct effects of food poisoning is the *Salmonella* bacterium. The condition called salmonellosis is characterized by severe gastrointestinal symptoms within 72 hours of ingestion, including nausea, vomiting, abdominal pain, and diarrhea. In addition, patients with salmonellosis may be systemically ill with fever and generalized weakness. Some people are carriers of certain bacteria; although they may not become ill themselves, they may transmit diseases, particularly if they work in the food services industry. Usually, proper cooking kills bacteria, and proper cleanliness in the kitchen prevents the contamination of uncooked foods.

The more common cause of food poisoning is the ingestion of powerful toxins produced by bacteria, often in leftovers. The bacterium *Staphylococcus*, a common culprit, is quick to grow and produce toxins in foods that have been prepared in advance and kept too long, even in the refrigerator. Foods prepared with mayonnaise, when left unrefrigerated, are a common vehicle for the development of staphylococcal toxins. Usually, staphylococcal food poisoning results in sudden gastrointestinal symptoms, including nausea, vomiting, and diarrhea. Although timeframes may vary from person to person, symptoms usually start within 2 to 3 hours after ingestion or as long as 8 to 12 hours after ingestion.

The most severe form of toxin ingestion is botulism. This often-fatal disease usually results from eating improperly canned food. The symptoms of botulism are neurologic: blurring of vision, weakness,

Geriatric Needs

In a geriatric patient, the liver may not be able to metabolize the poison as effectively or the kidneys may not be able to excrete the poison as quickly. In either case, the drug or poison remains in the body for a longer period, causing additional tissue damage. When a medication is not metabolized or excreted as quickly as before, the drug could accumulate to toxic levels and, ultimately, become fatal in lesser doses than in a younger person.

and difficulty speaking and breathing. Symptoms may develop as long as 4 days after ingestion or as early as the first 24 hours.

In general, you should not try to determine the specific cause of acute gastrointestinal problems. Instead, you should obtain as much history as possible from the patient and transport him or her promptly to the hospital. When two or more people in one group have the same illness, you should take along some of the suspected food. In advanced cases of botulism, you may have to assist ventilation and give basic life support.

Plant Poisoning

Several thousand cases of poisoning from plants occur each year, some severe. Many household plants are poisonous if ingested. Children will frequently nibble on the leaves of poisonous plants. Some poisonous plants cause local irritation of the skin; others can affect the circulatory system, the gastrointestinal tract, or the CNS. It is impossible for you to memorize every plant and poison, let alone their effects. To treat a patient with suspected plant poisoning:

1. Assess the patient's airway and vital signs.
2. Notify the regional poison center for assistance in identifying the plant.
3. Take the plant to the emergency department.
4. Provide prompt transport.

Irritation of the skin and/or mucous membranes is a problem with the common houseplant called dieffenbachia, which resembles "elephant ears." When chewed, a single leaf may irritate the lining of the upper airway enough to cause difficulty swallowing, breathing, and speaking. For this reason, dieffenbachia has been called "dumbcane." In rare circumstances, the airway may be completely obstructed. Emergency medical treatment of dieffenbachia poisoning includes maintaining an open airway, giving oxygen, and transporting the patient promptly to the hospital for respiratory support. You should continue to assess the patient for airway difficulties throughout transport. If necessary, provide positive pressure ventilation.

You are the Provider Summary

It is vital to recognize when ingestion has occurred and to seek prompt treatment before the poison has time to be absorbed into the system. This is especially true with children who may "taste" anything within reach. Do not be fooled by stable vital signs. These patients can rapidly deteriorate. Follow local protocols and call for ALS backup as soon as the need is recognized.

1. **What questions should you ask the mother?**
   - How many pills were in the bottle?
   - How many did she find on the floor?
   - Has the patient vomited?
   - Has the mother called poison control?
   - If so, what did they advise?
   - How long has it been since she was exposed?

2. **What is the primary treatment goal for this patient?**

   To rapidly remove as much of the poison as possible from the gastrointestinal tract

3. **How is this accomplished?**

   Through the use of activated charcoal if carried by your service and advised by medical control

4. **The patient is alert and in no apparent distress. How should she be treated?**

   With substance abuse and poisonings, do not be complacent that a conscious, alert, and oriented patient is in stable condition and has no apparent life threats. The patient may have a harmful or even lethal amount of poison in her system that has not had time to produce systemic reactions.

5. **What is the dose of activated charcoal for this patient?**

   1 g of activated charcoal per kilogram of body weight

6. **What do her vital signs suggest?**

   Many poisons have no outward indications of the seriousness of the exposure. Changes in mental status, pulse, respirations, blood pressure, and skin are more sensitive indicators that something is seriously wrong. The poison may not have been in her system long enough to produce changes in vital signs.

7. **What else might you consider if the transport time was longer?**

   Calling for ALS backup

8. **What should you take along to the hospital?**

   The prescription bottle, any partial pills, any vomitus

9. **What physical response may occur as a result of ingestion and how should you prepare?**

   Nausea and vomiting. Remember to keep the airway clear and suction available.

Substance Abuse and Poisoning

Scene Size-up	Body substance isolation precautions should include a minimum of gloves and eye protection. Ensure scene safety, and determine NOI/MOI. Consider the number of patients, the need for additional help/ALS, and cervical spine stabilization.
Initial Assessment	
■ General impression	Determine level of consciousness, and find and treat any immediate threats to life. Determine priority of care based on environment and patient's chief complaint.
■ Airway	Ensure patent airway.
■ Breathing	Provide high-flow oxygen at 15 L/min. Evaluate depth and rate of respirations, and provide ventilations as needed.
■ Circulation	Evaluate pulse rate and quality; observe skin color, temperature, and condition, and treat accordingly. Determine if bleeding is present and control if life threatening.
■ Transport decision	Consider decontamination before rapid transport.
Focused History and Physical Exam	*NOTE: The order of the steps in the focused history and physical exam differs depending on whether the patient is conscious or unconscious. The order below is for a conscious patient. For an unconscious patient, perform a rapid physical exam, obtain vital signs, and obtain the history.*
■ SAMPLE history	Ask SAMPLE and pertinent OPQRST questions. Be sure to ask if and what interventions were taken before your arrival, how many interventions, and at what time.
■ Focused physical exam	Perform focused physical exam on affected body systems and any affected area.
■ Baseline vital signs	Take vital signs, noting skin color and temperature. Use pulse oximetry if available.
■ Interventions	Support patient as needed. Consider the use of oxygen, positive pressure ventilation, adjuncts, and proper positioning.
Detailed Physical Exam	Consider a detailed physical exam.
Ongoing Assessment	Repeat the initial assessment and focused assessment, and reassess interventions performed. Reassess vital signs every 5 minutes for a patient in unstable condition, every 15 minutes for a patient in stable condition. Document treatment, and treat the patient as necessary.
■ Communication and documentation	Contact medical control with a radio report giving patient's condition, agent of exposure, and amount ingested or exposed to. Relay any significant changes, including level of consciousness or difficulty in breathing. Contact the regional poison center for information as determined by local protocol. Document any changes, the time they occurred, and any interventions performed.

NOTE: While the steps below are widely accepted, be sure to consult and follow your local protocol.

Substance Abuse and Poisoning

General Management

1. Have trained rescuers remove patient from any poisonous environment.
2. Establish and maintain airway, suctioning as needed. Provide high-flow oxygen.
3. Obtain SAMPLE history and vital signs. Ascertain which drug(s) have been taken.
4. Request ALS when available.
5. Take all containers, bottles, and labels of poisons to the receiving hospital.

For patients who have taken hallucinogens, provide calm, prompt transport.

For cholinergic agents, it is critical to take sufficient body substance isolation precautions.

For patients who have plant poisoning, notify the regional poison center for assistance in identifying the plant.

For patients who have food poisoning, if there are more than two patients with the same illness, transport the food suspected to be responsible for the poisoning.

Administer activated charcoal for poisonous ingestions according to local protocol. Follow these steps:
1. Do not give if the patient exhibits altered mental status, has ingested acids or alkalis, or is unable to swallow.
2. Obtain order from medical control, or follow protocol.
3. Shake container.
4. Place in cup with straw and have patient drink 12.5 to 25 g (for infants and children) or 25 to 50 g (for adults).

Prep Kit

Ready for Review

- Poisons act acutely or chronically to destroy or impair body cells.
- If you believe a patient may have taken a poisonous substance, you should notify medical control and begin emergency treatment at once.
- Collect any evidence of the type of poison that was used and take it to the hospital; if possible, dilute and physically remove the poisonous agent; provide respiratory support; and transport the patient promptly to the hospital.
- A poison can be introduced into the body in one of four ways:
  - Ingestion
  - Inhalation
  - Injection
  - Surface contact (absorption)
- Approximately 80% of all poisoning is by ingestion, including plants, contaminated food, and most drugs. In general, activated charcoal should be used to treat the patients.
- In the case of surface contact poisons, be sure to avoid contaminating yourself. You should remove all contaminated substances and clothing from the patient and flush the contaminated part of the patient with copious amounts of water, unless contraindicated.
- Move patients who have inhaled poison into the fresh air; be prepared to use supplemental oxygen via nonrebreathing mask and/or provide bag-mask ventilation.
- Take special care with patients who have used inhalants because the drugs may cause seizures or sudden death.
- Sympathomimetics, including cocaine, stimulate the CNS, causing hypertension, tachycardia, seizures, and dilated pupils. Patients who have taken these drugs may be paranoid, as may patients who have taken hallucinogens.
- Anticholinergic medications, often taken in suicide attempts, can cause a person to become hot, dry, blind, red-faced, and mentally unbalanced. An overdose of tricyclic antidepressants can lead to cardiac arrhythmias.
- The symptoms of cholinergic medications, which include organophosphate insecticides, can be remembered by the mnemonic DUMBELS or SLUDGE.
- Two main types of food poisoning cause gastrointestinal symptoms.
  - In one type, bacteria in the food directly cause disease, such as salmonellosis; in the other, bacteria such as *Staphylococcus* produce powerful toxins, often in leftover food.
  - The most severe form of toxin ingestion is botulism, which can produce the first neurologic symptoms as late as 4 days after ingestion.
- Plant poisoning can affect the circulatory system, the gastrointestinal system, and the CNS. Some plants, such as dieffenbachia, irritate the skin or mucous membranes and sometimes cause obstruction of the airway.

Vital Vocabulary

hallucinogens   Agents that produce false perceptions in any one of the five senses.

ingestion   Swallowing; taking a substance by mouth.

poison   A substance with a chemical action that could damage structures or impair function when introduced into the body.

stimulant   An agent that produces an excited state.

substance abuse   The misuse of any substance to produce some desired effect.

Technology

Refresher.EMSzone.com

- Interactivities
- Vocabulary Explorer
- Anatomy Review
- Web Links
- Online Review Manual

Assessment in Action

You are called to a residence for a "sick person." On arrival you find a 37-year-old man who is complaining of nausea, vomiting, and dizziness that started about an hour ago. He thinks it may have been something he ate at a family reunion.

1. Food poisoning is almost always caused by eating food that is contaminated with _____.
   - A. viruses
   - B. bacteria
   - C. botulism
   - D. shigella

2. A toxin is a poison produced by _____.
   - A. bacteria
   - B. animals
   - C. plants
   - D. all of the above

3. A common vehicle for staphylococcal toxins is _____.
   - A. vinegar
   - B. butter
   - C. mayonnaise
   - D. yogurt

4. Poisons may be introduced into the body by _____.
   - A. ingestion
   - B. inhalation
   - C. absorption
   - D. all of the above

5. What is the most severe form of toxin ingestion?
   - A. shellfish
   - B. staphylococcus
   - C. botulism
   - D. methyl alcohol

6. Severe gastrointestinal symptoms within 72 hours of ingestion, including nausea, vomiting, and diarrhea, are indicative of _____.
   - A. botulism
   - B. salmonellosis
   - C. staphylococcus
   - D. dieffenbachia

Challenging Questions

7. What is the proper treatment for possible dieffenbachia poisoning?

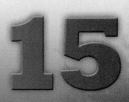

15

Environmental Emergencies

You are the Provider 1

You are called to the track at the local high school for a 15-year-old boy with severe leg cramps. It is a warm day (96°F) and they are getting ready for a big track meet. He is on the ground in a fetal position holding both calves when you arrive. The coach tells you that they tried to get him to walk but he said it hurt too badly to try and straighten his legs.

Initial Assessment	Recording Time: 0 Minutes
Appearance	Flushed, diaphoretic
Level of consciousness	Alert to person, place, and time
Airway	Open and clear
Breathing	Normal, deep
Circulation	Radials present, bounding

1. What is this patient's problem?
2. What is the first step in treating him?
3. Should the patient be cooled? If so, how?

Introduction

Environmental emergencies encompass a wide variety of situations including heat and cold exposure, drowning and near drowning situations, and diving emergencies.

Heat and cold emergencies can overwhelm temperature regulation mechanisms, particularly in children, the elderly, those with chronic illnesses, or young adults who overexert themselves. There is also a range of medical emergencies that arise from water recreation, including localized injuries and scuba diving emergencies. These can all be complicated by the cold.

This chapter reviews how the body regulates core temperature, and the ways in which body heat is lost to the environment. It then discusses heat and cold emergencies and water-related emergencies. We will also review assessment and treatment of hypothermia, frostbite, hyperthermia, and diving injuries.

Factors Affecting Exposure

There are a number of factors that affect how your patients are able to deal with a cold or hot environment:

1. **Physical condition.** Patients who are sick, have a significant medical history, or are in poor physical condition are not able to tolerate extreme temperatures. A well-trained athlete performs much better and is less likely to experience injury or illness than the "weekend warrior" who has not trained well.
2. **Age.** Patients who are very young or very old are more likely to experience an emergency due to heat or cold exposure. Infants have poor thermoregulation at birth and do not have the ability to shiver and generate heat when needed until about 12 to 18 months of age. Their larger surface area and smaller mass contribute to increased heat loss and heat gain. Older adults lose subcutaneous tissues, reducing the amount of insulation they have. Poor circulation contributes to increased heat loss and gain. Medications taken by older persons can also affect their body's thermostat, putting them at more risk.
3. **Nutrition and hydration.** Your body needs calories for your metabolism to function. Staying well hydrated provides water as a catalyst for much of this metabolism. A decrease will aggravate both hot and cold stress. Calories provide fuel to burn, creating heat during the cold, and water provides sweat for evaporation and removing heat. Alcohol use may increase fluid loss and place the patient at greater risk for temperature-related problems.
4. **Environmental conditions.** Conditions such as air temperature, humidity levels, and wind can complicate or improve environmental situations. Extremes in temperature and humidity are not needed to produce hot or cold injuries. Most heat stroke cases occur when the temperature is 80°F and the humidity is 80%. Be sure to examine the environmental temperature of your patient. Older patients may turn the heat down in the winter or neglect to use air conditioning because of financial concerns.

Cold Exposure

Normal body temperature must be maintained within a very narrow range for the body's chemistry to work efficiently. If the body, or any part of it, is exposed to cold environments, these mechanisms may be overwhelmed. Cold exposure may cause injury to individual parts of the body, such as the feet, hands, ears, or nose, or to the body as a whole. When the entire body temperature falls, the condition is called hypothermia.

Because heat always travels from a warmer place to a cooler place, the body tends to lose heat to the environment. The body loses heat in the following five ways:

- Conduction is the direct transfer of heat from a part of the body to a colder object by direct

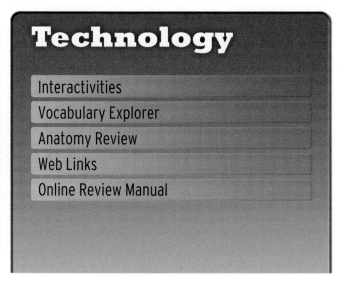

Technology

Interactivities

Vocabulary Explorer

Anatomy Review

Web Links

Online Review Manual

contact, as when a warm hand touches cold metal or ice, or is immersed in water with a temperature of less than 98°F (37°C). Heat passes directly from the body to the colder object. Heat can also be gained if the substance being touched is warm.

- Convection occurs when heat is transferred to circulating air, as when cool air moves across the body surface. The effects of the wind or a fan are good examples of heat transfer by convection. A person can also gain heat if the air moving across his or her body is hotter than his or her body temperature, such as in deserts or an industrial setting.

- Evaporation is the conversion of any liquid to a gas, a process that requires energy, or heat. Evaporation is the natural mechanism by which sweating cools the body. Individuals who exercise vigorously in a cool environment may sweat and feel warm at first, but later, as their sweat evaporates, they can become exceedingly cool. Measures should be taken to keep a person dry if he or she is too cold.

- Radiation is the transfer of heat by radiant energy. Radiant energy is a type of invisible light that transfers heat. The body can lose heat by radiation, such as when a person stands in a cold room. Heat can also be gained by radiation, for example, when a person stands by a fire.

- Respiration causes body heat to be lost as warm air in the lungs is exhaled into the atmosphere and cooler air is inhaled. In warm climates, the air temperature can be well above body temperature, causing an individual to gain heat with each breath.

The rate and amount of heat loss or gain by the body can be modified in three ways:

1. **Increase or decrease heat production.** One way for the body to increase its heat production is to increase the rate of metabolism of its cells, as occurs in shivering. Often people have a natural urge to move around when they are cold. If they are hot, you want to reduce their activity, thus reducing heat production.

2. **Move to an area where heat loss is decreased or increased.** The most obvious way to decrease heat loss from radiation and convection is to move out of a cold environment and seek shelter from wind. Just covering the head will minimize radiation heat loss by up to 70%. The same holds

EMT-B Safety

Remember to protect yourself from the environment. Dress in layers and use sweat-wicking materials near the skin.

true for a patient who is too hot. Simply moving into the shade can reduce the ambient temperature by 10 degrees or more. If you cannot move the patient to a cooler environment, provide shade if possible and air movement by fanning.

3. **Wear insulated clothing,** which helps to decrease heat loss in several ways. Layers of clothing that trap air provide good insulation. Protective clothing also traps perspiration and prevents evaporation. Sweating without evaporation will not result in cooling. To encourage heat loss, loosen or remove clothing, particularly around the head and neck.

Hypothermia

Hypothermia is diagnosed when the core temperature of the body—the temperature of the heart, lungs, and vital organs—falls below 95°F (35°C). The body can usually tolerate a drop in core temperature of a few degrees. However, below this critical point, the body loses the ability to regulate its temperature and to generate body heat.

To protect against heat loss, the body normally constricts blood vessels in the skin. The body also creates additional heat by shivering. If exposure to the cold continues, these mechanisms are overwhelmed and many body functions begin to slow down. Eventually, the functioning of key organs such as the heart begins to decrease.

Hypothermia can develop either quickly, as when someone is immersed in cold water, or more gradually, as when a lost person is exposed to the cold environment for several hours or more. The temperature does not have to be below freezing for hypothermia to occur. In winter, homeless people and those whose homes lack heating may develop hypothermia at temperatures above the freezing level. Even in summer, swimmers who remain in the water for a long time are at risk of hypothermia. Patients with burns, shock, head injury, stroke, infection, spinal cord injury,

Table 15-1 Characteristics of Systemic Hypothermia

Core Temperature	90° to 95°F (32° to 35°C)	89° to 92°F (32° to 33°C)	80° to 88°F (27° to 31°C)	<80°F (<27°C)
Signs and Symptoms	Shivering, foot stamping	Loss of coordination, muscle stiffness	Coma	Apparent death
Cardiorespiratory Response	Constricted blood vessels, rapid breathing	Slowing respirations, slow pulse	Weak pulse, arrhythmias, very slow respirations	Cardiac arrest
Level of Consciousness	Withdrawn	Confused, lethargic, sleepy	Unresponsive	Unresponsive

diabetes, and hypoglycemia are more prone to hypothermia, as are patients who have taken certain drugs.

Signs and Symptoms

Signs and symptoms of hypothermia become progressively more severe as the core temperature falls. Hypothermia progresses through four general stages, as shown in Table 15-1 . When you assess a patient in the field, you should be able to distinguish between mild and severe hypothermia.

To assess the patient's general temperature, pull back on your glove and place the back of your hand on the patient's skin on the abdomen. If the skin feels cool, the patient is likely experiencing a generalized cold emergency. If you work in a cold environment, you may carry a hypothermia rectal thermometer, which registers lower core temperatures. Remember that regular thermometers will not register the temperature of a patient who has significant hypothermia. Mild hypothermia occurs when the core temperature is between 90° and 95°F (32° and 35°C). The patient is usually alert and shivering in an attempt to generate more heat. Pulse rate and respirations are usually rapid. The skin in light-skinned individuals may be red, but may eventually appear pale, then cyanotic. Individuals in a cold environment may have blue lips or fingertips because of the body's constriction of blood vessels at the skin to retain heat.

More severe hypothermia occurs when the core temperature is less than 90°F (32°C). It is around this temperature that shivering stops and muscular activity decreases. At first, small, fine muscle activity such as coordinated finger motion ceases. Eventually, as the temperature falls further, all muscle activity stops.

You are the Provider 2

The patient is moved into the locker room where there is air conditioning and his excess clothing is removed. The coach places a moist towel around his neck. He is still unable to walk due to the cramps.

Vital Signs	Recording Time: 3 Minutes
Skin	Flushed, diaphoretic
Pulse	120 beats/min, bounding
Blood pressure	96/58 mm Hg
Respirations	18 breaths/min, deep

4. What else can you do for this patient?
5. Do you think the patient could be hypovolemic?
6. What vital sign might point towards hypovolemia?
7. What could be causing it?

As the core temperature drops toward 85°F (29°C), the patient becomes lethargic, usually losing interest in continuing to fight the cold. The level of consciousness decreases and the patient may try to remove his or her own clothes. Poor coordination and memory loss follow, along with reduced or complete loss of sensation to touch, mood changes, and impaired judgment. The patient becomes less communicative, experiences joint or muscle stiffness, and has trouble speaking. The muscles eventually become rigid, and the patient begins to appear stiff or rigid.

If the temperature continues to fall to 80°F (27°C), vital signs slow, the pulse becomes weaker, and respirations slow to shallow or become absent. Cardiac arrhythmias may occur as the blood pressure decreases or disappears.

At a core temperature of less than 80°F (27°C), all cardiorespiratory activity may cease, pupil reaction is slow, and the patient may appear dead. Never assume that a cold, pulseless patient is dead. Patients may survive severe hypothermia if proper emergency medical care is provided.

■ Assessment of Cold Injuries

Management of hypothermia in the field, regardless of the severity of the exposure, consists of stabilizing the ABCs and preventing further heat loss.

Scene Size-up

Your scene assessment begins with information provided by dispatch. This information helps you prepare for any conditions your patient may have, especially when dealing with environmental emergencies. Note air temperature, wind chill, and whether it is wet or dry outside.

Ensure that the scene is safe for you and other responders. Identify potential safety hazards, such as wet grass, mud, or icy streets. Cold environments may present special problems both for you and your patient. Use appropriate BSI precautions and consider the number of patients you may have. Request additional help, such as a search–and–rescue team, as quickly as possible.

Initial Assessment
General Impression

Determine whether a life threat exists, and if so, treat it. If the chief complaint is simply being cold, quickly assess how cold the patient is by feeling the patient's skin on the abdomen. This area of the body is usually well protected and insulated and will give you a general idea of the core body temperature. Assess the patient's environment and the position of the patient. This can give you an early indication of the severity of the problem.

Airway and Breathing

Your assessment of ABCs should take into account the physiologic changes that occur as a result of hypothermia. Ensure the patient has an adequate airway and is breathing. Consider spinal precautions based on your scene size-up and the chief complaint. If your patient's breathing is slow, shallow, or absent, provide ventilations with a bag-mask device. Use warmed, humidified oxygen if it is available.

Circulation

If you cannot feel a radial pulse in an unresponsive patient who is possibly hypothermic, palpate for a carotid pulse for 30 to 45 seconds before you decide that the patient is pulseless. The American Heart Association (AHA) recommends chest compressions immediately if there is no pulse. If you have any doubt about whether the pulse is present or not, start chest compressions. If CPR is started, you should also use the automated external defibrillator (AED). If the AED detects a shockable rhythm, you should shock the patient once and then immediately start CPR (starting with compressions). If there is still no pulse, you should continue CPR and transport the patient. In the hypothermic patient, the AHA recommends one shock only until the patient can be warmed.

Perfusion will be compromised based on the degree of cold the patient is experiencing. Assessment of the skin will not be helpful in determining shock. Assume shock is present and treat it appropriately. If the scene size-up, MOI, or chief complaint suggests the potential for bleeding, look for sources of the bleeding and treat accordingly based on your findings.

Documentation Tips

Document the patient's physical status, conditions on the scene, length of exposure, protective clothing, and any changes in mental status during treatment and transport.

Transport Decision

Even mild degrees of hypothermia can have significant complications including cardiac arrhythmias and problems with blood clotting. All patients with hypothermia require immediate transport for evaluation and treatment. Assess the scene for the safest way to quickly remove your patient from the cold environment. As you package your patient for transport, work quickly, safely, and gently. Rough handling of a hypothermic patient may cause a cold, slow, weak heart to fibrillate and the patient may become pulseless. Remove any wet garments and protect the patient from any further heat loss.

Focused History and Physical Exam

Try to get a SAMPLE history, perform a focused physical exam, and obtain baseline vital signs. If your patient is unresponsive, begin with a rapid physical exam.

SAMPLE History

Obtaining a patient's history in these situations may be difficult. If possible, determine how long your patient has been exposed to the cold environment (from the patient or bystanders). The SAMPLE history can provide important information to guide your treatment in the field and the treatment your patient will receive in the hospital. Medications your patient has taken and underlying medical conditions may have an impact on the way cold affects his or her metabolism. The patient's last oral intake and what the patient was doing prior to the exposure may help to determine the severity of the situation.

Focused Physical Exam

Your focused physical exam should concentrate on the severity of hypothermia and assessing the areas of the body directly affected by cold exposure. Is the whole body cold (hypothermia) or just parts (frostbite)? These determinations have important consequences for your treatment decisions. For example, shivering indicates that the body is using a protective mechanism to produce more heat because the body is cold. When shivering stops and the patient remains in a cold environment, the cold emergency is more severe.

Baseline Vital Signs

Remember that vital signs may be altered by the hypothermia and can be an indicator of its severity. Respirations may be slow and shallow, resulting in low oxygen levels in the body. Low blood pressure and a slow pulse rate also indicate moderate to severe hypothermia. Carefully assess your patient for changes in mental status.

Interventions

You should move the patient to a warmer environment to prevent further heat loss. To prevent further

You are the Provider 3

Once he drinks 8 ounces of a half-strength sports drink, he says he feels better and thinks he can walk. You and your partner assist him in standing and his legs start to buckle. You quickly lower him to a sitting position and reassess his vital signs.

Reassessment	Recording Time: 5 Minutes
Pulse	132 beats/min, thready
Blood pressure	88/40 mm Hg
Respirations	20 breaths/min, normal
Breath sounds	Clear bilaterally
Pulse oximetry	97% on room air

8. What caused the change in his vital signs?
9. How should this be treated?
10. What type of consent is used to treat this patient?
11. If the cramps do not subside, what are your options?

damage to the feet, do not allow the patient to walk. Remove any wet clothing, and place dry blankets over and under the patient. Handle the patient gently so that you do not cause any pain or further injury to the skin. Do not massage the extremities. Do not allow the patient to eat, drink coffee, tea, or cola, or to smoke or chew tobacco.

Administer warm, humidified oxygen if you have not already done so in the initial assessment. Begin passive rewarming, which includes wrapping the patient in blankets and turning up the heat in the patient compartment of the ambulance. If your protocol allows, you can apply heat packs to the groin, armpits, and behind the neck.

You must try to minimize further loss of body heat. However, when the patient has moderate or severe hypothermia, you should never try to rewarm the patient actively (placing heat on or into the body). Rewarming too quickly may cause a fatal cardiac arrhythmia. Active rewarming should be done in the hospital.

If you cannot get the patient out of the cold immediately, move him or her out of the wind and away from contact with any object that will conduct heat from the body. Place a protective cover on the patient, and remember that most heat is lost around the head and neck.

If the patient is alert and shivering, you may assume that the hypothermia is relatively mild. You can give warm fluids by mouth in this case, assuming that the patient can swallow without a problem. Remove all wet clothing, and cover the patient with a blanket. Notify the hospital of the patient's condition so that staff can prepare to start rewarming as soon as you arrive.

When the patient is not shivering and is lethargic, moderate or severe hypothermia is most likely present. Remove wet clothing, and protect the patient from the cold and wind with blankets in a warmer environment.

Detailed Physical Exam

Your detailed physical exam should be aimed at determining the degree and extent of cold injury, as well as any other injuries or conditions that may not have been initially detected. The numbing effect of cold, both on the brain and on the body, may affect your patient's ability to tell you about other injuries or illnesses. Therefore, a careful examination of your patient's entire body will help you avoid missing important clues to your patient's condition.

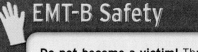

EMT-B Safety

Do not become a victim! Throw a rope or life preserver if the patient is responsive. If you are not trained for water rescue, wait for assistance to arrive on scene.

Ongoing Assessment

Closely monitor your patient's level of consciousness and vital signs. As the body rewarms, the sudden redistribution of fluids and the release of built-up chemicals can have harmful effects, including cardiac arrhythmias.

Communication and Documentation

Communicate all of the information you have gathered to the receiving facility. The conditions you found on scene, what your patient was wearing, and information gathered from bystanders may be essential in evaluating and treating your patient in the hospital. Document not only your patient's physical status, but also the conditions on scene, and carefully document changes in mental status during treatment and transport.

■ Management of Cold Exposure

All patients with significant trauma are at risk for hypothermia. Keep this in mind when you are assessing a patient with multiple injuries. A sick or injured person who has been trapped in a cold environment may experience hypothermia or may already have problems related to cold exposure. These patients are more susceptible than a healthy person to a cold injury. Remember these steps to prevent further cold injury:

1. **Remove wet clothing** and keep the patient dry.
2. **Prevent conduction heat loss.** Move the patient away from any wet or cold surfaces.
3. **Cover all exposed body parts,** especially the head, by wrapping them in a blanket or any other available dry, bulky material.
4. **Prevent convection heat loss** by limiting any wind exposure to the patient.
5. **Remove the patient from the cold** environment as quickly as possible.

Regardless of the nature or severity of the cold injury, remember that even an unresponsive patient may be able to hear you. Some patients have told of hearing themselves pronounced dead by someone who had forgotten the saying: "No one is dead unless they are warm and dead."

Local Cold Injuries

Most injuries from cold are confined to exposed parts of the body. The extremities, particularly the feet, and the exposed ears, nose, and face, are especially vulnerable to cold injury Figure 15-1 ▼. When exposed areas become very cold but are not frozen, the condition is called frostnip, chilblains, or immersion foot (trench foot). When areas become frozen, the injury is called frostbite.

There are several factors to consider as you assess for the severity of a local cold injury:

- The duration of the exposure
- The temperature to which the body part was exposed
- Exposure to wet conditions
- Inadequate insulation from cold or wind
- Restricted circulation from tight clothing or shoes or circulatory disease
- Alcohol or drug abuse
- Diabetes
- Cardiovascular disease
- Age of the patient

In hypothermia, blood is shunted away from the extremities in an attempt to maintain the core temperature. This shunting of blood increases the risk

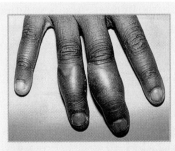
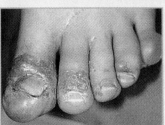
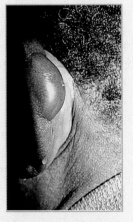

Figure 15-1 The extremities and the ears, nose, and face are particularly susceptible to frostbite.

of local cold injury to the extremities, ears, nose, and face. Patients with hypothermia should also be assessed for frostbite or other local cold injury. The reverse is also true. You must remember that both local and systemic cold exposure problems can occur in the same patient.

Frostnip and Immersion Foot

After prolonged exposure to the cold, the skin may be freezing while the deeper tissues are unaffected. This condition, which often affects the ears, nose, and fingers, is called frostnip. Because frostnip is usually not painful, the patient often is unaware that an injury has occurred. Immersion foot (trench foot) occurs after prolonged exposure to cold water. It is particularly common in hikers or hunters who stand for a long time in a river or lake. With frostnip and immersion foot, the skin is pale (blanched) and cold to the touch; capillary refill is delayed. In some cases, the skin of the foot will be wrinkled and may remain soft. The patient reports loss of feeling and sensation in the injured area.

The emergency treatment of these less severe local cold injuries consists of removing the patient from the cold, wet environment, but also rewarming the affected part. With frostnip, contact with a warm object may be all that is needed. During rewarming, the affected part will often tingle and become red. With immersion foot, remove wet shoes, boots, and socks, and rewarm the foot gradually, protecting it from further cold exposure.

Frostbite

Frostbite is the most serious local cold injury, because the tissues are actually frozen. Freezing permanently damages cells. The presence of ice crystals within the cells may cause physical damage. The change in the water content in the cells may also cause changes in the concentration of critical electrolytes, producing permanent changes in the chemistry of the cell. When the ice crystals thaw, further chemical changes occur in the cell, causing permanent damage or cell death, called gangrene Figure 15-2 ▶. If gangrene occurs, the dead tissue must be surgically removed, sometimes by amputation. Following less severe damage, the exposed part will become inflamed, tender to touch, and unable to tolerate exposure to cold.

Frostbite can be identified by the hard, frozen feel of the affected tissues. Most frostbitten parts are hard and waxy Figure 15-3 ▶. The injured part will feel firm to frozen. If the frostbite is only skin deep

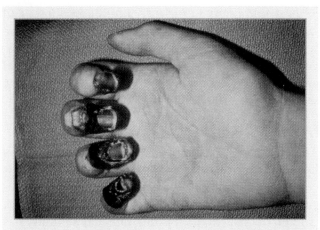

Figure 15-2 Gangrene, or permanent cell death, can occur when tissue is frozen and certain chemical changes occur in the cells.

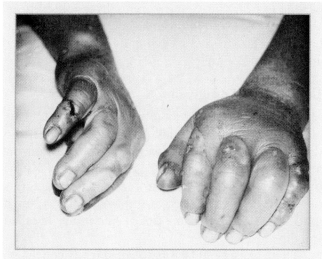

Figure 15-3 Frostbitten parts are hard and usually waxy to the touch.

it will feel leathery or thick, not hard and frozen all the way through. Blisters and swelling may be present. In light-skinned individuals with a deep injury that has thawed or partially thawed, the skin may appear red with purple and white, or it may be mottled and cyanotic.

As with a burn, the depth of skin damage will vary. With superficial frostbite, only the skin is frozen; with deep frostbite, the deeper tissues are frozen as well. You may not be able to tell superficial from deep frostbite in the field.

Emergency Medical Care for Local Cold Injury

Treatment of local cold injuries in the field should include the following steps:

1. **Remove the patient** from further exposure to the cold.
2. **Handle the injured part gently,** and protect it from further injury.
3. **Administer oxygen,** if this was not already done as part of the initial assessment.
4. **Remove any wet or restricting clothing** over the injured part.

With an early or superficial injury, such as frostnip or immersion foot, splint the extremity and cover it loosely with a dry, sterile dressing. Never rub or massage injured tissues as this causes further damage. Do not reexpose the injury to cold.

With a late or deep cold injury, such as frostbite, be sure to remove any jewelry from the injured part and cover the injury loosely with a dry, sterile dressing. Do not break blisters or rub or massage the area. Do not apply heat or rewarm the part. Unlike frost-

nip and trenchfoot, rewarming of the frostbitten extremity is best accomplished under controlled circumstances in the emergency department. You can cause a great deal of further injury to fragile tissues by attempting to rewarm a frostbitten part. Do not allow the patient to stand or walk on a frostbitten foot.

Evaluate the patient's general condition for signs or symptoms of hypothermia. Support the vital functions as necessary, and transport the patient promptly to the hospital.

If prompt hospital care is not available and medical control instructs you to begin rewarming in the field, use a warm-water bath. Immerse the frostbitten part in water with a temperature between 100° and 105°F (38° and 40°C). Check the water temperature with a thermometer before immersing the limb, and recheck it frequently during the rewarming process. The water temperature should never exceed 105°F (40°C). Stir the water continuously. Keep the frostbitten part in the water until it feels warm and sensation has returned to the skin. Cover the area with dry, sterile dressings, placing them also between injured fingers or toes. You should anticipate that the patient will report severe pain as the injured area thaws.

Never attempt rewarming if there is any chance that the part may freeze again before the patient reaches the hospital. Some of the most severe consequences of frostbite, including gangrene and amputation, have occurred when parts were thawed and then refrozen.

Geriatric Needs

Older adults undergo changes in their ability to compensate for low or high ambient temperatures. Because of reduced circulation to the skin, heat loss via conduction, convection, and radiation is significantly lower. Additionally, the aging process alters the patient's ability to perspire; therefore, heat loss through evaporation is reduced. Since the elderly patient cannot disperse heat effectively, classic heatstroke can develop rapidly. Typically, the older adult will not go through an initial stage of heat exhaustion. Factors that increase the possibility of heatstroke include medications, diabetes, alcohol abuse, malnutrition, parkinsonism, hyperthyroidism, and obesity.

Cold Exposure and the EMS Provider

As an EMT-B, you are also at risk for hypothermia if you work in a cold environment. You should be thoroughly familiar with local conditions. Be aware of existing and potential weather conditions, and stay on top of changes that are forecast for the area. Make sure proper clothing is available, and wear it whenever appropriate. Your vehicle should also be properly equipped and maintained for a cold environment. You cannot help others if you do not protect yourself.

■ Heat Exposure

The body's thermoregulatory systems keep the internal temperature constant, regardless of the temperature of the surrounding environment. In a hot environment or during vigorous physical activity, when the body itself produces excess heat, the body tries to rid itself of the excess heat. The two most efficient mechanisms are sweating (and evaporation of the sweat) and dilation of skin blood vessels, which brings blood to the skin surface to increase the rate of heat radiation.

Ordinarily, the heat-regulating mechanisms of the body work very well, and individuals are able to tolerate significant temperature changes. When the body is exposed to more heat energy than it can lose or the body generates more heat than it can lose, hyperthermia results. Hyperthermia is a high core temperature, usually 101°F (38.3°C) or higher.

High air temperature reduces the body's ability to lose heat by radiation; high humidity reduces the ability to lose heat through evaporation. Another contributing factor is vigorous exercise, during which the body can lose more than one liter of sweat an hour, causing loss of fluid and electrolytes. Heat exposure emergencies include:

- Heat cramps
- Heat exhaustion
- Heatstroke

All three forms of heat illness may be present in the same patient, since untreated heat exhaustion may progress to heatstroke. Heatstroke is a life-threatening emergency.

Persons at greatest risk for heat emergencies are children; geriatric patients; patients with heart disease, COPD, diabetes, dehydration, and obesity; and those with limited mobility. Older people, newborns, and infants exhibit poor thermoregulation. Newborns and infants often wear too much clothing. Alcohol and certain drugs, including medications that dehydrate the body or decrease the ability of the body to sweat, also make a person more susceptible to heat illnesses. When you are treating someone for a heat illness, always obtain a medication history.

Heat Cramps

Heat cramps are painful muscle spasms that occur after vigorous exercise. They do not occur only when it is hot outdoors. Sweat produced during strenuous exercise, particularly in a warm environment, causes a change in the body's electrolyte, or salt, balance. The result may be a loss of essential electrolytes from the cells. Dehydration may also play a role in the development of muscle cramps. Large amounts of water can be lost from the body as a result of excessive sweating. This loss of water may affect muscles that are being stressed and cause them to go into spasm.

Heat cramps usually occur in the leg or abdominal muscles. When the abdominal muscles are involved, the pain and muscle spasm may be so severe that the patient appears to have an acute abdominal problem. If a patient with a sudden onset of abdominal cramps has been exercising vigorously in a hot environment, you should suspect heat cramps.

Take the following steps to treat heat cramps in the field:

1. **Move the patient to a cooler environment** and loosen any tight clothing.
2. **Rest the cramping muscles.** Have the patient sit or lie down until the cramps subside.

3. **Replace fluids by mouth.** Use water or a diluted (half-strength) balanced electrolyte solution, such as Gatorade. In most cases, plain water is the most useful. Do not give salt tablets or solutions that have a high salt concentration.

If the cramps do not go away after these measures, transport the patient to the hospital. Most people will be able to resume activity once the cramps are gone. However, increased sweating may cause the cramps to recur. Hydration by drinking a lot of water is the best preventive and treatment strategy.

Heat Exhaustion

Heat exhaustion is the most common serious illness caused by heat. Heat exposure, stress, and fatigue are causes of heat exhaustion, which is due to hypovolemia as the result of the loss of water and electrolytes from significant sweating. For sweating to be an effective cooling mechanism, the sweat must be able to evaporate from the body. Otherwise, the body will continue to produce sweat, with further loss of body water. People standing in the hot sun and particularly those wearing several layers of clothing, such as football fans or parade watchers, may sweat profusely but experience little body cooling. High humidity also decreases the amount of evaporation that can occur. Individuals working or exerting themselves in poorly ventilated areas are unable to release heat through convection. People who work or exercise vigorously and those who wear heavy clothing in a warm, humid, or poorly ventilated environment are particularly prone to heat exhaustion.

Signs and symptoms of heat exhaustion include dizziness, weakness, or faintness with nausea or headache; pale, cold, clammy skin; dry tongue; and thirst. Vital signs are usually normal, although the pulse is often rapid and the diastolic blood pressure may be low. The patient's body temperature is normal or slightly elevated and on rare occasions, as high as 104°F (40°C).

To treat a patient with heat exhaustion, review the steps in Skill Drill 15-1 ▶:

1. **Remove any excessive layers of clothing,** particularly around the head and neck (**Step ①**).
2. **Move the patient promptly** from the hot environment, preferably into the back of the air-conditioned ambulance. If outdoors, move out of the sun.
3. **Give the patient oxygen** if not already done in the initial assessment.
4. **Encourage the patient to lie down** and elevate the legs (supine position). Loosen any tight clothing and fan the patient for cooling (**Step ②**).

5. **If the patient is fully alert,** encourage him or her to sit up and slowly drink up to a liter of water, as long as nausea does not develop. Never force fluids by mouth on a patient who is not fully alert, or allow drinking while supine, because the patient could aspirate the fluid into the lungs (**Step ③**). If the patient does become nauseated, transport on the side to prevent aspiration.

You should transport the patient to the hospital in the following circumstances:
- The symptoms do not clear up promptly.
- The level of consciousness decreases.
- The temperature remains elevated.
- The person is very young, older, or has any underlying medical condition, such as diabetes or cardiovascular disease.

6. **Transport the patient on his or her side** if the patient is nauseated, but make certain that the patient is secured (**Step ④**).

Heatstroke

Heatstroke, the least common but most serious illness caused by heat exposure, occurs when the body is subjected to more heat than it can handle. The body's normal mechanisms for getting rid of the excess heat are overwhelmed. Untreated heatstroke always results in death.

Heatstroke can develop in patients during vigorous physical activity or when they are outdoors or in a closed, poorly ventilated, humid environment. It also occurs during heat waves among individuals (particularly in geriatric patients) who live in buildings with no air conditioning or with poor ventilation. Heatstroke may also develop in children who are left unattended in a locked car on a hot day.

Many patients with heatstroke have hot, dry, flushed skin because their sweating mechanism is no longer working. However, early in the course of heatstroke, the skin may be moist or wet. Remember that a patient can have heatstroke even if he or she is still sweating. The body temperature rises rapidly to 106°F (41°C) or more in patients with heatstroke. As the core temperature rises, the patient's mental status becomes altered.

Often, the first sign of heatstroke is a change in behavior. Patients may become unresponsive very quickly. The pulse is usually rapid and strong at first, but as the patient becomes increasingly unresponsive, the pulse becomes weaker and the blood pressure falls.

Recovery from heatstroke depends on the speed with which treatment is administered, so you must be

Skill Drill   15-1   Treating for Heat Exhaustion

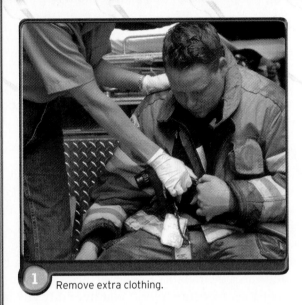

1 Remove extra clothing.

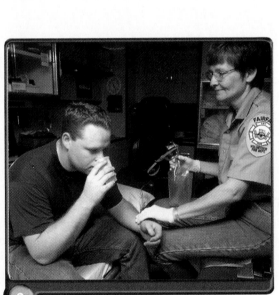

2 Move the patient to a cooler environment. Give oxygen. Place the patient in a supine position, elevate the legs, and fan the patient.

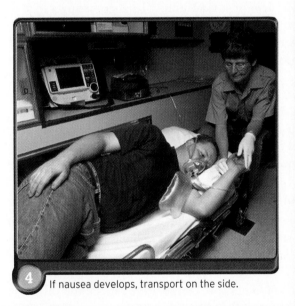

3 If the patient is fully alert, give water by mouth.

4 If nausea develops, transport on the side.

able to identify this patient quickly. Emergency treatment is aimed at getting the body temperature down by any means available. Review these steps when treating a patient with heatstroke:

1. **Move the patient out of the hot environment** and into an air-conditioned ambulance if possible.
2. **Remove the patient's clothing.**
3. **Administer oxygen** if not done as part of the initial assessment.
4. **Apply cool packs** to the patient's neck, groin, and armpits.
5. **Cover the patient with wet towels or sheets,** or spray the patient with cool water and fan.
6. **Provide immediate transport** to the hospital.

■ Assessment of Heat Emergencies

Scene Size-up

As part of your scene size-up, perform an environmental assessment. How hot is it outside? How hot is it in the room where your patient is? How well is the patient tolerating the heat? Dispatch may report the call initially as a medical or trauma problem. The heat illness may only be secondary. Approach the scene looking for hazards as well as clues as to what may have caused your patient's problem. If you anticipate a prolonged scene time, protect yourself from the heat. Use appropriate BSI precautions, including gloves and eye protection. Consider whether you need ALS backup. Intravenous fluids may need to be administered.

Initial Assessment

General Impression

As you approach your patient, observe how the patient interacts with you and the environment. Remember that a heat emergency may be the primary problem or it may simply be aggravating a medical or trauma condition. Use this initial interaction to guide you in assessing for immediate life threats and related problems.

Assess the patient's mental status using the AVPU scale. Heatstroke is a true life-threatening emergency. The severity of your patient's condition may be identified by gathering clues about his or her mental status. The more altered the patient's mental status is, the more serious the heat emergency.

Airway, Breathing, and Circulation

Assess the patient's ABCs and treat any life-threatening problems found. Nausea and vomiting are common in heat problems. Position the patient to protect the airway as necessary. Breathing will be fast depending on the patient's core temperature but should otherwise be adequate. Providing oxygen to the patient will assist with the perfusion of body tissues and may decrease nausea. If your patient is unresponsive, insert an airway and provide bag-mask ventilations.

Assess circulation by palpating for a radial pulse. If it is adequate, assess the patient for perfusion and bleeding. Hot, dry, or moist skin that appears red may indicate an elevated core-body temperature. Treat the patient aggressively for shock by removing the patient from the heat and positioning the patient to improve circulation.

Transport Decision

If your patient has any signs of heatstroke (high temperature; red, dry skin; altered mental status; tachycardia; poor perfusion), transport without delay.

Focused History and Physical Exam

If your patient is unresponsive, perform a rapid physical exam from head to toe. Obtain vital signs and gather any available history by talking to family or bystanders. If the patient is conscious, begin with getting a history and then perform a focused physical exam.

SAMPLE History

Obtain a SAMPLE history with emphasis on any activities, conditions, or medications that may predispose a patient to dehydration or heat-related problems. Patients with inadequate oral intake, or who are taking diuretics, may have difficulty tolerating exposure to heat. Many psychiatric medications used in geriatric patients affect their ability to tolerate heat. Determine your patient's exposure to heat and humidity and activities prior to the onset of symptoms.

Focused Physical Exam

Exposure to heat has significant effects on the metabolism, muscles, and cardiovascular system. Assess the patient's mental status and note skin vitals. If possible, take the patient's temperature.

Baseline Vital Signs

Patients who are hyperthermic have an increased respiratory rate and are tachycardic. As long as they maintain a normal blood pressure, their bodies are compensating for the fluid loss. Once their blood pressure begins to fall, it indicates they are no longer able to compensate for fluid loss and are going into shock. Your assessment of the patient's skin will help determine how significant the heat emergency is. In heat exhaustion, the skin temperature may be normal to cool and clammy. In heatstroke, the skin is hot.

Interventions

Remove your patient as quickly as possible from the hot environment. Patients with heat cramps or exhaustion usually respond well to passive cooling and fluids by mouth. Patients with symptoms of heatstroke should be transported immediately and actively cooled. Cover your patient with a wet sheet and fan him or her. Turn the ambulance air conditioner on high. Place cold packs to the neck, groin, and armpits.

Detailed Physical Exam

Perform a detailed physical exam if circumstances and time permits. Pay special attention to the patient's skin temperature. Perform a careful neurologic examination.

Ongoing Assessment

Monitor your patient's condition carefully. Any decline in level of consciousness is an ominous sign. Monitor the patient's vital signs at least every 5 minutes. Evaluate the effectiveness of your interventions. Be careful not to cause shivering when cooling down a patient that is overheated. Shivering generates more heat and can occur when cooling is not monitored closely.

Communication and Documentation

Notify the staff at the receiving facility early on that your patient is experiencing a heatstroke because additional resources may be required. Document the weather conditions and the activities prior to the emergency in your report.

◼ Drowning and Near Drowning

Drowning is death from suffocation after submersion in water. Near drowning is defined as survival, at least temporarily (24 hours), after suffocation in water. Drowning is often the last in a cycle of events caused by panic in the water (Figure 15-4 ▶). It can happen to anyone who is submerged in water for even a short period of time. Struggling toward the surface or the shore, the person becomes fatigued or exhausted, which leads him or her to sink even deeper. Drowning can also occur in mop buckets, puddles, bathtubs, and other places where the individual is not completely submerged. Small children can drown in only a few inches of water.

Inhaling very small amounts of either fresh or salt water can severely irritate the larynx, sending the muscles of the larynx and the vocal cords into spasm (laryngospasm). Laryngospasm prevents more water

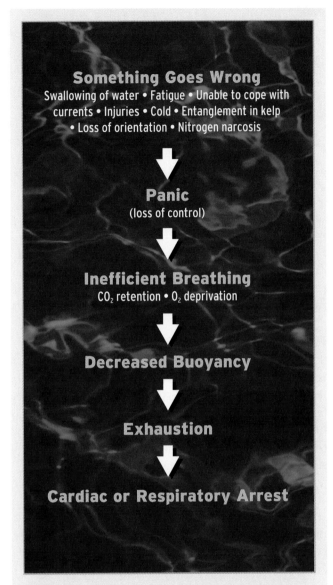

Figure 15-4 Panic in the water often precedes drowning.

Something Goes Wrong
Swallowing of water • Fatigue • Unable to cope with currents • Injuries • Cold • Entanglement in kelp • Loss of orientation • Nitrogen narcosis

⬇

Panic
(loss of control)

⬇

Inefficient Breathing
CO_2 retention • O_2 deprivation

⬇

Decreased Buoyancy

⬇

Exhaustion

⬇

Cardiac or Respiratory Arrest

from entering the lungs. In severe cases of drowning, you may have difficulty ventilating the patient because the patient may have a significant laryngospasm. Increasing hypoxia occurs until the patient becomes

You are the Provider 4

The patient's parents arrive on scene and he is feeling much better. After drinking approximately 32 ounces of fluid, his vital signs are within normal limits and he is walking around without assistance. The parents decide he does not need to be transported at this time and they sign your release form. They agree to call 9-1-1 or transport him to the emergency department immediately if anything changes.

Documentation Tips

Document the events regarding a drowning:

- How long was the patient submerged?
- What was the temperature of the water?
- What was the clarity of the water?
- Is there any possibility of cervical spine injury?

unconscious. At this point, the spasm relaxes, making rescue breathing possible. If the patient has not been removed from the water, the patient may now inhale deeply, and more water may enter the lungs. In 85% to 90% of cases, significant amounts of water enter the lungs of the drowning victim.

Spinal Injuries in Submersion Incidents

Submersion incidents may be complicated by spinal injuries. You must assume that a spinal injury exists when the incident is the result of a diving mishap or a fall, the patient is unconscious and there is little or no information available regarding the circumstances, or the patient is conscious and reports weakness, paralysis, or numbness in the arms or legs.

Most spinal injuries in diving incidents affect the cervical spine. When spinal injury is suspected, the spine must be protected from further injury. Review these steps to stabilize a suspected spinal injury if the patient is still in the water Skill Drill 15-2 ▶ :

1. **Turn the patient supine.** Two rescuers are usually required to turn the patient safely, although in some cases one rescuer will suffice. Always rotate the entire upper half of the patient's body as a single unit (**Step ①**).
2. **Manage the airway** and begin ventilation. Immediate ventilation is the primary treatment of all drowning and near-drowning patients as soon as the patient is face up in the water. Use a pocket mask if it is available. Have the other rescuer support the head and trunk as a unit while you open the airway and begin artificial ventilation (**Step ②**).
3. **Float a buoyant backboard** under the patient as you continue ventilation (**Step ③**).
4. **Secure the trunk and head** to the backboard (**Step ④**).
5. **Remove the patient from the water** on the backboard (**Step ⑤**).

6. **Cover the patient with a blanket.** Give oxygen if the patient is breathing spontaneously. Begin CPR if there is no pulse. Effective CPR is extremely difficult to perform when the patient is still in the water (**Step ⑥**).

Resuscitation Efforts

You should never give up on resuscitating a cold-water drowning victim. When a person is submerged in water that is colder than body temperature, heat will be conducted from the body to the water. The resulting hypothermia can protect vital organs from the lack of oxygen. In addition, exposure to cold water will occasionally activate certain primitive reflexes, which may preserve basic body functions for prolonged periods.

Whenever a person dives or jumps into very cold water, the diving reflex (slowing of the heart rate caused by submersion in cold water) may cause immediate bradycardia. Loss of consciousness and drowning may follow. However, the person may be able to survive for an extended period of time under water due to the lowering of the metabolic rate. For this reason, you should continue full resuscitation efforts no matter how long the patient has been submerged.

■ Diving Emergencies

Most serious water-related injuries are associated with dives, with or without scuba gear. Some of these problems are related to the nature of the dive; others result from panic. Panic is not restricted to the person who is frightened by water. It can happen even to the experienced diver or swimmer. Diving emergencies are separated into the three phases of the dive: descent, bottom, and ascent.

Descent Emergencies

Descent problems are usually due to the sudden increase in pressure on the body as the person dives deeper into the water. Some body cavities cannot adjust to the increased external pressure of the water, resulting in severe pain. The usual areas affected are the lungs, the sinus cavities, the middle ear, the teeth, and the area of the face surrounded by the diving mask. Usually, the pain caused by these "squeeze problems" forces the diver to return to the surface to equalize the pressures, and the problem clears up by itself. A diver who continues to report pain, particularly in the ear, after returning to the surface should be transported to the hospital.

Skill Drill   15-2   Stabilizing a Suspected Spinal Injury in the Water

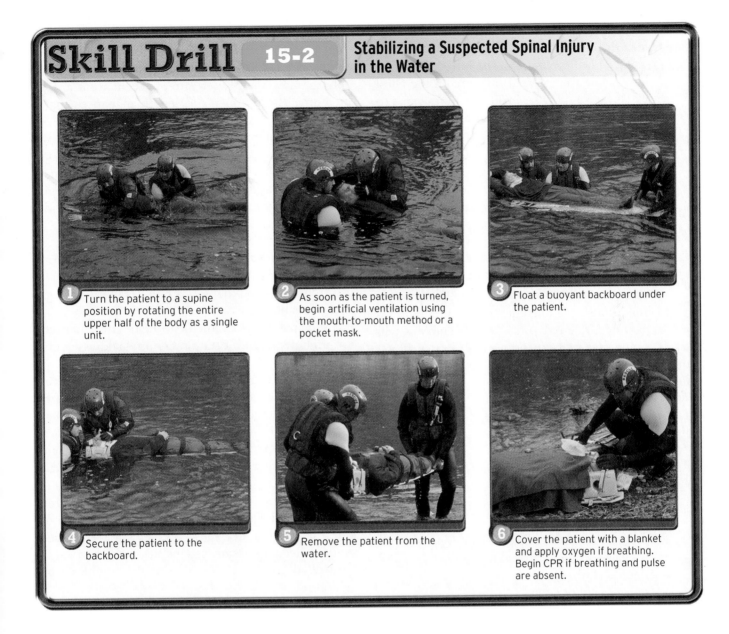

1 Turn the patient to a supine position by rotating the entire upper half of the body as a single unit.

2 As soon as the patient is turned, begin artificial ventilation using the mouth-to-mouth method or a pocket mask.

3 Float a buoyant backboard under the patient.

4 Secure the patient to the backboard.

5 Remove the patient from the water.

6 Cover the patient with a blanket and apply oxygen if breathing. Begin CPR if breathing and pulse are absent.

A person with a perforated tympanic membrane (ruptured eardrum) may develop a special problem while diving. If water enters the middle ear through a ruptured eardrum, the diver may lose his or her balance and orientation. The diver may then return too rapidly to the surface.

Emergencies at the Bottom

Problems related to the bottom of the dive are rarely seen. They include inadequate mixing of oxygen and carbon dioxide in the air the diver breathes and accidental mixing of poisonous carbon monoxide into the breathing apparatus. Both are the result of faulty connections in the diving gear. These situations can cause drowning or rapid ascent and require emergency resuscitation and transport.

Ascent Emergencies

Most injuries associated with diving are related to ascending from the bottom. These emergencies usually require aggressive resuscitation. Two particularly dangerous medical emergencies are air embolism and decompression sickness (also called "the bends").

Air Embolism

The most dangerous, and most common, emergency in scuba diving is <u>air embolism</u>, a condition involving bubbles of air in the blood vessels. Air embolism may occur on a dive as shallow as 6'. The problem starts when the diver holds his or her breath during a rapid ascent. The air pressure in the lungs remains at a high level while the external pressure on the chest decreases. As a result, the air inside the lungs expands rapidly, causing the alveoli in the lungs to rupture. The air released from this rupture can cause the following injuries:

- Air may enter the pleural space and compress the lungs (a pneumothorax).
- Air may enter the mediastinum (the space within the thorax that contains the heart and great vessels), causing a condition called pneumomediastinum.
- Air may enter the bloodstream and create bubbles of air in the vessels called air emboli.

Pneumothorax and pneumomediastinum both result in pain and severe dyspnea. An air embolus will act as a plug and prevent the normal flow of blood and oxygen to a specific part of the body. The brain and spinal cord are the organs most severely affected by air embolism.

The following are potential signs and symptoms of air embolism:

- Blotching (mottling of the skin)
- Froth (often pink or bloody) at the nose and mouth
- Severe pain in the muscles, joints, or abdomen
- Dyspnea and/or chest pain
- Dizziness, nausea, and vomiting
- Dysphasia (difficulty speaking)
- Vision disturbances
- Paralysis and/or coma
- Irregular pulse and even cardiac arrest

Decompression Sickness

Decompression sickness, commonly called the bends, occurs when bubbles of gas, especially nitrogen, obstruct the blood vessels. This condition results from too rapid an ascent from a dive. During the dive, inhaled nitrogen dissolves in the blood and tissues because it is under pressure. When the diver ascends, the external pressure is decreased, and the dissolved nitrogen forms small bubbles within those tissues. These bubbles can lead to problems similar to those that occur in air embolism (blockage of tiny blood vessels, depriving parts of the body of their normal blood supply). Severe pain in certain tissues or spaces in the body is the most common problem.

The most striking symptom is abdominal and/or joint pain so severe that the patient literally doubles up or "bends." Dive tables and computers are available to show the proper rate of ascent from a dive, including the number and length of pauses that a diver should make on the way up. However, even divers who stay within these limits can suffer the bends.

Even after a "safe dive," decompression sickness can occur from driving a car up a mountain or flying in an unpressurized airplane that climbs too rapidly to a great height. The risk of this diminishes after 24 to 48 hours. The problem is exactly the same as ascent from a deep dive: a sudden decrease of external pressure on the body and release of dissolved nitrogen from the blood that forms bubbles of nitrogen gas within the blood vessels.

You may find it difficult to distinguish between air embolism and decompression sickness. As a general rule, air embolism occurs immediately on return to the surface. The symptoms of decompression sickness may not occur for several hours after the dive. Emergency treatment of these conditions includes basic life support and transport to a facility with a hyperbaric chamber. A hyperbaric chamber is a chamber or a small room that is pressurized higher than atmospheric pressure. Recompression treatment allows the bubbles of gas to dissolve into the blood and equalizes the pressures inside and outside the lungs. Once these pressures are equalized, gradual decompression can be accomplished under controlled conditions to prevent the bubbles from reforming.

■ Assessment of Drowning and Diving Emergencies

Scene Size-up

In managing water emergencies, your BSI precautions should include gloves and eye protection. A mask may be necessary if aggressive airway management is necessary. Check for hazards to your crew. Never drive through moving water—a small amount can push the vehicle. Use extreme caution when driving through standing water. Never attempt a water rescue without proper training and equipment. If your patient is still in the water, look for the best, safest means of removal. This may require additional help from search-and-rescue teams or special extrication equipment. Trauma and spinal stabilization must be considered when the scene is a recreational setting. Check for additional patients based on where and how the problem occurred.

Initial Assessment
General Impression

Use the patient's chief complaint to guide you in your assessment of life threats and determine if spinal precautions are necessary. Pay particular attention to chest pain, dyspnea, and complaints related to sensory changes when a diving emergency is suspected. Determine their LOC using the AVPU scale. Remember that alcohol and drug use are known to be common with these types of emergencies.

Airway, Breathing, and Circulation

Begin with opening the airway and assessing breathing in any unresponsive patient. Use an airway adjunct to facilitate bag-mask ventilations as necessary. Suction if the patient has vomited or pink, frothy secretions are found in the airway. Provide bag-mask ventilations for breathing that is inadequate. Check for a pulse. It may be difficult to find a pulse because of constriction of the peripheral blood vessels and low cardiac output. If there is no pulse, start CPR.

If the patient is responsive, provide high-flow oxygen with a nonrebreathing mask and position the patient to protect the airway from aspiration in case of vomiting. Evaluate the patient for adequate perfusion and treat for shock by maintaining normal body temperature and improving circulation through positioning. If the chief complaint suggests trauma, assess for bleeding and treat appropriately.

Transport Decision

You should always transport near-drowning patients to the hospital. Inhalation of any amount of fluid can lead to delayed complications lasting for days or weeks. Patients with decompression sickness and air embolism must be treated in a recompression chamber. Perform all interventions en route.

Focused History and Physical Exam

If a drowning patient is responsive, assess the history first. On the basis of the chief complaint and the history obtained, perform a focused physical exam. This should include a thorough exam including breath sounds. For an unresponsive drowning patient, you should begin with a rapid physical exam to look for life threats and potential trauma, even if trauma is not suspected. After you perform a head-to-toe exam,

obtain the patient's baseline vital signs and a SAMPLE history.

Rapid Physical Exam

Perform a rapid physical exam on unresponsive medical patients. Look for signs of trauma or complications with the drowning. A diver with problems should be checked from head to toe for indications of the bends or an air embolism. Focus on pain in the joints and the abdomen. Pay attention to whether your patient is getting adequate ventilation and oxygenation, and check for signs of hypothermia.

Baseline Vital Signs

The vital signs are a good indicator of how your patient is tolerating the effects of drowning or diving complications. Check the patient's pulse rate, quality, and rhythm. Pulse and blood pressure may be difficult to palpate in the hypothermic patient. Check the respiratory rate, quality, and rhythm. Assess and document pupil size and reactivity.

SAMPLE History

Obtain a SAMPLE history, paying special attention to the length of time the drowning victim was under water or the time of onset of symptoms in relation to the last dive. Note any physical activity, alcohol or drug consumption, and other medical conditions. All of these may have an effect on the diving or drowning emergency. In diving emergencies, it is important to determine the dive parameters in your history, including depth, time, and previous diving activity.

Drowning Interventions

Treatment begins with rescue and removal from the water. When necessary, artificial ventilation should begin as soon as possible, even before the victim is removed from the water. Associated cervical spine injuries are possible, especially in diving accidents. If you do not suspect a spinal injury, you can turn the patient quickly to the left side to allow draining from the upper airway. Administer oxygen if this was not done as part of the initial assessment, either by mask for patients who are breathing spontaneously or via a bag-mask device for those requiring assisted ventilation.

Make sure that the patient is kept warm, especially after submersion in cold water. Make sure blankets and protection from the environment are provided as needed.

Diving Interventions

In treating patients who are suspected of having air embolism or decompression sickness, you should position the patient on his or her left side with the head down, or lower than the rest of the body. If local protocol allows, provide rapid transport to the closest hospital with a hyperbaric chamber.

Injury from decompression sickness is usually reversible with proper treatment. However, if the bubbles block critical blood vessels that supply the brain or spinal cord, permanent central nervous system injury may result. Therefore, the key in emergency management of these serious ascent problems is to recognize that an emergency exists and provide treatment as soon as possible. Administer oxygen and provide rapid transport.

Detailed Physical Exam

Time and personnel permitting, complete a detailed physical exam en route to the hospital. A careful head-to-toe exam may reveal additional injuries not initially observable. Examine the patient for respiratory, circulatory, and neurologic compromise. A careful distal circulatory, sensory, and motor function exam will be helpful in assessing the extent of the injury. Examine peripheral pulses, skin color and discoloration, itching, pain, and for any numbness and tingling.

Ongoing Assessment

The condition of patients who have experienced near drowning may deteriorate rapidly due to respiratory involvement, fluid shifts in the body, cerebral hypoxia, and hypothermia. Patients with air embolism or decompression sickness may decompensate quickly. Assess your patient's mental status constantly, and assess vital signs at least every 5 minutes, paying particular attention to respirations and lung sounds.

Communication and Documentation

Document the circumstances of the drowning and the events regarding the incident. The receiving facility personnel will need to know how long the patient was submerged, the temperature of the water, the clarity of the water, and whether there was any possibility of cervical spine injury.

The hospital will also need a complete dive profile to properly treat your patient. This may be available in a dive log or from diving partners. Small diving computers have become standard equipment for most divers, and they record information from the current as well as previous dives. If possible, bring any information and all of the diver's equipment to the hospital.

■ Other Water Hazards

You must pay close attention to the body temperature of a person who is rescued from cold water. Treat hypothermia caused by immersion in cold water the same way you treat hypothermia caused by cold exposure. Remove all wet clothing and prevent further heat loss from contact with the ground, stretcher, or air, and transport the patient promptly.

A person swimming in shallow water may experience breath-holding syncope, a loss of consciousness caused by a decreased stimulus for breathing. This happens to swimmers who breathe in and out rapidly and deeply before entering the water in an effort to expand their capacity to stay underwater. While increasing the oxygen level, this hyperventilation lowers the carbon dioxide level. Because an elevated level of carbon dioxide in the blood is the strongest stimulus for breathing, the swimmer may not feel the need to breathe even after using up all the oxygen in his or her lungs. The emergency treatment for a breath-holding syncope is the same as that for a drowning or near drowning.

Injuries caused by boat propellers, sharp rocks, water skis, or dangerous marine life may be complicated by immersion in cold water. In these cases, remove the patient from the water, taking care to protect the spine, and administer oxygen. Apply dressings and splints if indicated, and monitor the patient closely for any signs of immersion or cold injury.

You should be aware that a child who is involved in a drowning or near drowning may be the victim of child abuse. Although it may be difficult to prove, such incidents should be handled according to your protocols for suspected child abuse.

■ Prevention

Appropriate precautions can prevent most drowning incidents. Each year, many small children drown in residential pools. All pools should be surrounded by a fence that is at least 6' high, with slats no farther apart than 3" and self-closing, self-locking gates. The most common problem is lack of adult supervision. Half of all teenage and adult drownings are associated with the use of alcohol. As a health care professional, you should be involved in public education efforts to make people aware of the hazards of swimming pools and water recreation.

You are the Provider   Summary

Heat exhaustion is the most common of the serious heat emergencies and heat stroke is the most severe. Left untreated, this patient would have rapidly progressed to heat exhaustion. Move patients out of the hot environment and cool them down. Only give fluids by mouth if the patient is alert and able to swallow.

1. **What is this patient's problem?**

   Heat cramps

2. **What is the first step in treating him?**

   Move him out of the hot environment.

3. **Should the patient be cooled? If so, how?**

   Yes. He should be passively cooled but never to the point of shivering. Shivering is a means of generating heat and will defeat the purpose of cooling him.

4. **What else can you do for this patient?**

   He needs fluid for rehydration. Give water or a half-strength sports drink.

5. **Do you think the patient could be hypovolemic?**

   Yes.

6. **What vital sign might point toward hypovolemia?**

   His blood pressure is a little low for what you would expect for a 15-year-old boy.

7. **What could be causing it?**

   Excessive sweating due to the ambient temperature and his exertion

8. **What caused the change in his vital signs?**

   Orthostatic hypotension. Due to his dehydrated status, his change in position caused his blood pressure to drop and his heart rate to increase.

9. **How should this be treated?**

   As long as he is not nauseated, he can continue to drink fluids for rehydration. Only give fluids by mouth to those patients who are able to swallow and maintain their airway.

10. **What type of consent is used to treat this patient?**

    Implied consent. He is a minor and his parents are not on scene to give consent.

11. **If the cramps do not subside, what are your options?**

    He would need to be transported to the emergency department for IV fluid replacement and possible muscle relaxants to stop the cramping.

Assessment and Emergency Care

	Cold Injuries	Heat Injuries	Drowning and Diving Injuries
Scene Size-up	Body substance isolation precautions should include a minimum of gloves and eye protection. Ensure scene safety and determine NOI/MOI. Consider the number of patients, the need for additional help/ALS, and c-spine stabilization.	Body substance isolation precautions should include a minimum of gloves and eye protection. Ensure scene safety and determine NOI/MOI. Consider the number of patients, the need for additional help/ALS, and c-spine stabilization.	Body substance isolation precautions should include a minimum of gloves and eye protection. Ensure scene safety and determine NOI/MOI. Consider the number of patients, the need for additional help/ALS, and c-spine stabilization.
Initial Assessment			
■ General impression	Determine level of consciousness and find and treat any immediate threats to life. Determine priority of care based on environment and patient's chief complaint.	Determine level of consciousness and find and treat any immediate threats to life. Determine priority of care based on environment and patient's chief complaint.	Determine level of consciousness and find and treat any immediate threats to life. Determine priority of care based on environment and patient's chief complaint.
■ Airway	Ensure patent airway.	Ensure patent airway.	Ensure patent airway.
■ Breathing	Provide high-flow oxygen at 15 L/min. Evaluate depth and rate of respirations and provide ventilations as needed. Be prepared to suction.	Provide high-flow oxygen at 15 L/min. Evaluate depth and rate of respirations and provide ventilations as needed. Be prepared to suction.	Provide high-flow oxygen at 15 L/min. Evaluate depth and rate of respirations and provide ventilations as needed. Be prepared to suction.
■ Circulation	Evaluate pulse over a 30- to 45-second period for rate and quality; observe skin color, temperature, and condition and treat for any signs of shock. Determine if bleeding is present and control if life threatening.	Evaluate pulse rate and quality; observe skin color, temperature, and condition and treat aggressively for shock. If bleeding is present, control if life threatening.	Evaluate pulse rate and quality; observe skin color, temperature, and condition and treat for any sign of shock. Determine if bleeding is present and control if life threatening.
■ Transport decision	Rapid transport	Rapid transport	Rapid transport
Focused History and Physical Exam	NOTE: The order of the steps in the focused history and physical exam differs depending on whether the patient is conscious or unconscious. The order below is for a conscious patient. For an unconscious patient, perform a rapid physical exam, obtain vital signs, and obtain the history.		
■ SAMPLE history	Obtain SAMPLE history. Be sure to ask if and what interventions were taken before your arrival, how many interventions, and at what time.	Obtain SAMPLE history. Be sure to ask if and what interventions were taken before your arrival, how many interventions, and at what time. Determine patient's activities before onset of symptoms.	Obtain SAMPLE history. Determine if alcohol or recreational drugs have been consumed. Determine how long the patient was submerged and the water temperature and clarity.

	Cold Injuries	Heat Injuries	Drowning and Diving Injuries
■ Focused physical exam	Perform a focused physical exam on the affected area, looking for frostbite. Consider the possibility of hypothermia.	Perform focused physical exam on the respiratory drive, adequacy of ventilation, adequacy and effectiveness of the circulatory system, and the patient's mental status. Obtain core body temperature.	Perform focused physical exam on the respiratory drive, adequacy of ventilation, adequacy and effectiveness of the circulatory system, and the patient's mental status. Perform a rapid assessment and obtain a Glasgow Coma Scale score.
■ Baseline vital signs	Take vital signs for 60 seconds, noting skin color and temperature.	Take vital signs, noting skin color and temperature. Use pulse oximetry if available.	Take vital signs, noting skin color and temperature. Assess pupil size and reactivity.
■ Interventions	Handle the patient gently. Remove from cold environment/clothing and begin to rewarm the patient according to local protocol. Support patient as needed. Consider the use of humidified oxygen, positive pressure ventilations, adjuncts, and proper positioning.	Support patient as needed. Consider the use of oxygen, positive pressure ventilations, adjuncts, and proper positioning. Remove clothing, lay a wet sheet over the patient, and turn on air conditioner/fan. Place wrapped ice packs on groin and axillae. Request ALS for fluid therapy for patients suspected of having hypovolemia.	Continue spinal stabilization. Suction as needed. Consider the use of oxygen, positive pressure ventilations, and adjuncts. Make sure the patient is kept warm.
Detailed Physical Exam	Complete a detailed physical exam.	Complete a detailed physical exam.	Complete a detailed physical exam.
Ongoing Assessment	Repeat the initial assessment, focused assessment, and reassess interventions performed. Reassess vital signs every 5 minutes for the unstable patient, every 15 minutes for the stable patient. Note and treat the patient as necessary.	Repeat the initial assessment, focused assessment, and reassess interventions performed. Reassess vital signs every 5 minutes for the unstable patient, every 15 minutes for the stable patient. Note and treat the patient as necessary.	Repeat the initial assessment, focused assessment, and reassess interventions performed. Reassess vital signs every 5 minutes for the unstable patient, every 15 minutes for the stable patient. Note and treat the patient as necessary.
■ Communication and documentation	Contact medical control with a radio report that gives information on patient's condition. Relay any significant changes, including level of consciousness or difficulty in breathing. Note what the patient was wearing and pertinent bystander information. Add any changes in patient condition, at what time, and any interventions performed.	Contact medical control with a radio report that gives information on patient's condition. Relay any significant changes, including level of consciousness or difficulty in breathing. Be sure to document weather conditions and events leading up to the illness. Record any changes, at what time, and any interventions performed.	Contact medical control with a radio report that gives information on patient's condition. Relay any significant changes, including level of consciousness or difficulty in breathing. Be sure to document any changes, at what time, and any interventions performed. If the patient was on a diving expedition, include the patient's diving log and pertinent information from diving partners, as available.

Assessment and Emergency Care

Assessment and Emergency Care

NOTE: While the steps below are widely accepted, be sure to consult and follow your local protocol.

Cold Injuries	Heat Injuries	Drowning and Diving Injuries
1. Remove wet clothing and keep the patient dry.	1. Remove any excess layers of clothing.	1. Turn the patient to a supine position by rotating the entire upper half of the body as a single unit.
2. Prevent heat loss. Move the patient away from any wet or cold surface.	2. Move the patient promptly from the hot environment and out of the sun.	2. Begin artificial ventilation using the mouth-to-mouth method or a pocket mask.
3. Insulate all exposed body parts by wrapping them in a blanket or dry, bulky material.	3. Provide oxygen, if not already done during the initial assessment.	3. Float a buoyant backboard under the patient.
4. Prevent convection heat loss by erecting a wind barrier around the patient.	4. Encourage the patient to lie supine with legs elevated. Loosen any tight clothing and fan the patient.	4. Secure the patient to the backboard.
5. Remove the patient from the cold environment as promptly as possible.	5. If the patient is alert, encourage him or her to sit up and slowly drink a liter of water if nausea does not develop.	5. Remove the patient from the water.
	6. Transport patient in the left-lateral recumbent position.	6. Cover the patient with a blanket and apply oxygen if breathing. Begin CPR if breathing and pulse are absent.

Prep Kit

Ready for Review

- Local cold injuries include frostbite, frostnip, and immersion foot. Frostbite is the most serious because tissues actually freeze. All patients with a local cold injury should be removed from the cold and protected from further exposure.
- If instructed to do so by medical control, rewarm frostbitten parts by immersing them in water at a temperature between 100° and 105°F (38° and 40°C).
- The key to treating hypothermic patients is to stabilize vital functions and prevent further heat loss. Do not attempt to rewarm patients who have moderate to severe hypothermia, because they are prone to developing arrhythmias.
- Do not consider a patient dead until he or she is "warm and dead." Local protocol will dictate whether or not such patients receive CPR or defibrillation in the field.
- The body's regulatory mechanisms normally maintain body temperature within a very narrow range around 98.6°F (37°C). Body temperature is regulated by heat loss to the atmosphere via conduction, convection, evaporation, radiation, and respiration.
- Heat illness can take three forms: heat cramps, heat exhaustion, and heatstroke.
- Heat cramps are painful muscle spasms that occur with vigorous exercise. Treatment includes removing the patient from the heat, resting the affected muscles, and replacing lost fluids.
- Heat exhaustion is essentially a form of hypovolemic shock caused by dehydration. Symptoms include cold and clammy skin, weakness, confusion, headache, and rapid pulse. Body temperature can be high, and the patient may or may not still be sweating. Treatment includes removing the patient from the heat and treating for shock.
- Heatstroke is a life-threatening emergency, usually fatal if untreated. Patients with heatstroke are usually dry and have high body temperatures. Changes in mental status can include coma. Rapid lowering of the body temperature in the field is critical.
- The first rule in caring for drowning or near drowning victims is to be sure not to become a victim yourself. Protect the spine when removing patients from the water because spinal cord injuries often occur in drownings. Be aware of the possibility of hypothermia.
- Injuries associated with scuba diving may be immediately apparent or may show up hours later. Patients with air embolism or decompression sickness may have pain, paralysis, or altered mental status. Be prepared to transport such patients to a recompression facility with a hyperbaric chamber.

Vital Vocabulary

air embolism Air bubbles in the blood vessels.

conduction The loss of heat by direct contact (eg, when a body part comes into contact with a colder object).

convection The loss of body heat caused by air movement (eg, breeze blowing across the body).

drowning Death from suffocation by submersion in water.

evaporation Conversion of water or another fluid from a liquid to a gas.

frostbite Damage to tissues as the result of exposure to cold; frozen body parts.

heat cramps Painful muscle spasms usually associated with vigorous activity in a hot environment.

heat exhaustion A form of heat injury in which the body loses significant amounts of fluid and electrolytes because of heavy sweating; also called heat prostration or heat collapse.

heatstroke A life-threatening condition of severe hyperthermia caused by exposure to excessive natural or artificial heat, marked by warm, dry skin; severely altered mental status; and often irreversible coma.

hyperthermia A condition in which the core temperature rises to 101°F (38.3°C) or more.

hypothermia A condition in which the core temperature falls below 95°F (35°C) after exposure to a cold environment.

near drowning Survival, at least temporarily, after suffocation in water.

radiation The transfer of heat to colder objects in the environment by radiant energy, for example, heat gain from a fire.

respiration The loss of body heat as warm air in the lungs is exhaled into the atmosphere and cooler air is inhaled.

Technology

- Interactivities
- Vocabulary Explorer
- Anatomy Review
- Web Links
- Online Review Manual

Refresher.EMSzone.com

Assessment in Action

You work in the northeast where the humidity is high. Most of your calls consist of some type of cold-related problem during the winter and heat-related problems in the summer.

1. Cold emergencies can overwhelm temperature regulation mechanisms in which of the following populations?
   A. children
   B. elderly
   C. those with chronic illnesses
   D. all of the above

2. Most heat stroke cases occur when the temperature is _____.
   A. 70°F
   B. 80°F
   C. 90°F
   D. 100°F

3. The effect of the wind is a good example of heat transfer by _____.
   A. conduction
   B. convection
   C. evaporation
   D. radiation

4. How many times should a hypothermic patient in ventricular fibrillation be defibrillated with an AED?
   A. one
   B. two
   C. three
   D. six

5. What is the most common serious illness caused by heat?
   A. heat cramps
   B. heat exhaustion
   C. heat stroke
   D. heat prostration

Challenging Questions

6. Explain why shivering raises the body temperature.

7. Why do patients with heat stroke have hot, dry, flushed skin?

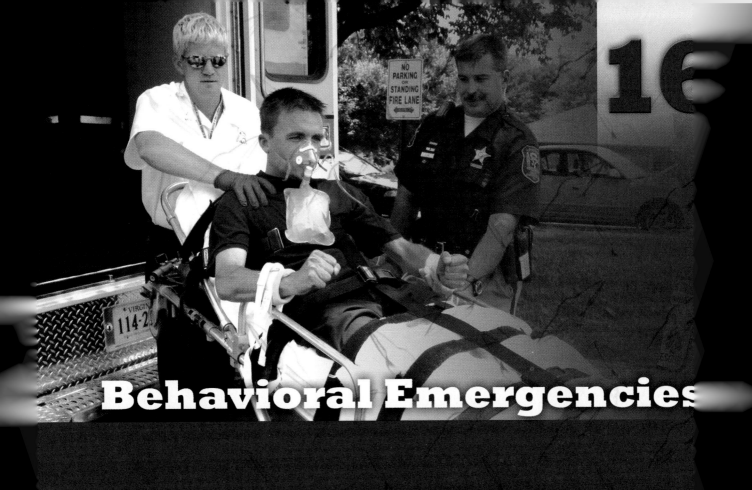

16

Behavioral Emergencies

You are the Provider 1

A 24-year-old woman with a psychiatric history has threatened to take a bottle of sleeping pills with a pint of vodka. She has written a suicide note stating that she is depressed because she lost her job and her boyfriend left her.

   You talk her into going willingly to the hospital for help, but she wants to gather a few things and use the bathroom before she goes.

Initial Assessment	Recording Time: 0 Minutes
Appearance	Anxious, otherwise normal
Level of consciousness	Alert to person, place, and time
Airway	Open and clear
Breathing	Normal
Circulation	Radials present, slightly tachycardic

1. What is significant about the method she has chosen to kill herself and the note she has written?
2. How should you handle her request?
3. Leaving the patient alone could result in what charges?

■ Introduction

As an EMT-B, you often deal with patients undergoing a psychological or behavioral crisis. The crisis may be due to many causes including the emergency situation, mental illness, mind-altering substances, or stress. This chapter discusses various kinds of behavioral emergencies, including those involving overdoses, violent behavior, and mental illness. We will review how to assess a person who exhibits signs and symptoms of a behavioral emergency and what kind of emergency care may be required in these situations. The chapter also covers legal concerns in dealing with disturbed patients. Finally, it describes how to identify and manage the potentially violent patient, including the use of restraints.

■ Myth and Reality

Everyone develops some symptoms of mental illness at some point in life, but that does not mean everyone develops mental illness. Perfectly healthy people may have some of the signs and symptoms of mental illness from time to time.

There are many normal reasons for feeling depressed, including divorce, loss of a job, and the death of a relative or friend. Temporarily withdrawing from ordinary activities and feeling down is a natural reaction to a crisis situation. Periodic, temporary depression is a normal part of life. However, when a person remains depressed week after week, he or she may indeed have a clinical disorder and need help.

As with all behavioral disorders, depression carries the potential for violence. It is not true that all depressed individuals are suicidal, nor are they all

dangerous. Seasoned EMTs know that only a small percentage of those with depression fall into these categories. You may be called to assist a depressed individual because family members or friends feel unable to manage the patient by themselves. This may be a result of drug or alcohol abuse which tends to worsen the depression. It may also be that the patient has a long history of mental illness and is reacting to a particularly stressful event. While you may not always be able to determine what has caused a person's depression, you may be able to predict whether the person will become violent. The ability to predict violence is an important assessment tool for you.

■ Defining Behavioral Emergencies

Behavior is what you can see of a person's response to the environment: his or her actions. Most of the time, individuals respond to the environment in reasonable ways. Over the years, they have learned to adapt to a variety of situations in daily life, including stresses and strains. This is called adjustment. There are times, however, when the stress is so great that the normal ways of adjusting do not work. When this happens, a person's behavior is likely to change, even if only temporarily. The new behavior may not be appropriate or considered normal.

The definition of a behavioral crisis or emergency is any reaction to events that interferes with the activities of daily living (ADL) or has become unacceptable to the patient, family, or community. For example, when someone experiences an interruption of the daily routine, such as bathing, dressing, and eating, chances are his or her behavior has become a problem. For that person, at that time, a behavioral emergency may exist. If the interruption of daily routine tends to recur on a regular basis, the behavior is also considered a mental health problem. It is then a pattern, rather than an isolated incident.

A person who experiences a panic attack after having a heart attack is not necessarily mentally ill. Likewise, you would expect a person who is fired from a job to have some sort of reaction, often sadness and depression. These problems are short-term and isolated events. However, a person who reacts with a fit of rage, attacking people and property or going on a "bender" for a week, has gone beyond what society considers appropriate or normal behavior. That person is clearly undergoing a behavioral emergency. Usually, if an abnormal or disturbing pattern of behavior lasts for at least a month, it is regarded as a matter of concern from a mental health standpoint. For example, chronic depression, a persistent feeling of sadness and despair, may be a symptom of a mental or physical disorder. This type of long-term problem would be labeled a mental health disorder.

When a psychiatric emergency arises, the patient may show agitation or violence or become a threat to himself, herself, or others. This is more serious than a more typical behavioral emergency that causes inappropriate behavior such as interference with ADL or bizarre behavior. An immediate threat to the person involved or to others in the immediate area, including family, friends, bystanders, and EMT-Bs should be considered a psychiatric emergency. For example, a person might respond to the death of a spouse by attempting suicide. On the other hand, although this is a major life disruption, it does not have to involve violence or harm to an individual. Disruption can take many forms; not all involve violence, nor are they all psychiatric emergencies.

The Magnitude of Mental Health Problems

According to the National Institutes of Mental Health, at one time or another, one in five Americans has some type of mental disorder, an illness with psychological or behavioral symptoms that may result in impaired functioning. It can be caused by a social, psychological, genetic, physical, chemical, or biologic disturbance.

Causes of Behavioral Emergencies

As an EMT-B, you are not responsible for diagnosing the underlying cause of a behavioral or psychiatric emergency. However, you should know the two basic categories of diagnosis a physician will use: organic (physical) and functional (psychological).

Organic brain syndrome is a temporary or permanent dysfunction of the brain caused by disturbance in the physical or physiologic functioning of brain tissue. Causes of organic brain syndrome include sudden illness, recent trauma, drug or alcohol intoxication, and diseases of the brain, such as Alzheimer's disease. Altered mental status can arise from low levels of blood glucose, lack of oxygen, inadequate blood flow to the brain, and excessive heat or cold.

A functional disorder is one in which the abnormal operation of an organ cannot be traced to an obvious change in the actual structure, or physiology, of the organ. Something has gone wrong, but the root cause cannot be identified as the working of the organ itself. Schizophrenia and depression are good examples of functional disorders. There may be a chemical or physical cause for these disorders, but it is not obvious or well understood.

These two types of disorders can present the same way. An altered mental status, or a change in the way a person thinks or behaves, is one indicator of central

You are the Provider 2

You explain to her that your policy will not allow her to be alone. Either your female partner or you must accompany her. She suddenly becomes very agitated. She does not want anyone in the bathroom with her. She says that if you will not allow her to go alone she will refuse to go to the hospital. She pleads her case and promises that she will be okay.

Vital Signs	Recording Time: 3 Minutes
Skin	Warm, flushed
Pulse	120 beats/min, regular
Blood pressure	140/90 mm Hg
Respirations	22 breaths/min, normal tidal volume

4. Should you allow her to go to the bathroom alone to ensure her cooperation?
5. What are your options?

nervous system diseases. A patient displaying bizarre behavior may actually have an acute medical illness that is the cause, or a partial cause, of the behavior. Recognizing this possibility may allow you to save a life.

Safe Approach to a Behavioral Emergency

All regular EMT-B skills—assessment, providing care, patient approach, obtaining the history, and patient communication—are used in behavioral emergencies. Other management techniques are also needed when dealing with a behavioral emergency. Review the general guidelines in ⟨ Table 16-1 ▾ ⟩ to ensure your safety at the scene of a behavioral emergency.

■ Assessment of a Behavioral Emergency

Scene Size-up

Dispatch may provide you with information that suggests a behavioral emergency. However, remember that

every situation has the potential for some component of a behavioral emergency. It may be a medical problem made worse by a behavioral issue, or it may be that a behavioral issue has led to trauma. Regardless, the first things to consider are your safety and the patient's response to the environment. Some situations may be more serious than others and, therefore, more threatening to your safety. Is the situation dangerous to you and your partner? Do you need immediate law enforcement backup? Does the patient's behavior seem typical or normal in the circumstances? Are there legal

✋ EMT-B Safety

Always leave yourself an out! Make sure the patient is not between you and the door. Call for law enforcement early when there is the potential for violence.

Table 16-1 Safety Guidelines for Behavioral Emergencies

Have a definite plan of action.	Who will do what? If restraint is needed, how will it be accomplished?
Identify yourself calmly.	Try to gain the patient's confidence. A low, calm voice is often a quieting influence.
Be direct.	State your intentions and what you expect of the patient.
Assess the scene.	If the patient is armed or has potentially harmful objects in his or her possession, have these removed by law enforcement personnel before you provide care.
Stay with the patient.	Do not let the patient leave the area, and do not leave it yourself unless law enforcement personnel can stay with the patient. The patient may obtain weapons or take pills if left alone.
Encourage purposeful movement.	Help the patient get dressed and gather appropriate belongings to take to the hospital.
Do not get too close to the patient.	Do not physically talk down to or directly confront the patient. A squatting, 45° angle approach is usually not confrontational but may hinder your movements. Do not allow the patient to get between you and the exit.
Avoid fighting with the patient.	You do not want to get into a power struggle. The patient may be wrestling with internal forces over which neither of you has control. If you can respond with understanding to the feeling that the patient is expressing, you may be able to gain his or her cooperation. If it is necessary to use force, be sure you have adequate help. Move toward the patient quietly and with assured firmness.
Be honest and reassuring.	If the patient asks whether he or she has to go to the hospital, the answer should be, "Yes, that is where you can receive medical help."

issues involved (crime scene, consent, refusal)? Take appropriate BSI precautions. Request any additional resources you may need (law enforcement, additional personnel) early. You can always send them away if they are not needed.

Initial Assessment
General Impression

Begin your assessment as you approach the patient. How does the patient appear? Calm? Agitated? Awake or sleepy? Begin with an introduction of who you are and let the patient know that you are there to help. Start talking to the patient by asking "What happened?" Allow the patient to tell what happened or how he or she feels. Is the patient alert and oriented? Use the AVPU scale for alertness.

Airway, Breathing, and Circulation

If your patient is in physical distress, assess the ABCs as for any other patient. Provide the appropriate interventions based on your assessment findings. Some behavioral situations may involve a compromised airway and inadequate breathing secondary to a suicide attempt from ingesting a handful of sleeping pills with alcohol. A depressed person may slit his or her wrists, causing bleeding. Almost every situation, medical or trauma, will have some behavioral component. It is just as important to treat the behavioral problem as it is to treat the medical or traumatic problem. Remember that the focus of the initial assessment is assessing and treating life threats.

Transport Decision

Unless your patient is unstable from a medical problem or trauma, prepare to spend time with him or her. Local protocols may allow for transporting a patient with a behavioral emergency to a specific facility.

In an unconscious medical patient, begin with a rapid physical exam to look for a reason for the unresponsiveness. Follow this rapid check for hidden life threats with a complete set of baseline vital signs and then gather what history you can.

When a medical patient is conscious, begin with asking the patient about health history and performing a focused physical exam as necessary; then obtain a full set of baseline vital signs. A focused physical exam for a behavioral problem may be difficult to perform but may provide clues to the patient's state of mind and thinking. Some patients welcome physical contact as reassuring, but others may feel acutely

threatened. Avoid touching the patient without permission.

Your assessment should consider three major areas:

- Is the patient's central nervous system functioning properly? Assess for a possible diabetic emergency (hypoglycemia), overdose, or trauma that could be causing the behavior.
- Are hallucinogens or other drugs or alcohol a factor? Does the patient see strange things? Is everything distorted? Do you smell alcohol on the patient's breath?
- Are psychogenic circumstances, symptoms, or illness (caused by mental rather than physical factors) involved? These might include the death of a loved one, severe depression, a history of mental illness, threats of suicide, or some other major interruption of ADL.

Focused History and Physical Exam
SAMPLE History

A complete and careful SAMPLE history will be helpful in treating your patient and passing on information to personnel at the receiving facility. You may be able to elicit information not available to the hospital staff. Ask specifically about previous episodes, treatments, hospitalizations, and medications related to behavioral problems Table 16-2 ▼.

Table 16-2 Questions to Ask in Evaluating a Behavioral Crisis

- Does the patient answer your questions appropriately?
- Does the patient's behavior seem appropriate?
- Does the patient seem to understand you and the surroundings?
- Is the patient withdrawn or detached? Hostile or friendly? Elated or depressed?
- Are the patient's vocabulary and expressions what you would expect under the circumstances?
- Does the patient seem aggressive or dangerous to you or others?
- Is the patient's memory intact? Check orientation to time, place, person, and event: What day, month, and year is it? Who am I?
- Does the patient express disordered thoughts, delusions, or hallucinations?

Is Alzheimer's disease or another type of dementia a possible cause? In geriatric patients, consider Alzheimer's disease and dementia as possible causes of abnormal behavior. In these cases, it is essential to obtain information from relatives, friends, or extended care facility staff. Determining the patient's baseline mental status will be essential in guiding your treatment and transport decisions.

Family, friends, and observers may be of great help in answering these questions. Together with your observations and interaction with the patient, they should provide enough data for you to assess the situation. This assessment has two primary goals: recognizing major threats to life and reducing the stress of the situation as much as possible.

Reflective listening is a technique frequently used by mental health professionals to gain insight into a patient's thinking. It involves repeating, in question form, what the patient has said, encouraging the patient to expand on the thoughts. Although it often requires more time to be effective than is available in an EMS setting, it may be a helpful tool for you to use when other techniques are unsuccessful at gathering the patient's history.

Focused Physical Exam

Sometimes even a patient who is conscious in a behavioral or psychiatric emergency will not respond at all to your questions. In those cases, you may be able to tell quite a lot about the patient's emotional state from facial expressions, pulse, and respirations. Tears, sweating, and blushing may be significant indicators of state of mind. Also, make sure that you look at the patient's eyes; a patient who has a blank gaze or rapidly moving eyes may be experiencing central nervous system dysfunction.

A behavioral crisis puts tremendous stress on a person's coping mechanisms. The person is actually incapable of responding reasonably to the demands of the environment. This state may be temporary, as in an acute illness, or longer lived, as in a complex,

Teamwork Tips

Separate family members and bystanders from the patient to de-escalate a potentially violent situation. One EMT-B should talk to the patient alone while the second EMT-B talks to others in a separate area.

chronic mental illness. In either case, the patient's perception of reality may be compromised or distorted.

Baseline Vital Signs

Obtain vital signs when doing so will not exacerbate your patient's emotional distress. Make every effort to assess blood pressure, pulse, respirations, skin, and pupils. Remember that behavioral emergencies can be caused or precipitated by physiologic problems, and they can exacerbate preexisting conditions.

Interventions

There often is little you will be able to do for the patient during the short time you will be treating him or her. Your job is to diffuse and control the situation and safely transport your patient to the hospital. Intervene only as much as it takes to accomplish these tasks. Be caring and careful. If you have determined that it is necessary to restrain your patient, release the restraints only if necessary to provide patient care.

Detailed Physical Exam

Unless there is an accompanying physical complaint, the detailed physical exam is rarely called for in a patient with a behavioral problem. This may, in fact, be detrimental to gaining the patient's trust.

Ongoing Assessment

Never let your guard down. Most patients you are called to treat and transport with emotional complaints pose no danger to you or others on your crew, but it is impossible to determine this on scene. Remember that many patients experiencing behavioral problems will act spontaneously. Be prepared to intervene quickly. If restraints are necessary, reassess and document respirations, as well as pulse and motor and sensory function in all restrained extremities, every 5 minutes. Respiratory and circulatory problems have been known to occur in combative patients who are restrained. When available, have additional personnel such as law enforcement officers or fire fighters accompany you in the back of the ambulance during transport. This provides additional assistance should the patient's behavior change rapidly.

Communication and Documentation

Try to give the receiving hospital advance warning when a behavioral emergency patient is coming. Many hospitals require extra preparation to ensure appropriate staff or rooms are available. Report whether restraints will be required when the patient arrives at the hospital. Document thoroughly and carefully. Think about what you are going to write before you write it, so that you can describe what are often confusing scenes as clearly as possible. Behavioral emergencies can often involve legal matters; be sure to document everything that occurred on the call, particularly situations that required restraint. When restraints are required to protect you or the patient from harm, include why and what type of restraints were used. This information is essential if the case is reviewed for medicolegal reasons.

■ Suicide

The single most significant factor that contributes to suicide is depression. Any time you encounter an emotionally depressed patient, you must consider the possibility of suicide. Risk factors for suicide are listed in Table 16-3 ▶.

It is a common misconception that people who threaten suicide never commit it. This is not correct. Suicide is a cry for help. Threatening suicide is an indication that someone is in a crisis he or she cannot handle. Immediate intervention is necessary.

Whether or not the patient has any of these risk factors, you must be alert to the following warning signs:

- Does the patient exhibit sadness, deep despair, or hopelessness that suggests depression?
- Does the patient avoid eye contact, speak slowly or haltingly, and project a sense of vacancy, as if he or she really isn't there?

Table 16-3 Risk Factors for Suicide

- Depression, any age
- Previous suicide attempt (80% of successful suicides are preceded by at least one unsuccessful attempt.)
- Current expression of wanting to commit suicide or a sense of hopelessness
- Family history of suicide
- Age older than 40 years, particularly for single, widowed, divorced, alcoholic, or depressed individuals. Men in this category who are older than age 55 years have an especially high risk.
- Recent loss of spouse, significant other, family member, or support system
- Holidays
- Chronic debilitating illness or recent diagnosis of serious illness
- Financial setback, loss of job, police arrest, imprisonment, or some sort of social embarrassment
- Substance abuse, particularly with increasing usage
- Children of an alcoholic parent
- Severe mental illness
- Anniversary of death of loved one, job loss, marriage, etc.
- Unusual gathering or new acquisition of things that can cause death, such as purchase of a gun, a large volume of pills, or a large amount of alcohol

You are the Provider 3

Your partner steps outside to call medical control who advises to go ahead and restrain the patient and transport. There is no one on scene except you and your partner, so you call for law enforcement assistance. While waiting for them to arrive, you ask about her medications. She tells you that she is not crazy and she wants you to leave her house. When you tell her that you cannot leave her alone she becomes even more upset and calls 9-1-1, crying hysterically, and tells the dispatcher that she is being assaulted by the people who were supposed to help her.

Reassessment	Recording Time: 5 Minutes
Skin	Flushed, diaphoretic
Pulse	136 beats/min, bounding
Blood pressure	152/94 mm Hg
Respirations	26 breaths/min, good tidal volume

6. Why is law enforcement needed for assistance?
7. What type of consent is used to treat this patient?
8. What else might you try to calm her down?

- Does the patient seem unable to talk about the future? Ask the patient whether he or she has any vacation plans. Suicidal people consider the future so uninteresting that they do not think about it.
- Is there any suggestion of suicide? Even vague suggestions should not be taken lightly, even if presented as a joke. If you think that suicide is a possibility, do not hesitate to bring the subject up. You will not "give the patient ideas" if you ask directly, "Are you considering suicide?"
- Does the patient have any specific plans relating to death? Has the patient recently prepared a will? Given away significant possessions or advised close friends what he or she would like done with them? Arranged for a funeral service? These are critical warning signs.

Consider also the following additional risk factors for suicide:

- Are there any unsafe objects in the patient's hands or nearby (for example, a sharp knife, glass, a gun)?
- Is the environment unsafe (for example, an open window in a high-rise building, a patient standing on a bridge)?
- Is there evidence of self-destructive behavior (for example, partially cut wrists, large alcohol or drug intake)?
- Is there an imminent threat to the patient or others?
- Is there an underlying medical problem?

Remember, the suicidal patient may be homicidal as well. Do not jeopardize your life or the lives of your fellow EMT-Bs. If you have reason to believe that you are in danger, you must obtain police intervention. In the meantime, try not to frighten the patient or make him or her suspicious.

■ Medicolegal Considerations

The medical and legal aspects of emergency medical care become more complicated when the patient is undergoing a behavioral or psychiatric emergency. Nevertheless, legal problems are greatly reduced with an emotionally disturbed patient who consents to care. Gaining the patient's confidence is a critical task.

Mental incapacity can take many forms: unconsciousness (as a result of hypoxia, alcohol, or drugs), temporary but severe stress, or depression. Once you have determined that a patient has impaired mental capacity, you must decide whether he or she requires

Documentation Tips

Documentation should always be *objective*. Include only those things that can be seen, measured, or are told to you by the patient. Do not add your own opinions.

immediate emergency medical care. A patient with a mentally unstable condition may resist your attempts to provide care. Nevertheless, you must not leave this patient alone. Doing so may result in harm to the patient and expose you to civil action for abandonment or negligence. In such situations, you should request that law enforcement handle the patient. Another reason for seeking law enforcement support is for the patient who resists treatment; such a patient often threatens EMT-Bs and others. Violent or dangerous people must be taken into custody by the police before emergency care can be rendered.

Consent

When a patient is not mentally competent to grant consent for emergency medical care, the law assumes that there is implied consent. In a situation that is not immediately life threatening, emergency medical care or transportation may be delayed until the proper consent is obtained. If you are not sure, you should request the assistance of law enforcement personnel.

Limited Legal Authority

As an EMT-B, you have limited legal authority to require or force a patient to undergo emergency medical care when no life-threatening emergency exists. Patients have the right to refuse care. However, most states have legal statutes regarding the emergency care of mentally ill and drug-impaired individuals. These statutory provisions permit law enforcement personnel to place such a person in protective custody so that emergency care can be given. You should be familiar with your local and state laws regarding these situations.

The general rule of law is that a competent adult has the right to refuse treatment, even if lifesaving care is involved. In psychiatric cases, however, a court of law would probably consider your actions in providing lifesaving care to be appropriate, particularly if you have a reasonable belief that the patient would harm himself, herself, or others without your inter-

Geriatric Needs

As the population ages, you will begin to see more patients older than 65 years. In responding to an increasing number of geriatric patients, you will probably notice some behavioral or mental health problems, including depression, dementia, and delirium. These mental status changes can affect your ability to thoroughly assess and treat an ill or injured geriatric patient.

As the EMT-B responding to a call for help, you should accept the possibility of depression in a geriatric patient. Do not discount the patient's feelings or devalue his or her emotions. Be alert for a suicidal gesture, and pay attention to any statements about death. To get the patient's cooperation, you can elicit his or her help in providing care for the acute illness or injury. A smile and a touch can go a long way in alleviating fear in all of your patients, especially older adults.

vention. In addition, a patient who is in any way impaired, whether by mental illness, medical condition, or intoxication, may not be considered competent to refuse treatment or transportation. When in doubt, consult your supervisor, police, or medical control. Err on the side of treatment and transport.

Restraint

If you restrain a person without authority in a non-emergency situation, you expose yourself to a possible lawsuit and to personal danger. Legal actions against you can involve charges of assault, battery, false imprisonment, and violation of civil rights. You may use restraints only to protect yourself or others from bodily harm or to prevent the patient from causing injury to himself or herself. In either case, you may use only reasonable force as necessary to control the patient. For this reason, you should always consult medical control and contact law enforcement personnel for help before restraining a patient.

You should always involve law enforcement personnel if you are called to assist a patient in a severe behavioral or psychiatric crisis. They will provide physical backup in managing the patient and serve as the necessary witnesses and legal authority to restrain the patient. A patient who is restrained by law enforcement personnel is in their custody.

Always try to transport the patient without restraints if possible. Once the decision has been made to restrain a patient, however, you should carry it out quickly. Be aware of BSI precautions. If the patient is spitting, place a surgical mask over his or her mouth.

Make sure you have adequate help to restrain a patient safely. At least four people should be present to carry out the restraint, each being responsible for one extremity. Before you begin, discuss the plan of action.

In subduing a disturbed patient, use the minimum force necessary. You should avoid acts of physical force that may cause injury to the patient. The level of force will vary, depending on the following factors:

- The degree of force that is necessary to keep the patient from injuring himself, herself, or others
- A patient's gender, size, strength, and mental status
- The type of abnormal behavior the patient is exhibiting

Remember to treat the patient with dignity and respect at all times. Also, monitor the patient for vomiting, airway obstruction, and cardiovascular stability. Drug or alcohol intoxication may cause violent behavior but can also lead to medical emergencies. Never place your patient facedown because it is impossible to adequately monitor the patient and this position may inhibit the breathing of an impaired or exhausted patient. Be careful not to place restraints in such a way that the patient's airway and breathing are compromised. Reassess airway and breathing continuously. You should make frequent checks of circulation on all

You are the Provider 4

Two deputies arrive on scene and she agrees to go willingly without being restrained. She is transported to the emergency department where laboratory work shows that her psychiatric medication levels are low. Her medication is adjusted and she is released from the hospital after 2 days with continuing appointments set up for outpatient counseling.

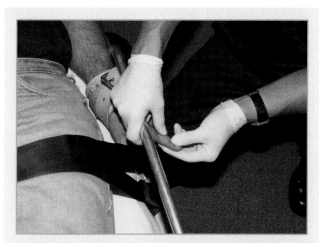

Figure 16-1 Assess circulation frequently while a patient is restrained.

restrained extremities, regardless of the patient's position Figure 16-1▲. Document the reason for the restraint and the technique that was used. Be especially careful if a combative patient suddenly becomes calm and cooperative. This is the time not to relax but to secure the situation. The patient may suddenly become combative again and injure someone. Keep in mind that you may use reasonable force to defend yourself against an attack by an emotionally disturbed patient. It is extremely helpful to have (and document) witnesses in attendance even during transport to protect against false accusations.

■ The Potentially Violent Patient

Violent patients make up only a small percentage of those undergoing a behavioral or psychiatric crisis. However, the potential for violence by such a patient is always an important consideration Figure 16-2 ▶.

Use the following list of risk factors to assess the level of danger:

- **History.** Has the patient previously exhibited hostile, overly aggressive, or violent behavior? Ask individuals at the scene, or request this information from law enforcement personnel or family.
- **Posture.** How is the patient sitting or standing? Is the patient tense, rigid, or sitting on the edge of his or her seat? Such physical tension is often a warning signal of impending violence.
- **The scene.** Is the patient holding or near potentially lethal objects such as a knife, gun, glass, or bat (or near a window or glass door)?

- **Vocal activity.** What kind of speech is the patient using? Loud, obscene, erratic, and bizarre speech patterns usually indicate emotional distress. Someone using quiet, ordered speech is not as likely to strike out as someone who is yelling and screaming.
- **Physical activity.** The motor activity of a person undergoing a psychiatric crisis may be the most telling factor of all. The patient who has tense muscles, clenched fists, or glaring eyes; is pacing; cannot sit still; or is fiercely protecting personal space requires careful watching. Agitation may predict a quick escalation to violence.

Other factors to consider in assessing a patient's potential for violence include the following:

- Poor impulse control
- A history of truancy, fighting, and uncontrollable temper
- Low socioeconomic status, unstable family structure, or inability to keep a steady job
- Tattoos, especially those with gang identification or statements such as "Born to Kill" or "Born to Lose"
- Substance abuse
- Depression, which accounts for 20% of violent attacks
- Functional disorder (If the patient says that voices are telling him or her to kill, believe it.)

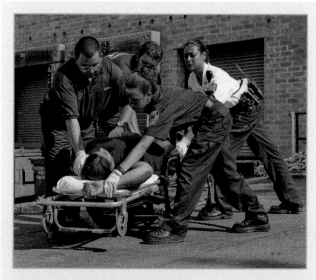

Figure 16-2 The potential for violence is an important consideration for EMT-Bs.

You are the Provider | Summary

Psychiatric patients are often difficult to deal with, especially if they have not taken their medication properly or if the dose is incorrect. When in doubt, always call medical control for direction and follow local protocols for properly restraining a patient.

1. **What is significant about the method she has chosen to kill herself and the note she has written?**

   She has a plan and has written a note. These are signs that she will probably follow through with her threat.

2. **How should you handle her request?**

   Do not leave her alone. A suicidal patient may lock themselves in another room and carry out their plans. Offer for your partner or a family member to gather her belongings, or offer to help her pack them.

3. **Leaving the patient alone could result in what charges?**

   Abandonment and negligence. This is especially true if something happens to her.

4. **Should you allow her to go to the bathroom alone to ensure her cooperation?**

   No. The patient should not be left alone for any reason.

5. **What are your options?**

   Explain the situation to her and tell her that you cannot allow her to be alone for her personal safety. Call for law enforcement. Call medical control for orders to restrain the patient.

6. **Why is law enforcement needed for assistance?**

   You must have four persons to restrain a patient. There should be one for each extremity.

7. **What type of consent is used to treat this patient?**

   Implied. Even though she is alert and oriented, she is not capable of making rational decisions.

8. **What else might you try to calm her down?**
   - Have your partner talk to her.
   - Explain again that she needs help.
   - Offer to help her gather her clothes. By giving her a task to take her mind off of the situation, she may be more receptive to your presence.

Assessment and Emergency Care

Behavioral Emergencies

Scene Size-up	Body substance isolation should include a minimum of gloves and eye protection. Ensure scene safety and determine NOI/MOI. Consider the number of patients, the need for additional help/ALS, and c-spine stabilization.
Initial Assessment	
■ General impression	Begin assessing from a distance. Determine level of consciousness and find and treat any immediate threats to life. Determine priority of care based on environment and patient's chief complaint.
■ Airway	Ensure patent airway.
■ Breathing	Consider high-flow oxygen at 15 L/min. Evaluate depth/rate of the respirations and provide ventilations as needed. Be prepared to suction.
■ Circulation	Evaluate pulse for rate and quality; observe skin color, temperature, and condition and treat accordingly. Evaluate and treat external bleeding. Treating any sign of shock.
■ Transport decision	Transport to appropriate facility.
Focused History and Physical Exam	*NOTE: The order of the steps in the focused history and physical exam differs depending on whether the patient is conscious or unconscious. The order below is for a conscious patient. For an unconscious patient, perform a rapid physical exam, obtain vital signs, and obtain the history.*
■ SAMPLE history	Obtain SAMPLE history, eliciting answers from family members/friends when possible.
■ Focused physical exam	Perform focused physical on the central nervous system, recent use of drugs, including alcohol and hallucinogens, and whether psychogenic circumstances, symptoms, or illness is involved.
■ Baseline vital signs	Take a full set of vital signs, noting skin color and temperature.
■ Interventions	Diffuse and control the situation and safely transport. Intervene only as much as it takes to accomplish these tasks.
Detailed Physical Exam	Without suspicion of physical injury, a detailed physical exam may be deferred.
Ongoing Assessment	Never let your guard down. Repeat the initial assessment, focused assessment, and reassess interventions performed. Reassess vital signs every 5 minutes for the unstable patient, every 15 minutes for the stable patient. When possible, have other authorized personnel ride in back of the ambulance with you for your own safety.
■ Communication and documentation	Contact medical control with a radio report that gives information on the patient's condition. Relay any significant changes, including level of consciousness or difficulty breathing. Document everything that occurred on the call, particularly situations that required restraint. Include why and what type of restraints were used.

NOTE: While the steps below are widely accepted, be sure to consult and follow your local protocol.

Behavioral Emergencies

The main task is to diffuse and control the situation and safely transport the patient. Risk factors to assess the level of danger include:
1. **History**—Has the patient previously exhibited hostile, overly aggressive, or violent behavior?
2. **Posture**—Physical tension is often a warning signal of impending hostility.
3. **The scene**—Is the patient holding or near potentially lethal objects?
4. **Vocal activity**—What kind of speech is the patient using? Loud, obscene, erratic, and bizarre speech patterns usually indicate emotional distress.
5. **Physical activity**—The patient who has tense muscles, clenched fists, or glaring eyes; is pacing; cannot sit still; or is fiercely protecting personal space requires careful watching. Agitation may predict a quick escalation to violence.

Prep Kit

Ready for Review

- Your major responsibility in behavioral emergencies is to defuse potentially life-threatening incidents and reduce the impact of the stressful condition without exposing yourself to unnecessary risks.
- There are a number of warning signs of violent behavior, including a history of hostile behavior, rigidity, loud and erratic speech patterns, agitation, and depression.
- A behavioral emergency is any reaction to events that interferes with activities of daily living. A person who is no longer able to respond appropriately to the environment may be having a more serious psychiatric emergency.
- Underlying causes of behavioral emergencies fall into two categories: organic brain syndrome and functional disorders.
- Assessing a person who may be having a behavioral crisis involves observing the person, talking with the person, and talking with witnesses to the person's behavior. Look for indications that the person's thoughts, feelings, and reactions are inappropriate for the circumstances.
- Consider contributing factors in three areas: central nervous system functioning, drug or alcohol use, and psychogenic circumstances.
- The threat of suicide requires immediate intervention. Depression is the most significant risk factor for suicide.
- You have limited legal authority to require a patient to undergo emergency medical care in the absence of a life-threatening emergency. However, most states have provisions allowing law enforcement personnel to place mentally impaired persons in custody so that care can be provided. Involve law enforcement personnel any time you are called to assist a patient in a severe behavioral or psychiatric crisis.
- Always consult medical control and contact law enforcement personnel for help before restraining a patient. If restraints are required, use the minimum force necessary. Assess the airway and circulation frequently while the patient is restrained.
- In providing emergency medical care for a patient having a behavioral emergency, be direct, honest, and calm; have a definite plan of action; stay with the patient at all times, but don't get too close. Always treat such patients with respect.

Vital Vocabulary

behavior How a person functions or acts in response to his or her environment.

behavioral crisis The point at which a person's reactions to events interfere with activities of daily living; this becomes a psychiatric emergency when it causes a major life interruption, such as attempted suicide.

depression A persistent mood of sadness, despair, and discouragement; may be a symptom of many different mental and physical disorders, or it may be a disorder on its own.

mental disorder An illness with psychological or behavioral symptoms and/or impairment in functioning caused by a social, psychological, genetic, physical, chemical, or biologic disturbance.

Technology

Interactivities

Vocabulary Explorer

Anatomy Review

Web Links

Online Review Manual

Assessment in Action

It is late January and your unit is called to a wooded area outside of a shopping mall where an 82-year-old man was found wandering along the dirt roadway. He is disoriented and wearing only flannel pajamas and house slippers. He does not know his name or where he lives. Police on scene are calling to see if an elderly man has been reported missing. They find out that Mr. Jones, an Alzheimer's patient, was noticed missing 12 hours ago from a personal care home about 2.5 miles away. There is a light rain/sleet mix falling.

1. What is your first concern for this patient?
   A. changing his clothes
   B. assessing ABCs
   C. listening to breath sounds
   D. calling the personal care home

2. Other than the Alzheimer's, what else might cause his altered mental status?
   A. hyperthermia
   B. normal glucose levels
   C. hypothermia
   D. eupnea

3. Under what type of consent is this patient treated?
   A. implied
   B. expressed
   C. informed
   D. direct

4. Treatment for this patient should include:
   A. oxygen.
   B. warming.
   C. checking for medic alert bracelets.
   D. all of the above.

5. You should do all of the following EXCEPT:
   A. call the patient by name.
   B. start an IV and draw blood for baseline labs.
   C. speak in a calming tone.
   D. assess his glucose level.

Challenging Questions

6. How should a hypothermic patient be treated?

7. What is the best source of information to determine the patient's *normal* mental status?

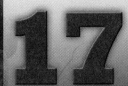

Obstetric and Gynecologic Emergencies

17

You are the Provider 1

You are called to the local shopping mall for a woman in active labor. On arrival you find a 25-year-old woman in the dressing room of a large department store. She is pregnant and complaining of severe intermittent abdominal pain. She is lying on a couch and panting.

Initial Assessment	Recording Time: 0 Minutes
Appearance	Pale, diaphoretic
Level of consciousness	Alert to person, time, and place
Airway	Open and clear
Breathing	A little fast and shallow
Circulation	Radials present, regular

1. What questions should you ask in relation to her pregnancy?
2. What questions should you ask about the pain/contractions?

Introduction

Most infants in the United States are delivered in a hospital. Occasionally, the birth process moves faster than the mother expects, and you will find yourself with a decision to make: Should you stay on the scene and deliver the infant or transport the patient to the hospital? This chapter reviews this decision-making process and how to proceed if on-scene delivery is necessary. It describes the normal process of childbirth and discusses common complications so that you will be prepared to handle normal and abnormal deliveries. We will also review the assessment and care of the newborn infant and gynecologic emergencies.

Anatomy of the Female Reproductive System

The <u>uterus</u>, or womb, is the muscular organ where the <u>fetus</u> grows (Figure 17-1 ▶). It is responsible for contractions during labor and ultimately helps to push the infant through the birth canal. The birth canal is made up of the vagina and the lower part, or neck of the uterus, called the <u>cervix</u>. The cervix contains a mucous plug that seals the uterine opening, preventing contamination from the outside world. When the cervix begins to dilate, this plug is discharged and appears as pink-tinged mucus. This is referred to as a <u>bloody show</u>. There is usually a small amount of blood at the vagina and may signal the first stage of labor.

The <u>vagina</u> is the outermost cavity of a woman's reproductive system and forms the lower part of the birth canal. It is about 8 to 12 cm in length, begins at the cervix, and ends as an external opening of the

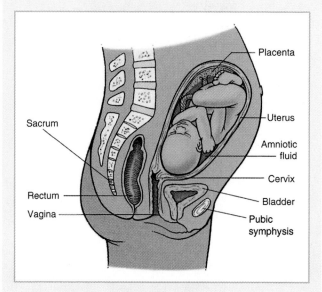

Figure 17-1 Anatomic structures of the pregnant woman.

body. The vagina completes the passageway from the uterus to the outside world for the infant. The <u>perineum</u> is the area of skin between the vagina and the anus. As the infant moves through the birth canal, the perineum will begin to bulge significantly.

The <u>placenta</u> (afterbirth) is a disk-shaped structure that attaches to the inner lining of the wall of the uterus and is connected to the fetus by the umbilical cord. There is normally no mixing of blood between the fetus and the mother. The placental barrier consists of two layers of cells, keeping the circulation of the mother and fetus separated but allowing nutrients, oxygen, waste, carbon dioxide, and many toxins and most medications to pass between the fetus and mother. After delivery, the placenta separates from the uterus and is expelled from the vagina. The <u>umbilical cord</u> is the infant's lifeline, connecting mother and infant through the placenta. The umbilical cord contains two arteries and one vein. These vessels supply blood to the fetus: The vein carries blood toward the heart (baby), and the arteries carry blood away from the heart (baby). Oxygen and other nutrients cross from the mother's circulation through the placenta and then along the umbilical cord to support the fetus as it grows. Carbon dioxide and waste products travel the same route in the opposite direction. The mother's blood and that of the fetus do not mix during the process.

The fetus develops inside a fluid-filled, baglike membrane called the <u>amniotic sac</u>, or bag of waters.

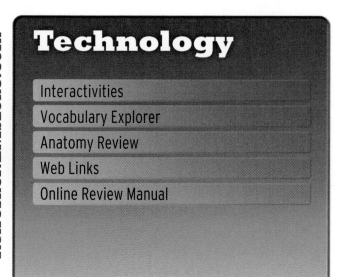

Technology

Interactivities

Vocabulary Explorer

Anatomy Review

Web Links

Online Review Manual

The sac contains about 500 to 1,000 mL of amniotic fluid, which helps insulate and protect the floating fetus as it develops. Released in a gush when the sac ruptures, usually at the onset of labor, this fluid helps to lubricate the birth canal and remove bacteria.

A full-term pregnancy is from 36 to 40 weeks, counting from the first day of the last menstrual cycle. The pregnancy is divided into three trimesters of about 3 months each. Deliveries before 36 weeks are considered premature. Toward the end of the third trimester, the head of the fetus normally descends into the mother's pelvis to position itself for delivery.

Stages of Labor

There are three stages of labor: dilation of the cervix, delivery of the baby, and delivery of the placenta. The first stage begins with the onset of contractions and ends when the cervix is fully dilated. Because the cervix has to be stretched thin by uterine contractions until the opening is large enough for the infant to pass through into the vagina, the first stage is usually the longest, lasting an average of 16 hours for a first delivery. You will usually have time to transport the mother during the first stage of labor.

Other signs of the beginning of labor are the bloody show and the rupture of the amniotic sac. These events may occur before the first contraction or later in the first stage of labor. Initially, contractions may not occur at regular intervals. The frequency and intensity of contractions in true labor increase with time. Contractions become more regular and last about 30 to 60 seconds each. The length of time the mother is in labor varies greatly. As a general rule, labor is longer for a woman who is experiencing her first pregnancy, and shorter for a woman who has experienced previous pregnancies. Table 17-1 ▶ reviews how to tell when true labor is occurring.

The second stage of labor begins when the cervix is fully dilated and ends when the infant is born. During this stage, you will have to make a decision about helping the mother to deliver on the scene or providing transport to the hospital. Because the infant has to move through the birth canal during this stage, the uterine contractions are usually closer together and last longer. Pressure on the rectum may make the mother feel as if she needs to have a bowel movement. Under no circumstances should you let the mother sit on the toilet. She may also have the uncontrollable urge to push or bear down. The perineum will begin to bulge significantly, and the top of the infant's head

TABLE 17-1 General Signs and Symptoms of Labor

False Labor and Braxton-Hicks Contractions	Real or True Labor
Contractions are not regular and do not increase in intensity or frequency. Contractions come and go.	Contractions, once started, consistently get stronger and closer together. Change in position does not relieve contractions.
Pain is in the lower abdomen. Contractions start and stay in the lower abdomen.	Pains and contractions start in the lower back and "wrap around" to the lower abdomen.
Activity or changing position will alleviate the pain and contractions.	Activity may intensify the contractions. Pain and contractions are consistent in any position.
If there is any bloody show, it is brownish.	The bloody show will be pink or red and generally accompanied by mucus.
There may be some leakage of fluid, but it is usually urine and will be in small amounts and smell of ammonia.	The bag of waters may have broken just before the contractions started or during contractions and will be of a moderate amount, may smell sweet, and will continue to leak.

should begin to appear at the vaginal opening. This is called crowning.

The third stage begins with the birth of the infant and ends with the delivery of the placenta. It may take up to 30 minutes for the placenta to deliver. If the mother is at this stage, you will need to stay on scene and assist with the delivery. It is important that you always follow BSI precautions, to protect yourself, the baby, and the mother from exposure to body fluids. There is a high potential of exposure because of body fluids released during the childbirth process.

Emergencies Before Delivery

Most pregnant women are healthy, but some may be ill when they become pregnant or become ill during pregnancy.

As the pregnancy progresses, there is an increased chance that the mother may develop complications related to the pregnancy. One of these is preeclampsia, or <u>pregnancy-induced hypertension</u>. This condition can develop after the 20th week of pregnancy and is most common in women who are pregnant for the first time. This condition is characterized by high blood pressure, headaches, swelling in the hands and feet, anxiety, and vision problems (seeing spots).

Another condition is <u>eclampsia</u>, or seizures that result from severe hypertension. To treat eclampsia, lay the mother on her side (left side preferred), maintain an airway, and provide supplemental oxygen. You should rapidly transport a pregnant patient with seizures. Perform your initial assessment, history, and physical exam, and assess the baseline vital signs. Provide treatment based on signs and symptoms.

If the patient is hypotensive, transport her on her left side. Transporting the mother in this position can prevent <u>supine hypotensive syndrome</u>, a problem due to compression by the uterus on the inferior vena cava when the mother lies supine, resulting in low blood pressure. As a general rule, you should transport all pregnant patients in this position and maintain this position whenever she is lying, except during delivery. Patients in the third trimester should not be in the supine position.

Internal bleeding may be the sign of an <u>ectopic pregnancy</u>, a pregnancy that develops outside the uterus, most often in a fallopian tube. Ectopic pregnancy occurs about once in every 200 pregnancies. The leading cause of maternal death in the first trimester is internal hemorrhage into the abdomen following rupture of an ectopic pregnancy. For this reason, you should consider the possibility of an ectopic pregnancy in women who have missed a menstrual cycle and complain of sudden stabbing and usually unilateral pain in the lower abdomen. A history of pelvic inflammatory disease, tubal ligation (tubes tied), or previous ectopic pregnancies should increase your suspicion of a possible ectopic pregnancy.

Hemorrhage from the vagina that occurs before labor begins may be very serious; consider calling for ALS backup. In early pregnancy, this may be a sign of a spontaneous <u>abortion</u>, or <u>miscarriage</u>. In the later stages of pregnancy, vaginal hemorrhage may indicate complications with the placenta. In <u>placenta abruptio</u>, the placenta separates prematurely from the wall of the uterus [Figure 17-2 ▶]. In <u>placenta previa</u>, the placenta develops over and covers the cervix [Figure 17-3 ▶].

Many women who did not have diabetes before pregnancy develop diabetes during pregnancy. This is called gestational diabetes and for most women will clear up after delivery. The mother may control her blood glucose level with diet and exercise or may take medication. In some cases, the mother needs to take insulin. A mother experiencing hyperglycemia or hypoglycemia should be cared for in the same manner as any diabetic. If a pregnant woman is found with an altered level of consciousness, your history should include questions about diabetes, and you should check the blood glucose level if local protocols allow. Remember that labor is hard work. Many mothers experience nausea before labor and may not have eaten. These factors can lead to hypoglycemia and weakness in the mother and fetus. Consult with medical control if delivery is imminent. Rapid transport to the hospital is usually preferred to out-of-hospital delivery.

Any bleeding from the vagina in a pregnant woman is significant and should be treated in the hospital promptly. If the mother shows signs of shock, have her lie on her left side during transportation, and

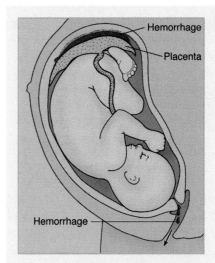

Figure 17-2 In placenta abruptio, the placenta separates prematurely from the wall of the uterus.

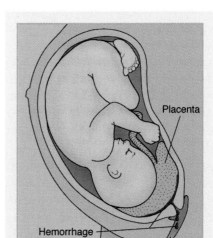

Figure 17-3 In placenta previa, the placenta develops over and covers the cervix.

give her high-flow oxygen. Place a sterile pad or sanitary napkin over the vagina, and replace it as often as necessary. Save the pads so that hospital personnel can estimate how much blood she has lost. Also save any tissue that may be passed from the vagina. Do not put anything into the vagina.

When a pregnant woman is involved in an automobile crash, severe hemorrhage may occur from injuries to the pregnant uterus. The resulting oxygen deprivation can cause life-threatening injuries to the fetus. Promptly evaluate and transport a pregnant crash victim; support the airway, and if there is any sign of bleeding, administer high-flow oxygen and call for ALS backup. Have the mother lie on her left side rather than on her back. Pregnant women have an increased amount of blood volume. Therefore, a pregnant trauma patient may have a significant amount of blood loss before showing signs of shock. Remember that the infant may be in distress well before the mother displays any signs or symptoms of shock. If the mother has significant trauma, the blood supply to the fetus is reduced so that the body can supply an adequate amount of blood to the mother. The only chance to save the infant is to resuscitate the mother.

■ Assessment

Scene Size-up

When EMS is called for a maternity case, dispatch protocols usually include simple questions to determine whether birth in imminent. Hopefully, this information is relayed to you to help you prepare for the situation. Contractions may be caused by trauma or medical conditions. It may just be "time" to deliver. Because a pregnant woman's balance is altered by the weight and position of the fetus and hormones that relax the musculature, falls and spinal stabilization must be considered.

Your first preparation for delivery should be to take appropriate BSI precautions. Gloves and eye protection should be a minimum when delivery has already begun or has occurred. If time allows, a mask and gown should also be used. Do not be complacent in your safety observations and precautions because the delivery is in progress or the family is anxious. Rushing around may hurt not only you, but also the child and mother. Remain calm and professional.

Initial Assessment
General Impression

The general impression is a good across-the-room assessment that should tell you whether the mother is in active labor or you have time to assess for imminent delivery. Evaluate the chief complaint and ask the mother if she feels like the baby is on its way. When trauma or other medical problems are the presenting complaint, assess these first and then assess the impact of these problems on the fetus. Use the AVPU scale to determine the level of consciousness.

You are the Provider 2

This is her second pregnancy and her due date is in 3 days. Her water broke while she was shopping and the contractions started almost immediately afterwards. She had preeclampsia with the first pregnancy but has had no problems with this one. She has had regular prenatal care and is taking her vitamins as prescribed. She takes no other medications. Contractions are regular and barely 2 minutes apart. She tells you she feels like she needs to push.

Vital Signs	Recording Time: 2 Minutes
Skin	Pale, diaphoretic
Pulse	112 beats/min, regular
Blood pressure	138/92 mm Hg
Respirations	28 breaths/min, shallow with contractions

3. What is the next step?
4. Should she be transported or prepared for delivery?
5. In what position should she be placed?

Airway, Breathing, and Circulation

During an uncomplicated childbirth, the ABCs are not usually an issue. However, a motor vehicle crash, an assault, or other medical conditions in a pregnant woman may lead to a complicated delivery. In these situations, evaluate the airway, breathing, and circulation to ensure they are adequate and provide treatment, including the administration of oxygen.

Transport Decision

If delivery is imminent, prepare to deliver on scene. The ideal place to deliver an infant is in the security of your ambulance or the privacy of the home. If possible, the area should be warm and private with plenty of room to move around.

If the delivery is not imminent, prepare the patient for transport. Pregnant women in the last two trimesters of pregnancy should be transported lying on the left side when possible. If a spinal injury is suspected, place a towel roll under the right side of the backboard to prevent supine hypotensive syndrome.

Focused History and Physical Exam

If the mother is unconscious, perform a rapid physical exam to locate injuries and other problems, then obtain vital signs and as much history as is available. Most of this can be performed en route to the hospital. If the mother is conscious, begin with asking history

questions, perform a focused physical exam, and then obtain vital signs.

SAMPLE History

Many women who have a significant medical history become pregnant. Some women do not experience medical problems that require medications until they become pregnant. Do not just focus on the pregnancy history. Ask the patient specifically about prenatal care. Identify any complications she may have had during the pregnancy or that her physician has discussed with her about the delivery. Determine the due date, frequency of contractions, and history of previous pregnancies and deliveries and if she had complications in the past. Determine whether there is a possibility of twins and whether the mother has taken any drugs or medications. If the patient tells you her water has broken, ask about the color of the fluid. Green fluid is due to <u>meconium</u> (fetal stool). The presence of meconium can indicate distress in the infant and it is possible for the infant to aspirate meconium during delivery. Any of these are risk factors for fetal distress and indicate the possible need for neonatal resuscitation.

Focused Physical Exam

Your focused physical exam should focus on the abdomen and delivery of the fetus. Assess the length and frequency of contractions by feeling the abdo-

---

You are the Provider 3

Your partner also applies oxygen via a nonrebreathing mask at 15 L/min. You ask your partner to prepare the OB kit while you assist the patient in lying on a blanket and check for crowning. You see the head begin to emerge from her vagina. She screams as she bears down and the head clears the birth canal.

Reassessment	Recording Time: 5 Minutes
Pulse	136 beats/min, regular
Blood pressure	132/90 mm Hg
Respirations	16 breaths/min, deep
Breath sounds	Clear bilaterally
Pulse oximetry	97% on oxygen via nonrebreathing mask

6. What should you do as the head emerges?
7. How should you instruct the mother?
8. What should you look for?
9. What should you do if there is a nuchal cord?

men. Compare what you feel with what the woman experiences in pain with each contraction. When appropriate and according to local protocol, inspect the vaginal opening for rupture of the amniotic sac, bloody show, and crowning if you suspect delivery is imminent. Be sure to protect the woman's privacy during the examination. If the woman has other complaints, such as difficulty breathing, a focused physical exam of her breathing should be performed. The focus of your physical exam should be based on her chief complaint.

Baseline Vital Signs

Assess baseline vital signs. Pay special attention to tachycardia and hypotension (which could mean hemorrhage or compression of the vena cava) or hypertension (possibly indicating preeclampsia). It is common for a woman's blood pressure to drop slightly during pregnancy. Compare your findings with previous blood pressures in prenatal visits. Hypertension may indicate more significant concern.

Detailed Physical Exam

If delivery is imminent or other assessments or treatments require your attention, defer the detailed physical exam.

Ongoing Assessment

Your ongoing assessment should center on reassessing the woman's ABCs, particularly vaginal bleeding after delivery. Repeat the vital signs and compare those to the baseline set from earlier in your assessment. Frequent reassessment of vital signs may identify hypoperfusion from excessive blood loss due to delivery.

Documentation Tips

Document any pertinent history, medications, and whether or not the patient has received prenatal care. Also include the following:
- EDC (Estimated date of confinement)—due date
- GPA
  - Gravida—Number of pregnanacies
  - Para—Number of viable births
  - Abortus—Number of miscarriages, stillbirths, or surgical abortions

Recheck interventions and treatments to see whether they were effective.

Communication and Documentation

Be sure to notify the receiving hospital of all relevant information so that they will be prepared when you arrive. What you tell them may determine whether your patient will be seen in the emergency department or whether you will go directly to the labor and delivery department. Document very carefully, especially on your assessment and condition of the baby.

■ Emergency Care

Preparing for Delivery

To determine whether delivery will occur within a few minutes and to evaluate for any potential complications, ask the pregnant woman these questions:
- When are you due?
- Is this your first baby?
- Are you having contractions? How far apart are the contractions? How long do the contractions last?
- Do you feel as though you have to strain or move your bowels?
- Have you had any spotting or bleeding?
- Has your water broken?
- Were any of your previous children delivered by cesarean section?
- Have you had a complicated pregnancy in the past?
- Do you use drugs, drink alcohol, or take any medications?
- Is there any possibility that this is a multiple birth?
- Does your doctor expect any complications?

If this is not the patient's first child, she may be able to tell you whether she is about to deliver. If she says that she is, make immediate preparations for delivery. Otherwise, does she have an extremely firm abdomen? Does she say that she has to move her bowels or feels the need to push? If so, the infant's head is probably pressing on the rectum, and delivery is about to occur. You should assess for crowning which is a reliable sign that delivery is imminent. In general, do not touch the vaginal area except during delivery (under certain circumstances) and when your partner is present. Be sure to explain everything you are doing to the patient.

Once labor has begun, there is no way it can be slowed or stopped. Never attempt to hold the woman's legs together. Do not let her go to the bathroom. Instead, reassure her that the sensation of needing to move her bowels is normal and that it means she is about to deliver.

Remember that you are only assisting the woman with the delivery. Your part is to help, guide, and support the baby as it is born. Remember to use BSI precautions at all times. You want to appear calm and reassuring while protecting the woman's modesty. Most important, recognize when the situation is beyond your level of training. If delivery is imminent with crowning, contact medical control for a decision to deliver on the scene or to transport. Always recognize your own limitations, and when you are unsure about what to do, transport the patient even if delivery must occur during transport.

Your sterile emergency obstetric (OB) kit should contain the following items **Figure 17-4 ▼** :

- Surgical scissors or a scalpel
- Umbilical cord clamps
- Umbilical tape
- Bulb syringe
- Towels
- 4" × 4" gauze sponges
- Sterile gloves
- Infant blanket
- Sanitary napkins
- Protective eyewear or shield
- A plastic bag

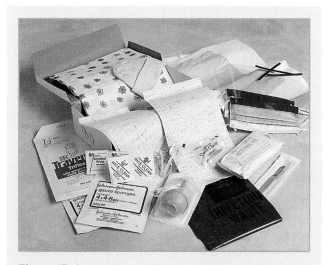

Figure 17-4 Your unit should contain a sterile OB kit.

Patient Position

You must expose the patient's lower body to assist with childbirth. Remember to preserve her modesty as much as you can while helping her to move into a comfortable position. Place the patient on a firm surface that is padded with blankets, folded sheets, or towels. Put a pillow or blankets beneath her hips to elevate them a few inches. It is sometimes more comfortable to put a pillow under one hip to allow the patient to turn to one side. This may also make it easier to suction the baby once it is born. Support the mother's head, neck, and upper back with pillows and blankets.

If the delivery is occurring at home, you should move the patient to a sturdy, flat surface. You will find it easier to work with the patient on a firm surface rather than on a bed. Elevate the patient's hips, and support her head with one or two pillows. Have her keep her legs and hips flexed, with her feet flat on the surface beneath her and her knees spread apart. Track the progression of the delivery closely at all times; you do not want an abrupt delivery to occur, when the crowning head pops out uncontrollably.

Preparing the Delivery Field

Take the following steps to prepare the area where the infant will be born:

1. As time allows, place towels or sheets on the floor around the delivery area to help soak up the amniotic fluid that will be released when the amniotic sac ruptures and/or when delivery occurs **Figure 17-5A ▶** . Note that the amniotic sac may have ruptured before you arrived.
2. Open the OB kit carefully so that its contents remain sterile and put on the sterile gloves.
3. Use the sterile sheets and towels from the OB kit to make a sterile delivery field. Place one sheet or towel under the patient's buttocks, and unfold it toward her feet. The other sheet should be draped over her abdomen and upper legs. You can also use three sheets: one sheet under the buttocks, one sheet wrapped behind the patient's back and draped over each thigh, and one sheet draped across the abdomen **Figure 17-5B ▶** .

Delivering the Baby

Your partner should be at the patient's head to comfort, soothe, and reassure her during the delivery. It is common for mothers to become nauseated, and

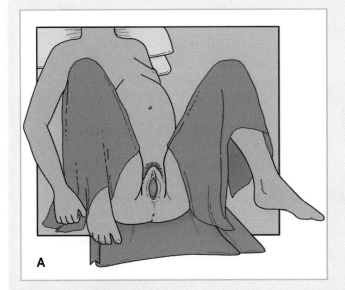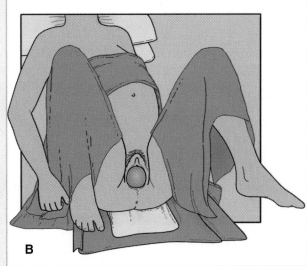

Figure 17-5 Preparing the delivery field. **A.** Place sheets or towels under the mother, elevate the mother's hips, and support her head with one or two pillows. **B.** Use sterile sheets and towels from the OB kit to make a clean delivery field. Place one sheet under her buttocks, drape the other over her abdomen, and wrap a third sheet behind her back with either end draped over the thighs.

some may vomit. If this occurs, have your partner turn the mother's head to the side so that her mouth and airway can be cleared manually or with suction if needed.

You must continually assess the mother for crowning. Do not allow an abrupt delivery to occur. Position yourself so that you can see the vagina at all times. Time the patient's contractions from the beginning of one to the beginning of the next to determine the frequency of the contractions. In addition, time the duration of each contraction. You do this by feeling the patient's abdomen from the moment the contraction begins (uterus and abdomen tightening) to the moment it ends (uterus and abdomen relaxing). Remind the patient to take quick, short breaths during each contraction but not to strain. Between contractions, encourage the mother to rest and breathe deeply through her mouth.

Review the steps in Skill Drill 17-1 ▶ to assist with delivery:

1. Allow the mother to push the head out. Support it as it emerges, placing your gloved hand over its bony parts. Suction fluid from the mouth first, then the nostrils (**Step ①**).
2. Feel at the neck to see if the cord is wrapped around it. If it is, gently lift it over the baby's head without pulling hard on the cord.

3. Once the head is delivered, the upper shoulder will be visible. Guide the head down slightly, if needed, to help that shoulder deliver (**Step ②**).
4. Support the head and upper body as the shoulders deliver. You may need to guide the head up slightly to deliver the lower shoulder (**Step ③**).
5. Once the body is delivered, handle the infant firmly but gently. It will be slippery. Make sure the baby's neck is in a neutral position to keep the airway open (**Step ④**).
6. Place the umbilical cord clamps about 2" to 4" apart, approximately 4" to 6" from the infant's body. Cut the cord between the clamps once the clamps are in place (**Step ⑤**). Local protocols vary on when to cut the cord—right after clamping, after delivery of placenta, or possibly not at all. Be sure to review and know your own local protocol.
7. The placenta delivers itself, usually within 30 minutes of birth. Never pull on the umbilical cord in an attempt to speed delivery of the placenta (**Step ⑥**).

Considerations When the Head Is Delivering

Support the baby's head as it begins to exit the vagina. It may take several contractions for the delivery of the head to occur from the time it begins to crown.

Skill Drill   17-1   Delivering the Baby

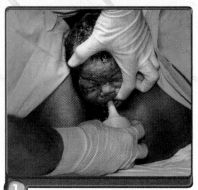

1 Support the bony parts of the head with your hands as it emerges. Suction fluid from the mouth, then nostrils.

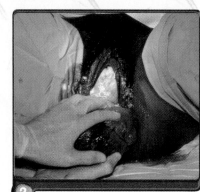

2 As the upper shoulder appears, guide the head down slightly, if needed, to deliver the shoulder.

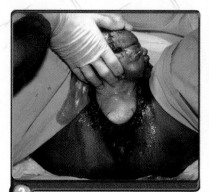

3 Support the head and upper body as the lower shoulder delivers, guiding the head up if needed.

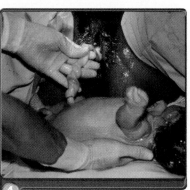

4 Handle the slippery, delivered infant firmly but gently, keeping the neck in neutral position to maintain the airway.

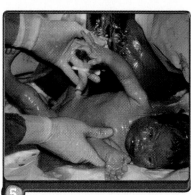

5 Place the umbilical cord clamps 2" to 4" apart, and cut between them.

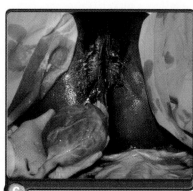

6 Allow the placenta to deliver itself. Do not pull on the cord to speed delivery.

Once it is obvious that the head is coming out farther with each contraction, you should place your gloved hand over the emerging bony parts of the head and exert very gentle pressure on it, decreasing the pressure slightly between contractions. This will allow the head to come out smoothly and prevent it and the rest of the infant from suddenly popping out during a strong contraction, possibly causing injury. Be careful that you do not poke your fingers into the infant's eyes or into the soft spots, called fontanels, on the head. One fontanel is located on the top of the head, near the brow, and one is near the back of the head. The brain is covered only by skin and membranes at these spots.

Methods of reducing the risk of perineal tearing during labor include applying gentle pressure horizontally across the perineum with a sterile gauze pad, or applying gentle pressure to the head while gently stretching the perineum. Consult your local proto-

Documentation Tips

Be sure to record the EXACT time of birth along with the APGAR score at 1 minute and 5 minutes after birth.

col regarding the methods used in your area. Also be prepared for the possibility that the mother may have a bowel movement because of the pressure on her rectum.

Unruptured Amniotic Sac and Meconium

The amniotic sac will usually break or rupture at the beginning of labor. The sac may also rupture during contractions. If the amniotic sac has not ruptured, it will appear as a fluid-filled sac (like a water balloon) emerging from the vagina. This situation is serious because the sac will suffocate the baby if it is not removed. You should puncture the sac with a clamp, away from the baby's face, only as the head is crowning, not before. As the sac is punctured, amniotic fluid will gush out. Push the ruptured sac away from the infant's face as the head is delivered. Clear the baby's mouth and nose immediately, using the bulb syringe and gauze.

If the amniotic fluid is greenish (meconium staining) instead of clear or has a foul odor, you will need to aggressively suction the baby's mouth before delivery of the body. This may prevent the baby from aspirating the meconium and developing respiratory distress. Meconium is a sign that the baby may be in distress. Thick meconium can obstruct or clog the airway of the newborn. Make sure that you tell the hospital in your radio report if meconium was present.

Umbilical Cord Around the Neck

As soon as the head is delivered, you should feel whether the umbilical cord is wrapped around the baby's neck. This commonly is called a nuchal cord. A nuchal cord that is wound tightly around the neck could cause the infant to strangle. It must be released from the neck immediately. Usually, you can slip the cord gently over the infant's delivered head (or over the shoulder, if necessary). If not, you must cut it by placing two clamps about 2" apart on the cord and cutting the cord between the clamps. In the rare event that the cord is wrapped more than once around the neck, you have to clamp and cut only once; then you can unwrap the cord from around the neck. Handle the cord very carefully; it is fragile, easily torn, and could bleed significantly. Do not let the clamps come off until the ends of the cord have been tied. However, you must always check for a nuchal cord.

After the head has delivered, you will need to suction the fluids from the infant's airway. You should

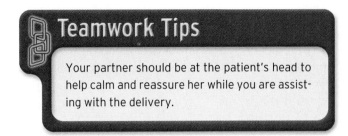

Teamwork Tips

Your partner should be at the patient's head to help calm and reassure her while you are assisting with the delivery.

ask the mother not to push while you are doing this. While supporting the infant's head with one hand, quickly and efficiently suction the fluid from the mouth first and then the nostrils. If you suction the nostrils first, you may stimulate the infant to aspirate the fluid in the mouth or pharynx. Infants are nose breathers and any stimulation of the nose may cause a gasping response. Remember to fully compress the bulb syringe before it is inserted 1" to 1½" into the infant's mouth. Release the bulb to suction fluids and mucus into the syringe. Make sure the syringe does not touch the back of the mouth. Discard the fluid into a towel, and repeat the procedure, suctioning the mouth and nostrils two or three times each, or until they are clear.

Delivering the Body

By the time you are finished suctioning, the mother will most likely be pushing again, and the upper shoulder will be visible. Because the infant's head is the largest part of the body, once it has delivered, the rest of the infant usually delivers easily. Support the head and upper body as the shoulders deliver. Do not pull on the infant. Support the baby's torso as it delivers. Grasp the infant's feet as they are born. Handle the infant firmly but carefully. It will be slippery and covered with a white, cheesy substance, called vernix caseosa.

Postdelivery Care

Immediately dry the baby off and wrap it in a blanket or towel. Place the baby on its side, with the head slightly lower than the rest of its body. Wrap the baby so that only the face is exposed, making sure that the top of the head is covered. Also make sure that the baby's neck is in a neutral position so the airway remains open. Newborn babies are very sensitive to cold, so if it is at all possible, use a warm blanket or towel. Use a sterile gauze pad to wipe the infant's mouth, and once again suction the mouth and nose. Suctioning the nose is particularly important. If you prefer, you can pick up and cradle the infant in your arm at the level of the mother's vagina while doing this, but always keep the head slightly downward to help prevent aspiration. After suctioning, keep the infant at the same level as the mother's vagina until the umbilical cord is cut. If the infant is higher than the vagina, blood will be siphoned from the infant through the umbilical cord back into the placenta.

A newborn's body temperature can drop very quickly, so dry and wrap the infant as soon as possible.

Once the infant is born, the umbilical cord is of no further use to the mother or infant. Postdelivery care of the umbilical cord is important because infection is easily transmitted through the cord to the baby. Use two clamps to clamp the cord about 2" to 4" apart. Cut the cord between the clamps with sterile scissors or a scalpel. Remember, the cord is fragile. If handled too roughly, the cord could be torn from the infant's abdomen, resulting in a fatal hemorrhage. Once the clamps are in place, there is no need to rush.

After you have cut the cord, tie the end coming from the infant. Do not use ordinary string or twine, which will cut through the soft, fragile tissues of the cord. Place a loop of the special umbilical tape around the cord about 1" nearer to the infant than to the clamp. Tighten the tape slowly so that it does not cut the cord and tie it firmly with a square knot. Cut the ends of the tape, but do not remove either clamp. The part of the cord that is coming out of the mother's vagina is attached to the placenta and will be delivered when the placenta delivers.

By now, the infant should be pink and breathing on his or her own. You can give the infant to the mother if the mother is alert and in stable condition. The mother may want to begin breastfeeding at this time. You need to return your attention to the mother and the delivery of the placenta.

Delivery of the Placenta

The placenta is attached to the end of the umbilical cord that is coming out of the vagina. Like the infant, the placenta delivers itself, usually within a few minutes of the birth, although it may take as long as 30 minutes. You do not have to stay on scene to wait for the placenta to deliver. However, you should monitor the patient and be prepared to assist with the delivery of the placenta should you decide to transport. Never pull on the end of the umbilical cord in an attempt to speed delivery of the placenta. You may tear the cord,

the placenta, or both and cause serious, perhaps life-threatening, hemorrhage.

The normal placenta has one side that is smooth and covered with a shiny membrane; the other surface is rough and divided into lobes. Wrap the entire placenta and cord in a towel, place them into a plastic bag, and take them to the hospital. Hospital personnel will examine the placenta and the cord to make certain that the entire placenta has been delivered. If a piece of the placenta has been retained inside the mother, it could cause persistent bleeding or infection.

After delivery of the placenta and before transport, place a sterile pad or sanitary napkin over the vagina and let the mother get into a comfortable position. You can help to slow bleeding by gently massaging the mother's abdomen with a firm, circular motion Figure 17-6 ▼ . You should be able to feel a firm, grapefruit-sized mass in the lower abdomen. This is called the fundus. As you massage the fundus, the uterus contracts and becomes firmer. You can also place the infant at the mother's breast to nurse, which stimulates the uterus to contract. Both massaging the uterus and having the baby stimulate the mother's nipples causes a production of oxytocin, which is a hormone that helps to contract the uterus and slow bleeding. Before transporting, take a minute to congratulate the mother and thank anyone who assisted. In writing your patient care report, be sure to record the time of birth for the birth certificate.

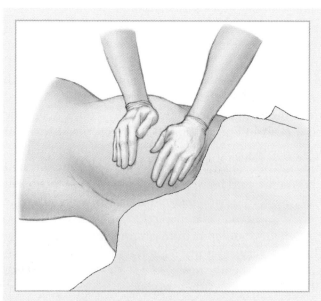

Figure 17-6 After delivery, massage the mother's abdomen in a firm, circular motion.

Some bleeding, usually less than 500 mL, occurs before the placenta delivers. If there is more than 500 mL of bleeding before delivery of the placenta or there is significant bleeding after the delivery of the placenta, transport the mother and infant to the hospital promptly. Place a sterile pad or sanitary napkin over the mother's vagina, place her in the shock position, administer oxygen, and monitor her vital signs closely. Never put anything into the vagina to try to control the bleeding.

■ Newborn Assessment and Resuscitation

You should complete an initial assessment as soon as the infant is born. A newborn infant will usually begin breathing spontaneously within 15 to 20 seconds after birth. If not, gently tap or flick the soles of the feet or rub the baby's back to stimulate breathing. If the baby does not breathe after 10 to 15 seconds, begin resuscitation efforts. You should use the Apgar score to assess the status of the infant. This system assigns a number value (0, 1, or 2) to each of five areas of activity of the newborn:

- **Appearance.** Shortly after birth, the skin of a light-skinned newborn infant and the mucous membranes of a dark-skinned infant should turn pink. Newborn infants often have cyanosis of the extremities for a few minutes after birth, but hands and feet should "pink up" quickly. Blue skin all over or blue mucous membranes signal a central cyanosis.

- **Pulse.** If a stethoscope is unavailable, you can measure pulsations with your fingers in the umbilical cord or at the brachial artery. Obviously, the infant with no pulse requires immediate CPR.

- **Grimace** or irritability. Grimacing, crying, or withdrawing in response to stimuli is normal in a newborn and indicates that the newborn infant is doing well. The way to test this is to snap a finger against the sole of the infant's foot.

- **Activity** or muscle tone. The degree of muscle tone indicates the oxygenation of the newborn infant's tissues. Normally, the hips and knees are flexed at birth, and, to some degree, the infant will resist attempts to straighten them out. A newborn should not be floppy or limp.

- **Respirations.** Normally, the newborn's respirations are regular and rapid, with a good strong cry. If the respirations are slow, shallow, or labored, or if the cry is weak, the newborn infant may have respiratory insufficiency and need assistance with ventilation. Complete absence of respirations or crying is obviously a very serious sign; in addition to assisted ventilation, CPR may be necessary.

The total of the five numbers is the Apgar score. A perfect score is 10. The Apgar score should be calculated at 1 minute and 5 minutes after birth. Most newborn infants will have a score of 7 or 8 at one minute and a score of 8 to 10 four minutes later. Table 17-2 ▼ shows how to calculate an Apgar score.

TABLE 17-2 Apgar Scoring System

Area of Activity	Score		
	2	1	0
Appearance	Entire infant is pink.	Body is pink, but hands and feet remain blue.	Entire infant is blue or pale.
Pulse	More than 100 beats/min	Fewer than 100 beats/min	Absent pulse
Grimace or irritability	Infant cries and tries to move foot away from finger snapped against its sole.	Infant gives a weak cry in response to stimulus.	Infant does not cry or react to stimulus.
Activity or muscle tone	Infant resists attempts to straighten hips and knees.	Infant makes weak attempts to resist straightening.	Infant is completely limp, with no muscle tone.
Respiration	Rapid respirations	Slow respirations	Absent respirations

Follow these steps to assess the newborn infant:

1. **Quickly calculate the Apgar score** to establish a baseline for the newborn. If your initial assessment reveals that the infant is in distress, you should not waste time to measure the Apgar score, begin emergency care immediately.

2. **Suctioning and stimulation** should result in an immediate increase in respirations. If they do not, you must begin artificial ventilation. Newborns in distress usually have respiratory problems. It is essential to keep the infant ventilating and oxygenating well.

3. **If the newborn is breathing adequately,** you should next check the pulse rate by feeling the brachial pulse or the pulsations in the umbilical cord. The pulse rate should be at least 100 beats/min. If it is not, begin artificial ventilation. This alone may increase the newborn infant's heart rate. Reassess respirations and heart rate at least every 30 seconds to make sure that the pulse rate is increasing and that respirations are adequate.

4. **Assess the newborn's skin color.** If the infant's torso is cyanotic, administer high-flow oxygen (10 to 15 L/min) through oxygen tubing held close to the newborn infant's face.

5. **Remember, you now have two patients.** You should request a second unit as soon as possible if you determine that the newborn infant will require resuscitation.

To assess a newborn's breathing, note whether or not the newborn is crying. Crying is proof that the infant is breathing. The newborn's breathing may be slightly irregular; this is normal. Gasping and grunting are usually signs of increased work of breathing and respiratory distress.

If the baby's breathing is not visible, he or she requires immediate intervention. Sometimes you can stimulate breathing simply by touching the newborn and suctioning. If the baby is still gasping after being dried and suctioned, further stimulation is not likely to improve ventilation. If stimulation is not effective or the baby continues to gasp, assisted ventilation is required.

In situations in which assisted ventilation is required, you should use an infant bag-mask device (Figure 17-7 ▶). Cover the newborn infant's mouth and nose with the mask and begin ventilation with high-flow oxygen at a rate of 40 to 60 breaths/min. Make sure you have a good mask-to-face seal. Ventilate just enough so that you see good chest rise. Initially, it may

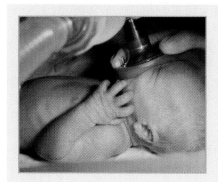

Figure 17-7 Use an infant bag-mask device and ventilate with high-flow oxygen at a rate of 40 to 60 breaths/min.

be necessary to bypass the pop-off valve to accomplish this.

After 30 seconds of adequate ventilations, assess the heart rate. If the heart rate is at least 100 beats/min and the newborn infant is breathing spontaneously, you can stop the assisted ventilation. Do not stop suddenly. Instead, gradually decrease the rate and pressure of the assisted ventilation to determine whether the newborn infant will continue to breathe adequately on its own. If not, continue assisting ventilations. You may find that gently stimulating the newborn infant by rubbing it will help it to maintain its respirations.

If the heart rate is less than 80 beats/min and not increasing with ventilation, continue assisted ventilation and start cardiac compressions. Even though this newborn infant has a pulse, the rate and blood output from the heart are not adequate for the needs of a newborn. There are two ways to give chest compressions to an infant. For the preferred method, follow the steps in (Skill Drill 17-2 ▶):

1. **Find the proper position:** one fingerbreadth below an imaginary line drawn between the nipples on the middle third of the sternum (**Step ①**).

2. On a normal, full-term-sized infant, **place both hands around the infant so that your thumbs are side by side,** resting on the middle third of the sternum, and the rest of your fingers encircle the thorax. In premature or very small infants, you may have to place one thumb over the other to perform chest compressions (**Step ②**).

3. **Press your thumbs gently against the sternum.** The newborn's chest is easy to compress. Use only enough force to compress the sternum ½" to ¾" (**Step ③**).

Ventilation with a bag-mask device is performed during the pause after every third compression. The compression-to-ventilation ratio for newborns is 3:1.

Skill Drill 17-2 Giving Chest Compressions to an Infant

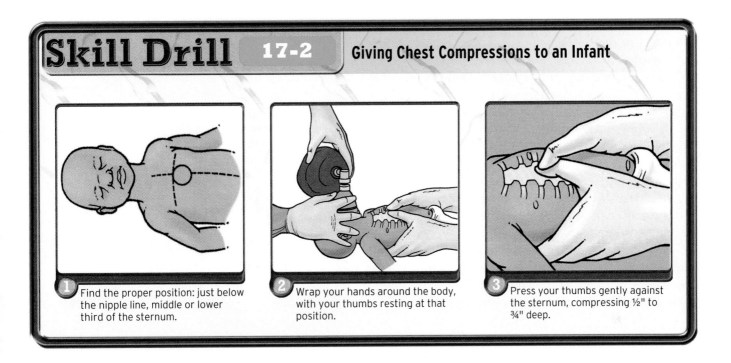

1. Find the proper position: just below the nipple line, middle or lower third of the sternum.

2. Wrap your hands around the body, with your thumbs resting at that position.

3. Press your thumbs gently against the sternum, compressing ½" to ¾" deep.

You should deliver a combined total of 120 events per minute (90 compressions to 30 ventilations every minute). Remember that ventilation is absolutely crucial to the successful resuscitation of the neonate.

If the infant does not begin breathing on its own or does not have an adequate heart rate, continue CPR on the way to the hospital. Once CPR has been started, do not stop until the infant responds with adequate respirations and heart rates or is pronounced dead by a physician. Many infants have survived without brain damage after prolonged periods of effective CPR.

■ Abnormal or Complicated Delivery Emergencies

Breech Delivery

The presentation is the position in which an infant is born, the part of the body that comes out first. Most infants are born head first, in what is called a vertex presentation. Occasionally, there is a breech presentation in which the buttocks come out first Figure 17-8 ▶ . With a breech presentation, the infant is at great risk for delivery trauma. Prolapsed cords are more common with a breech delivery. Breech deliveries are usually slow, so there is time to get the mother to the hospital. However, if the buttocks have already passed through the vagina, you should follow emergency procedures and call for ALS backup.

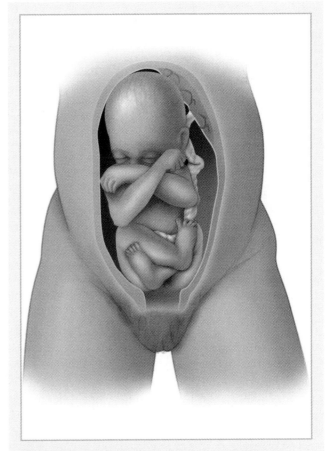

Figure 17-8 In a breech presentation, the buttocks are delivered first. Breech deliveries are usually slow, so you will often have time to transport the mother to the hospital.

In general, if the mother does not deliver within 10 minutes of the buttocks presentation, provide rapid transport.

The preparations for a breech delivery are the same as those for normal delivery. Allow the buttocks and legs to deliver spontaneously, supporting them with your hand to prevent rapid expulsion. The buttocks will usually come out easily. Let the legs dangle on either side of your arm while you support the trunk and chest as they are delivered. The head is almost always facedown and should be allowed to deliver on its own. As the head is delivering, you should keep the infant's airway open. Make a "V" with your gloved fingers, and then place them into the vagina to keep the walls of the vagina from compressing the airway. This is one of only two circumstances in which you should put your fingers into the vagina.

Rare Presentations

On very rare occasions, there may be a <u>limb presentation</u> in which the presenting part is a single arm, leg, or foot Figure 17-9 ▶ . These infants must be delivered by caesarean section and cannot be delivered in the field. If you are faced with a limb presentation, you must transport the mother to the hospital immediately. If a limb is protruding, cover it with a sterile towel. Never try to push it back in, and never pull on it. Administer high-flow oxygen to the mother and place her on her back, with her head down and pelvis elevated.

A <u>prolapsed cord</u> is a situation in which the umbilical cord comes out of the vagina before the infant Figure 17-10 ▶ . This is another life-threatening, rare presentation that must be handled in the hospital because the infant's head will compress the cord during birth and cut off circulation to the infant, depriving it of oxygenated blood. Do not attempt to push the cord back into the vagina. Prolapse of the umbilical cord usually occurs early in labor when the amniotic sac ruptures. As a result, there is time to get the mother to the hospital. Your focus is to try to keep the infant's head from compressing the cord.

Place the mother on a backboard in the Trendelenburg position, with her hips elevated on a pillow or folded sheet or in the knee-chest position (kneeling and bent forward, facedown). Both of these positions will help keep the weight of the infant off the prolapsed cord. Carefully insert your sterile gloved hand into the vagina, and gently push the infant's head away from the umbilical cord. Note that this is

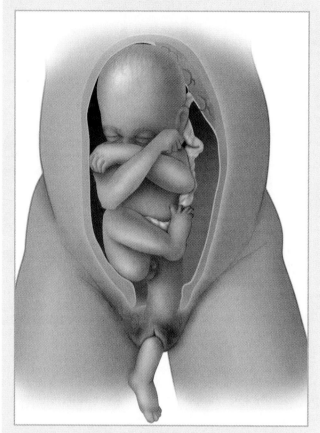

Figure 17-9 In very rare instances, an infant's limb, usually a single arm or leg, presents first. This is a very serious situation, and you must provide prompt transport for hospital delivery.

the only other occasion on which you should actually place a hand into the vagina. Wrap a sterile towel, moistened with saline, around the exposed cord. Give the mother high-flow oxygen and provide rapid transport.

Excessive Bleeding

Some bleeding always occurs with delivery. However, bleeding that exceeds approximately 500 mL is considered excessive. Although up to 500 mL of blood loss is tolerated, you should continue to massage the uterus after delivery to help control the bleeding. Be sure to check your massage technique if bleeding continues. If the mother appears to be in shock, treat her accordingly and transport, massaging the uterus en route. There are several other possible causes of excessive bleeding, all of which may be serious and require emergency care. Treat this condition by covering the vagina with a sterile pad, changing the pad as often as necessary. Do not discard these blood-soaked

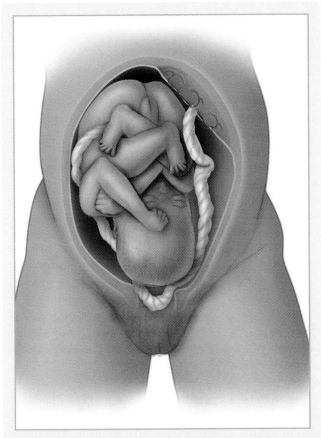

Figure 17-10 A prolapsed umbilical cord, another rare situation, is very dangerous and must be cared for at the hospital.

pads; hospital personnel will use them to estimate the amount of blood that the mother has lost. Also save any tissue that may have passed from the vagina.

Place the mother in the shock position, administer oxygen, monitor vital signs frequently, and transport her immediately to the hospital. Never hold the mother's legs together in an effort to stop the bleeding, and never pack the vagina with gauze pads in an attempt to control bleeding.

Spina Bifida

Spina bifida is a developmental defect in which a portion of the spinal cord or meninges may protrude outside of the vertebrae and possibly even outside of the body. This is very easily seen on the newborn's back and usually occurs in the lower third of the back in the lumbar area. It is extremely important to cover the open area of the spinal cord with a sterile, moist compress immediately after birth. This helps to prevent the newborn from getting a fatal infection. Mainte-

nance of body temperature is very important when applying a sterile, moist compress because the moisture can lower the newborn's body temperature. To prevent this, have someone hold the newborn against his or her body.

Abortion (Miscarriage)

Delivery of the fetus and placenta before 20 weeks is called abortion, or miscarriage. Abortions may be spontaneous, without any obvious known cause, or deliberate. Deliberate abortions may be self-induced, by the mother herself or by someone else, or planned and performed in a hospital or clinic. Regardless of the reasons for the abortion, it may cause complications that you may be called on to treat.

The most serious complications of abortion are bleeding and infection. Bleeding can result from portions of the fetus or placenta being left in the uterus (incomplete abortion) or from injury to the wall of the uterus (perforation of the uterus and possibly the adjacent bowel or bladder). Infection can result from this perforation and from the use of unsterile instruments. If the mother is in shock, treat and transport her promptly to the hospital. Collect and bring to the hospital any tissue that passes through the vagina. Never try to pull tissue out of the vagina. If tissue is present, cover the area with a sterile pad.

Twins

Twins occur about once in every 80 births. Sometimes, there is a family history of twins. The mother may suspect that she is having twins because she has an unusually large abdomen. Usually, twins are diagnosed early in pregnancy with modern ultrasound techniques. With twins, always be prepared for more than one resuscitation, and call for additional assistance.

Twins are smaller than single infants, and delivery is typically not difficult. Consider the possibility that you are dealing with twins any time the first infant is small or the mother's abdomen remains fairly large after the birth. If twins are present, the second one will usually be born within 45 minutes of the first. About 10 minutes after the first birth, contractions will begin again, and the birth process will repeat itself.

The procedure for delivering twins is the same as that for single infants. Clamp and cut the cord of the first infant as soon as it has been born and before the second infant is delivered. The second infant may deliver before or after the first placenta. There may be only one placenta, or there may be two. When the placenta has been delivered, check whether there is one umbilical cord or two. If two cords are coming out of one placenta, the twins are identical. If only one cord is coming out of the placenta, then the twins are fraternal, and there will be two placentas. Occasionally, the two placentas of fraternal twins are fused, so you might think that you are dealing with identical twins. Remember, if you see only one umbilical cord coming out of the first placenta, there is still another placenta to be delivered. However, if both cords are attached to one placenta, the delivery is over. Identical twins are of the same sex; fraternal twins may be of different sexes, or they may be the same.

Record the time of birth of each twin separately. Twins may be so small that they look premature; handle them very carefully, and keep them warm.

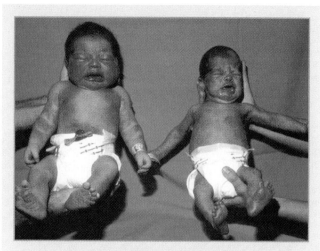

Figure 17-11 Premature infants (right) are smaller and thinner than full-term infants.

Delivering an Infant of an Addicted Mother

Unfortunately, more and more infants are being born to mothers who are addicted to drugs or alcohol. These mothers often have had little or no prenatal care. The effects of the addiction on the infants include prematurity, low birth weight, and severe respiratory depression. Some of these infants will die. Fetal alcohol syndrome is the term used to describe the condition of infants born to mothers who have abused alcohol.

If you are called to handle a delivery of a drug- or alcohol-addicted mother, pay special attention to your own safety. As with all other cases, follow BSI precautions. Wear goggles and sterile gloves at all times. Clues that you are dealing with an addicted mother may include the presence of drug paraphernalia, empty wine or liquor bottles, and statements made by others or by the mother herself. You should be prepared to support the infant's respirations and administer oxygen during transport. Do not judge or lecture the mother. Your job is to help deliver the infant as best you can and to transport both infant and mother to the hospital.

Premature Infant

The usual gestational period, the period of prenatal development, is 9 calendar months, or 40 weeks. A normal, single infant will weigh approximately 7 lb at birth. Any infant that delivers before 8 months (36 weeks of gestation) or weighs less than 5 lb at birth is considered premature. This determination is not always easy to make. Often, the exact gestation time cannot be determined. Because you probably have no scale to weigh the infant, you will have to use physical guidelines. A premature infant is smaller and thinner than a full-term infant, and its head is proportionately larger in comparison with the rest of its body Figure 17-11 ▲. The vernix caseosa, a cheesy white coating on the skin that is found on the full-term infant, will be missing on the premature infant or will be very minimal. There will also be less body hair.

You are the Provider 4

The amniotic fluid is clear, but the umbilical cord is wrapped around the neck. It is very loose and you are able to slip the cord over the head without difficulty. With one more push the body is delivered. You quickly dry, stimulate, and assess the baby. It is a healthy baby girl who is pink and crying vigorously. She is wrapped in a blanket and handed over to the mother. They are loaded onto the stretcher and transported to labor and delivery at the local hospital. They both are doing well and are sent home the next day.

Premature infants often require resuscitation, which should be done unless it is physically impossible. With such care, infants as small as 1 lb have survived and developed normally.

If possible, keep the temperature of the ambulance at 90°F to 95°F (32.2°C to 35.0°C) while the infant and mother are being transported to the hospital. If a special carrier is not available, you must keep the premature infant warm with additional blankets, thermal packets, and warmed patient compartments. Any delays will lower the infant's body temperature.

Fetal Demise

Unfortunately, you may find yourself delivering an infant who died in the mother's uterus before labor. This will be a true test of your medical, emotional, and social abilities. Grieving parents will be emotionally distraught and perhaps even hostile, requiring all your professionalism and support skills.

The onset of labor may be premature, but labor will otherwise progress normally in most cases. If an intrauterine infection has caused the demise, you may note an extremely foul odor. The delivered infant may have skin blisters, skin sloughing, and a dark discoloration, depending on the stage of decomposition. The head will be soft and perhaps grossly deformed.

Do not attempt to resuscitate an obviously dead infant. However, do not confuse such an infant with those who have had a cardiopulmonary arrest as a complication of the birthing process. You should attempt to resuscitate normal-appearing infants.

Delivery Without Sterile Supplies

On rare occasions, you may have to deliver an infant without a sterile OB kit. Even if you do not have an OB kit, you should always have goggles and gloves with you. These are for your own protection and for that of the mother and infant. Carry out the delivery as if sterile supplies were on hand. If you can, use clean sheets and towels that have not been used since they were laundered. As soon as the infant is born, wipe the inside of its mouth with your finger to clear away blood and mucus. Without the OB kit, you should not cut or tie the umbilical cord. Instead, as soon as the placenta delivers, wrap it in a clean towel or put it in a plastic bag and transport it with the infant and mother to the hospital. Always keep the placenta and the infant at the same level, or elevate the placenta slightly if possible, so that blood does not drain from the infant into the placenta. Be sure to keep the infant warm.

Gynecologic Emergencies

Occasionally, women who are not pregnant will have significant gynecologic conditions requiring emergency medical care. These include excessive bleeding and soft-tissue injuries to the external genitalia. The genitalia have a rich nerve supply, making injuries very painful.

Treat lacerations, abrasions, and tears with moist, sterile compresses, using local pressure to control bleeding and a diaper-type bandage to hold the dressings in place. Leave any foreign bodies in place after stabilizing them with bandages. Under no circumstances should you ever pack or place dressings in the vagina. Continue to assess these patients while transporting them to the emergency department.

Although you might not know the exact cause of a gynecologic emergency, you should treat these individuals as you would any other victim of blood loss: Observe BSI precautions, ensure maintenance of the airway, give oxygen, take and document vital signs, and treat for shock.

You are the Provider   Summary

You must recognize the need for delivery on scene versus transporting the patient. If it is not the first pregnancy for the patient she should be able to tell you when the baby is coming. Assess vital signs and time contractions. If the mother feels the need to push or crowning is present, prepare for delivery immediately. Most deliveries occur without complications; however, knowledge and preparation are key when dealing with those rare emergencies.

1. **What questions should you ask in relation to her pregnancy?**
   - When are you due?
   - Is this your first baby? Gravida, Para, Abortus?
   - Has your water broken?
   - Do you use drugs, drink alcohol, or take any medications?
   - Is there any possibility that this is a multiple birth?
   - Does your doctor expect any complications?
   - Were any of your previous children delivered by cesarean section?

2. **What questions should you ask about the pain/contractions?**
   - How far apart are the contractions?
   - How long do the contractions last?
   - Do you feel as though you have to strain or move your bowels?
   - Have you had any spotting or bleeding?

3. **What is the next step?**

   Prepare the OB kit and check for crowning.

4. **Should she be transported or prepared for delivery?**

   Prepare for delivery. She is having contractions less than 2 minutes apart, it's her second child, and she feels the need to push.

5. **In what position should she be placed?**

   She should be placed in the lithotomy position—on her back with her knees spread.

6. **What should you do as the head emerges?**

   Apply a slight downward pressure with the palm of your hand to prevent an explosive delivery. Suction the mouth and then the nose while supporting the head.

7. **How should you instruct the mother?**

   Keep telling her not to push as you suction the baby.

8. **What should you look for?**

   Meconium staining, the umbilical cord around the neck

9. **What should you do if there is a nuchal cord?**

   If the cord is loose enough, you can slip it over the head. If not, the cord should be clamped in two places and cut between the clamps.

Obstetric and Gynecologic Emergencies

Scene Size-up

Body substance isolation precautions should include a minimum of gloves, eye protection, mask, and gown. Ensure scene safety and determine NOI/MOI. Consider the number of patients, the need for additional help/ALS, and c-spine stabilization.

Initial Assessment

■ General impression

Determine level of consciousness and find and treat any immediate threats to life. Determine priority of care based on environment and patient's chief complaint.

■ Airway

Ensure patent airway.

■ Breathing

Provide high-flow oxygen at 15 L/min. Evaluate depth and rate of respirations and provide ventilations as needed.

■ Circulation

Evaluate pulse rate and quality; observe skin color, temperature, and condition and treat accordingly. Treat for any signs of shock.

■ Transport decision

If delivery of a baby is not imminent, provide rapid transport.

Focused History and Physical Exam

NOTE: The order of the steps in the focused history and physical exam differs depending on whether the patient is conscious or unconscious. The order below is for a conscious patient. For an unconscious patient, perform a rapid physical exam, obtain vital signs, and obtain the history.

■ SAMPLE history

Obtain SAMPLE history. If patient is pregnant, determine the due date, frequency of contractions, and history of previous pregnancies and deliveries and complications, if any. Determine whether there is a possibility of twins and whether the patient has taken any drugs or medications. If patient's water has broken, ask whether the fluid was green.

■ Focused physical exam

Your focused physical exam should include the abdomen and assessing the length and frequency of contractions. When appropriate and according to local protocol, inspect the vaginal opening for rupture of the amniotic sac, bloody show, and crowning if you suspect delivery is imminent.

■ Baseline vital signs

Take vital signs, noting skin color and temperature. Use pulse oximetry if available. Watch for increases in blood pressure.

■ Interventions

Support patient as needed. Consider the use of oxygen, positive pressure ventilations, adjuncts, and proper positioning of the patient.

Detailed Physical Exam

If delivery is imminent or other assessments or treatments require your attention, defer the detailed physical exam.

Ongoing Assessment

Repeat the initial assessment and focused assessment, and reassess interventions performed. Reassess vital signs every 5 minutes for the unstable patient and every 15 minutes for the stable patient. Note and treat the patient as necessary.

■ Communication and documentation

Contact medical control with a radio report that gives information on patient's and newborn's condition. Relay any significant changes, including level of consciousness or difficulty in breathing. Record any changes, at what time, and any interventions performed.

Assessment and Emergency Care

Assessment and Emergency Care

NOTE: While the steps below are widely accepted, be sure to consult and follow your local protocol.

Delivering the Baby	Giving Chest Compressions to an Infant	Premature Infant
1. Support the bony parts of the head with your hands as it emerges. Suction fluid from the baby's mouth, then nostrils.	1. Find the proper position—just below the nipple line, middle or lower third of the sternum.	1. Keep the infant warm. Keep the infant in a place where the temperature is between 90°F and 95°F (between 32.2°C and 35°C).
2. As the upper shoulder appears, guide the head down slightly, if needed, to deliver the shoulder.	2. Wrap your hands around the body, with your thumbs resting at that position.	2. Keep the mouth and nose clear of mucus with a bulb syringe.
3. Support the head and upper body as the lower shoulder delivers, guiding the head up if needed.	3. Press the two thumbs against the sternum, compressing ½" to ¾" deep.	3. Inspect the cut end of the cord attached to the infant for bleeding.
4. Handle the slippery, delivered infant firmly but gently, keeping the neck in neutral position to maintain the airway.		4. Administer oxygen.
5. Place the umbilical cord clamps 2" to 4" apart, and cut between them.		5. Do not infect the infant. Wear a mask to help prevent you from breathing on the infant.
6. Allow the placenta to deliver itself. Do not pull on the cord to speed delivery.		6. Notify the hospital of a neonatal transport.

Prep Kit

Ready for Review

- Inside the uterus, the developing fetus floats in the amniotic sac. The umbilical cord connects mother and infant through the placenta.
- The first stage of labor, dilation, begins with the onset of contractions and ends when the cervix is fully dilated. The second stage, expulsion of the baby, begins when the cervix is fully dilated and ends when the infant is born. The third stage, delivery of the placenta, begins with the birth of the infant and ends with the delivery of the placenta.
- Once labor has begun, it cannot be slowed or stopped. There is usually time to transport the patient to the hospital during the first stage. During the second stage, you must decide whether to deliver the baby at the scene or transport the mother. During the third stage, once the infant has been born, you will probably not transport until the placenta has delivered.
- Use an infant BVM device to assist ventilation, starting with high-flow oxygen at a rate of 40 to 60 breaths/min. If the infant starts to breathe on its own, give oxygen and watch for signs of adequate oxygenation. If the heart rate is less than 80 beats/min, start cardiac compressions to compress the sternum ½" to ¾". Perform a combination of 90 compressions to 30 ventilations per minute.
- Abnormal or complicated deliveries include breech deliveries, limb presentations (arm, leg, or foot first), and prolapse of the umbilical cord (umbilical cord first). Quickly transport the patient with a limb presentation or prolapsed umbilical cord to the hospital.
- The only times you should place a finger or hand into the vagina are to keep the walls of the vagina from compressing the infant's airway during a breech presentation or to push the infant's head away from the cord when a prolapsed cord is present.
- Excessive bleeding is a serious emergency. Cover the vagina with a sterile pad; change the pad as often as necessary, and take all used pads to the hospital for examination.
- Be prepared to support respirations during transport in an infant delivered by a drug- or alcohol-addicted mother. Also use oxygen with premature infants, and keep the temperature of the ambulance at 90°F (32.2°C) or more during transport.

Vital Vocabulary

abortion   The delivery of the fetus and placenta before 20 weeks; miscarriage.

amniotic sac   The fluid-filled, baglike membrane in which the fetus develops.

Apgar score   A scoring system for assessing the status of a newborn that assigns a number value to each of five areas of assessment.

bloody show   A small amount of blood at the vagina that appears at the beginning of labor and may include a plug of pink-tinged mucus that is discharged when the cervix begins to dilate.

breech presentation   A delivery in which the buttocks come out first.

cervix   The lower third, or neck, of the uterus.

crowning   The appearance of the infant's head at the vaginal opening during labor.

eclampsia   Seizures (convulsions) resulting from severe hypertension in a pregnant woman.

ectopic pregnancy   A pregnancy that develops outside the uterus, typically in a fallopian tube.

fetus   The developing, unborn infant inside the uterus.

limb presentation   A delivery in which the presenting part is a single arm, leg, or foot.

meconium   A dark green material in the amniotic fluid that can indicate disease in the newborn; the meconium can be aspirated into the infant's lungs during delivery; the baby's first bowel movement.

miscarriage   The delivery of the fetus and placenta before 20 weeks; spontaneous abortion.

perineum   The area of skin between the vagina and the anus.

placenta   The tissue attached to the uterine wall that nourishes the fetus through the umbilical cord.

placenta abruptio   A premature separation of the placenta from the wall of the uterus.

placenta previa   A condition in which the placenta develops over and covers the cervix.

preeclampsia   A condition of late pregnancy that involves headache, visual changes, and swelling of

Technology

- Interactivities
- Vocabulary Explorer
- Anatomy Review
- Web Links
- Online Review Manual

the hands and feet; also called pregnancy-induced hypertension.

pregnancy-induced hypertension A condition of late pregnancy that involves headache, visual changes, and swelling of the hands and feet; also called preeclampsia.

prolapsed cord A situation in which the umbilical cord comes out of the vagina before the infant.

supine hypotensive syndrome Low blood pressure resulting from compression of the inferior vena cava by the weight of the pregnant uterus when the mother is supine.

umbilical cord The conduit connecting mother to infant via the placenta; contains two arteries and one vein.

uterus The muscular organ where the fetus grows, also called the womb; responsible for contractions during labor.

vagina The outermost cavity of a woman's reproductive system; the lower part of the birth canal.

Assessment in Action

Even though deliveries are a natural occurrence, occasionally medical intervention is required. Once the baby delivers, assessment and the neonate's progression will direct your course of care.

1. Following stimulation, begin resuscitation efforts if the baby does not begin to breathe after how many seconds?
   A. 5 to 10
   B. 10 to 15
   C. 15 to 20
   D. 20 to 25

2. The "G" in APGAR stands for:
   A. gravida.
   B. grand multipara.
   C. grimace.
   D. grunting.

3. When should the APGAR score be assessed?
   A. once resuscitation efforts have been performed
   B. at 5 minutes and 10 minutes after delivery
   C. at 1 minute and 5 minutes after delivery
   D. after the placenta delivers

4. During resuscitation, if the heart rate is less than 60 beats/min and not increasing with ventilations, you should:
   A. dry, warm, and stimulate the baby.
   B. change oxygen delivery devices.
   C. increase the rate of ventilations.
   D. start chest compressions.

5. Some bleeding with delivery is normal; however, bleeding is considered excessive when it exceeds approximately how many milliliters?
   A. 250
   B. 500
   C. 750
   D. 1,000

6. The most serious complications of abortion are bleeding and _____.
   A. bronchoconstriction
   B. infection
   C. tachycardia
   D. tachypnea

Challenging Questions

7. Explain the procedure for caring for a prolapsed cord.

Trauma

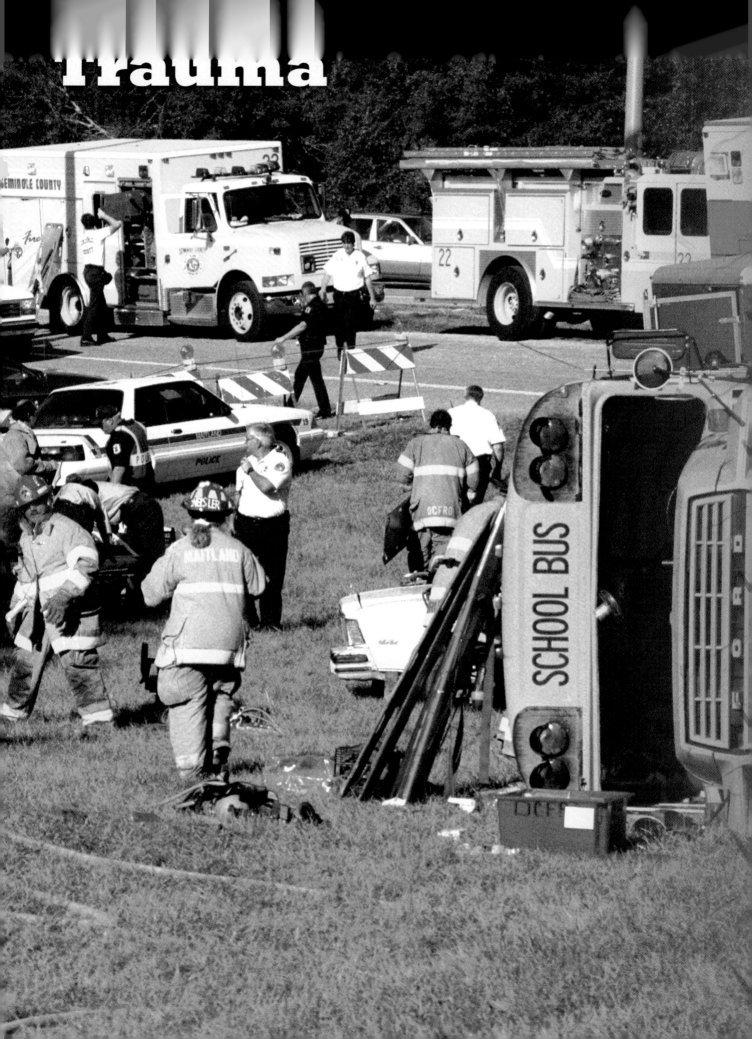

Section 5

Cognitive Objectives

1. Provide care to a patient with shock (hypoperfusion). (Chapter 19, p 366)
   - State methods of emergency medical care of external bleeding.
   - List signs and symptoms of shock (hypoperfusion).
   - State the steps in the emergency medical care of the patient with signs and symptoms of shock (hypoperfusion).
2. Provide care to a patient with suspected spinal injury. (Chapter 20, p 389)
   - State the signs and symptoms of a potential spine injury.
   - Describe how to stabilize the spine.
3. Provide care to a patient with a suspected head injury. (Chapter 20, p 384)
   - Relate mechanism of injury to potential injuries of the head and spine.
4. Provide care to a patient with a soft-tissue injury. (Chapter 21, p 414)
   - Describe the emergency medical care of the patient with a closed soft-tissue injury.
   - Describe the emergency medical care of the patient with an open soft-tissue injury.
5. Perform a rapid extrication of a trauma patient. (Chapter 20, p 386)
   - Describe the indications for the use of rapid extrication.
   - List steps in performing rapid extrication.

Affective Objectives

1. Explain the sense of urgency to transport patients that are bleeding and show signs of hypoperfusion. (Chapter 19, p 349)
2. Explain the rationale for splinting at the scene versus load and go. (Chapter 21, p 430)
3. Explain the rationale for using rapid extrication approaches only when they will make the difference between life and death. (Chapter 20, p 386)

Psychomotor Objectives

1. Demonstrate care of the patient experiencing external bleeding. (Chapter 19, p 352)
2. Demonstrate care of the patient exhibiting signs and symptoms of shock (hypoperfusion). (Chapter 19, p 366)
3. Demonstrate the steps in the care of open and closed soft-tissue injuries. (chest injuries, abdominal injuries, burns and amputations). (Chapters 21 and 22)
4. Demonstrate the steps in the care of a patient with a head or spine injury. (Chapter 20, p 385)
5. Demonstrate the procedure for rapid extrication. (Chapter 20, p 386)

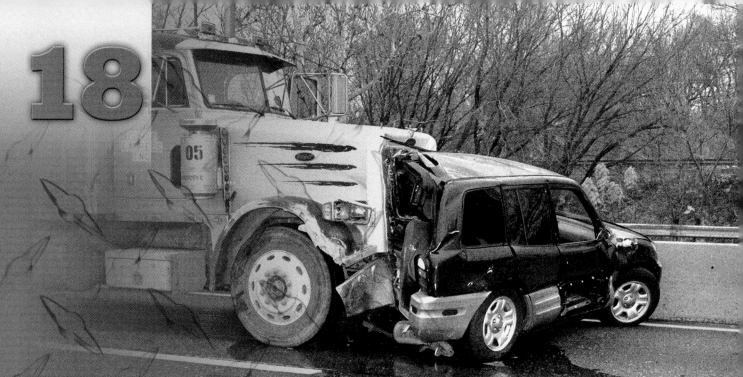

18

Kinematics of Trauma

■ Introduction

Injuries are the leading cause of death and disability in the United States among children and young adults (ages 1 to 34 years), claiming 140,000 lives annually—more than all other diseases combined. Each year, one person in three sustains an injury that requires medical treatment. Proper prehospital assessment and care can do much to minimize suffering, long-term disability, and death from trauma.

This chapter reviews the basic physical concepts regarding the way injuries occur and how they affect the human body. EMS providers who understand these concepts are better able to size up a trauma scene and use that information as a vital part of patient assessment and emergency medical care.

This section begins with a basic discussion of energy and trauma. Next, different types of crashes and their impact on the body are explained. By assessing a vehicle that has crashed, you can often determine what happened to the passengers at the time of impact, which may allow you to predict what injuries the passengers sustained at the time of impact. Evaluation of the mechanism of injury for the trauma patient will provide you with an index of suspicion for serious underlying injuries. The index of suspicion is your concern for potentially serious underlying and unseen injuries. Certain injury patterns occur with certain types of injury events. Answers to simple questions will provide you with information on how to identify life-threatening and potentially life-threatening injuries.

■ Energy and Trauma

Traumatic injury occurs when the body's tissues are exposed to energy levels beyond their tolerance Figure 18-1 ▼. The mechanism of injury (MOI) is the way in which injuries from trauma occur. The MOI describes the forces (or energy transmission) acting on the body that cause injury. Three concepts of energy are typically associated with injury (not including thermal energy, which causes burns): potential energy, kinetic energy, and work. In considering the effects of energy on the human body, it is important to remember that energy can be neither created nor destroyed, but can only be converted or transformed. It is not the objective of this section to help you to reconstruct the scene of a motor vehicle crash. Rather, you should have a sense of the effects of work on the body and understand, in a broad sense, how that work is related to potential and kinetic energy. For example, when you are assessing a patient who fell, you need not calculate the speed at which the person hit the ground. However, it is important to estimate the height from which he or she fell and to appreciate the injury potential of the fall.

Work is defined as force acting over a distance. For example, the force needed to bend metal multiplied by the distance over which the metal is bent is the work that crushes the front end of an automobile that is involved in a frontal impact. Similarly, forces that bend, pull, or compress tissues beyond their inherent limits result in the work that causes injury to the human body.

Technology

Interactivities

Vocabulary Explorer

Anatomy Review

Web Links

Online Review Manual

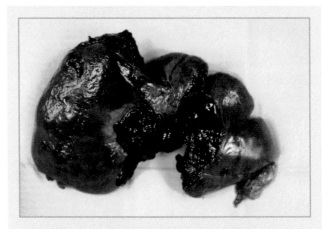

Figure 18-1 Traumatic injury occurs when the body's tissues are exposed to energy levels beyond their tolerance. This photo shows a ruptured spleen.

The energy of a moving object is called <u>kinetic energy</u> and is calculated as:

$$\text{Kinetic energy} = \tfrac{1}{2}mv^2$$

m = mass (weight) and v = velocity (speed)

Remember that energy cannot be created or destroyed, only converted. In the case of a motor vehicle crash, the kinetic energy of the speeding car is converted into the work of stopping the car, usually by crushing the car's exterior Figure 18-2 ▾ . Similarly, the passengers in the car have kinetic energy because they were traveling at the same speed as the car. Their kinetic energy is converted to the work of bringing them to a stop. It is this work on the passengers that results in injury. Remember that speed has a greater impact on injury than weight. In the equation for kinetic energy, the energy that is available to cause injury doubles when an object's weight doubles but *quadruples* when its speed doubles. Consider the debate over raising the speed limit. Increasing a car's speed from 50 to 70 mph quadruples the energy that is available to cause injury. This point is even easier to understand in considering gunshot wounds. The speed of the bullet (high-velocity compared with low-velocity) has a greater impact on producing injury than the mass (size) of the bullet. This is why it is so important to report to the hospital the type of firearm that was used in a shooting. The amount of kinetic energy that is converted to do work on the body dictates the severity of the injury. High-energy injuries often produce more severe damage to the patient.

Potential energy is the product of mass (weight), force of gravity, and height, and is mostly associated with the energy of falling objects. A worker on a scaffold has some potential energy because he or she is some height above the ground. If the worker falls, potential energy is converted into kinetic energy. As the worker hits the ground, the kinetic energy is converted into work. It is the work of bringing the body to a stop that results in injury.

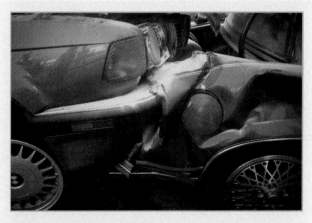

Figure 18-2 The kinetic energy of a speeding car is converted into the work of stopping the car, usually by crushing the car's exterior.

You are the Provider 2

Your general impression of the patient shows an anxious, confused teenager with a series of small lacerations across his forehead. The windshield is spider-webbed and you note that he was only wearing a lap belt. The shoulder belt was pushed behind him. The airbag has not deployed. You ask a first responder on scene to hold c-spine control as you continue with your assessment.

Vital Signs	Recording Time: 2 Minutes
Skin	Pale
Pulse	116 beats/min, regular
Blood pressure	122/78 mm Hg
Respirations	20 breaths/min, deep

4. What collisions has the patient experienced?
5. What type of injury might you suspect from the spider-webbed windshield and altered level of consciousness?
6. What type of injuries may result from the improperly worn restraints?
7. At what point should oxygen be applied to the patient? How should it be administered?

Documentation Tips

Be sure to describe the scene well and document the kinetic energy involved: speed, distance of fall, etc.

Traumatic injuries are described in the two categories of <u>blunt trauma</u> and <u>penetrating trauma</u>. Either type may occur from a variety of MOIs. It is important for you to consider unseen as well as visible, obvious injuries with either type of trauma. Blunt trauma is the result of force (or energy transmission) to the body that causes injury primarily without penetrating the soft tissues or internal organs and cavities. Penetrating trauma causes injury by objects that primarily pierce and penetrate the surface of the body and cause damage to soft tissues, internal organs, and body cavities.

As you know, different MOIs will produce many types of injuries. Some mechanisms involve only one body system but many MOIs result in injury to more than one body system. Therefore, you should always maintain a high index of suspicion for serious unseen injuries. Common types of MOI patterns that injure trauma patients are falls, motor vehicle collisions, auto versus pedestrian (or bicycle), gunshot wounds, and stabbings.

■ Blunt Trauma

Blunt trauma results from an object making contact with the body. Motor vehicle crashes and falls are two of the most common MOIs for blunt trauma. Any object, for example a baseball bat, can cause blunt trauma if it is moving fast enough. You should pay attention to signs of skin discoloration or complaints of pain because these may be the only signs of blunt trauma. You also should maintain a high index of suspicion during patient assessment for hidden injuries in patients with blunt trauma.

Vehicular Collisions

Motor vehicle crashes are classified traditionally as frontal (head-on), lateral (T-bone), rear-end, rotational (spins), and rollovers. The principal difference among these collision types is the direction of the force of impact. There is an increased possibility of multiple impacts when the collision involves a spin or a rollover.

Motor vehicle crashes typically consist of a series of three collisions. The three collisions in a frontal impact are as follows:

1. **The collision of the car against another car, a tree, or some other object.** Damage to the car is perhaps the most dramatic part of the collision, but it does not directly affect patient care, except possibly to make extrication difficult. However, it does provide information about the severity of the collision and has an indirect effect on patient care. The greater the damage to the car, the greater the energy that was involved and, therefore, the greater the potential to cause injury to the patient. By assessing the damage to the vehicle, you may be able to predict what injuries may have happened to the passengers at the time of impact. When you arrive on scene and perform your scene size-up, quickly inspect the severity of damage to the vehicle(s). If there is significant damage to a vehicle, your index of suspicion for the presence of life-threatening injuries should automatically increase. A great amount of force is required to crush and deform a vehicle, cause intrusion into the passenger compartment, tear seats from their mountings, and collapse steering wheels. Such damage suggests the presence of high-energy trauma.

2. **The collision of the passenger against the interior of the car.** Just as the kinetic energy produced by the car's mass and velocity is converted into the work of bringing the car to a stop, the kinetic energy produced by the passenger's weight and speed is converted into the work of stopping his or her body `Figure 18-3 ▶`. Just like the obvious damage to the car, the injuries that result are often dramatic and immediately apparent during your initial assessment. Common injuries include lower extremity fractures (knees into the dashboard), flail chest (rib cage into the steering wheel), and head trauma (head into the windshield). Such injuries occur more frequently if the passenger is not restrained. Even when the passenger is properly restrained, injuries can occur.

3. **The collision of the passenger's internal organs against the solid structures of the body.** The injuries that occur during the third collision may not be as obvious as external injuries, but they are often the most life threatening. For example, as the passenger's head hits the windshield, the brain continues to move forward until it

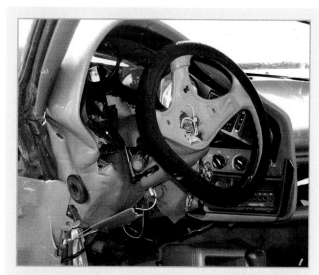

Figure 18-3 The second collision in a frontal impact is that of the passenger against the interior of the car. The appearance of the interior of the car can provide you with information about the severity of the patient's injuries.

comes to rest by striking the inside of the skull. This results in compression injury (or bruising) to the anterior portion of the brain and stretching (or tearing) of the posterior portion of the brain Figure 18-4 ▼. This is an example of a coup-contrecoup brain injury. Similarly, in the chest, the heart may slam forward into the sternum, occasionally rupturing the aorta and causing fatal bleeding.

Understanding the relationship among the three collisions will help you make the connections between the amount of damage to the exterior of the car and potential injury to the passenger. For example, in

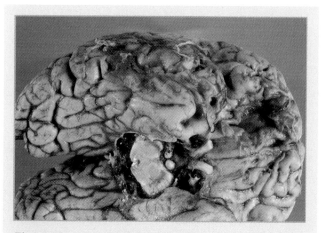

Figure 18-4 A brain with contusions.

a high-speed collision that results in massive damage to the car, you should suspect serious injuries to the passengers, even if the injuries are not readily apparent. Your quick initial assessment of the patient and the evaluation of the MOI can help direct lifesaving care.

The amount of damage that is considered significant varies, depending on the type of collision, but any substantial deformity of the vehicle should be enough cause for you to consider transporting the patient to a trauma center. Significant mechanisms of injury include the following:

- Severe deformities of the frontal part of a vehicle, with or without intrusion into the passenger compartment
- Moderate intrusions from a lateral (T-bone) type of accident
- Severe damage from the rear
- Collisions in which rotation is involved (rollover and spins)

Damage to the vehicle and information from your patient assessment are not the only clues to crash severity. Clearly, if one or more of the passengers are dead, you should suspect that the other passengers have also sustained potentially life-threatening injuries, even if the injuries are not obvious. Because these passengers have likely experienced the same amount of force that caused the death of the other patient, you should focus on treating life-threatening injuries and providing transport to a trauma center.

Frontal Collisions

Understanding the MOI after a frontal collision first involves evaluation of the supplemental restraint system (seat belts and air bags). Identifying the types of restraints used and whether air bags were deployed will help you identify injury patterns related to the supplemental restraint systems.

When properly applied, seat belts are successful in restraining the passengers in a vehicle and preventing a second collision inside the motor vehicle. In addition, they may decrease the severity of the third

EMT-B Safety

Be alert for undeployed airbags. Severed lines may still hold a charge, allowing airbags to deploy and thus injuring you and the patient.

collision. The very presence of air bags allows seat belts to provide even more "ride down," or the gentle cushioning of the occupant as the body slows, or decelerates. Air bags provide the final capture point of the passengers and again decrease the severity of <u>deceleration</u> injuries by cushioning the occupant as he or she moves forward.

Remember that air bags decrease injury to the chest, face, and head very effectively. However, you should still suspect that other serious injuries to the extremities (resulting from the second collision) and to internal organs (resulting from the third collision) have occurred. Because a rear-facing car seat is in proximity to the dashboard, rapid inflation of the air bag could cause serious injury or death to an infant. Children should ride in the rear seat.

When you are providing care to an occupant inside a motor vehicle, it is important to remember that if the air bag did not inflate, it may deploy during extrication. If this occurs, you may be seriously injured or even killed. Extreme caution must be used when extricating a patient in a vehicle with an air bag that has not deployed.

You should also remember that supplemental restraint systems can cause harm whether they are used properly or improperly. For example, some older models have seat belts that buckle automatically at the shoulder but require the passengers to buckle the lap portion; these can result in the body "submarining" forward underneath the shoulder restraint when the lap portion is not attached. This movement of the body can cause the lower extremities and the pelvis to crash into the dashboard because that part of the body is unrestrained. In addition, individuals of short stature can sustain significant neck and facial injuries caused by the belting systems when their lower torso is unrestrained.

When passengers are riding in vehicles equipped with air bags but are not restrained by seat belts, they are often thrown forward. As a result, they come into

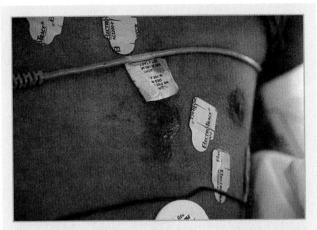

Figure 18-5 Air bags can cause injury in frontal collisions, specifically, abrasions and traction-type injuries to the face, neck, and chest.

contact with the air bag and/or the doors at the time of deployment. This MOI is also responsible for some severe injuries to children who are riding unrestrained in the front seats of vehicles. You should assess for abrasions and/or traction-type injuries on the face, lower part of the neck, and chest Figure 18-5▲.

Rear-End Collisions

Rear-end impacts are known to cause whiplash-type injuries, particularly when the head and/or neck is not restrained by an appropriately placed headrest. As the body is propelled forward, the head and neck (due to the relative weight of the head) are left behind and then are whipped back into position relative to the torso. As the vehicle comes to rest, the unrestrained passenger moves forward, striking the dashboard. In this type of collision, the cervical spine and surrounding area may be injured. The cervical spine is less tolerant of damage when it is bent back. Headrests decrease extension during a collision and help reduce injury. Other parts of the spine and the pelvis may also be at risk for injury. In addition, the patient may sustain an acceleration-type injury to the brain as the brain collides within the skull.

Lateral Collisions

Lateral impacts (T-bone collisions) are probably now the number one cause of death associated with motor vehicle crashes. When a vehicle is struck from the side, it is typically struck above its center of gravity and begins to rock away from the side of the impact. This results in a lateral whiplash injury Figure 18-6▶.

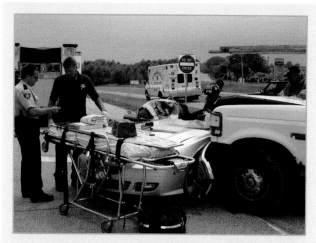

Figure 18-6 In a lateral collision, the car is typically struck above its center of gravity and begins to rock away from the side of impact.

The movement is to the side, and the passenger's shoulders and head whip toward the intruding vehicle. This action may thrust the shoulder, thorax, and upper extremities, and, more important, the skull against the doorpost or the window. The cervical spine has little tolerance for lateral bending.

If there is substantial intrusion into the passenger compartment, you should suspect lateral chest and abdominal injuries on the side of the impact, as well as possible fractures of the lower extremities, pelvis, and ribs. In addition, the organs within the abdomen are at risk because of a possible third collision. Approximately 25% of all severe injuries to the aorta that occur in motor vehicle crashes are a result of lateral collisions.

Rollover Crashes

Certain vehicles, such as large trucks and sport utility vehicles, are more prone to rollover crashes because of their high center of gravity. Injury patterns associated with rollover crashes differ, based on whether the passenger was restrained. The most unpredictable are rollover crashes in which an unrestrained passenger may have sustained multiple strikes within the interior of the vehicle as it rolled. The most common life-threatening event in a rollover is ejection or partial ejection of the passenger from the vehicle ▶Figure 18-7▶. Passengers who have been ejected may have struck the interior of the vehicle many times before ejection. The passenger may also have struck several objects, such as trees or a guardrail, before landing. Passengers who have been partially ejected may have struck both the interior and exterior of the vehicle and may have been sandwiched between the exterior of the vehicle and the environment as the vehicle rolled.

Even when restrained, passengers can sustain severe injuries during a rollover crash. A passenger on the outboard side of a vehicle that rolls over is at high risk for injury because of the centrifugal force (the patient is pinned against the door of the vehicle). When

You are the Provider 3

Your partner enters the vehicle from the passenger side and applies oxygen via a nonrebreathing mask at 15 L/min. He talks to the patient to try and calm him. Other than the aforementioned injuries, you find nothing else that appears to be significant.

Reassessment	Recording Time: 5 Minutes
Pulse	108 beats/min, regular
Blood pressure	122/78 mm Hg
Respirations	20 breaths/min, deep
Breath sounds	Clear bilaterally
Pulse oximetry	96% on oxygen via nonrebreathing mask

8. Is this a load-and-go patient? Why or why not?
9. How should the patient be removed from the vehicle?
10. Based on his presentation, how often should this patient be reassessed?

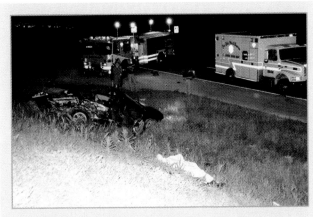

Figure 18-7 Passengers who have been ejected or partially ejected may have struck the interior of the car many times before ejection.

was wearing a helmet, you should inspect the helmet for damage. You should suspect head and spinal injuries and immobilize the patient accordingly.

Falls

The injury potential of a fall is related to the height from which the patient fell. The greater the height of the fall, the greater the potential for injury. A fall from more than 15' or 3 times the patient's height is considered significant. The patient lands on the surface just as an unrestrained passenger smashes into the interior of a vehicle. The internal organs travel at the speed of the patient's body before it hits the ground and stop by smashing into the interior of the body. Again, it is these internal injuries that are the least obvious during assessment but pose the gravest threat to life. You

the roof hits the ground during a rollover, a passenger who is restrained can still move far enough toward the roof to make contact and sustain a spinal cord injury. Therefore, rollover crashes are particularly dangerous for both restrained and, to a greater degree, unrestrained passengers because these crashes provide multiple opportunities for second and third collisions.

Auto-Versus-Pedestrian Collisions

Auto-versus-pedestrian collisions often present with graphic and apparent injuries. You must also maintain a high index of suspicion for unseen injuries. Multisystem injuries are common after this type of event. A thorough evaluation of the MOI is critical. When evaluating the MOI, you should attempt to estimate the speed of the vehicle, determine whether the patient was thrown through the air and the distance traveled, and whether the patient was pulled under the vehicle. You should evaluate the vehicle for structural damage that might indicate contact points with the patient and alert you to potential injuries.

In an auto-versus-bicycle collision, you should evaluate the MOI with particular attention to the damage to and the position of the bicycle. If the patient

You are the Provider 4

The patient is removed from the vehicle directly onto a backboard with the c-spine controlled. He is transported to the local trauma center where he is found to have a mild concussion and a bruised liver. He is kept over the weekend for observation and released on Monday morning.

344 Section 5 Trauma

should suspect internal injuries in a patient who has fallen from a significant height, just as you would in a patient who has been in a high-speed motor vehicle crash. Always consider syncope or other underlying medical causes of the fall.

Patients who fall and land on their feet may have less severe internal injuries because their legs may have absorbed much of the energy of the fall. As a result, they may have severe injuries to the lower extremities and pelvis and spinal injuries from energy that the legs do not absorb. Patients who fall onto their heads, as in diving accidents, will likely have serious head and/or spinal injuries. In either case, a fall from a significant height has a great injury potential, and the patient should be evaluated thoroughly. Take the following factors into account:

- The height of the fall
- The surface struck
- The part of the body that hit first

Many falls, especially those by older persons, are not considered "true" trauma, even though bones may be broken. Often, these falls occur as a result of a fracture. Older patients often have osteoporosis, a condition in which the musculoskeletal system can fail under relatively low stress. Because of this condition, an older patient can sustain a fracture while in a standing position and then fall as a result. Therefore, an older patient may have actually sustained a fracture before the fall. These cases do not constitute true high-energy trauma unless the patient fell from a significant height.

■ Penetrating Trauma

Penetrating trauma is the second largest cause of death in the United States after blunt trauma. Low-energy penetrating trauma may be caused accidentally by impalement or intentionally by a knife, ice pick, or other weapon (Figure 18-8 ▶). Many times it is difficult to determine entrance and exit wounds in a prehospital setting (unless you can determine an obvious exit wound). Determine the number of penetrating inju-

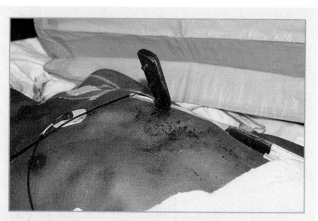
Figure 18-8 Injuries from low-energy penetrations, such as a stab wound, are caused by the sharp edges of the object moving through the body.

ries and combine that with the important things you already know about the potential pathway of penetrating projectiles to form an index of suspicion about unseen life-threatening injuries.

With low-energy penetrations, injuries are caused by the sharp edges of the object moving through the body and are close to the object's path. Weapons such as knives may have been deliberately moved around internally, causing more damage than the external wound might suggest.

In medium- and high-velocity penetrating trauma, the path of the object (usually a bullet) may not be as easy to predict. The bullet may flatten out, tumble, or even ricochet within the body before exiting. Also, because of its speed, pressure waves emanate from the bullet, causing damage remote from its path (Figure 18-9 ▼). This phenomenon, called <u>cavitation</u>,

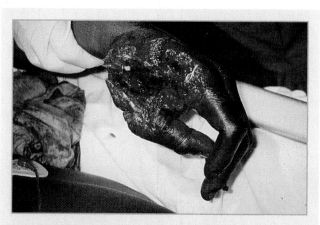
Figure 18-9 The area damaged by high-velocity projectiles, such as bullets, can be many times larger than the diameter of the projectile itself.

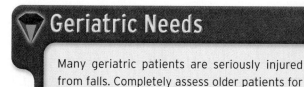

◆ Geriatric Needs

Many geriatric patients are seriously injured from falls. Completely assess older patients for all possible injuries, even from low-impact falls.

can result in serious injury to internal organs distant to the actual path of the bullet. Much like a boat moving through water, the bullet disrupts not only the tissues that are directly in its path but also those in its wake. Therefore, the area that is damaged by medium- and high-velocity projectiles can be many times larger than the diameter of the projectile itself. This is one reason that exit wounds are often many times larger than entrance wounds. As with motor vehicle crashes, the energy available for a bullet to cause damage is more a function of its speed than its mass (weight). If the mass of the bullet is doubled, the energy that is available to cause injury is doubled. If the speed (velocity) of the bullet is doubled, the energy that is available to cause injury is *quadrupled*. For this reason, it is important for you to try to determine the type of weapon that was used. Although not always possible, any information regarding the type of weapon that was used should be relayed to the hospital. Police at the scene may be a useful source of information regarding the caliber of weapon.

You are the Provider Summary

Occult injuries may mean the difference in a stable or critical patient. Failure to recognize the potential for these injuries may result in improper care and possible morbidity or mortality. Learn to "read" the mechanism of injury and apply that information to the care of the patient.

1. **What questions should you ask as you approach the patient?**
   - General impression, level of consciousness?
   - Was the patient restrained?
   - Have the airbags deployed?
   - Do I see any exsanguinating hemorrhage?
   - What type of damage is there to the vehicle?

2. **How should first responders on scene be used?**
   - Stabilizing the vehicle
   - C-spine control
   - Bleeding control
   - Assistance removing the patient from the vehicle

3. **What other personal safety issues might concern you with this type of collision?**
   If the airbag has not deployed, it is a potential hazard to the patient and rescuers. Never position yourself in front of an undeployed airbag.
   Is there any leaking fuel or smoke coming from the vehicle?

4. **What collisions has the patient experienced?**
   - Car versus tree
   - Body versus car
   - Organs versus body

5. **What type of injury might you suspect from the spider-webbed windshield and altered level of consciousness?**
   His head struck the windshield and he has probably experienced a coup-contrecoup injury.

6. **What type of injuries may result from the improperly worn restraints?**
   He is thrown forward into the steering wheel, windshield, etc. The result may be head, chest, upper extremity, and abdominal injuries.

7. **At what point should oxygen be applied to the patient? How should it be administered?**
   As soon as there is access to the patient. Since he has good tidal volume, a nonrebreathing mask is appropriate.

8. **Is this a load-and-go patient? Why or why not?**
   Yes, he is a load-and-go. He has a significant mechanism of injury as well as an altered mental status.

9. **How should the patient be removed from the vehicle?**
   There is no apparent danger to the rescuers, but the patient is a load-and-go. C-spine should be controlled while he is removed to a long spine board and packaged for transport.

10. **Based on his presentation, how often should this patient be reassessed?**
    Every 5 minutes. He is considered unstable based on the mechanism of injury and the altered mental status.

Prep Kit

Ready for Review

- Determine the MOI as quickly as possible; this will assist you in developing an index of suspicion for the significance of unseen injuries.
- Communicate MOI findings in the written patient report and verbally to hospital staff; this will ensure that appropriate treatment continues for the patient at the hospital for potential serious injuries.
- In every crash there are three collisions that occur:
  - The collision of the vehicle against some type of object
  - The collision of the passenger against the interior of the vehicle
  - The collision of the passenger's internal organs against the solid structures of the body
- Maintain a high index of suspicion for serious injury in the patient who has been involved in a car crash with significant damage to the vehicle, has fallen from a significant height, or has sustained penetrating trauma to the body.

Vital Vocabulary

blunt trauma   An impact on the body by objects that cause injury without penetrating soft tissues or internal organs and cavities.

cavitation   A phenomenon in which speed causes a bullet to generate pressure waves, which cause damage distant from the bullet's path.

coup-contrecoup brain injury   A brain injury that occurs when force is applied to the head and energy transmission through brain tissue causes injury on the opposite side of original impact.

deceleration   The slowing of an object.

index of suspicion   Awareness that unseen life-threatening injuries may exist when determining the mechanism of injury.

kinetic energy   The energy of a moving object.

mechanism of injury (MOI)   The forces or energy transmission applied to the body that cause injury.

penetrating trauma   Injury caused by objects, such as knives and bullets, that pierce the surface of the body and damage internal tissues and organs.

Technology

Interactivities

Vocabulary Explorer

Anatomy Review

Web Links

Online Review Manual

Assessment in Action

Evaluation of the mechanism of injury can lead you in the right direction to recognize the potential for occult injuries. You should have a basic understanding of the mechanism of injury as well as possible injuries created by the direction of travel associated with the mechanism of injury. Assessing damage to a vehicle may allow you to predict injuries sustained at the time of impact.

1. Which of the following may reduce deceleration injuries?
   A. frontal impacts
   B. air bags
   C. lap belts
   D. rollovers

2. The _____ is your concern for occult injuries.
   A. index of suspicion
   B. occult factor
   C. trauma index
   D. mechanism of injury

3. The most significant factor in a fall is the _____.
   A. surface struck
   B. weight of the patient
   C. height of the fall
   D. part of the body that hit first

4. Whiplash injuries most often occur with what type of impacts?
   A. rollovers
   B. frontal collisions
   C. lateral impacts
   D. rear-end collisions

5. Aorta injuries are associated with what type of impact?
   A. rollovers
   B. frontal collisions
   C. lateral impacts
   D. rear-end collisions

6. Pressure waves resulting from a projectile are known as _____.
   A. yaw
   B. cavitation
   C. tumbling
   D. kinetic energy

Challenging Questions

7. Explain why rollover crashes have such a high potential for serious injuries.

19

Bleeding and Shock

You are the Provider 1

You arrive on scene of a motor vehicle crash to find a 35-year-old woman who was a restrained driver and has t-boned a large pickup. First responders tell you that the driver of the pickup is uninjured and that there were no other passengers in either vehicle.

As you approach your patient's car you see massive damage to the front driver's side. The patient is still sitting in the driver's seat with her seatbelt fastened and another rescuer is holding c-spine control and talking to her.

Initial Assessment	Recording Time: 0 Minutes
Appearance	Pale, diaphoretic
Level of consciousness	Alert but a little confused
Airway	Open and clear
Breathing	A little fast
Circulation	Radials present, regular, rapid

1. Is this a load-and-go patient? Why or why not?
2. How should you approach your assessment?

Introduction

Recognizing bleeding and understanding how it affects the patient's body is critical in assessment and care. Bleeding can be external and obvious or internal and hidden. Either way it can cause shock and death if left uncontrolled.

Shock is the result of hypoperfusion to the cells of the body that causes organs and then organ systems to fail. Unless treated successfully, this process will ultimately result in the death of the organism. In the early stages of shock, the body will attempt to maintain homeostasis (a balance of all systems of the body). As shock progresses, blood circulation slows and eventually ceases. If not treated promptly, shock (hypoperfusion) can be fatal. Shock can occur because of several medical or traumatic events such as a heart attack, severe allergic reaction, an automobile crash, or a gunshot wound. To manage these patients effectively, EMS providers must be able to anticipate, recognize, and treat shock.

This chapter will review how the cardiovascular system reacts to blood loss. It begins with a brief review of the anatomy and function of the cardiovascular system, then describes the signs, symptoms, and emergency medical care of both external and internal bleeding. Next it looks at the physiologic causes of shock and describes each of its major forms. Finally, it discusses the emergency treatment of shock.

Anatomy and Physiology of the Cardiovascular System

The cardiovascular system circulates blood to all of the body's cells and tissues, delivering oxygen and nutrients and carrying away metabolic waste products. Certain parts of the body, such as the brain, spinal cord, and heart, require a constant flow of blood to live. The cells in these organs cannot tolerate a lack of blood for more than a few minutes. Other organs, such as the lungs and kidneys, can survive for short periods without adequate blood flow. Inadequate blood flow to the tissues will cause the cells to begin to die. Untreated, this can lead to a permanent loss of function or death.

The cardiovascular system consists of three parts:

- The pump (the heart)
- A container (the blood vessels that reach every cell in the body)
- The fluid (blood and body fluids)

The Heart

The heart is a hollow muscular organ about the size of a clenched fist. It is an involuntary muscle that is under the control of the autonomic nervous system, but it has its own regulatory system. It can function even if the nervous system shuts down.

All organs depend on the heart to provide a rich blood supply. For this reason, it has a number of special features that other muscles do not. First, because the heart cannot tolerate a disruption of its blood supply for more than a few seconds, the heart muscle needs a rich and well-distributed blood supply. Second, the heart works as two paired pumps Figure 19-1 ▶ . Each side of the heart has an upper chamber (atrium) and a lower chamber (ventricle) to pump blood. Blood leaves each chamber through a one-way valve that keeps the blood moving in the proper direction by preventing backflow.

The right side of the heart receives oxygen-poor (deoxygenated) blood from the veins of the body. Blood enters the right atrium from the vena cava, then fills the right ventricle. After the right ventricle contracts, blood flows into the pulmonary artery and the pulmonary circulation. The now oxygen-rich (oxygenated) blood returns to the left side of the heart from the lungs through the pulmonary veins. Blood enters the left atrium, then passes into the left ventricle. This side of the heart is more muscular than the other because it must pump blood into the aorta and on to the arteries throughout the body. It is important to remember that the left ventricle is responsible for providing 100% of the body with oxygen-rich blood.

Technology

Interactivities

Vocabulary Explorer

Anatomy Review

Web Links

Online Review Manual

Refresher.EMSzone.com

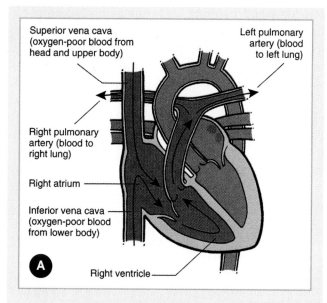

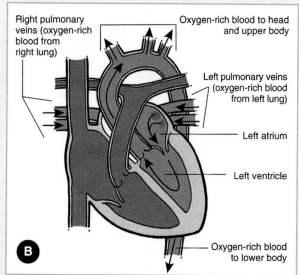

Figure 19-1 A. The right side of the heart circulates blood from the body to the lungs. **B.** The left side of the heart circulates oxygen-rich blood to all parts of the body. It is the more muscular of the two pumps because it must pump blood into the aorta and into the arteries.

Blood Vessels and Blood

There are five types of blood vessels:

- Arteries
- Arterioles
- Capillaries
- Venules
- Veins

As blood flows out of the heart, it passes into the <u>aorta</u>, the largest artery in the body. The arteries become smaller as they move away from the heart. The smaller vessels that connect the arteries and capillaries

are called arterioles. <u>Capillaries</u> are small tubes, with the diameter of a single red blood cell, that pass among all the cells in the body, linking the arterioles and the venules. Blood leaving the other side of the capillaries flows into the venules. These small, thin-walled vessels empty into the <u>veins</u>, and the veins then empty into the vena cava. Oxygen and nutrients easily pass from the capillaries into the cells, and waste and carbon dioxide move out of the cells and into the capillaries. This transportation system allows the body to rid itself of waste products.

The arterial ends of the capillaries and the arteries have circular muscular walls, which constrict and dilate automatically under the control of the autonomic nervous system. When these muscles open (dilate), blood passes into the capillaries in proximity to each cell of the surrounding tissue; when the muscles are closed (constricted), there is no capillary blood flow. The muscles dilate and constrict in response to conditions such as fright, heat, cold, a specific need for oxygen, and the need to dispose of metabolic waste. In a healthy individual, all the vessels are never fully dilated or fully constricted at the same time.

The last part of the cardiovascular system is the contents of the container, or the blood. Blood contains red cells, white cells, platelets, and plasma. Red blood cells are responsible for the transportation of oxygen to the cells and for transporting carbon dioxide (a waste product of cellular metabolism) away from the cells to the lungs where it is exhaled and removed from the body. Platelets are responsible for forming blood clots. In the body, a blood clot forms depending on one of the following principles: the rate of the flow of the blood (blood that moves too slow or that is not moving will clot), changes in the vessel wall (such as a wound), and the blood's ability to clot (due to a disease process or medication). When injury occurs to tissues in the body, platelets will begin to collect at the site of injury; this causes red blood cells to become sticky and clump together. As the red blood cells begin to clump, another substance in the body called fibrinogen reinforces the red blood cells. This is the final step in formation of a blood clot. Blood clots are an important response from the body to control blood loss.

The autonomic nervous system constantly monitors the body's needs and adjusts the blood flow by changing the tone in the blood vessels. During emergencies, the autonomic nervous system automatically redirects blood away from other organs to the heart, brain, lungs, and kidneys. The cardiovascular system is dynamic and constantly adapting to changing conditions in the body to maintain homeostasis and perfusion. When the system fails to provide sufficient circulation for every body part to perform its function the result is hypoperfusion, or shock.

Pathophysiology and Perfusion

Blunt force trauma may cause injury and significant bleeding that is unseen inside a body cavity or region, such as an injury to the liver or the spleen. These injuries cause the patient to lose significant amounts of blood, causing hypoperfusion without visible bleeding. In penetrating trauma, the patient may have only a small amount of bleeding that is visible; however, the patient may have sustained injury to internal organs that will produce significant bleeding that is unseen by you and may cause death quickly.

Perfusion is the circulation of blood within an organ or tissue in adequate amounts to meet the cells' current needs for oxygen, nutrients, and waste removal. Blood enters an organ or tissue first through the arterial system and the capillary beds. While passing through the capillaries, the blood delivers nutrients and oxygen to the surrounding cells and picks up the wastes they have generated. The blood leaves the capillary beds through the venous system, which takes the blood back to the heart.

Blood must pass through the cardiovascular system at a speed that is fast enough to maintain adequate circulation throughout the body and slow enough to allow each cell time to exchange oxygen and nutrients for carbon dioxide and other waste products. Although some tissues, such as the lungs and kidneys, never rest and require a constant blood supply, most require circulating blood only intermittently, especially when active. Muscles are a good example. When you sleep, they are at rest and require a minimal blood supply. However, during exercise, they need a very large blood supply. The gastrointestinal tract requires a high flow of blood after a meal, but after digestion, functions with a small fraction of that flow.

All organs and organ systems of the human body are dependent on adequate perfusion to function properly. Some of these organs receive a very rich supply of blood and do not tolerate interruption of blood supply for very long. If perfusion is interrupted to these organs and damage occurs to the organ tissue, dysfunction and failure of that organ system will oc-

Documentation Tips

In order to alert the physician to any potential internal injuries, carefully document any damage to the vehicle, direction of travel of a weapon (knife), distance of a fall and the surface struck, or any other mechanism of injury.

cur. Death of an organ system can quickly lead to the patient's death. Emergency medical care is designed to support adequate perfusion to these organ systems.

The heart requires constant perfusion to function properly. The brain and spinal cord can be damaged after 4 to 6 minutes without perfusion. It is important to remember that cells of the central nervous system do not have the capacity to regenerate. Kidneys can be damaged after 45 minutes of inadequate perfusion. Skeletal muscle demonstrates evidence of injury after 2 hours of inadequate perfusion. The gastrointestinal tract can tolerate slightly longer periods of inadequate perfusion. These times are based on a normal body temperature (98.6°F [37.0°C]). An organ or tissue that is considerably colder may be better able to resist damage from hypoperfusion.

External Bleeding

The Significance of Bleeding

When patients have significant external blood loss, it is often difficult to determine the amount of blood that the patient has actually lost. This is because blood looks different on different surfaces, such as when it is absorbed in clothing or when it has been diluted when mixed in water. Always attempt to determine the amount of external blood loss, but remember that the presentation and your patient assessment will direct your care and treatment.

The body will not tolerate an acute blood loss of greater than 20% of blood volume. The typical adult has approximately 70 mL of blood per kilogram of body weight, or 6 L (10 to 12 pints) in a body weighing 80 kg (175 lb). If the typical adult loses more than 1 L of blood (a little less than 3 cans of pop), significant changes in vital signs will occur, including increasing heart and respiratory rates and decreasing blood pressure. Because infants and children have less blood volume to begin with, the same effect is seen with smaller amounts of blood loss. For example, a 1-year-old infant has a total blood volume of about 800 mL. Significant symptoms of blood loss will occur after only 100 to 200 mL of blood loss. To put this in perspective, a soft drink can holds roughly 345 mL of liquid.

How well patients compensate for blood loss is related to how rapidly they bleed. A healthy adult can comfortably donate 1 unit (500 mL) of blood during a period of 15 to 20 minutes and adapts well to this decrease in blood volume. However, if a similar blood loss occurs in a much shorter period, the person may rapidly develop <u>hypovolemic shock</u>, a condition in which low blood volume results in inadequate perfusion and even death. The body simply cannot compensate for such a rapid blood loss.

You should consider bleeding to be potentially life-threatening if the following conditions are present:

- It is associated with a significant mechanism of injury.
- The patient has a poor general appearance.
- Assessment reveals signs and symptoms of shock (hypoperfusion).
- You note a significant amount of blood loss.
- The blood loss is rapid.
- You cannot control the bleeding.

In any situation, blood loss is an extremely serious problem. It demands your immediate attention as soon as you have cleared the airway and managed the patient's breathing.

Characteristics of Bleeding

Injuries and some illnesses can disrupt blood vessels and cause bleeding. Typically, bleeding from an open artery is brighter red (high in oxygen) and spurts in time with the pulse. The pressure that causes the blood to spurt also makes this type of bleeding difficult to control. As the amount of blood circulating in the body drops, so does the patient's blood pressure and, eventually, the arterial spurting.

Blood from an open vein is darker (low in oxygen) and flows steadily. Because it is under less pressure, most venous blood does not spurt and is easier to manage. Bleeding from damaged capillary vessels is dark red and oozes from a wound steadily but slowly. Venous and capillary blood is more likely to clot spontaneously than arterial blood.

Bleeding tends to stop on its own rather quickly, within about 10 minutes, in response to internal mechanisms and exposure to air. When we are cut, blood flows rapidly from the open vessel. Soon afterward, the cut ends of the vessel begin to narrow, reducing the amount of bleeding. A clot then forms that plugs the hole and seals the injured portions of the vessel. This process is called <u>coagulation</u>. Bleeding will never stop if a clot does not form, unless the injured vessel is completely cut off from the main blood supply. Direct contact with body tissues and fluids or the external environment commonly triggers the blood's clotting factors.

Despite the efficiency of this system, it may fail in certain situations. A number of medications, including aspirin and blood thinners, interfere with normal clotting. With a severe injury, the damage to the vessel may be so large that a clot cannot completely block the hole. Sometimes only part of the vessel wall is cut, preventing it from constricting. In these cases, bleeding will continue unless it is stopped by external means. Occasionally, blood loss occurs very rapidly. In these cases, the patient might die before the body's defenses, such as clotting, can help.

A very small portion of the population lacks one or more of the blood's clotting factors (hemophilia). There are several forms of hemophilia, most of which are hereditary and some of which are severe. Sometimes bleeding may occur spontaneously in hemophilia. Because the patient's blood does not clot, all injuries, no matter how trivial, are potentially serious. A patient with hemophilia should be transported immediately.

Emergency Medical Care

As you begin to care for a patient with obvious external bleeding, remember to follow BSI precautions. As

EMT-B Safety

Use appropriate PPE/BSI when there is bleeding. Be alert for splashing and use goggles and a gown.

Documentation Tips

Document any history of bleeding abnormalities, such as hemophilia. Also include the use of any medications that may interfere with clotting such as aspirin or other anticoagulants.

with all patient care, make sure that the patient has an open airway and is breathing adequately. Provide high-flow oxygen to the patient and then focus on controlling the bleeding. In some cases, obvious life-threatening bleeding may be present and should be addressed as an immediate life threat and controlled as quickly as possible.

Several methods are available to control external bleeding. Starting with the most commonly used, these methods include:

- Direct pressure and elevation
- Pressure dressings
- Pressure points (for upper and lower extremities)
- Splints
- Air splints
- Pneumatic antishock garment
- Tourniquets (last resort)

Basic Methods

Skill Drill 19-1 ▾ reviews the basic techniques to control external bleeding.

1. The most effective way to control external bleeding is with direct pressure. Almost all external bleeding can be controlled simply by **applying direct pressure to the bleeding site.** Pressure stops the flow of blood and permits normal coagulation to occur. You may apply pressure with your gloved fingertip or hand over the top of a sterile dressing if one is immediately available. If there is an object protruding from the wound, apply bulky dressings to stabilize the object in place, and apply pressure as best you can. Never remove an impaled object from a wound. Hold *uninterrupted pressure* for at least 5 minutes.

2. **Elevating a bleeding extremity** by as little as 6" often stops venous bleeding. In most cases, direct pressure and elevation will stop the bleeding. Remember to never elevate an open fracture to control bleeding. Fractures can be elevated after splinting, and splinting will also help control bleeding (**Step 1**).

3. **Once you have applied a dressing to control the bleeding,** you can create a pressure dressing to maintain the pressure by firmly wrapping a sterile, self-adhering roller bandage around the entire wound. Use 4" × 4" sterile gauze pads for small wounds and sterile universal dressings for larger wounds.

Cover the entire dressing above and below the wound. Stretch the bandage tight enough to control bleeding but not so tight as to decrease blood flow to the extremity. If you were able to palpate a distal pulse before applying the dressing, you should still be able to palpate a distal pulse on the injured extremity after applying the pressure dressing. If bleeding continues, the

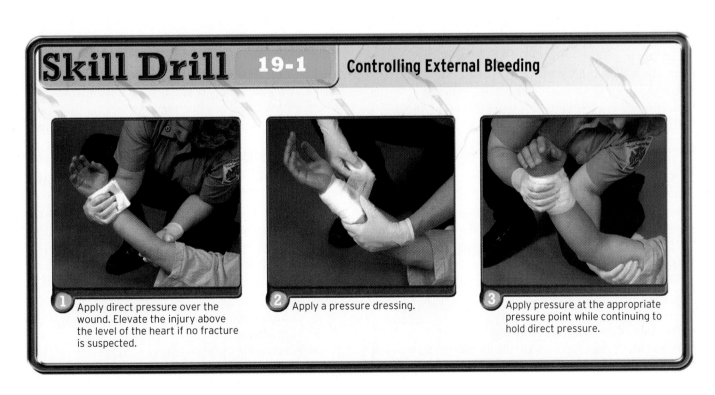

Skill Drill   19-1   Controlling External Bleeding

1 Apply direct pressure over the wound. Elevate the injury above the level of the heart if no fracture is suspected.

2 Apply a pressure dressing.

3 Apply pressure at the appropriate pressure point while continuing to hold direct pressure.

dressing is probably not tight enough. Do not remove a dressing until a physician has evaluated the patient. Instead, apply additional manual pressure through the dressing. Then add more gauze pads over the first dressing, and secure them both with a second, tighter roller bandage.

Bleeding will almost always stop when the pressure of the dressing exceeds arterial pressure. This will assist in controlling bleeding and helping blood to clot (**Step ②**).

4. **If a wound continues to bleed** despite direct pressure and elevating the extremity, try placing additional pressure over a proximal <u>pressure point</u>. A pressure point is a spot where a blood vessel lies near a bone. This technique is also useful if you have no material on hand to use for a dressing. Because a wound usually draws blood from more than one major artery, proximal compression of a major artery rarely stops bleeding completely, but it helps to slow the loss of blood. You must be familiar with the location of the pressure points for this to work Figure 19-2 ▶ (**Step ③**).

Special Techniques

Much of the bleeding associated with broken bones occurs because the sharp ends of the bones cut muscles and other tissues. As long as a fracture remains unstable, the bone ends will move and continue to injure partially clotted vessels. Therefore, stabilizing a fracture and decreasing movement is a high priority in the prompt control of bleeding. Often, simple splints will quickly control bleeding associated with a fracture. If not, you may need to use another splinting device, such as an air splint, pneumatic antishock garment, or a tourniquet.

Air Splints

Air splints can control the bleeding associated with severe soft-tissue injuries, such as large lacerations or fractures. An air splint acts like a pressure dressing applied to an entire extremity rather than to a small, local area. Once you have applied an air splint, be sure to monitor circulation in the distal extremity. Use only BSI-approved, clean, or disposable valve stems when orally inflating air splints.

Pneumatic Antishock Garments

If a patient has injuries to the lower extremities or pelvis, you may be able to use a <u>pneumatic antishock</u>

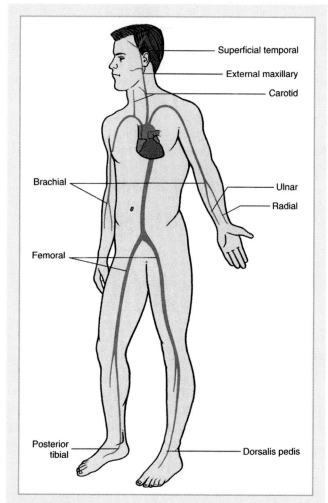

Figure 19-2 You should be familiar with the locations of arterial pressure points.

<u>garment (PASG)</u> as a splinting device, if local protocol allows. The following are the few specific purposes for which a PASG may be effective:

- To stabilize fractures of the pelvis and proximal femurs
- To control significant internal bleeding associated with fractures of the pelvis and proximal femurs
- To control massive soft-tissue bleeding of the lower extremities when direct pressure is not effective

Do not use the PASG if any of the following conditions exist:

- Pregnancy
- Pulmonary edema
- Acute heart failure
- Penetrating chest injuries
- Groin injuries

- Major head injuries
- A transport time of less than 30 minutes

In these situations, the PASG may worsen or complicate the patient's condition. The PASG works by compressing the abdomen and lower extremities, increasing peripheral resistance in the circulatory system. This increases the amount of blood that is available to perfuse the vital organs. When applying the PASG, you should carefully inflate the device in increments. As a general rule, gradually inflate the legs of the PASG before inflating the abdominal portion. If you are using the device to stabilize a possible pelvic fracture, you must inflate all compartments. Always document all obvious injuries or deformities before application of the PASG. Follow these steps to apply the PASG for bleeding control Skill Drill 19-2 ▶ :

1. **Apply the garment.** If you will immobilize or move the patient on a backboard, lay the PASG out on the board before rolling the patient onto it. Position the top of the abdominal section of the PASG below the lowest rib to ensure that it does not compromise chest expansion (**Step ①**).
2. **Close and fasten both leg compartments** and the abdominal compartment (**Step ②**).
3. **Open the stopcocks (valves)** to the compartments you are preparing to inflate. You will inflate both leg compartments or all three compartments together (**Step ③**).
4. **Inflate the compartments** with the foot pump. Do not increase the pressure any more than necessary. A PASG is adequately inflated when the Velcro crackles. Higher pressures may cause local tissue damage. Always stop inflating the PASG once the patient's systolic blood pressure exceeds 100 mm Hg (**Step ④**).
5. **Check the patient's blood pressure** during inflation, and continue to monitor vital signs at least every 5 minutes afterward. Remember that the pressure gauges of the PASG measure the air pressure in the device, they do not reflect the patient's blood pressure. Be aware of temperature extremes or external pressure changes that can significantly affect the pressure exerted by the PASG, thus requiring frequent monitoring and adjustment (**Step ⑤**).

Do not remove a PASG in the field. It must be deflated gradually in the hospital under careful supervision by a physician and only after appropriate intravenous solutions have been given.

Tourniquets

A tourniquet is rarely needed to control bleeding. Applying a tourniquet is considered a last resort because it is rarely necessary and is effective for only a very limited number of injuries. A tourniquet often creates, rather than solves, problems. Application of a tourniquet can cause permanent damage to nerves, muscles, and blood vessels, resulting in the loss of an extremity. In addition, tourniquets are often improperly applied.

If you cannot control bleeding from a major vessel in an extremity in any other way, a properly applied tourniquet may save a patient's life. Specifically, the tourniquet is useful if a patient is bleeding severely from a partial or complete amputation or from an explosion or blast injury to an arm or leg.

Whenever you apply a tourniquet, make sure you observe the following precautions:

- Do not apply a tourniquet directly over any joint. Keep it as close to the injury as possible.
- Use the widest bandage possible. Make sure that it is tightened securely.
- Never use wire, rope, a belt, or any other narrow material. It could cut into the skin.
- Use wide padding under the tourniquet if possible. This will protect the tissues and help with arterial compression.
- Never cover a tourniquet with a bandage. Leave it open and in full view.
- Do not loosen the tourniquet after you have applied it. Hospital personnel will loosen it once they are prepared to manage the bleeding.

Bleeding from the Nose and Ears

Several conditions can result in bleeding from the nose, ears, and/or mouth:

- Skull fracture
- Facial injuries, including those caused by a direct blow to the nose
- Sinusitis, infections, nose drop use and abuse, dried or cracked nasal mucosa, or other abnormalities
- High blood pressure
- Clotting disorders
- Digital trauma (nose picking)

Epistaxis, or nosebleed, is a common emergency. Occasionally, it can cause enough of a blood loss to send a patient into shock. Keep in mind that the blood you see may be only a small part of the total blood loss. Much of the blood may pass down the throat into the stomach as the patient swallows. A person who swallows a large amount of blood may become

Skill Drill   19-2   Applying a Pneumatic Antishock Garment

1 Apply the garment so that the top is below the lowest rib.

2 Enclose both legs and the abdomen.

3 Open the stopcocks.

4 Inflate with the foot pump, and close the stopcocks when the patient's systolic blood pressure reaches 100 mm Hg or the Velcro crackles.

5 Check the patient's blood pressure again. Monitor the vital signs.

nauseated and start vomiting the blood, which may be confused with internal bleeding. Most nontraumatic nosebleeds occur from sites in the septum, the tissue dividing the nostrils. You can usually handle this type of bleeding effectively by pinching the nostrils together. Most often, failure to stop a nosebleed is the result of releasing the pressure too soon. You or the patient should pinch the nostrils for about 15 minutes. Keep the patient calm and quiet, especially if he or she has high blood pressure or is anxious. Anxiety tends to increase blood pressure, which could worsen the nosebleed. If you cannot control the bleeding, if the patient has a history of frequent nosebleeds, or if there is a significant amount of blood loss, transport

the patient immediately. Assess the patient for signs and symptoms of shock and treat accordingly.

Bleeding from the nose or ears following a head injury may indicate a skull fracture. In these cases, you should not attempt to stop the blood flow. This bleeding may be difficult to control. Applying excessive pressure to the injury may force the blood leaking through the ear or nose to collect within the head. This could increase the pressure on the brain and possibly cause permanent damage. If you suspect a skull fracture, loosely cover the bleeding site with a sterile gauze pad to collect the blood and help keep contaminants away from the site. There is always a risk of infection to the brain. Apply light compression

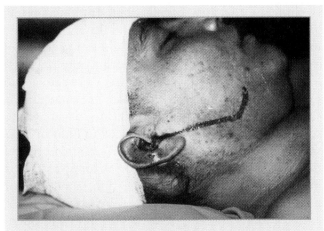

Figure 19-3 Bleeding from the ear after a head injury may indicate a skull fracture. Loosely cover the bleeding site with a sterile gauze pad, and apply light compression by wrapping the dressing loosely around the head.

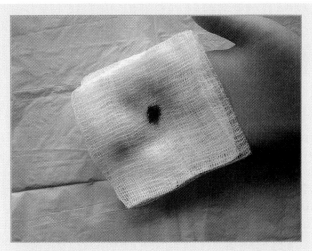

Figure 19-4 When cerebrospinal fluid is present in blood or drainage, a stain in the shape of a target or halo will appear.

by wrapping the dressing loosely around the head **Figure 19-3 ▲**. If blood or drainage contains cerebrospinal fluid, a characteristic staining of the dressing, much like a target or halo, will occur **Figure 19-4 ▶**.

■ Internal Bleeding

Internal bleeding can be very serious, especially because you might not be aware that it is happening. Injury or damage to internal organs commonly results in extensive internal bleeding, which can cause hypovolemic shock before you realize the extent of blood loss. A person with a bleeding stomach ulcer may lose a large amount of blood very quickly. Similarly, a person who has a lacerated liver or a ruptured spleen may lose a considerable amount of blood within the abdomen even though the patient has no outward signs of bleeding.

Broken bones, especially broken ribs, also may cause serious internal blood loss. Sometimes this bleeding extends into the chest cavity and the soft tissues of the chest wall. A broken femur can easily result in the loss of 1 L or more of blood into the soft tissues of the thigh. Often the only signs of such bleeding are

You are the Provider 2

You begin your assessment by looking for any exsanguinating hemorrhage and checking ABCs. Her airway is open and clear, and she is breathing with good depth. She has radial pulses that are a little weak, and her skin is pale and clammy. Her only complaint is that her "stomach hurts."

Vital Signs	Recording Time: 3 Minutes
Skin	Pale, diaphoretic
Pulse	112 beats/min, regular
Blood pressure	104/62 mm Hg
Respirations	22 breaths/min, adequate depth

3. What type of oxygen does she need? Why?
4. Should you focus only on her complaint?
5. How should she be removed from the vehicle?

Documentation Tips

If you must use a tourniquet, write "TK" and the time applied in dark ink on adhesive tape and fasten to the patient's forehead.

local swelling and bruising due to the accumulation of blood. Pelvic fractures may result in life-threatening hemorrhage.

You must always be alert to the possibility of internal bleeding and assess the patient for related signs and symptoms, particularly if the mechanism of injury is severe. If you suspect that a patient is bleeding internally, you should promptly transport him or her to the hospital.

Mechanism of Injury

A high-energy mechanism of injury (MOI) should increase your index of suspicion for the possibility of serious unseen injuries such as internal bleeding in the abdominal cavity. Internal bleeding is possible whenever the MOI suggests that severe forces (blunt and penetrating trauma) affected the body. Internal bleeding commonly occurs as a result of falls, blast injuries, and automobile or motorcycle crashes. You should always suspect internal bleeding in a patient who has a penetrating injury or blunt trauma.

Nature of Illness

Internal bleeding is not always caused by trauma. Many illnesses can cause internal bleeding. Some of the more common causes of nontraumatic internal bleeding include bleeding ulcers, bleeding from the colon, ruptured ectopic pregnancy, and aneurysms.

Abdominal pain and distention are frequent in these situations but are not always present. In older patients, dizziness, faintness, or weakness may be the first sign of nontraumatic internal bleeding. Ulcers or other gastrointestinal problems may cause vomiting of blood or bloody diarrhea.

It is not as important for you to know the specific organ involved as it is to recognize that the patient is in shock and respond appropriately.

Signs and Symptoms

The most common symptom of internal bleeding is pain. Significant internal bleeding will generally cause swelling in the area of bleeding. Intra-abdominal bleeding will often cause pain and distention. Bruising is a sign of internal bleeding and can be a sign of significant abdominal trauma. Bleeding into the chest may cause dyspnea in addition to tachycardia and hypotension. A hematoma, a mass of blood in the soft tissues beneath the skin, indicates bleeding into soft tissues and may be the result of a minor or a severe injury. Bruising may not be present initially, and the only sign of severe pelvic or abdominal trauma may be a reddened area on the skin, abrasions, or pain.

Bleeding, however slight, from any body opening is serious. It usually indicates internal bleeding that is not easy to see or control. Bright red bleeding from the mouth or rectum or blood in the urine (hematuria) may suggest serious internal injury or disease. Nonmenstrual vaginal bleeding is always significant.

Other signs and symptoms of internal bleeding in both trauma and medical patients include the following:

- Hematemesis. This is vomited blood. It may be bright red or dark red, or, if the blood has been partially digested, it may look like coffee-grounds vomitus.
- Melena. This is a black, foul-smelling, tarry stool that contains digested blood.
- Hemoptysis. This is bright red blood that is coughed up by the patient.
- Pain, tenderness, bruising, guarding, or swelling. These signs and symptoms may mean that a closed fracture is bleeding.
- Broken ribs, bruises over the lower part of the chest, or a rigid, distended abdomen. These signs and symptoms may indicate a lacerated spleen or liver. Patients with an injury to either organ may have referred pain in the right shoulder (liver) or left shoulder (spleen).

The first sign of hypovolemic shock (hypoperfusion) is a change in mental status, such as anxiety, restlessness, or combativeness. In nontrauma patients, weakness, faintness, or dizziness on standing is another early sign. Changes in skin color or pallor (pale skin) are seen often in both trauma and medical patients. Later signs of hypoperfusion suggesting internal bleeding include the following:

- Tachycardia
- Weak, rapid (thready) pulse
- Weakness, fainting, or dizziness at rest
- Thirst

- Nausea and vomiting
- Cold, moist (clammy) skin
- Shallow, rapid breathing
- Dull eyes
- Slightly dilated pupils that are slow to respond to light
- Capillary refill in infants and children of more than 2 seconds
- Decreasing blood pressure
- Altered level of consciousness

Emergency Medical Care

Controlling internal bleeding or bleeding from major organs usually requires surgery or other procedures that are performed in the hospital. It is important for you to calm and reassure the patient. Keeping the patient as still and quiet as possible assists the body's clotting process. Next, if spinal injury is not suspected, place the patient in the shock position. Provide high-flow oxygen and keep the patient warm. You can usually control internal bleeding in the extremities simply by splinting the extremity. You should never use a tourniquet to control the bleeding from closed, internal, soft-tissue injuries.

Follow these steps to care for patients with possible internal bleeding:

1. **Follow BSI precautions.**
2. **Maintain the airway** with cervical spine immobilization if the mechanism of injury suggests the possibility of spinal injury.
3. **Administer high-flow oxygen** and provide artificial ventilation as necessary.
4. **Control all obvious external bleeding.**
5. **Treat suspected internal bleeding** in an extremity by applying a splint.
6. **Monitor and record vital signs** at least every 5 minutes.
7. **Give the patient nothing** (not even small sips of water) by mouth.
8. **Elevate the legs 6" to 12" in nontrauma patients** to increase blood return to the vital organs.
9. **Keep the patient warm.**
10. **Provide immediate transport** for all patients with signs and symptoms of shock (hypoperfusion). Report any changes in the patient's condition to emergency department personnel.

■ Shock

Perfusion is the cardiovascular system's circulation of blood and oxygen to all cells in different tissues and organs in the body. Perfusion is also an important part of the process by which waste products made by the cells are removed. Shock, or hypoperfusion, refers to a state of collapse and failure of the cardiovascular system that leads to inadequate circulation. Like internal bleeding, shock is an unseen underlying life threat caused by a medical disorder or traumatic injury. Inadequate circulation can lead to cell death. To protect vital organs, the body attempts to compensate by directing blood flow from organs that are more tolerant of low flow (such as the skin and intestines) to organs that cannot tolerate low blood flow (such as heart, brain, and lungs). If the conditions causing shock are not promptly addressed, the patient will soon die.

The cardiovascular system consists of three parts: a pump (the heart), a set of pipes (the blood vessels), and the contents of the container (the blood). When a patient is in shock, one or more of these components is not working properly.

Blood is the vehicle for carrying oxygen and nutrients through the vessels to the capillary beds, where these supplies are exchanged for waste products. The blood keeps moving as a result of pressure that is generated by the contractions of the heart and affected by the dilating and constricting of the vessels. This pressure (blood pressure) is usually carefully controlled by the body so that there is always sufficient circulation, or perfusion, in the various tissues and organs. Blood pressure is a rough measure of perfusion.

Remember that blood pressure is really the pressure of blood within the vessels at any one time. The systolic pressure is the peak arterial pressure, or pressure generated every time the heart contracts; the diastolic pressure is the pressure maintained within the arteries while the heart rests between beats.

Blood flow through the capillary beds is regulated by the capillary sphincters, circular muscular walls that constrict and dilate. These sphincters are under the control of the autonomic nervous system. Capillary sphincters also respond to other stimuli such as heat, cold, the need for oxygen, and the need for waste removal. Under normal circumstances, not all cells have the same needs at the same time.

Thus, regulation of blood flow is determined by cellular need and is accomplished by vessel constriction or dilation, together with sphincter constriction or dilation. Maintenance of blood flow, or perfusion, is accomplished by the heart, blood vessels, and blood working together.

Perfusion requires more than just having a working cardiovascular system. It also requires adequate oxygen exchange in the lungs, adequate nutrients in the form of glucose in the blood, and adequate waste removal, primarily through the lungs. Carbon dioxide is one of the primary waste products of cellular work (metabolism) in the body and is removed from the body by the lungs. This is the reason adequate ventilation and oxygenation is one of your primary concerns. The body has mechanisms in place to help support the respiratory and cardiovascular systems when the need for perfusion of vital organs is increased. These mechanisms, including the autonomic nervous system and certain hormones, are triggered when the body senses that the pressure in the system is falling. The sympathetic side of the autonomic nervous system, which is responsible for the fight-or-flight response, assumes more control of the body's functions during a state of shock. This response by the autonomic nervous system causes the release of hormones such as epinephrine. These hormones cause changes in certain body functions such as an increase in heart rate and in the strength of cardiac contractions and vasoconstriction in nonessential areas, primarily in the skin and gastrointestinal tract (peripheral vasoconstriction). Together, these actions are designed to maintain pressure in the system and perfusion of all vital organs.

Eventually, there is also a shifting of body fluids to help maintain pressure within the system. However, the response of the autonomic nervous system and hormones comes within seconds. It is this response that causes all the signs and symptoms of shock in a patient.

■ Causes of Shock

Shock can result from many conditions but with all causes of shock, the damage is due to lack of perfusion to the organs and tissues. As soon as perfusion stops or becomes impaired, tissues start to die. If not promptly treated, death soon follows.

Reviewing the basic physiologic causes of shock will better prepare you to treat your patients Figure 19-5 ▶ . There are cardiovascular and noncardiovascular causes of shock. Cardiovascular causes of shock include heart attack, disease, and injury. Noncardiovascular causes include respiratory insufficiency and anaphylaxis.

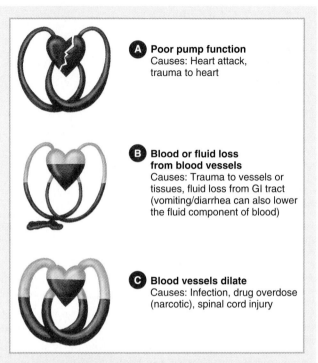

A **Poor pump function**
Causes: Heart attack, trauma to heart

B **Blood or fluid loss from blood vessels**
Causes: Trauma to vessels or tissues, fluid loss from GI tract (vomiting/diarrhea can also lower the fluid component of blood)

C **Blood vessels dilate**
Causes: Infection, drug overdose (narcotic), spinal cord injury

Figure 19-5 There are three basic causes of shock and impaired tissue perfusion. **A.** Pump failure occurs when the heart is damaged by disease or injury. The heart may not generate enough energy to move the blood through the system. **B.** Decreased blood volume, often a result of bleeding, leads to inadequate perfusion. **C.** The blood vessels can dilate excessively so that the blood within them, even though it is of normal volume, is inadequate to fill the system and provide efficient perfusion.

Cardiovascular Causes of Shock
Pump Failure

Cardiogenic shock is caused by inadequate function of the heart, or pump failure. Circulation of blood throughout the vascular system requires the constant pumping action of a normal and vigorous heart muscle. Many diseases can cause destruction or inflammation of this muscle. Within certain limits, the heart can adapt to these problems. After a heart attack however, there may be too much damage to the heart muscle and the heart will no longer function well. Because the heart is no longer pumping efficiently, there is a backup of blood into the lungs. The resulting buildup of fluid within the pulmonary tissue is called pulmonary edema. Edema is the presence of abnormally large amounts of fluid between cells in body tissues, causing swelling of the affected area Figure 19-6 ▶ . Pulmonary edema leads to impaired ventilation, which you may assess in your patient as shortness of breath, increased respiratory rate, and abnormal lung sounds.

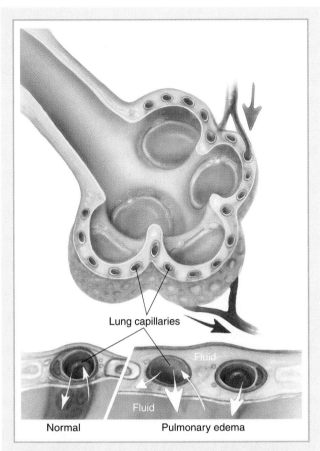

Lung capillaries

Fluid

Normal

Fluid

Pulmonary edema

Figure 19-6 Pulmonary edema develops as a result of fluid buildup within the pulmonary tissue. The edema leads to impaired ventilation.

For blood to circulate efficiently throughout the entire system, there must be the right amount of pressure and an adequate number of heartbeats. For this reason, the heart has its own electrical system that initiates and regulates its beating. Disease or injury can damage or destroy this system, causing irregular and uncoordinated beats, beats that are too slow (less than 60/min), or beats that are too fast (more than 150/min).

Cardiogenic shock develops when the heart muscle can no longer generate enough pressure to circulate the blood to all organs or when the regularity of the heartbeat is so disrupted that the volume of blood within the system can no longer be handled efficiently. In either case, direct pump failure is the cause of shock.

Poor Vessel Function

Damage to the spinal cord, particularly at the upper cervical levels, may cause significant injury to the part of the nervous system that controls the size and muscular tone of the blood vessels (neurogenic shock). Although not as common, there are also medical causes that result in poor vessel function such as brain conditions, tumors, pressure on the spinal cord, and spina bifida. In neurogenic shock, the muscles in the walls of the blood vessels are cut off from the nerve impulses that cause them to contract. Therefore, all vessels below the level of the spinal injury dilate widely, increasing the size and capacity of the vascular system and causing blood to pool. The available 6 L of blood in the body can no longer fill the enlarged vascular system. Even though no blood or fluid has been lost, perfusion of organs and tissues becomes inadequate, and shock occurs. In this condition, a radical change in the size of the vascular system has caused shock. A characteristic sign of this type of shock is the absence of sweating below the level of injury.

With this type of injury, many other functions that are under the control of the same part of the nervous system are also lost. The most important of them, in an acute injury setting, is the ability to control body temperature. Body temperature in a patient with neurogenic shock can rapidly fall to match that of the environment. In many situations, significant hypothermia occurs, severely complicating the situation. Maintenance of body temperature is always an important element of treatment for a patient in shock.

Content Failure

Following trauma, shock is often a result of fluid or blood loss (hypovolemic shock). Hypovolemic shock caused by bleeding is known as hemorrhagic shock. The loss may be due to external bleeding, which is common in patients with severe lacerations or fractures. Or it may be due to internal bleeding, such as rupture of the liver or the spleen, lacerations of the great vessels in the abdomen or the chest, or GI bleeds.

Documentation Tips

Document the amount of blood loss as well as the color and characteristics.
- Bright red/spurting
- Dark red/oozing

Hypovolemic shock also occurs with severe thermal burns. In this case, it is intravascular plasma (the colorless part of the blood) that is lost, leaking from the circulatory system into the burned tissues that lie adjacent to the injury. Likewise, crushing injuries may result in the loss of blood and plasma from damaged vessels into injured tissues. Dehydration, the loss of water from body tissues, aggravates shock. In these circumstances, the common factor is an insufficient volume of blood within the vascular system to provide adequate circulation to the organs of the body.

Combined Vessel and Content Failure

In some patients who have severe infections, usually bacterial, toxins (poisons) generated by the bacteria or by infected body tissues result in septic shock. In this condition, the toxins damage the vessel walls, causing them to become leaky and unable to contract well. Widespread dilation of vessels, in combination with plasma loss through the injured vessel walls, results in shock.

Initially in septic shock, there is an insufficient volume of fluid in the container because much of the plasma has leaked out of the vascular system (hypovolemia). Second, the fluid that has leaked out often collects in the respiratory system, interfering with ventilation. Third, there is a larger-than-normal vascular bed to contain the smaller-than-normal volume of intravascular fluid. Septic shock is almost always a complication of a significant illness or injury or a surgery and is more frequently seen in older patients.

Noncardiovascular Causes of Shock

There are two causes of shock that do not result from disturbances of the cardiovascular system: respiratory insufficiency and anaphylaxis.

Respiratory Insufficiency

A patient with a severe chest injury or obstruction of the airway may be unable to breathe in an adequate amount of oxygen.

An insufficient concentration of oxygen in the blood can produce shock as rapidly as vascular causes, even if the volume of blood, the volume of the vessels, and the action of the heart are all normal. Without oxygen, the organs in the body cannot survive.

This is why the first two steps in resuscitation are always securing an airway and restoring respirations. Circulation of nonoxygenated blood will not benefit the patient.

You are the Provider 3

You place the patient on a nonrebreathing mask at 15 L/min. A cervical collar is applied and she is removed onto a long back board and loaded into the ambulance for transport. While en route you continue with your head-to-toe assessment. Her mental status has decreased and she is asking repetitive questions. Other than some abrasions to her arms from the airbag and across the right side of her abdomen from the seatbelt, you do not find anything significant. Her abdomen is soft but tender on palpation.

Reassessment	Recording Time: 7 Minutes
Pulse	138, very weak radials
Blood pressure	92/p mm Hg
Respirations	24 breaths/min, adequate depth
Pupillary response	Equal and reactive to light
Pulse oximetry	96% on oxygen via nonrebreathing mask

6. What occult injury might you suspect?
7. Would this explain the change in vital signs?
8. Do you suspect a head injury? Why or why not?
9. What definitive care does this patient need?
10. What other treatment can you provide?

Anaphylactic Shock

Anaphylaxis, or anaphylactic shock, occurs when a person has an exaggerated reaction to a substance to which he or she has been sensitized. Sensitization means becoming sensitive to a substance that did not initially cause a reaction. Do not be misled by a patient who reports no history of allergic reaction to a substance on first or second exposure. Each subsequent exposure after sensitization tends to produce a more severe reaction.

Severe allergic reactions commonly fall into four categories of exposure:

- Injections (tetanus antitoxin, penicillin)
- Stings (honeybee, wasp, yellow jacket, hornet)
- Ingestion (shellfish, fruit, medication)
- Inhalation (dusts, pollens)

Anaphylactic reactions can develop in minutes or even seconds after contact with the substance to which the patient is allergic. The signs of such allergic reactions are very specific and not seen with other forms of shock. Table 19-1 ▶ shows the signs of anaphylactic shock in the order in which they typically occur.

In anaphylactic shock, there is no loss of blood, no mechanical vascular damage, and only a slight possibility of direct cardiac muscular injury. Instead, there is widespread vascular dilation. The combination of poor oxygenation and poor perfusion in anaphylactic shock may easily prove fatal.

Psychogenic Shock

A patient in psychogenic shock has had a sudden reaction of the nervous system that produces a temporary, generalized vascular dilation, resulting in fainting, or syncope. Blood pools in the dilated vessels, reducing the blood supply to the brain. As a result, the brain ceases to function normally, and the patient faints. Potentially life-threatening causes of syncope include an irregular heartbeat or a brain aneurysm. Other non-life-threatening events that cause syncope may be the receipt of bad news or experiencing fear or unpleasant sights (like the sight of blood).

■ The Progression of Shock

The early stage of shock, while the body can still compensate for blood loss, is called compensated shock Table 19-2 ▶. The late stage, when blood pressure is falling, is called decompensated shock. The last stage,

Table 19-1 Signs and Symptoms of Anaphylactic Shock

Skin
- Flushing, itching, or burning, especially over the face and upper chest
- Urticaria (hives), which may spread over large areas of the body
- Edema, especially of the face, tongue, and lips
- Cyanosis about the lips

Circulatory System
- Dilation of peripheral blood vessels
- A drop in blood pressure
- A weak, barely palpable pulse
- Pallor
- Dizziness
- Fainting and coma

Respiratory System
- Sneezing or itching in the nasal passages
- Tightness in the chest, with a persistent dry cough
- Wheezing and dyspnea
- Secretions of fluid and mucus into the bronchial passages, alveoli, and lung tissue
- Bronchoconstriction; difficulty drawing air into the lungs
- Forced expiration, requiring exertion and accompanied by wheezing
- Respiratory arrest

when shock has progressed to a terminal stage, is called irreversible shock.

Remember that blood pressure may be the last measurable factor to change in shock. The body has several automatic mechanisms to compensate for initial blood loss and to help maintain blood pressure. By the time you detect a drop in blood pressure, shock is well developed. This is particularly true in infants and children, who can maintain their blood pressure until they have lost more than half their blood volume. By the time blood pressure drops in infants and children who are in shock, they are close to death.

You should anticipate shock in many emergency medical situations. For example, you would expect shock to accompany massive external or internal

Table 19-2 Progression of Shock

Compensated Shock

- Agitation
- Anxiety
- Restlessness
- Feeling of impending doom
- Altered mental status
- Weak, rapid (thready), or absent pulse
- Clammy (pale, cool, moist) skin
- Pallor, with cyanosis about the lips
- Shallow, rapid breathing
- Air hunger (shortness of breath), especially if there is a chest injury
- Nausea or vomiting
- Capillary refill in infants and children of longer than 2 seconds
- Marked thirst

Decompensated Shock

- Falling blood pressure (systolic blood pressure of 90 mm Hg or lower in an adult)
- Labored or irregular breathing
- Ashen, mottled, or cyanotic skin
- Thready or absent peripheral pulses
- Dull eyes, dilated pupils
- Poor urinary output

bleeding. You should also expect shock if a patient has any one of the following conditions:

- Multiple severe fractures
- Abdominal or chest injury
- Spinal injury
- A severe infection
- A major heart attack
- Anaphylaxis

◼ Assessment of Shock

Scene Size-up

As you approach the scene, be alert to potential hazards to your safety. When you first see the patient, observe the scene and patient for clues to determine the nature of the illness or the mechanism of injury. Medical complaints typically involve only one patient, but always ensure that you only have one patient to care

for. Trauma incidents commonly involve more than one patient.

Initial Assessment

General Impression

When you first see your patient, quickly form a general impression. This includes age, sex, signs of distress, obvious life-threatening injuries, abnormal positioning, and skin color. These observations will help you develop an early sense of urgency for care of a patient who appears "sick."

Once you are close to the patient, determine the need for manual spinal immobilization and assess the patient's level of consciousness using the AVPU scale. A patient who has an altered level of consciousness may need emergency airway management. If the patient is awake and alert, determine the chief complaint.

Airway and Breathing

Quickly assess the airway to ensure it is patent. Be alert to abnormal airway sounds such as gurgling (suction the airway) or stridor, indicating partial airway obstruction. Consider an airway adjunct (oral or nasal airway) for a patient with an altered LOC.

Next, you must quickly assess breathing in the patient. You must inspect and palpate the chest wall for DCAP-BTLS. Observe the patient for signs of accessory muscle use such as the muscles of the neck, intercostal retractions, or abnormal use of the abdominal muscles. Increased respiratory rate is often an early sign of impending shock. You should assess the patient's breath sounds for wheezes or other abnormal breath sounds. Administer high-flow oxygen, or, if needed, assist respirations with a bag-mask device.

Circulation

Assess the patient's circulatory status. Check for a radial pulse. Make a rapid determination if the pulse is fast, slow, weak, strong, or altogether absent. A rapid pulse suggests compensated shock. In shock or compensated shock, the skin may be cool, clammy, or ashen. If the patient has no pulse and is not breathing, immediately begin CPR. In trauma patients, ensure you have assessed for and identified any life-threatening bleeding and provided treatment. You must also quickly assess skin temperature, condition, and color.

Transport Decision

After the ABCs have been assessed and treated, you can determine whether the patient should be treated as high priority, whether ALS is needed, and to which facility to transport. Trauma patients with shock, or a significant MOI, generally should go to a trauma center. Sometimes, local protocols dictate that a patient should be transported to the nearest hospital for stabilization prior to transfer to a definitive treatment center.

Focused History and Physical Exam

Once you have determined that the initial assessment is complete and any life threats found during that assessment have been addressed, begin the focused history and physical exam based on the patient's complaint and the extent of trauma incurred. Obtain a history, and perform a continued assessment specific to the patient's chief complaint and the body region(s) affected.

Rapid or Focused Physical Exam

If your patient is a trauma patient with a significant MOI or multiple injuries, one who gives you a poor general impression, or you found problems in the initial assessment, perform a rapid physical exam. If your patient has a medical problem but is not responsive or problems were noted in the initial assessment, perform a rapid physical exam. These rapid assessments should be performed quickly but thoroughly to ensure that you do not miss any significant or life-threatening problems or delay needed care.

If your patient has only a simple MOI, such as a twisted ankle, perform a focused physical exam on the area affected. Whether you perform a rapid or a focused exam, if a life-threatening problem is found, treat it immediately. The focused physical exam and the rapid physical exam will also help you to identify injuries that must be addressed when packaging the patient for transport.

Baseline Vital Signs

Obtain a complete set of baseline vital signs. If the patient's condition is unstable or could become unstable, reassess vital signs every 5 minutes. If the patient is in stable condition, reassess vital signs every 10 to 15 minutes.

SAMPLE History

You should quickly obtain a SAMPLE history from the patient. Remember, if the patient has a significant change in LOC before arrival at the hospital, you will be able to provide the hospital personnel with this important information.

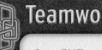

Teamwork Tips

One EMT can continue with the assessment while the second EMT actually performs interventions, such as using a bag-valve-mask device (BVM).

Interventions

You must determine what interventions are needed at this point based on your assessment findings. You should focus on supporting the cardiovascular system. Treating for shock early and aggressively will help to prevent inadequate perfusion from harming your patient. Provide oxygen and put the patient in the shock position.

Detailed Physical Exam

When time permits and the patient's condition is stable, perform a detailed physical exam. Perform a thorough head-to-toe assessment of the patient. This includes a complete neurologic assessment. If the patient is critically ill and problems are found in the initial assessment, you may not have the opportunity to perform a detailed physical exam.

Ongoing Assessment

This part of the patient assessment is very important in patient care. The rule of thumb is assess, then intervene, then reassess. This portion of the assessment revisits the initial assessment, the vital signs, and any treatment performed on the patient, including oxygen administration. You must assess the patient to determine whether the interventions performed are having any effect on the patient.

Communication and Documentation

Patients who are in decompensated shock will need rapid interventions to restore adequate perfusion.

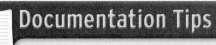

Documentation Tips

Document the presence or absence of pulses before and after splinting. Also include the time the PASG is applied, especially if it is fully inflated.

Determine, based on the signs and symptoms found in your assessment, whether your patient is in compensated or decompensated shock. Document these findings after you have treated for shock.

■ Emergency Medical Care

You must begin immediate treatment for shock as soon as you realize that the condition may exist. Follow the steps in Skill Drill 19-3 ▾:

1. **Begin by following BSI precautions,** making sure the patient has an open airway, and checking breathing and pulse. In general, keep the patient in a supine position. Patients who have had a severe heart attack or who have lung dis-

ease may find it easier to breathe in a sitting or semisitting position (**Step** ①).

2. **Next, control all obvious external bleeding.** Use dry, sterile dressings as you apply direct pressure (**Step** ②).

3. **Splint any bone or joint injuries.** This minimizes pain, bleeding, and discomfort, all of which can aggravate shock. It also prevents the broken bone ends from further damaging adjacent soft tissue. Splinting also makes it easier to move the patient. Handle the patient gently and no more than is necessary (**Step** ③).

There is some controversy surrounding the use of the PASG. When used improperly, the device can increase bleeding from chest injuries,

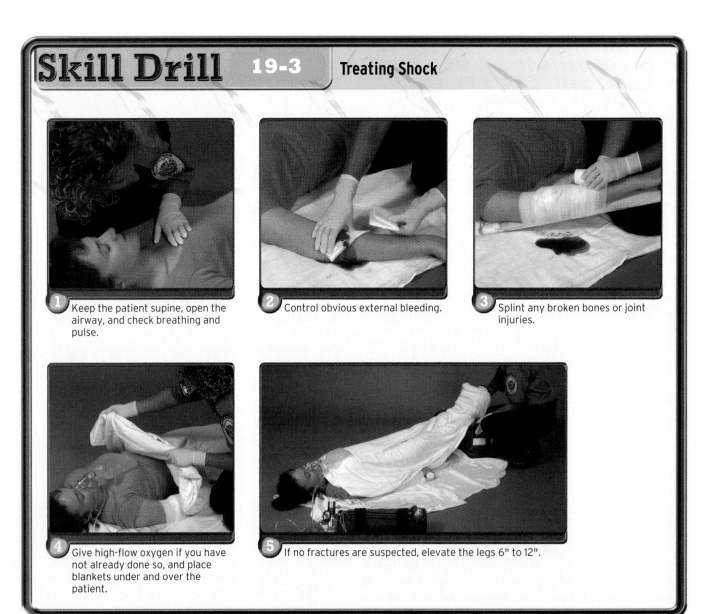

Skill Drill   19-3   Treating Shock

① Keep the patient supine, open the airway, and check breathing and pulse.

② Control obvious external bleeding.

③ Splint any broken bones or joint injuries.

④ Give high-flow oxygen if you have not already done so, and place blankets under and over the patient.

⑤ If no fractures are suspected, elevate the legs 6" to 12".

interfere with adequate air exchange, and promote cardiovascular collapse. When used properly, it can effectively control bleeding from fractures and massive soft-tissue wounds. In general, the PASG should not be used without the approval of medical control or established local protocols.

4. Remember that inadequate ventilation may be the primary cause of shock or a major factor in its development. **Always provide oxygen,** assist with ventilations as needed, and continue to monitor the patient's breathing. To prevent the loss of body heat, place blankets under and over the patient (**Step ④**).

5. Once you have positioned the patient on a backboard or a stretcher, **place the patient in the Trendelenburg position.** This technique is easily accomplished by raising the foot of the backboard or stretcher about 6" to 12". If the patient is not on a backboard and no lower extremity fractures are suspected, place the patient in the shock position (elevate the patient's legs 6" to 12" by propping them up on a several blankets or other stable objects) (**Step ⑤**).

Accurately record the patient's vital signs approximately every 5 minutes throughout treatment and transport. It is essential to transport trauma patients to the hospital as rapidly as possible for definitive treatment. The Golden Hour refers to the first 60 minutes after injury, which is thought to be a critically important period for the early resuscitation and treatment of severely injured trauma patients. The goal of EMS is to limit on-scene time (time on-scene until transport to hospital is started) to 10 minutes or less. Remember to speak calmly and reassuringly to a conscious patient throughout assessment, care, and transport.

Treating Cardiogenic Shock

The patient who is in shock as a result of a heart attack does not require a transfusion of blood, intravenous fluids, elevation of the legs, or a PASG. There is already a greater volume of blood in circulation than the heart can handle. The damaged heart muscle simply cannot generate the necessary power to pump blood throughout the circulatory system.

Remember that chronic lung disease will aggravate cardiogenic shock. If the patient has COPD and heart disease, oxygenation of the blood passing through the lungs is impaired. Because fluid is collecting in the

> ## Documentation Tips
>
> It is important to include baseline vital signs and subsequent vital signs to follow the progression of shock.

lungs, this patient is often able to breathe better in a sitting or semisitting position.

Patients with cardiogenic shock usually do not have any injury, but they may be complaining of chest pain. Such a patient may have taken nitroglycerin before your arrival and may want to take more. You will need to perform an accurate assessment to ensure that the patient's blood pressure meets the criteria for nitroglycerin administration. If the blood pressure is already low, nitroglycerin may increase the problem. Remember that patients in cardiogenic shock usually have a low blood pressure.

Treatment of cardiogenic shock should begin by placing the patient in the position in which breathing is easiest as you give high-flow oxygen. Be ready to assist ventilations as necessary, and have suction nearby in case the patient vomits. Remember also to approach a patient who has had a suspected heart attack with calm reassurance.

Treating Neurogenic Shock

Shock that accompanies spinal cord injury is treated with supportive measures. The patient who has sustained this kind of injury usually will require hospitalization for a long time. Emergency treatment must be directed at obtaining and maintaining a proper airway, providing spinal immobilization, assisting inadequate breathing as needed, conserving body heat, and providing the most effective circulation possible.

This patient usually is not losing blood. However, the capacity of his or her blood vessels has become significantly larger than the volume of blood they contain. Slight elevation of the foot end of the spine board will help bring the blood that is pooling in the vessels of the legs to the vital organs. Be sure to monitor the patient for any breathing problems, and, if they appear, lower the spine board. Supplemental oxygen will increase the concentration of oxygen in the blood. If respirations are weak or inadequate, provide assisted ventilations. Keep the patient as warm as possible with blankets because the injury may have disabled the body's normal temperature controls. Transport promptly.

Treating Hypovolemic Shock

The emergency treatment of hypovolemic or hemorrhagic shock includes the control of all obvious external bleeding. You should use direct pressure to control obvious external bleeding, splint any bone and joint injuries, and ensure that you use great care to handle the patient gently. If there are no fractured extremities, you should place the patient in the Trendelenburg position, raising the legs 6" to 12". This will increase blood flow to the heart from the lower body and keep unwanted pressure off the diaphragm.

Although you cannot control internal bleeding in the field, you must recognize its existence and provide aggressive general support. Secure and maintain an airway, and provide respiratory support, including supplemental oxygen and, if needed, assisted ventilations. Start the oxygen as soon as you suspect shock, and continue it during transport; with too little circulating blood, additional oxygen may be lifesaving. Be sure the patient does not aspirate blood or vomitus. Most important, you must transport the patient as rapidly as possible.

Treating Septic Shock

The proper treatment of septic shock requires complex hospital management, including antibiotics. If you suspect that a patient has septic shock, you must use appropriate BSI precautions and transport as promptly as possible. Use high-flow oxygen during transport. Ventilatory support may be necessary to maintain adequate tidal volume. Use blankets to conserve body heat.

Treating Respiratory Insufficiency

In treating the patient who is in shock as a result of inadequate respiration, you must immediately secure and maintain the airway. Clear the mouth and throat of anything obstructing the air passages, including mucus, vomitus, and foreign material. If necessary, provide ventilations with a bag-valve-mask device. Give supplemental oxygen, and transport the patient promptly.

Treating Anaphylactic Shock

Effective treatment for a severe, acute allergic reaction is to administer epinephrine. Patients with a history of severe allergic reactions may carry their own EpiPen autoinjector. If the patient is unable to inject the medication, you may have to do so if you are allowed by local protocol. If the patient's signs and symptoms recur or the patient's condition deteriorates, you should repeat the injection after consulting with medical control.

Promptly transport the patient while providing all possible support, primarily supplemental oxygen and ventilatory assistance. You should also try to find out what agent caused the reaction (for example, a drug, an insect bite or sting, a food item) and how it was received (for example, by mouth, by inhalation, or by injection). The severity of allergic reactions can vary greatly, with symptoms ranging from mild itching to profound coma and rapid death. Keep in mind that a mild reaction may worsen suddenly or over time. Consider requesting advanced life support backup, if available.

Treating Psychogenic Shock

In an uncomplicated case of fainting, once the patient collapses and becomes supine, circulation to the brain is usually restored and the patient recovers. If the syncope has caused the patient to fall, you must check for injuries, especially in older patients. You should also assess the patient thoroughly for any other conditions. If, after regaining consciousness, the patient is unable to walk without weakness, dizziness, or pain, you should suspect another problem. You should transport this patient promptly.

Be sure to record your initial set of vital signs and level of consciousness. In addition, ask bystanders whether the patient complained of anything before fainting and how long he or she was unconscious.

You are the Provider 4

You treat her for shock and call medical control to alert the trauma team. On arrival at the emergency department, she is rapidly assessed and taken to surgery where a tear is found in her liver. It is treated and she spends a week in the hospital before going home to complete her recovery.

You are the Provider   Summary

Shock occurs in stages. In order to provide optimal care, you must keep a high index of suspicion when there is a significant mechanism of injury and recognize subtle changes in mental status and vital signs that indicate progressive stages of shock.

1. **Is this a load-and-go patient? Why or why not?**
   Yes. Your decision should be based on the mechanism of injury and the alteration in mental status.

2. **How should you approach your assessment?**
   She should receive a rapid trauma assessment starting with ABCs.

3. **What type of oxygen does she need? Why?**
   Nonrebreathing mask. She has an adequate rate and depth.

4. **Should you focus only on her complaint?**
   No. Her complaint should be addressed as part of your assessment, but she has a significant mechanism of injury and should receive a complete assessment.

5. **How should she be removed from the vehicle?**
   You should apply a cervical collar and remove her with controlled movements onto a long spine board.

6. **What occult injury might you suspect?**
   Damage to the liver or spleen. Particularly the liver since indications point to the right side.

7. **Would this explain the change in vital signs?**
   Yes. If she is bleeding internally, her signs and symptoms will change as she becomes more hypovolemic. Pulse and respirations increase, skin is pale and diaphoretic, and blood pressure will start to drop.

8. **Do you suspect a head injury? Why or why not?**
   No. She has no indication of hitting her head, her pupils are reacting properly, and her vital signs do not indicate increasing intracranial pressure (increased blood pressure, decreased pulse, and irregular respirations).

9. **What definitive care does this patient need?**
   Control of internal bleeding is necessary to help stabilize this patient's condition. Such control is not possible in the pre-hospital setting. Options for achieving control include surgery and angiography for emobilization of bleeding vessels.

10. **What other treatment can you provide?**
    Treat for shock. Elevate the foot of the backboard, cover the patient, administer high-flow oxygen, and if there is time, call for ALS backup for fluid resuscitation.

Assessment and Emergency Care

	External Bleeding	Internal Bleeding
Scene Size-up	Wear a minimum of gloves and eye protection to protect from bleeding.	Use appropriate BSI. Consider the need for manual spinal immobilization.
	Consider if additional resources are needed.	Consider if additional resources are needed.
	If incident involved violence, ensure that police are on scene.	
Initial Assessment		
■ General impression	Check for responsiveness.	Ask the patient what happened. Determine level of consciousness.
	Ask the patient about the chief complaint, if responsive.	
■ Airway and breathing	Ensure a patent airway, check for breath sounds, provide high-flow oxygen.	Ensure a patent airway, provide high-flow oxygen, or assist ventilation with a BVM device.
■ Circulation	Control significant bleeding.	Assess pulse rate and quality, skin color, and temperature.
	Consider shock in patients with blood loss. Assess for pale, cool, clammy skin or dizziness. Apply oxygen for significant blood loss.	Treat patient for shock if needed—apply oxygen, improve circulation, maintain normal body temperature.
■ Transport decision	Transport quickly if breathing problem or significant bleeding exists.	Transport quickly if signs of shock are present.
Focused History and Physical Exam	*NOTE: The order of the steps in the focused history and physical exam differs depending on whether or not the patient has a significant MOI. The order below is for a patient with a significant MOI. For a patient without a significant MOI, perform a focused trauma assessment, obtain vital signs, and obtain the history.*	
■ Focused physical exam or rapid physical exam	Type of exam will depend on the type of patient.	Type of exam will depend on the type of patient.
	Perform the focused physical exam if the patient is responsive and has an isolated injury.	Perform the focused physical exam on a responsive medical patient.
	Perform a rapid physical exam if the patient has significant mechanism of injury. Look for DCAP-BTLS. Treat life-threatening problems immediately.	Perform a rapid physical exam if the patient has significant mechanism of injury. Look for DCAP-BTLS. Treat life-threatening problems immediately.
■ Baseline vital signs	Assess baseline vital signs. Look for signs of hypoperfusion (shock).	Assess baseline vital signs. Look for signs of shock: systolic BP less than 100 mm Hg with weak, rapid pulse and cool, moist skin.
■ SAMPLE history	Obtain via bystanders or medic alert tags if patient is unresponsive.	For a responsive medical patient, use the OPQRST mnemonic.
■ Interventions	Provide high-flow oxygen if significant bleeding is suspected.	Treat for shock if not yet done.
	Control significant bleeding if it is visible.	
	If signs of shock are present, treat aggressively for shock. Rapidly transport to hospital.	
Detailed Physical Exam	Perform detailed physical exam during transport. If time allows, help to identify all injuries.	If patient is stable, problems persist from initial assessment, and time permits, perform detailed physical exam.
Ongoing Assessment	Reassess patient. In cases of severe bleeding, take vital signs at least every 5 minutes.	Reassess vital signs. Determine whether patient's condition is improving or deteriorating. Assess effectiveness of interventions.
■ Communication and documentation	Report approximate amount of blood lost. Report all injuries and how patient has responded to care.	Communicate with hospital regarding findings, interventions, and patient's response. Include the MOI in your report.

NOTE: While the steps below are widely accepted, be sure to consult and follow your local protocol.

External Bleeding

Follow BSI precautions—minimum of gloves and eye protection.

Ensure that patient has open airway.

Maintain the cervical stabilization if MOI suggests possible spinal injury.

Provide high-flow oxygen.

Control bleeding using one of the following methods:
- Direct pressure and elevation
- Pressure dressings
- Pressure points
- Splints
- Air splints
- PASG
- Tourniquets

Controlling External Bleeding
1. Apply direct local pressure to bleeding site.
2. Elevate the bleeding extremity.
3. Create a pressure dressing.
4. Apply pressure at the appropriate pressure point while continuing to hold direct pressure.
5. If the wound continues to bleed, elevate extremity and place additional pressure over proximal pressure point.

Using PASG for Control of Massive Soft-tissue Bleeding in the Extremities
1. Apply the garment.
2. Close and fasten both leg compartments and the abdominal compartment.
3. Open the stopcocks.
4. Inflate the compartments similar to an air splint.
5. Check the patient's circulation, motor function, and sensation in distal lower extremities.

Applying a Tourniquet
1. Fold a triangular bandage.
2. Wrap the bandage around the extremity twice.
3. Tie one knot in the bandage. Place a stick or rod on top of the knot. Tie the ends of the bandage on the stick in a square knot.
4. Use the stick as a handle and twist it to tighten the tourniquet until bleeding has stopped.
5. Secure the stick in place with another triangular bandage.
6. Write "TK" and the exact time the tourniquet was applied on a piece of adhesive tape. Fasten the tape to the patient's forehead.
7. As an alternative, use a blood pressure cuff. Inflate enough to stop bleeding.

Treating Epistaxis
1. Follow BSI precautions.
2. Help the patient to sit, leaning forward.
3. Apply direct pressure for at least 15 minutes by pinching nostrils together.
4. Keep the patient calm and quiet.
5. Apply ice over the nose.
6. Maintain the pressure until bleeding is completely controlled.
7. Provide prompt transport.
8. If bleeding cannot be controlled, transport patient immediately. Treat for shock and administer oxygen via mask if necessary.

Internal Bleeding

Steps to Caring for Patient With Internal Bleeding
1. Follow BSI precautions.
2. Maintain the airway with cervical immobilization if MOI suggests possible spinal injury.
3. Administer high-flow oxygen.
4. Control all obvious external bleeding.
5. Apply a splint to an extremity where internal bleeding is suspected.
6. Monitor and record vital signs at least every 5 minutes.
7. Give the patient nothing by mouth.
8. Elevate the legs 6" to 12" in nonsignificant trauma patients.
9. Keep the patient warm.
10. Provide immediate transport for patients with signs and symptoms of shock. Report changes in condition to hospital personnel.

Using PASG for Treatment of Shock
1. Apply the garment.
2. Close and fasten both leg compartments and the abdominal compartment.
3. Open the stopcocks.
4. Contact medical control for specific verbal orders to inflate or use standing orders specific to inflation of PASG.
5. Inflate the compartments based on the patient's blood pressure.
6. Recheck the patient's blood pressure and inflate more based on patient response and blood pressure.

Shock	
Scene Size-up	Body substance isolation precautions should include a minimum of gloves and eye protection. Ensure scene safety and determine NOI/MOI. Consider the number of patients, the need for additional help/ALS, and c-spine stabilization.

Initial Assessment

■ General impression	Determine level of consciousness and find and treat any immediate threats to life. Determine priority of care based on environment and patient's chief complaint.
■ Airway	Ensure patent airway.
■ Breathing	Listen for abnormal breath sounds and evaluate depth and rate of the respirations. Maintain ventilations as needed. Provide high-flow oxygen at 15 L/min.
■ Circulation	Evaluate distal pulse rate and quality; observe skin color, temperature, and condition and treat accordingly. Consider external bleeding based on chief complaint and MOI.
■ Transport decision	Rapid transport based on a poor general impression or problems with ABCs.

Focused History and Physical Exam	*NOTE: The order of the steps in the focused history and physical exam differs depending on whether or not the patient has a significant MOI. The order below is for a patient with a significant MOI. For a patient without a significant MOI, perform a focused trauma assessment, obtain vital signs, and obtain the history.*
■ Significant MOI	Reevaluate the mechanism of injury(s). Perform rapid trauma assessment to identify hidden injuries.
■ No significant MOI	Reevaluate the mechanism of injury. If the patient is alert and oriented, perform a focused assessment on the body system or affected area.
■ Baseline vital signs	Take vital signs, noting skin color and temperature and patient's level of consciousness. Use pulse oximetry if available.
■ SAMPLE history	Ask pertinent SAMPLE and OPQRST. Be sure to ask if and what interventions were taken before your arrival, how many interventions, and at what time.
■ Interventions	Support patient and cardiovascular system as needed. Consider the use of oxygen, eliminate the cause of the shock, maintain normal body temperature, and use proper positioning of the patient to improve circulation.

Detailed Physical Exam	Complete a detailed physical exam.

Ongoing Assessment	Repeat the initial assessment, focused assessment, and reassess interventions performed. Reassess vital signs every 5 minutes for the unstable patient, and every 15 minutes for the stable patient. Reassure and calm the patient.
■ Communication and documentation	Contact medical control with a radio report. Relay any change in level of consciousness or difficulty breathing. Be sure to document physician's orders and changes in patient's condition, and at what time they occurred.

Prep Kit

Ready for Review

- Perfusion is the circulation of blood in adequate amounts to meet each cell's current needs for oxygen, nutrients, and waste removal.
- The three components that must be functioning to meet this demand are a working pump (heart), a set of intact pipes (blood vessels), and fluid volume (enough oxygen-carrying blood).
- Hypoperfusion, or shock, occurs when one or more of these components is not working properly and the cardiovascular system fails to provide adequate perfusion.
- Both internal and external bleeding can cause shock. You must know how to recognize and control both.
- The six methods to control bleeding are:
  - Direct local pressure
  - Elevation
  - Pressure dressing
  - Pressure points
  - Splinting device
- Use of a tourniquet is always a last resort and should be avoided if possible.
- Bleeding from the nose and ears may indicate a skull fracture. Other causes of nosebleeds include high blood pressure and sinus infection.
- Bleeding around the face always presents a risk for airway obstruction or aspiration. Maintain a clear airway by positioning the patient appropriately and using suction when indicated.
- If bleeding is present at the nose and a skull fracture is suspected, place a gauze pad loosely under the nose.
- If bleeding from the nose is present and a skull fracture is not suspected, pinch both nostrils together for 15 minutes. If the patient is awake and has a patent airway, place a gauze pad inside the upper lip against the gum.
- Any patient you suspect of having internal bleeding or significant external bleeding should be transported promptly.
- If the MOI is significant, be alert to signs of unseen bleeding in the chest or abdomen (such as serious bruising or symptoms or complaints of difficulty breathing or abdominal pain).
- Signs of significant internal bleeding include the following:
  - Vomiting blood (hematemesis)
  - Black tarry stools (melena)
  - Coughing up blood (hemoptysis)
  - Distended abdomen
  - Broken ribs
  - Pain
  - Patient is restless and can't get in a comfortable position
- Signs of compensated shock include anxiety or agitation; tachycardia; pale, cool, moist skin; increased respiratory rate; nausea and vomiting; and increased thirst. If there is any question, treat for shock. It is never wrong to treat for shock.
- Signs of decompensated shock include labored or irregular respirations, ashen gray or cyanotic skin color, weak or absent distal pulses, dilated pupils, and profound hypotension.
- Remember, by the time a drop in blood pressure is detected, shock is usually in an advanced stage.
- Anticipate shock in patients who have the following conditions:
  - Severe infection
  - Significant blunt force trauma or penetrating trauma
  - Massive external bleeding or index of suspicion for major internal bleeding
  - Spinal injury
  - Chest or abdominal injury
  - Major heart attack
  - Anaphylaxis
- Treatment for all patients suspected to be in shock includes:
  - Open and maintain the airway.
  - Provide high-flow oxygen and as needed, provide bag-mask-assisted ventilations.
  - Control all obvious external bleeding.
  - Place the patient in the shock position or, if on a backboard or stretcher, in the Trendelenburg position.
  - Maintain normal body temperature with blankets.
  - Provide prompt transport.

Vital Vocabulary

anaphylactic shock Severe shock caused by an allergic reaction.
anaphylaxis An unusual or exaggerated allergic reaction to foreign protein or other substances.
aorta The main artery, which receives blood from the left ventricle and delivers it to all the other arteries that carry blood to the tissues of the body.

Technology

- Interactivities
- Vocabulary Explorer
- Anatomy Review
- Web Links
- Online Review Manual

autonomic nervous system   The part of the nervous system that regulates involuntary functions, such as heart rate, blood pressure, digestion, and sweating.

capillaries   The small blood vessels that connect arterioles and venules; various substances pass through capillary walls, into and out of the interstitial fluid, and then on to the cells.

cardiogenic shock   Shock caused by inadequate function of the heart, or pump failure.

coagulation   The formation of clots to plug openings in injured blood vessels and stop blood flow.

compensated shock   The early stage of shock, in which the body can still compensate for blood loss.

cyanosis   A bluish-gray skin color that is caused by reduced levels of oxygen in the blood.

decompensated shock   The late stage of shock when blood pressure is falling.

dehydration   Loss of water from the tissues of the body.

dyspnea   Shortness of breath or difficulty breathing.

edema   The presence of abnormally large amounts of fluid between cells in body tissues, causing swelling of the affected area.

epistaxis   A nosebleed.

hematoma   A mass of blood in the soft tissues beneath the skin.

hemorrhage   Bleeding.

homeostasis   A balance of all systems of the body.

hypovolemic shock   A condition in which low blood volume, due to massive internal or external bleeding or extensive loss of body water, results in inadequate perfusion.

irreversible shock   The final stage of shock, resulting in death.

neurogenic shock   Circulatory failure caused by paralysis of the nerves that control the size of the blood vessels, leading to widespread dilation; seen in spinal cord injuries.

perfusion   Circulation of blood within an organ or tissue in adequate amounts to meet the current needs of the cells.

pneumatic antishock garment (PASG)   An inflatable device that covers the legs and abdomen; used to splint the lower extremities or pelvis or to control bleeding in the lower extremities, pelvis, or abdominal cavity.

pressure point   A point where a blood vessel lies near a bone; useful when direct pressure and elevation do not control bleeding.

psychogenic shock   Shock caused by a sudden, temporary reduction in blood supply to the brain that causes fainting (syncope).

septic shock   Shock caused by severe infection, usually a bacterial infection.

shock   A condition in which the circulatory system fails to provide sufficient circulation to enable every body part to perform its function; also called hypoperfusion.

syncope   Fainting.

tourniquet   The bleeding control method of last resort that occludes arterial flow; used only when all other methods have failed and the patient's life is in danger.

veins   The blood vessels that carry blood from the tissues to the heart.

Assessment in Action

Shock can result from many conditions, but ultimately the damage is due to lack of perfusion to the organs and tissues. Early recognition and prompt treatment may mean the difference between life and death.

1. Noncardiovascular causes of shock include respiratory insufficiency and _____.
   A. heart attack
   B. anaphylaxis
   C. disease
   D. all of the above

2. Cardiogenic shock is caused by _____.
   A. edema
   B. container problems
   C. volume depletion
   D. pump failure

3. Hypovolemic shock may be caused by _____.
   A. bleeding
   B. burns
   C. vomiting
   D. all of the above

4. Severe infections may result in what type of shock?
   A. cardiogenic
   B. neurogenic
   C. septic
   D. hypovolemic

5. What type of shock results in syncope?
   A. neurogenic
   B. spinal
   C. psychogenic
   D. anaphylactic

6. What is the primary treatment for anaphylactic shock?
   A. respiratory maintenance
   B. pharmacologic
   C. early defibrillation
   D. sensitization

Challenging Questions

7. What is the cause of pulmonary edema for a patient in cardiogenic shock?

20

Head and Spine Injuries

You are called to the scene of an altercation. Dispatch tells you that police are on the scene and the scene is safe. Upon arrival you find a 24-year-old man lying on the kitchen floor in a puddle of blood. There is a bloody baseball bat beside him.

Initial Assessment	Recording Time: 0 Minutes
Appearance	Pale, covered in blood
Level of consciousness	Does not appear to be alert
Airway	You hear gurgling
Breathing	Fast and irregular
Circulation	Radials present, strong

1. What should you do first?
2. How will you accomplish this?
3. Should you call for backup? Why or why not?

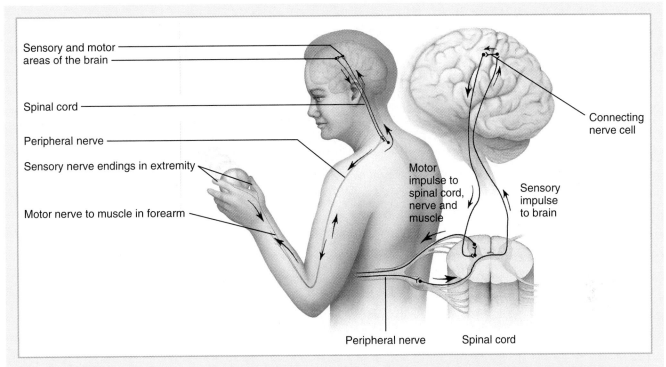

Sensory and motor areas of the brain

Spinal cord

Peripheral nerve

Sensory nerve endings in extremity

Motor nerve to muscle in forearm

Connecting nerve cell

Motor impulse to spinal cord, nerve and muscle

Sensory impulse to brain

Peripheral nerve

Spinal cord

Figure 20-1 The nervous system has two anatomic components: the central nervous system and the peripheral nervous system. The central nervous system is composed of the brain and the spinal cord. The peripheral nervous system conducts sensory and motor impulses from the skin and other organs to the spinal cord and brain.

■ Introduction

The nervous system is a complex network of nerve cells that enables all parts of the body to function. It includes the brain, the spinal cord, and several billion nerve fibers that carry information to and from all parts of the body. Because the nervous system is so vital, it is well protected. The brain lies within the skull, and the spinal cord is inside the bony spinal canal. Despite this protection, serious injuries can damage the nervous system.

This chapter first briefly reviews the anatomy and function of the nervous and skeletal systems. Review of specific head and spinal injuries follows, including signs, symptoms, assessment, and treatment.

■ Anatomy and Physiology of the Nervous System

The nervous system is composed of the central nervous system and the peripheral nervous system Figure 20-1▲. The <u>central nervous system (CNS)</u> includes the brain and the spinal cord. Long nerve fibers link the nerve cells of the brain and spinal cord to the body's various organs through openings in the spinal column. These cables of nerve fibers make up the <u>peripheral nervous system</u>.

Central Nervous System

The brain is the organ that controls the body and is the center of consciousness. It is divided into three major areas: the cerebrum, the cerebellum, and the brain stem Figure 20-2▶.

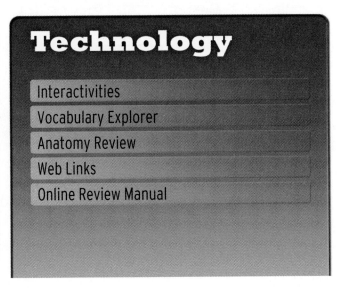

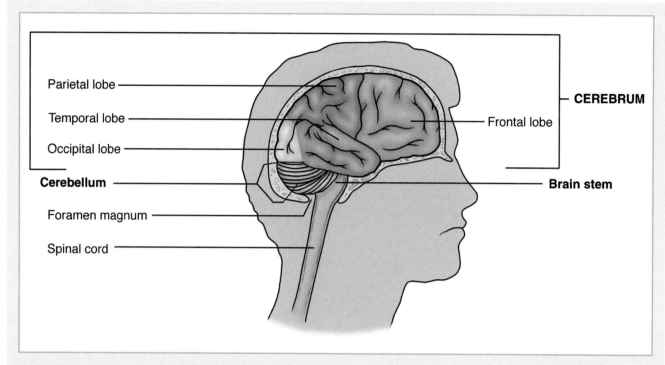

Figure 20-2 The brain is part of the central nervous system and is the organ that controls the body. It is divided into three major areas: the cerebrum, the cerebellum, and the brain stem.

The <u>cerebrum</u>, which contains about 75% of the brain's total volume, controls a wide variety of activities, including most voluntary motor function and conscious thought. Underneath the cerebrum lies the <u>cerebellum</u>, which coordinates body movements. The most primitive part of the CNS, the <u>brain stem</u>, controls virtually all the functions that are necessary for life, including the cardiac and respiratory systems. Deep within the cranium, the brain stem is the best-protected part of the CNS.

The spinal cord is made up mostly of fibers that extend from the brain's nerve cells. The spinal cord carries messages between the brain and the body.

Protective Coverings

The cells of the brain and spinal cord are soft and easily injured. Once damaged, they cannot be regenerated or reproduced. Therefore, the entire CNS is contained within a protective framework.

The thick, bony structures of the skull and spinal canal withstand injury very well. The skull is covered by a layer of muscle fascia and above that is the scalp. The spinal canal is also surrounded by a thick layer of skin and muscles.

The CNS is further protected by the <u>meninges</u>, three distinct layers of tissue that suspend the brain

and the spinal cord within the skull and the spinal canal (Figure 20-3 ▼). The outer layer, the dura mater, is a tough, fibrous layer that closely resembles leather. This layer forms a sac to contain the CNS, with small openings through which the peripheral nerves exit.

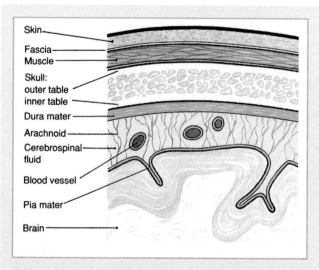

Figure 20-3 The central nervous system has several layers of protective coverings: the skin, muscles and their fascia, bone, and the meninges. The three layers of the meninges are the dura mater, the arachnoid, and the pia matter.

The inner two layers of the meninges, called the arachnoid and the pia mater, are much thinner than the dura mater. They contain the blood vessels that nourish the brain and spinal cord. Cerebral spinal fluid (CSF) is produced in a chamber inside the brain, called the third ventricle. CSF fills the spaces between the meninges and acts as a shock absorber. The brain and spinal cord essentially float in this fluid. The brain depends on a rich supply of oxygenated blood to function properly. When this supply is interrupted, even for short periods, serious brain damage may occur.

When an injury penetrates all these protective layers, clear, watery CSF may leak from the nose, the ears, or an open skull fracture. Therefore, if a patient with a head injury has what looks like a runny nose or has a salty taste at the back of the throat, you should assume that the fluid is CSF.

Ironically, the closed bony structure of the skull (which is similar to a vault) and the meninges, the very layers of tissue that isolate and protect the CNS, can lead to serious problems in closed head injuries. Severe injury may cause bleeding within the skull, referred to as intracranial hemorrhage. Such bleeding causes increased pressure inside the skull and compresses softer brain tissue. In many cases, only prompt surgery can prevent permanent brain damage.

Peripheral Nervous System

The peripheral nervous system has two anatomic parts: 31 pairs of spinal nerves and 12 pairs of cranial nerves Figure 20-4 . The 31 pairs of spinal nerves conduct sensory impulses from the skin and other organs to the spinal cord. They also conduct motor impulses from the spinal cord to the muscles. Because the arms and legs have so many muscles, the spinal nerves serving the extremities are arranged in complex networks. The brachial plexus controls the arms, and the lumbosacral plexus controls the legs.

Cranial nerves are the 12 pairs of nerves that pass through holes in the skull and transmit information directly to or from the brain. For the most part, they perform special functions in the head and face, including sight, smell, taste, hearing, and facial expressions.

There are two major types of peripheral nerves. The sensory nerves, with endings that can perceive only one type of information, carry that information from the body to the brain via the spinal cord. The motor nerves, one for each muscle, carry information from the CNS to the muscles. The connecting nerves, found only in the brain and spinal cord, connect the

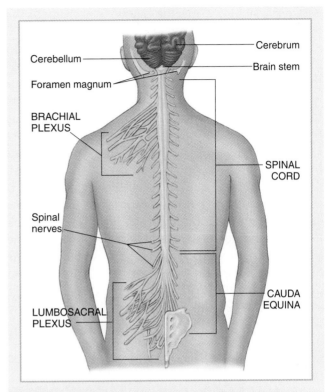

Figure 20-4 The peripheral nervous system is a complex network of motor and sensory nerves. The brachial plexus controls the arms, and the lumbosacral plexus controls the legs.

sensory and motor nerves with short fibers, which allow the cells on either end to exchange simple messages.

How the Nervous System Works

The nervous system controls virtually all of our body's activities, including reflex, voluntary, and involuntary activities. In connecting the sensory and motor nerves of the limbs, the connecting nerves in the spinal cord form a reflex arc. If a sensory nerve in this arc detects an irritating stimulus, such as heat, it will bypass the brain and send a message directly to a motor nerve to initiate a response.

The part of the nervous system that regulates or controls our voluntary activities, including almost all coordinated muscular activities, is called the somatic (voluntary) nervous system. The brain interprets the sensory information that it receives from the peripheral and cranial nerves and responds by sending signals to the voluntary muscles.

The body functions that occur without conscious effort are regulated by the much more primitive autonomic (involuntary) nervous system. The autonomic nervous system controls the functions of many of the body's vital organs.

The autonomic nervous system is divided into the sympathetic nervous system and the parasympathetic nervous system. Confronted with a threatening situation, the sympathetic nervous system reacts to the stress with the fight-or-flight response. This response causes the pupils to dilate, smooth muscle in the lungs to dilate, heart rate to increase, and blood pressure to rise. This response will also cause the body to shunt blood to vital organs and to skeletal muscle. During this time of stress, a hormone called epinephrine (adrenaline) is released, which is responsible for many of these activities inside the body. The parasympathetic nervous system has the opposite effect on the body, causing blood vessels to dilate, slowing the heart rate, and relaxing the muscle sphincters. When this portion of the autonomic nervous system is activated, the body shunts blood to the organs of digestion. As the body attempts to maintain homeostasis (balance), these two divisions of the autonomic nervous system tend to balance each other so that basic body functions remain stable and effective.

■ Anatomy and Physiology of the Skeletal System

The skull has two layers of bone, the outer and inner tables, both of which protect the brain. It is divided into two large structures: the cranium and the face Figure 20-5 ▾ . The cranium is occupied by 80% brain tissue, 10% blood supply, and 10% CSF. The mandible (lower jaw), the only movable facial bone, is connected to the cranium at the temporomandibular joint just in front of each ear.

The spinal column is the body's central supporting structure. It has 33 bones (vertebrae) and is divided into five sections: cervical, thoracic, lumbar, sacral, and coccygeal Figure 20-6 ▶ . Injury to the vertebrae, depending on the level at which the injury occurs, can result in paralysis if the underlying spinal cord is also damaged.

The front part of each vertebra consists of a round, solid block of bone called the vertebral body; the back part forms a bony arch. From one vertebra to the next, the series of arches form a tunnel running the length of the spinal column. This tunnel is the spinal canal, which encases and protects the spinal cord.

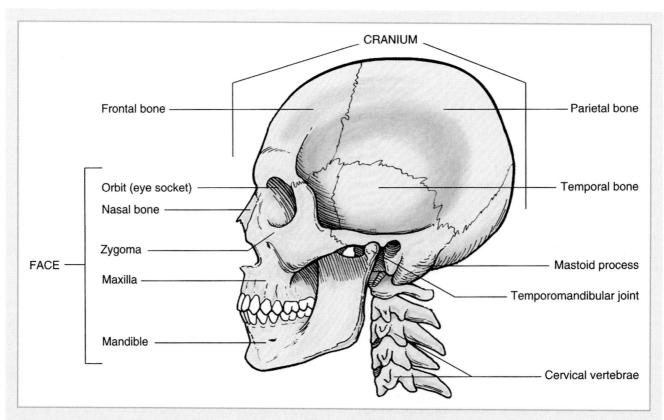

Figure 20-5 The skull includes two large structures: the cranium and the face.

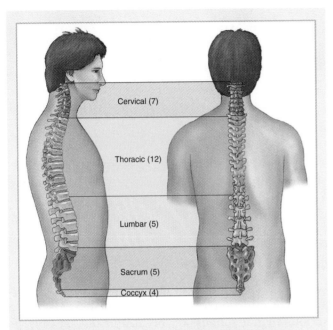

Figure 20-6 The spinal column is the body's central supporting system and consists of 33 bones divided into five sections. Injury to the vertebrae can cause paralysis.

The vertebrae are connected by ligaments and separated by cushions, called intervertebral disks. While allowing the trunk to bend forward and back, these ligaments and disks also limit motion so that the spinal cord is not injured. When the spine is injured or fractured, the spinal cord and its nerves are left unprotected. Therefore, until the spine is stabilized, you must keep it aligned as best you can to prevent further injury to the spinal cord.

The spinal column itself is almost entirely surrounded by muscles. However, you can usually palpate the posterior spinous process of each vertebra, which lies just under the skin in the midline of the back. The most prominent and most easily palpable spinous process is at the seventh cervical vertebra at the base of the neck.

■ Head Injuries

Any head injury is potentially serious. If not properly treated, suspected minor head injuries may end up becoming life threatening. Severe scalp lacerations or skull fractures may occur with little or no brain injury and may lead to minimal or no long-term consequences.

There are two general types of head injuries. A closed head injury, usually associated with blunt trauma, is one in which the brain has been injured but there is no opening into the brain. An open head injury is one in which an opening from the brain to the outside world exists. Obvious skull deformity is a sign of an open head injury, which is often caused by penetrating trauma. There may be bleeding and exposed brain tissue.

Scalp Lacerations

Scalp lacerations can be minor or very serious. Because the face and the scalp have unusually rich blood supplies, even small lacerations can quickly lead to significant blood loss   Figure 20-7 ▾ . Occasionally, this blood loss may be severe enough to cause hypovolemic shock, particularly in children. In any patient with multiple injuries, bleeding from scalp or facial lacerations may contribute to hypoperfusion. Scalp lacerations are usually the result of direct blows to the head and often a sign of a more significant injury.

Skull Fracture

Significant force applied to the head may cause a skull fracture. A skull fracture may be open or closed, depending on whether there is a scalp laceration. Injuries from bullets or other penetrating trauma frequently result in fracture of the skull. The diagnosis of a skull fracture is usually made in the hospital by computed tomography (CT) scan, but you should maintain a high index of suspicion that a fracture is present if the patient's head appears or feels deformed or if there is a visible crack in the skull within a scalp laceration. Additional signs of skull fracture that you may see include raccoon eyes (bruising that develops

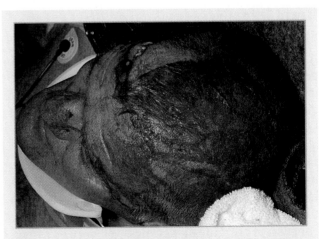

Figure 20-7 The scalp has an unusually rich blood supply; therefore, even small lacerations can result in significant blood loss.

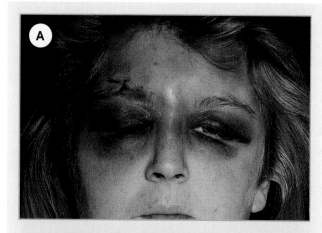

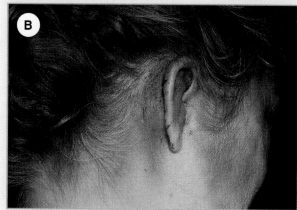

Figure 20-8 Signs of skull fracture include ecchymosis **A.** under the eyes (raccoon eyes) or **B.** behind one ear over the mastoid process (Battle's sign).

Patients with symptoms consistent with a concussion can also have a serious underlying brain injury. You should always assume that a patient with signs or symptoms of concussion has a more serious injury until proven otherwise.

Contusion

Like any other soft tissue in the body, the brain can sustain a contusion, or bruise. A contusion is far more serious than a concussion because it involves physical injury to the brain tissue, which may result in permanent damage. With contusions, there is associated bleeding and swelling from injured blood vessels. Injury of brain tissue or bleeding inside the skull will cause an increase of pressure within the skull.

Intracranial Bleeding

Laceration or rupture of a blood vessel inside the brain or in the meninges will produce intracranial bleeding in one of three areas (Figure 20-9 ▶):

- Beneath the dura but outside the brain: a subdural hematoma
- Within the substance of the brain tissue itself: an intracerebral hemorrhage
- Outside the dura and under the skull: an epidural hematoma

A hematoma may develop rapidly such as with an epidural hematoma, which is caused by a tear or laceration of an artery above the dura mater. Or it may develop slowly, as with a subdural hematoma when a vein is lacerated or torn beneath the dura mater. In any case, because the brain occupies nearly the entire space inside the skull, the result is increased pressure inside the skull, leading to compression of the brain tissue. The expanding hematoma will cause progressive loss of brain function and, if not treated properly, death.

Other Brain Injuries

Brain injuries are not always a result of trauma. Certain medical conditions, such as blood clots or hem-

under the eyes) and <u>Battle's sign</u> (bruising behind the ear) (Figure 20-8 ▲).

Brain Injuries

Concussion

A blow to the head or face may cause a <u>concussion</u>. In general, a concussion is a temporary loss or alteration of part or all of the brain's abilities to function without demonstrable physical damage to the brain. A concussion may result in unconsciousness and even the inability to breathe for short periods.

A patient with a concussion may be confused or have amnesia (loss of memory). Usually, a concussion lasts only a short time and is often resolved by the time you arrive. You should ask about symptoms of concussion (dizziness, weakness, or visual changes) in any patient who has sustained an injury to the head.

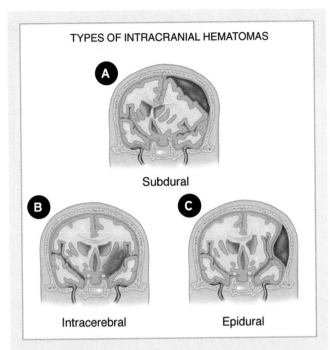

Figure 20-9 Intracranial bleeding can occur in one of three areas. **A.** Beneath the dura but outside the brain (subdural hematoma). **B.** Within the substance of the brain tissue (intracerebral hemorrhage). **C.** Outside the dura and under the skull (epidural hematoma).

orrhages, can also cause brain injuries that produce significant bleeding or swelling. Problems with the blood vessels themselves, high blood pressure, or any number of other problems may cause spontaneous bleeding into the brain, affecting the patient's level of consciousness. The signs and symptoms are often the same as those of traumatic brain injuries, except that there is no obvious mechanism of injury or any signs of trauma.

Complications of Head Injury

Cerebral edema, or swelling of the brain, is one of the most common complications of any head injury. It is also one of the most serious because swelling in the skull compresses the brain tissue, resulting in a loss of brain function.

Cerebral edema is aggravated by a low oxygen level in the blood and improved by a high level. In fact, the brain consumes more oxygen than any other organ in the body. For this reason, you must make sure that the airway is open and that adequate ventilations and high-flow oxygen are given to any patient with a head injury. This is especially true if the patient is unconscious.

Seizures are common in head-injured patients (owing to the excessive excitability of the brain) caused by direct injury or the accumulation of fluid within the brain (edema). You should be prepared to manage seizures in all patients with a head injury. Other effects of cerebral edema and increased intracranial pressure may be increased blood pressure, decreased pulse rate, and irregular respirations. This triad of signs is called the Cushing reflex.

Signs and Symptoms of Head Injury

Open and closed head injuries have essentially the same signs and symptoms. Following an injury, any patient who exhibits one or more of these signs or symptoms has potentially sustained an underlying brain injury:

- Lacerations, contusions, or hematomas to the scalp
- Soft area or depression noted by palpation
- Visible fractures or deformities of the skull
- Bruising around the eyes or behind the ear over the mastoid process
- Clear or pink CSF leakage from a scalp wound, the nose, or the ear
- Pupils that do not respond to light
- Unequal pupil size
- Loss of sensation and/or motor function
- A period of unconsciousness
- Amnesia
- Seizures
- Numbness or tingling in the extremities
- Irregular respirations
- Dizziness
- Visual complaints
- Combative or other abnormal behavior
- Nausea or vomiting

■ Spine Injuries

The cervical, thoracic, and lumbar portions of the spine can be injured in a variety of ways. Compression injuries can occur as a result of a fall, regardless of whether the patient landed on his or her feet, coccyx, or on the top of the head. Motor vehicle crashes or other types of trauma can overextend, flex, or rotate the spine. Any one of these unnatural motions, as well as excessive lateral bending, can result in fractures and/or a neurologic deficit.

Assessment of Head and Spine Injuries

You should always suspect a possible spinal injury with the following mechanisms of injury (MOIs):

- Motor vehicle crashes
- Pedestrian–motor vehicle collisions
- Falls
- Blunt or penetrating trauma to the head, neck, or torso
- Motorcycle crashes
- Hangings
- Diving accidents

Motor vehicle crashes, direct blows, falls from heights, assault, and sports injuries are common causes of spinal injury. A patient who has experienced any of these events also may have sustained a head injury. It is especially important to assess and constantly monitor the level of consciousness in patients with suspected head injuries.

Scene Size-up

Motor vehicle collisions are a common cause of head and spinal injuries. These situations have the potential to cause injury to rescuers and bystanders as well. Evaluate every scene for hazards. Patients with head and spinal injuries can be in critical condition. When preparing to care for these patients, expect to encounter airway, breathing, and circulation problems. Have

resuscitation and spinal stabilization equipment available. As you evaluate information from dispatch or information you obtain as you arrive on scene, quickly evaluate the MOI. Be prepared with appropriate body substance isolation (BSI) precautions before you approach the patient, before you are tempted by the seriousness of the injuries to intervene without proper protection. Because the patients can have very complicated injuries, call for advanced life support as soon as possible when a serious MOI or complicated presentation is evident. Law enforcement personnel may be needed to control traffic or crowds.

Initial Assessment
General Impression

Begin your initial assessment with a general impression of your patient based on the MOI and his or her

EMT-B Safety

Be prepared with appropriate body substance isolation precautions before you approach the patient—before you are tempted by the seriousness of the injuries to intervene without proper protection.

You are the Provider 2

Your partner provides c-spine stabilization and you roll the patient to a supine position. Fire department personnel are en route and arrive as you are assessing the patient's airway. Your partner asks one of the fire fighters to radio the dispatcher to send ALS backup for a rendezvous.

As your partner opens the airway with a jaw thrust without a head tilt you hear gurgling. You also note clear fluid draining from the nose. Your partner tells you there are multiple depressions that he can feel in the skull. You also note bruising around both eyes.

Vital Signs	Recording Time: 2 Minutes
Skin	Pale, diaphoretic
Pulse	68 beats/min, strong
Blood pressure	172/110 mm Hg
Respirations	Cheyne-Stokes respirations

4. What is your next priority?
5. What do the vital signs tell you?
6. What signs back up your thoughts about the vital signs?

level of consciousness. Patients with head injuries frequently also have spinal injuries. When assessing a patient for possible head or spinal injury, you should begin by asking the responsive patient these questions to determine the chief complaint:

1. What happened?
2. Where does it hurt?
3. Does your neck or back hurt?
4. Can you move your hands and feet?
5. Did you hit your head?

Confused or slurred speech, repetitive questioning, or memory loss in responsive patients indicate a head injury. Although other medical conditions may cause similar symptoms, with trauma, assume a head injury exists until your assessment proves otherwise.

If the patient is found unresponsive, first responders, family members, or bystanders may have helpful information, including when the patient lost consciousness and his or her previous level of consciousness. Unresponsive patients with any trauma should be assumed to have a spinal injury. Patients with a decreased level of responsiveness on the AVPU scale should also be considered to have a head and spine injury. Unless the patient is absolutely clear in his or her thinking and is lacking other injuries that may distract the patient, you should immobilize the spine.

Airway and Breathing

With head- and spine-injured patients, airway and breathing problems are common and may result in death if not recognized and treated immediately. When a spinal injury is suspected, how you open and assess the airway is important. Begin by manually holding the head still while you assess the airway. Use a jaw-thrust maneuver to open the airway. When performed correctly, this will prevent movement of the cervical spine. Remember that maintaining an airway in a trauma patient is a high priority. If you cannot open and maintain the airway with a jaw thrust, use a head tilt–chin lift maneuver. An oral or nasal airway may assist in maintaining an airway; however, the best way to protect the airway adequately is to use advanced airway techniques, usually by EMT-Intermediates and paramedics. The decision to use an oropharyngeal or nasopharyngeal airway is based on the patient's ability to maintain his or her own airway, the presence of a gag reflex, and the extent of facial injuries.

Vomiting may occur in a patient with a head injury. With large amounts of emesis, the patient may

need to be log rolled to the side and the mouth cleared of secretions. When necessary, roll the patient in as straight a position as possible to minimize spinal injuries. Suctioning should be performed immediately to remove smaller amounts of secretions.

Apply a cervical spine immobilization device as soon as you have assessed the airway and breathing and provided necessary treatments. A cervical collar may help maintain spinal stabilization as you treat the airway and breathing. The key to managing spinal injuries and airway and breathing problems is to move the patient as little and as carefully as possible, maintaining spinal alignment throughout. Place an appropriately sized cervical-spine immobilization device on the patient when appropriate.

Breathing difficulty may result from a high cervical spinal cord injury or from increased pressure on the brain because of bleeding or swelling. In either situation, determine if breathing is present and adequate. Oxygen, delivered at a rate of 15 L/min by nonrebreathing mask or by bag-mask ventilation, is always indicated for patients with head and spinal injuries. A single episode of hypoxia in a patient with a head injury increases the risk of death or permanent disability significantly. Pulse oximeter values should be maintained at more than 95%. Positive-pressure ventilation is not always necessary; however, if the patient's breathing rate is too slow or too fast and shallow, provide positive-pressure ventilation using a bag-mask device. Ventilate at an age-appropriate rate. Do not panic and hyperventilate the patient because his or her condition appears severe. Hyperventilation should be reserved for specific conditions and performed under specific guidelines—follow local protocol.

Circulation

When approaching an unconscious patient, check for a pulse after assessing and treating the airway and breathing. A pulse that is too slow in a patient with

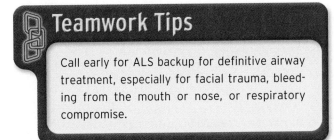

Teamwork Tips

Call early for ALS backup for definitive airway treatment, especially for facial trauma, bleeding from the mouth or nose, or respiratory compromise.

a possible head injury can indicate a potentially life-threatening injury.

A single episode of hypoperfusion in a head-injured patient can lead to significant brain damage and death. Assess for signs and symptoms of shock, and treat appropriately. In some patients with head and spinal injuries, blood pressure control will be difficult. The result can be hypotension and hypoperfusion. Bleeding may also be present from the same injury that caused the spine and/or head injury. That injury may involve blunt or penetrating forces. Consider again the MOI and the effects it has had on your patient. Control any external bleeding.

Transport Decision

A majority of head injuries are considered mild and result in no or limited permanent disability. Only a small percentage of head injuries are considered severe. Many patients with severe head injuries die before reaching the hospital or end up in a permanent vegetative state. There will be a number of patients with head or spine injuries that will not require much intervention other than a thorough assessment and continued observation while being transported to the hospital. In these cases, you should take time on scene to provide careful spine stabilization before transport. If the patient has significant problems with the ABCs or has been injured from a significant MOI, stabiliza-tion of the spine and rapid transport to the trauma center are indicated. If your patient has been involved in a motor vehicle crash and your initial assessment identifies life-threatening injuries, you should use the rapid extrication technique to remove the patient from the vehicle. See **Skill Drill 4-4** to review the steps of rapid extrication.

Focused History and Physical Exam

Remember that the ability to walk, move the extremities, and feel sensation does not necessarily rule out a spinal cord injury. Similarly, the absence of pain does not always indicate that a spinal injury has not occurred. Do not ask patients with possible spinal injuries to move their necks as a test for pain.

Rapid Physical Exam for Significant Trauma

Patients with moderate or severe head injuries associated with a significant MOI should receive lifesaving medical or surgical intervention at the hospital without delay. In these situations, a spinal injury should be suspected and appropriate measures taken regardless of your physical assessment findings. Perform a rapid physical exam using DCAP-BTLS to identify injuries. If immediate threats to the patient's life are found, they should be treated immediately. Minor injuries can be treated en route to the hospital. Extremities can be stabilized by using a long backboard and individual

You are the Provider 3

The patient is responsive to pain. You suction the airway and, after assessing his breathing, insert an oral adjunct. A fire fighter assists in ventilating the patient with the bag-mask device while you continue with your assessment.

You find multiple fractures, contusions, abrasions, and lacerations on his body. He is rapidly packaged and transferred to the ambulance for transport by an ALS unit. By the time he is loaded into the ambulance he is completely unresponsive.

Reassessment	Recording Time: 5 Minutes
Pulse	64 beats/min, irregular
Blood pressure	178/112 mm Hg
Respirations	Cheyne-Stokes respirations
Breath sounds	Slight rales bilaterally
Pulse oximetry	92% on oxygen via bag-mask ventillation

7. Is there anything else you can do to assist this patient?
8. How often should the patient be reassessed?
9. What does deterioration of neurologic signs in this case indicate?

splinting while in the back of the ambulance as time and conditions permit.

The rapid trauma exam should be a quick check of the head, chest, abdomen, extremities, and back. If a spinal injury is suspected, check perfusion, motor function, and sensation in all extremities before moving the patient. Determine whether the strength in each extremity is equal by asking the patient to squeeze your hands and to gently push each foot against your hands. Also compare the right and left limbs for equality of strength.

Decreased level of consciousness is the most reliable sign of a head injury. Monitor the patient for changes in level of consciousness, including signs of confusion, disorientation, or a decreasing mental status. Is the patient unresponsive or repeating questions? Experiencing seizures? Nauseated or vomiting? Next, determine if there is decreased movement and/or numbness and tingling in the extremities. Assess the vital signs carefully. Patients with head injuries may have irregular respirations, depending on which region of the brain is affected. Look for blood or CSF leaking from the ears, nose, or mouth and for bruising around the eyes and behind the ears.

You should also evaluate the patient's pupils, especially if he or she has a decreased level of consciousness. Unequal pupil size after a head injury in an unconscious patient is a critical finding. Developing blood clots may be compressing the brain and third cranial nerve, causing one pupil to dilate; unequal pupil size indicates a traumatic brain injury.

Do not probe open scalp lacerations with your gloved finger because this action may push bone fragments into the brain. Do not remove an impaled object from an open head injury.

Focused Physical Exam for Nonsignificant Trauma

A focused physical exam is used when the MOI or injuries are not considered significant. For example, a person falls to the ground while standing or is restrained in a low-speed motor vehicle collision in which the air bag has deployed but his or her only complaint is head, neck, or back pain. No other problems or conditions exist. The patient is alert and responds to questions appropriately. In these situations, you have the time necessary to focus your assessment on the spine and head. Change in the level of consciousness is the single most important observation that you can make in assessing the severity of brain

injury. Level of consciousness usually corresponds to the extent of loss of brain function. As soon as you determine that a head injury is present, you should perform a baseline assessment using the AVPU scale and record the time. Reevaluate the patient and record your observations every 15 minutes if the patient's condition is stable and at least every 5 minutes if the patient's condition is unstable.

Sometimes, the patient's mental status will fluctuate—improving, deteriorating, and then improving again over time. On other occasions, there may be a gradual, progressive deterioration in the patient's response to stimuli; this decline usually indicates a significant brain injury. The physicians who treat the patient will need to know when loss of consciousness occurred. They will want to compare their neurologic evaluation findings with yours from the evaluation performed in the field.

With a head injury, you should use the Glasgow Coma Scale (GCS) instead of the AVPU scale for a focused exam of the neurologic system Figure 20-10 ▶. The GCS helps you identify the patient's verbal response, eye opening, and ability to follow commands (motor response). Whether using the GCS or AVPU, always use simple, easily understood terms when reporting the level of consciousness, such as "does not remember events immediately before the injury" or "confused about date and time." Terms such as "obtunded" or "dazed" have different meanings to different people and should not be used in written or verbal reports.

When a head injury has not occurred but a spine injury is suspected, focus on assessing the spine and back. Inspect for DCAP-BTLS and check the extremities for circulation, motor, and sensory problems. Pain or tenderness when you palpate the spinal area is a warning sign that a spinal injury may exist. Patients with spinal injuries may complain of constant or intermittent pain along the spinal column or in their extremities. A spinal cord injury may also produce pain independent of movement or palpation.

Other signs and symptoms of spinal injury include an obvious deformity as you gently palpate the spine; numbness, weakness, or tingling in the extremities; and soft-tissue injuries in the spinal region. Patients with severe spinal injury may lose sensation or experience paralysis below the suspected level of injury or be incontinent (loss of urinary or bowel control). Obvious injury to the head and neck may indicate injury to the cervical spine. Injury to the shoulders, back, or abdomen (including penetrating trauma) may indicate

GLASGOW COMA SCALE

Eye Opening

Spontaneous	4
To Voice	3
To Pain	2
None	1

Verbal Response

Oriented	5
Confused	4
Inappropriate Words	3
Incomprehensible Words	2
None	1

Motor Response

Obeys Command	6
Localizes Pain	5
Withdraws (pain)	4
Flexion (pain)	3
Extension (pain)	2
None	1
Glasgow Coma Score Maximum Total	**15**
Glasgow Coma Score Minimum Total	**3**

Figure 20-10 The Glasgow Coma Scale is one method of evaluating level of consciousness. Note that the lower the score, the more severe the extent of brain dysfunction.

injury to the thoracic or lumbar spine. Injuries of the lower extremities may indicate a problem with the lumbar spine or sacrum.

Documentation Tips

Change in the LOC is the single most important observation that you can make in assessing the severity of brain injury. Record LOC, Glasgow Coma Scale score, and vital signs every 5 minutes for unstable patients and every 15 minutes for stable patients. Trending can provide valuable information that may direct further treatment in the emergency department.

Baseline Vital Signs

A complete set of baseline vital signs is essential in patients with head and spine injuries. Significant head injuries may cause the pulse to slow and the blood pressure to rise. With spinal shock, the blood pressure may drop and the heart rate may increase to compensate. Respirations may become irregular and inadequate with complications from head and spine injuries.

In head injuries, assess pupil size and reaction to light. The brain controls the diameter of pupils and how quickly they react. If an injury has occurred on one side of the brain, just one pupil will dilate. The pupils are windows to the brain and should be assessed as soon as possible to establish a baseline from which to monitor changes.

As soon as you have assessed the patient's level of consciousness, determine the reaction of each pupil to light. Continue to monitor the pupils. Any change in their reactions over time may indicate progressive brain damage.

SAMPLE History

The history may be difficult to obtain when a person is confused from a head injury or has sustained a spinal injury. Obtain as much of the SAMPLE history as you can while preparing for transport. In less urgent situations, you should have enough time to obtain a complete SAMPLE history without compromising patient care.

Interventions

You can almost always control bleeding from a scalp laceration by applying direct pressure over the wound. Remember to follow BSI precautions. Use a dry, sterile dressing, folding any torn skin flaps back down onto the skin bed before applying pressure. In some cases, you will have to apply firm compression for several minutes to control bleeding. If you suspect a skull fracture, do not apply excessive pressure to the open wound. Otherwise, you may increase intracranial pressure or push bone fragments into the brain.

If the dressing becomes soaked, do not remove it. Instead, place a second dressing over the first. Continue applying manual pressure until the bleeding has been controlled, and then secure the dressing in place with a soft, self-adhering roller bandage.

Rapid deterioration of neurologic signs following a head injury is an indication of an expanding intracranial hematoma or rapidly progressing brain swelling. The trauma patient with signs and symptoms of head injury who also displays signs of shock has lost blood into another body cavity if hemorrhage is not seen externally. Infants may lose enough blood into the skull region to produce shock, but this is not the case with older children and adults. Provide oxygen, monitor the airway, treat for shock, and provide immediate transport.

A common response to head injuries, even among children with only very slight head injuries, is vomiting. This is sometimes the result of increased intracranial pressure. In managing such vomiting, you should pay particular attention to protecting the airway.

As discussed earlier, the appearance of clear or pink watery CSF from the nose, the ear, or an open scalp wound indicates that the dura and the skull have been penetrated. You should make no attempt to pack the wound, ear, or nose in this situation. Cover the scalp wound, if there is one, with sterile gauze to prevent further contamination, but do not bandage it tightly.

Detailed Physical Exam

A thorough detailed exam should be performed if there is time and if the patient is in stable condition. This is a good time to ask the OPQRST questions about specific injuries. Because this exam is thorough and time-intensive, it is not often performed when attention is required to treat the ABCs. This exam should be performed only if time allows.

Ongoing Assessment

The ongoing assessment should focus on three key elements—reassessing the ABCs, interventions, and vital signs. Patients with head or spine injuries can lose an airway or stop breathing without warning. Careful reassessment after moving patients and after providing interventions will help identify these situations before they have a chance to lead to serious problems.

Multiple interventions may be necessary. The effectiveness of positive-pressure ventilation, spinal stabilization, and treatments for shock can be determined only with immediate and continuous observation after providing the intervention. If something is not working, try something else.

You have already established baseline vital signs as part of your assessment. Now is the time to compare the baseline vital signs with repeated vital signs. These changes will often tell you if treatments have been effective. Watch carefully for changes in pulse, blood pressure, and respirations. If the pressure in the head increases, the pulse may slow, blood pressure may rise, and respirations may become irregular. Document changes in level of consciousness.

Communication and Documentation

Hospitals may better prepare for seriously injured patients with more advanced warning and a description of the most significant findings in your assessment. Additional resources can be made available when you arrive. Trauma centers will activate their trauma team.

Your documentation should include the history you were able to obtain on scene, your findings during your assessment, and treatments you provided and how the patient responded to them. How frequently you document repeated vital signs depends on the condition of your patient. For patients in unstable condition, you should document vital signs every 5 minutes, whereas for patients in more stable condition, you should document vital signs every 15 minutes.

■ Emergency Medical Care of Spinal Injuries

Emergency medical care of a patient with a possible spinal injury begins, as does all patient care, with your protection; therefore, you must remember to follow BSI precautions. Next, you must maintain the

You are the Provider 4

You make the rendezvous with the ALS unit. En route to the trauma center the patient is intubated and his oxygen saturation increases. His mental status does not improve, however. He is treated for his head injury at the trauma center and placed in the neurologic intensive care unit. After several weeks he is transferred to a rehabilitation center. His prognosis is unsure, but there has been definite improvement.

patient's airway while keeping the spine in the proper position, assess respirations, and give supplemental oxygen.

Managing the Airway

Knowing that improper handling of a spinal injury can leave a patient permanently paralyzed must not prevent you from properly addressing an airway obstruction. Remember, all patients without an airway will die. If a patient with a spinal injury has an airway obstruction, you should perform the jaw-thrust maneuver to open the airway. If you cannot open and maintain the airway in a critically injured trauma patient, use a head tilt–chin lift maneuver. Once the airway is open, maintain the head and spine in a neutral, in-line position until it can be fully immobilized.

After you open the airway, consider inserting an oropharyngeal airway. If your patient accepts an oropharyngeal airway, be sure to monitor the airway closely; have a suctioning unit available because you will often need to clear away blood, saliva, or vomitus. Provide high-flow oxygen to any patient with suspected head or spine injury.

Stabilization of the Cervical Spine

Stabilizing the airway is your first priority. You must then stabilize the head and trunk so that bone fragments do not cause further damage. Even small movements cause significant injury to the spinal cord.

Once the patient's head and neck have been manually immobilized, assess the pulse, motor functions, and sensation in all extremities. Then assess the cervical spine area and neck. Keep in mind that the cervical collar is used to provide increased stability to the neck. It is used *in addition to*, not instead of, manual cervical spine stabilization. An improperly fitting collar will do more harm than good. If you do not have the proper size, place a rolled towel around the head and tape it to the backboard as you immobilize the patient on the board. In any case, maintain manual support until the patient has been fully secured to a backboard.

You should never force the head into a neutral, in-line position. Do not move the head any farther if the patient complains of the following:

- Muscle spasms in the neck
- Substantial increased pain

- Numbness, tingling, or weakness in the arms or legs
- Compromised airway or ventilations

In these situations, stabilize the patient in the position found.

Emergency Medical Care of Head Injuries

Patients with head injuries often have injuries to the cervical spine as well. Therefore, when treating a patient with a head injury, you must keep in mind the need to protect and stabilize the cervical spine at all times. Avoid moving the neck.

Beyond this, you should treat the patient with a head injury according to three general principles:

1. **Establish an adequate airway.** If necessary, begin and maintain ventilation and always provide high-flow supplemental oxygen.
2. **Control bleeding,** and support circulation to maintain cerebral perfusion.
3. **Assess the patient's baseline level of consciousness,** and continuously monitor it.

As you continue to treat the patient, do not apply pressure to an open or depressed skull injury. In addition, you must assess and treat other injuries, dress and bandage open wounds, splint fractures, anticipate and deal with vomiting to prevent aspiration, be prepared for seizures and changes in the patient's condition, and transport the patient promptly.

Managing the Airway

The most important step in the treatment of patients with head injury, regardless of the severity, is to establish an adequate airway. If the patient has an airway obstruction, you should perform the jaw-thrust maneuver to open the airway. Once the airway is open, maintain the head and cervical spine in a neutral, in-line position until the patient can be fully immobilized with a cervical collar and backboard. Remove any foreign bodies, secretions, or vomitus from the airway.

Once you have cleared the airway, check ventilation. If the respiratory control center of the brain has been injured, the rate and/or depth of breathing may be ineffective. Ventilation may also be limited by chest injuries or, if the spinal cord is injured, by paralysis of some or all of the muscles of respiration. Give high-flow oxygen to any patient with suspected head injury. The oxygen reduces hypoxia and possible cerebral edema. An injured brain is even less tolerant of hypoxia than a healthy brain, and studies have shown that supplemental oxygen can reduce brain damage; for this to be effective, it must be started as soon as possible. Continue to assist ventilations and administer supplemental oxygen until the patient reaches the hospital.

Circulation

Active blood loss aggravates hypoxia by reducing the available number of oxygen-carrying red blood cells. Although scalp lacerations rarely cause shock except in infants and children, they often cause the loss of large volumes of blood, which must be controlled. Bleeding inside the skull may cause intracranial pressure to rise to life-threatening levels, even though the actual volume of blood lost inside the skull is relatively small.

Shock that develops in a patient with a head injury is usually due to hypovolemia caused by bleeding from other injuries. As with other trauma patients, shock in these cases indicates that the situation is critical and patients must be transported immediately to a trauma center. Maintain the airway while you protect the patient's cervical spine, ensure adequate ventilation, administer 100% oxygen, control obvious bleeding with direct pressure, place the patient supine on a spine board, keep the patient warm, and provide immediate transport.

■ Preparation for Transport

Supine Patients

A patient who is supine can be effectively immobilized to a long backboard. The ideal procedure for moving a patient from the ground to a backboard is the four-person log roll. This procedure is recommended any time you suspect a spinal injury. The patient's condition, the scene, and the available resources will dictate the method you choose.

Direct the team from a kneeling position at the patient's head so that you can maintain manual in-line immobilization. Your job is to ensure that the head, torso, and pelvis move as a unit, with your teammates controlling the movement of the body. If necessary, you may recruit bystanders to the team, but be sure to instruct them fully before moving the patient. To immobilize a patient on a backboard, follow the steps in **Skill Drill 20-1 ▶** :

1. **Maintain in-line stabilization** at the patient's head. The EMT-B at the head will direct the log roll.
2. **Assess pulse, motor, and sensory function** in each extremity (**Step ①**).
3. **Apply an appropriately sized cervical collar** (**Step ②**).
4. The other team members should **position the immobilization device (backboard)** and place their hands on the far side of the patient to increase their leverage. Instruct them to use their body weight and their shoulder and back muscles to ensure a smooth, coordinated pull, concentrating their pull on the heavier portions of the patient's body (**Step ③**).
5. **On command from the EMT-B at the head,** the rescuers roll the patient toward themselves. One rescuer quickly examines the back while the patient is rolled on the side, and then slides the backboard behind and under the patient. The team rolls the patient back onto the board, avoiding independent rotation of the head, shoulders, or pelvis (**Step ④**).
6. **Ensure the patient is centered** on the board (**Step ⑤**).
7. **Secure the upper torso to the board** (**Step ⑥**). Consider padding voids between the patient and the backboard to make transport more comfortable and to protect the patient.
8. **Secure the pelvis and upper legs,** using padding as needed. For the pelvis, use straps over the iliac crests and/or groin loops (**Step ⑦**).
9. **Begin to immobilize the head to the board** by positioning a commercial immobilization device or towel rolls (**Step ⑧**).
10. **Secure the head by taping** the head immobilization device or towels across the forehead. To prevent airway problems and leave access to the airway, do not tape over the throat or chin (**Step ⑨**).

Teamwork Tips

When rolling a patient the person holding c-spine should call the move. Before rolling, decide on the count:

"Roll on 3" or "We're going to count to 3 and then roll."

Skill Drill 20-1   Immobilizing a Patient to a Long Backboard

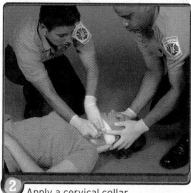

1 Apply and maintain cervical stabilization. Assess distal functions in all extremities.

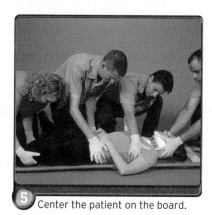

2 Apply a cervical collar.

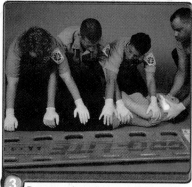

3 Rescuers kneel on one side of the patient and place hands on the far side of the patient.

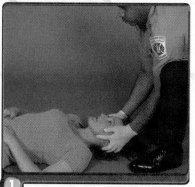

4 On command, rescuers roll the patient toward themselves, quickly examine the back, slide the backboard under the patient, and roll the patient onto the board.

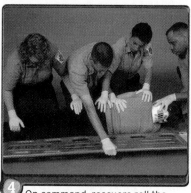

5 Center the patient on the board.

6 Secure the upper torso first.

11. **Check and readjust straps** as needed to ensure that the entire body is snugly secured and will not slide during patient movement.
12. **Reassess pulse and motor and sensory function** in each extremity (**Step 10**).

Sitting Patients

Some patients with a possible spinal injury will be in a sitting position, such as after an automobile crash. With these patients, you should use a short backboard or other short spinal extrication device to immobilize the cervical and thoracic spine. The short board is then secured to the long board.

The exceptions to this rule are situations in which you do not have time to first secure the patient to the short board, including the following situations:

- You or the patient is in danger.
- You need to gain immediate access to other patients.
- The patient's injuries justify urgent removal.

Review the steps in **Skill Drill 20-2 ▶** to use an extrication (vest-type) device or a short board to immobilize a sitting patient:

1. As with the supine patient, you must **first stabilize the head** and then maintain manual in-line stabilization.

Skill Drill 20-1 Continued

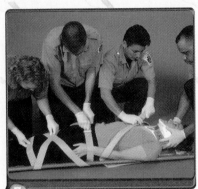
7 Secure the chest, pelvis, and upper legs.

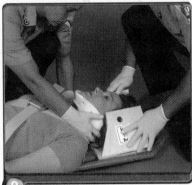
8 Begin to secure the patient's head using a commercial immobilization device or rolled towels.

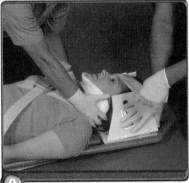
9 Place tape across the patient's forehead.

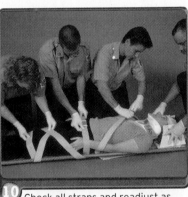
10 Check all straps and readjust as needed. Reassess distal functions in all extremities.

2. **Assess pulse and motor and sensory function** in each extremity.
3. **Apply the cervical collar** (**Step 1**).
4. **Insert a short spine immobilization device** between the patient's upper back and the seat back (**Step 2**).
5. **Open the board's side flaps (if present),** and position them around the patient's torso and snug to the armpits (**Step 3**).
6. Once the board has been properly positioned, **secure the straps around the torso** (**Step 4**).
7. **Position and fasten the leg straps.** Check all torso straps to make sure they are secure. Make any

adjustments necessary without excessive movement of the patient (**Step 5**).
8. **Pad any space between the patient's head** and the board as necessary.
9. **Secure the forehead strap,** and then fasten the lower head strap around the cervical collar (**Step 6**).
10. **Place the long backboard** next to the patient's buttocks, perpendicular to the trunk (**Step 7**).
11. **Turn the patient parallel to the long board,** and slowly lower him or her onto it.
12. **Lift the patient** (without rotating him or her), and slip the long board under the short board (**Step 8**).

Skill Drill   20-2   Immobilizing a Patient Found in a Sitting Position

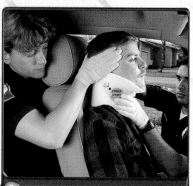

1. Stabilize the head and neck in a neutral, in-line position. Assess pulse, motor, and sensory function in each extremity. Apply a cervical collar.

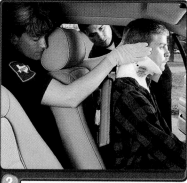

2. Insert a short spine immobilization device between the patient's upper back and the seat.

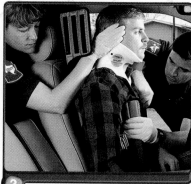

3. Open the side flaps, and position them around the patient's torso, snug around the armpits.

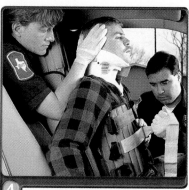

4. Secure the upper torso flaps, then the midtorso straps.

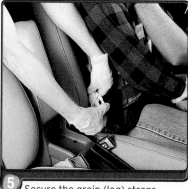

5. Secure the groin (leg) straps. Check and adjust torso straps.

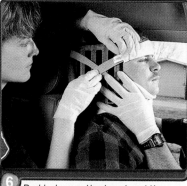

6. Pad between the head and the device as needed. Secure the forehead strap and fasten the lower head strap around the collar.

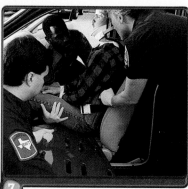

7. Wedge a long backboard next to the patient's buttocks.

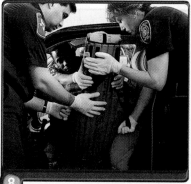

8. Turn and lower the patient onto the long board. Lift the patient, and slip the long board under the spine device.

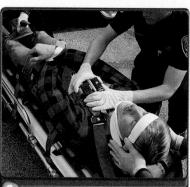

9. Secure the immobilization devices to each other. Reassess pulse, motor, and sensory functions in each extremity.

13. **Reassess the pulse, motor function, and sensation** in all four extremities. Note your findings, and prepare for immediate transport (**Step** ⑨).

Standing Patients

When you arrive on scene, you may find a patient standing or wandering around after an accident or injury. If the MOI suggests that there may be head or spinal injuries, you should immobilize the patient to a long backboard. Follow the steps in Skill Drill 20-3 ▾ for a standing backboard maneuver:

1. **Establish manual, in-line stabilization,** apply a cervical collar, and instruct the patient to remain still.

2. **Position the board upright** directly behind the patient (**Step** ①).
3. **Two EMT-Bs stand on either side** of the patient, and the third is directly behind the patient, maintaining immobilization.
4. **The two EMT-Bs grasp the handholds at shoulder level** or slightly above by reaching under the patient's arms (high up in the armpit) while standing at either side (**Step** ②).
5. **Prepare to lower the patient** to the ground (**Step** ③).
6. **Carefully lower the patient as a unit** under the direction of the EMT-B at the head. This EMT-B will have to make sure the head stays against the board and carefully rotate his or her hands as the patient is being lowered to maintain in-line stabilization (**Step** ④).

Skill Drill 20-3 — Immobilizing a Patient Found in a Standing Position

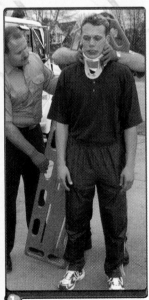

① While manually stabilizing the head and neck, apply a cervical collar. Position the board behind the patient.

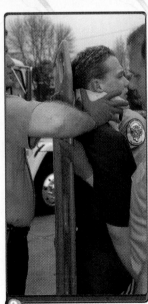

② Position EMT-Bs at sides and behind the patient. Side EMT-Bs reach under patient's arms and grasp handholds at or slightly above shoulder level.

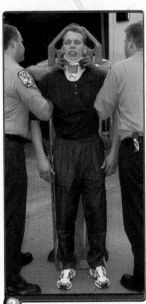

③ Prepare to lower the patient. EMT-Bs on the sides should be facing the EMT-B at the head and wait for his or her direction.

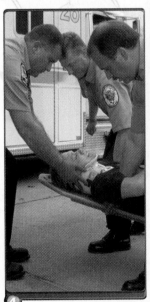

④ On command, lower the backboard to the ground.

Helmet Removal

As you plan care for a patient wearing a helmet, ask yourself the following questions:

- Is the patient's airway clear?
- Is the patient breathing adequately?
- Can you maintain the airway and assist ventilations if the helmet remains in place?
- Can the face guard easily be removed to allow access to the airway without removing the helmet?
- How well does the helmet fit?
- Can the patient move within the helmet?
- Can the spine be immobilized in a neutral position with the helmet on?

A helmet that fits well prevents the patient's head from moving and should be left on, provided:

- there are no impending airway or breathing problems,
- it does not interfere with assessment and treatment of airway or ventilation problems, and
- you can properly immobilize the spine.

You should also leave the helmet on if there is any chance that removing it will further injure the patient.

Remove a helmet if it makes assessing or managing airway problems difficult and removal of a face guard to improve airway access is not possible, it prevents you from properly immobilizing the spine, or it allows excessive head movement. Finally, always remove a helmet from a patient who is in cardiac arrest.

Sports helmets are typically open in the front and may or may not include an attached face mask. The mask can be removed without affecting helmet position or function by simply removing or cutting the straps that hold it to the helmet. In this way, sports helmets allow easy access to the airway. A patient who is involved in full contact sports may be wearing bulky pads to protect various body regions, such as shoulder pads. Leaving a helmet in place whenever possible is preferred so the body will maintain an in-line neutral position. If the helmet must be removed, be sure to provide padding to compensate for shoulder pads and maintain the in-line position of the body. Motorcycle helmets often have a shield covering the face. This, too, can be unbuckled to allow access to the airway Figure 20-11 ▶ . If a shield cannot be removed, the helmet must be removed.

Preferred Method

The technique for helmet removal depends on the actual type of helmet worn by the patient. Follow the steps in Skill Drill 20-4 ▶ to remove a helmet:

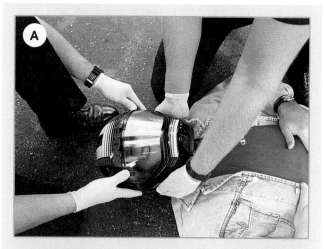

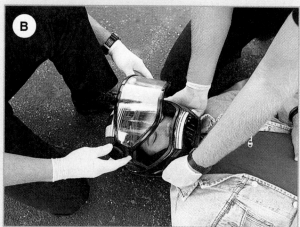

Figure 20-11 Motorcycle helmets often have a shield covering the face that can be removed. **A.** Stabilize the neck in a neutral, in-line position. **B.** Unbuckle or snap off the face shield to access the airway.

1. **Begin by kneeling at the patient's head.** Your partner should kneel on one side of the patient, at the shoulder area.
2. **Open the face shield,** if there is one, and assess the patient's airway and breathing. Remove eyeglasses if the patient is wearing them (**Step ①**).
3. **Stabilize the helmet** by placing your hands on either side of it, with your fingers on the patient's lower jaw to prevent movement of the head. Once your hands are in position, your partner can loosen the face strap (**Step ②**).
4. **Once the strap has been loosened,** your partner should place one hand on the patient's lower jaw at the angle of the jaw and the other behind the head at the occipital region. Once your partner's hands are in position, you may pull the sides of the helmet away from the patient's head (**Step ③**).

Skill Drill   20-4   Removing a Helmet

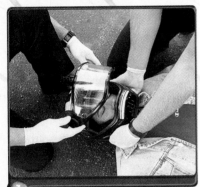

1 Kneel down at the patient's head with your partner at one side. Open the face shield to assess airway and breathing. Remove eyeglasses if present.

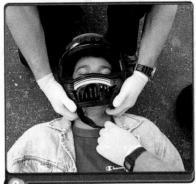

2 Prevent head movement by placing your hands on either side of the helmet and fingers on the lower jaw. Have your partner loosen the strap.

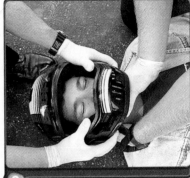

3 Have your partner place one hand at the angle of the lower jaw and the other at the occiput.

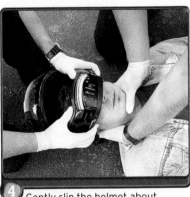

4 Gently slip the helmet about halfway off, then stop.

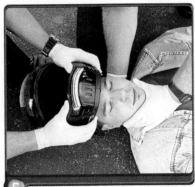

5 Have your partner slide the hand from the occiput to the back of the head to prevent it from snapping back.

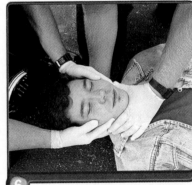

6 Remove the helmet and stabilize the cervical spine. Apply a cervical collar and secure the patient to a long backboard. Pad as needed to prevent neck flexion or extension.

5. **Gently slip the helmet** halfway off the patient's head, stopping when the helmet reaches the halfway point (**Step ④**).

6. **Your partner then slides his or her hand** from the neck up to the back of the head. This will prevent the head from snapping back once the helmet has been completely removed (**Step ⑤**).

7. With your partner's hand in place, **remove the helmet,** and immobilize the cervical spine.

8. **Apply the cervical collar,** and then secure the patient to the backboard.

9. **With large helmets** or small patients, you may need to pad under the shoulders to prevent flexion of the neck. If shoulder pads or heavy clothing are in place, you may need to pad behind the patient's head to prevent extension of the neck (**Step ⑥**). Current standards state that shoulder pads should always be removed when the helmet is removed.

Remember, you do not need to remove a helmet if you can access the patient's airway by removing the face shield, the head is snug inside the helmet, and the helmet can be secured to an immobilization device.

Alternative Method

An alternative method for removal of football helmets has also been used. The advantage of this method is that it allows the helmet to be removed with application of less force, therefore reducing the likelihood of motion occurring at the neck. The disadvantage of this method is that it is slightly more time-consuming. First, remove the chin strap by cutting or unsnapping it. Be careful during removal of the chin strap to avoid jarring the neck or head and causing excessive motion. Next, remove the face mask. The face mask is anchored to the helmet by plastic clips (loop straps) secured by screws. Current guidelines state that you should never use a screwdriver to remove the screws. Instead, you should use a *Trainer's Angel* (most athletic trainers will have these) or a set of pruning shears to cut the loop straps. It is recommended that you practice this technique before having to use it on a patient. The National Athletic Trainer's Association recommends that athletic trainers work with their local EMS providers to train on these techniques and work together to treat patients in whom a helmet must be removed.

After the face mask has been removed, the cheek pads can be popped out of place. This can be accomplished with the use of a tongue depressor. The fingers can then be placed inside the helmet, allowing greater control of the helmet during removal as the helmet is gently rocked back off the top of the head. One person controls the head by holding the jaw with one hand and the occiput with the other. Padding is inserted behind the occiput to prevent neck extension. If the

▲ Pediatric Needs

You are likely to find infants and children who have been in automobile crashes and are still in their car seats. Your best course of action is to immobilize the child using an appropriately sized pediatric immobilization device, or to consider using a rigid short board device instead. These allow you to completely assess and conduct the ongoing assessment of the injured child while transporting to the hospital. Whenever you apply a cervical collar, make sure it is properly sized. If a properly fitting collar is not available a rolled towel may be used as a substitution. If the child is not in a car seat or was removed before your arrival, use an appropriately sized immobilization device. If the cervical immobilization device does not fit, use a rolled towel, and tape it to the board and manually support the head.

shoulder pads are in place, appropriate padding must be applied behind the head to prevent hyperextension. As with the previously described method, the person over the patient's chest is responsible for making sure that the head and neck do not move during removal of the helmet. After the football helmet is removed, the shoulder pads should be removed using the six-person lift technique.

You are the Provider Summary

Good oxygenation is key for head injury patients. Hyperventilation should be avoided and ventilations should be performed once every 5 seconds for adults unless there are signs of cerebral herniation. Rapid transport and ALS intervention is key to patient survival in serious injuries.

1. **What should you do first?**
   The patient should be rolled to a supine position to assess airway.

2. **How will you accomplish this?**
   One rescuer should take c-spine control while the second grasps the shoulder and hip. The roll should be accomplished on the head man's count.

3. **Should you call for backup? Why or why not?**
   Yes. Fire department or first responders should be called if they are not already en route. They may be needed to assist with airway control, ventilations, and CPR.
   Consideration should also include a possible rendezvous with an ALS unit. There is gurgling indicating fluid in the airway. Definitive airway control may be needed to prevent aspiration.

4. **What is your next priority?**
   The airway must be cleared. Suction the airway and then assess breathing and decide on the appropriate oxygen amount and delivery.

5. **What do the vital signs tell you?**
   He has a head injury. He has the vital signs that make up Cushing's triad—increased blood pressure, decreased pulse, and irregular respirations.

6. **What signs back up your thoughts about the vital signs?**
   He has periorbital ecchymosis, cerebrospinal fluid draining from the nose, and depressed skull fractures.

7. **Is there anything else you can do to assist this patient?**
   Raise the head of the board to help decrease pressure. Tend to secondary injuries—splint fractures, and bandage lacerations.

8. **How often should the patient be reassessed?**
   Every 5 minutes. His condition is critical.

9. **What does deterioration of neurologic signs in this case indicate?**
   Possible increasing intracranial pressure or swelling in the brain.

Head and Spine Injuries

Scene Size-up

Body substance isolation precautions should include a minimum of gloves, mask, and eye protection. Ensure scene safety and determine NOI/MOI. Consider the number of patients, the need for additional help/ALS, and c-spine stabilization.

Initial Assessment

■ General impression

Determine level of consciousness and treat any immediate threats to life. Determine priority of care based on environment and patient's chief complaint.

■ Airway

Ensure patent airway.

■ Breathing

Listen for abnormal breath sounds and evaluate depth and rate of the respirations. Look for symmetric chest rise and fall. Maintain ventilations as needed. Provide high-flow oxygen at 15 L/min.

■ Circulation

Evaluate pulse rate and quality; observe skin color, temperature, and condition, and treat accordingly.

■ Transport decision

Prompt transport

Focused History and Physical Exam

NOTE: The order of the steps in the focused history and physical exam differs depending on whether or not the patient has a significant MOI. The order below is for a patient with a significant MOI. For a patient without a significant MOI, perform a focused trauma assessment, obtain vital signs, and obtain the history.

■ Rapid trauma assessment

Reevaluate the mechanism of injury. Perform a rapid trauma assessment, treating all life threats immediately. Log roll and secure patient to backboard for all patients with a suspected spinal injury.

■ SAMPLE history

Obtain SAMPLE history. If the patient is unresponsive, attempt to obtain information from family members, friends, or bystanders. Consider obtaining pertinent OPQRST information for patients with minor injuries.

■ Baseline vital signs

Take vital signs noting skin color/temperature as well as patient's level of consciousness. Use pulse oximetry if available.

■ Interventions

Provide complete spinal immobilization early if you suspect that your patient has spinal injuries. Maintain an open airway and suction as needed. Treat signs of shock and any other life threats.

Detailed Physical Exam

Complete a detailed physical exam.

Ongoing Assessment

Repeat the initial assessment, rapid/focused assessment, and reassess interventions performed. Reassess vital signs every 5 minutes for the unstable patient, every 15 minutes for the stable patient.

■ Communication and documentation

Contact medical control with a radio report. Relay any change in level of consciousness or difficulty breathing. Describe the MOI and any interventions you performed. Be sure to document any physician's orders and changes in the patient's condition and at what time they occurred.

NOTE: While the steps below are widely accepted, be sure to consult and follow your local protocol.

Head and Spine Injuries

Performing Manual In-line Stabilization
1. Kneel behind the patient and place your hands firmly around the base of the skull on either side.
2. Support the lower jaw with your index and long fingers, and the head with your palms. Gently lift the head into a neutral, eyes-forward position, aligned with the torso. Do not move the head or neck excessively, forcefully, or rapidly.
3. Continue to support the head manually while your partner places a rigid cervical collar around the neck. Maintain manual support until you have secured the patient to a backboard.

Immobilizing a Patient to a Long Backboard
1. Apply and maintain cervical stabilization. Assess distal functions in all extremities.
2. Apply a cervical collar.
3. Rescuers kneel on one side of the patient and place hands on the far side of the patient.
4. On command, rescuers roll the patient toward themselves, quickly examine the back, slide the backboard under the patient, and roll the patient onto the board.
5. Center the patient on the board.
6. Secure the upper torso first.
7. Secure the chest, pelvis, and upper legs.
8. Begin to secure the patient's head using a commercial immobilization device or rolled towels.
9. Place tape across the patient's forehead.
10. Check all straps and readjust as needed. Reassess distal functions in all extremities.

Immobilizing a Patient Found in a Sitting Position
1. Stabilize the head and neck in a neutral, in-line position. Assess pulse, motor, and sensory function in each extremity. Apply a cervical collar.
2. Insert a short spine immobilization device between the patient's upper back and the seat.
3. Open the side flaps, and position them around the patient's torso, snug around the armpits.
4. Secure the upper torso flaps, then the midtorso flaps.
5. Secure the groin (leg) straps. Check and adjust torso straps.
6. Pad between the head and the device as needed. Secure the forehead strap and fasten the lower head strap around the collar.
7. Wedge a long backboard next to the patient's buttocks.
8. Turn and lower the patient onto the long board. Lift the patient, and slip the long board under the spine device.
9. Secure the immobilization devices to each other. Reassess pulse, motor, and sensory functions in each extremity.

Immobilizing a Patient Found in a Standing Position
1. After manually stabilizing the head and neck, apply a cervical collar. Position the board behind the patient.
2. Position EMT-Bs at sides and behind the patient. Side EMT-Bs reach under patient's arms and grasp handholds at or slightly above shoulder level.
3. Prepare to lower the patient. EMT-Bs on the sides should be facing the EMT-B at the head and wait for his or her direction.
4. On command, lower the backboard to the ground.

Application of a Cervical Collar
1. Apply in-line stabilization.
2. Measure the proper collar size.
3. Place the chin support first.
4. Wrap the collar around the neck and secure the collar.
5. Assure proper fit and maintain neutral, in-line stabilization.

Removing a Helmet
1. Kneel down at the patient's head with your partner at one side. Open the face shield to assess airway and breathing. Remove eyeglasses if present.
2. Prevent head movement by placing your hands on either side of the helmet and fingers on the lower jaw. Have your partner loosen the strap.
3. Have your partner place one hand at the angle of the lower jaw and the other at the occiput.
4. Gently slip the helmet about halfway off, then stop.
5. Have your partner slide the hand from the occiput to the back of the head to prevent it from snapping back.
6. Remove the helmet and stabilize the cervical spine. Apply a cervical collar and secure the patient to a long backboard. Pad as needed to prevent neck flexion or extension.

Prep Kit

Ready for Review

- The nervous system is divided into two parts: the central nervous system (CNS) and the peripheral nervous system.
- The CNS consists of the brain and the spinal cord; the peripheral nervous system consists of a network of nerve fibers that transmit information to and from the body's organs and to and from the brain.
- The brain is protected by the skull, and the spinal cord is protected by the bones of the spinal column.
- The CNS is also covered and protected by three layers of tissue called the meninges. The layers are called the dura mater, arachnoid, and pia mater.
- The peripheral nervous system has two major types of nerves: sensory and motor.
- The nervous system can also be divided into the voluntary nervous system (under conscious control) and the autonomic nervous system (automatic processes that are not under conscious control).
- The autonomic nervous system is comprised of the sympathetic (fight-or-flight) system and the parasympathetic (rest and recovery) system. Both systems work together to maintain balance in the body systems and processes.
- The cervical, thoracic, and lumbar portions of the spinal column can be injured through compression such as in a fall, unnatural motions such as overextension from trauma, distraction such as from a hanging, or a combination of mechanisms. Each of these can also cause injury to the spinal cord encased in these regions of bone, causing permanent neurologic injury or death.
- Always begin patient assessment with a high index of suspicion for spinal injury in trauma patients and the need for manual spinal stabilization. Quickly assess the level of consciousness and perform the initial assessment.
- Conduct a rapid trauma assessment or focused history and physical exam (based on the MOI and potential injuries). During the assessment, be alert to the possibility of neurologic deficits.

- During the SAMPLE history or the focused history, ask these questions: "Do you have neck or back pain?" "What happened to you?" "Where do you have pain?" "Can you move your hands and feet?" Also, touch the patient's fingers and toes and ask, "Can you feel me touching you? Where?"
- Be alert to complaints of tingling in the upper or lower extremities, numbness, weakness, and paralysis (loss or diminished motor function).
- When applying manual immobilization and immobilizing the patient to a long backboard, keep the head in an in-line neutral position. Assess for signs of inadequate breathing and vomiting. Use the jaw-thrust maneuver to gain access to the airway. Provide high-flow oxygen.
- Common head injuries include scalp and facial lacerations and fractures of the skull. Brain injuries are also common (concussions, contusions, intracranial bleeding).
- Examples of MOIs that cause these head injuries are falls, motor vehicle crashes, assaults, gunshot wounds, and sport injuries.
- Brain swelling (cerebral edema), seizures, and vomiting are common complications of closed and open head injuries. CSF may also leak as a result of head injury.
- During the physical assessment, be alert for signs of deformity of the skull and for bruising around the eyes or behind the ear (both late signs). Assess for unequal pupil size or reaction, or failure to react to light, loss of sensation and function, and visual complaints.
- Patients with serious head injury have an increase in intracranial pressure from brain swelling and may have increased blood pressure (hypertension), decreased heart rate (bradycardia), and irregular respirations. This triad of signs is termed Cushing's reflex and indicates life-threatening pressure within the skull.
- One of the most important signs of head injury is a change in the patient's level of consciousness. Be alert to these changes. Reassess using the AVPU scale or the Glasgow Coma Scale every 5 minutes in a patient in unstable condition and every 15 minutes in a patient in stable condition.

Vital Vocabulary

autonomic (involuntary) nervous system The part of the nervous system that regulates functions that are not controlled by conscious will, such as digestion and sweating.

Battle's sign Bruising behind an ear over the mastoid process that may indicate skull fracture.

brain stem The part of the central nervous system that controls virtually all functions that are necessary for life, including the cardiac and respiratory systems.

Technology

- Interactivities
- Vocabulary Explorer
- Anatomy Review
- Web Links
- Online Review Manual

central nervous system (CNS) The brain and spinal cord.

cerebellum The part of the brain that coordinates body movements.

cerebral edema Swelling of the brain.

cerebrum The largest part of the brain, containing about 75% of the brain's total volume.

closed head injury An injury in which the brain has been injured but the skin has not been broken and there is no obvious bleeding.

concussion A temporary loss or alteration of part or all of the brain's abilities to function without actual physical damage to the brain.

four-person log roll The recommended procedure for moving a patient with a suspected spinal injury from the ground to a long backboard.

Glasgow Coma Scale (GCS) A method of evaluating level of consciousness that uses a scoring system for neurologic responses to specific stimuli.

meninges Three distinct layers of tissue that surround and protect the brain and the spinal cord within the skull and the spinal canal.

motor nerves The nerves that carry information from the central nervous system to the muscles.

open head injury An injury to the head often caused by a penetrating object in which there may be bleeding and exposed brain tissue.

peripheral nervous system The 31 pairs of spinal nerves and 12 pairs of cranial nerves that link the body to the central nervous system.

raccoon eyes Bruising under the eyes that may indicate skull fracture.

sensory nerves The nerves that transmit sensory input, such as touch, taste, heat, cold, and pain, from the periphery to the central nervous system.

somatic (voluntary) nervous system The part of the nervous system that regulates voluntary activities, such as walking, talking, and writing.

Assessment in Action

Your topic of refresher training for the month at your EMS service is head and spine injuries. Severe head and spine injuries often result in death. Continuing education is imperative to provide the ultimate care for your patient. You and your partner look over your material prior to class day.

1. The part of the nervous system that controls voluntary activities is known as the _____.
   - **A.** autonomic nervous system
   - **B.** somatic nervous system
   - **C.** central nervous system
   - **D.** parasympathetic nervous system

2. The components of Cushing's triad include:
   - **A.** irregular respirations.
   - **B.** increased blood pressure.
   - **C.** decreased pulse rate.
   - **D.** all of the above.

3. _____ is a common response to head injuries.
   - **A.** Tachycardia
   - **B.** Hypotension
   - **C.** Vomiting
   - **D.** Hemoptysis

4. The outer layer of the meninges is the _____.
   - **A.** dura mater
   - **B.** pia mater
   - **C.** arachnoid membrane
   - **D.** fascia

5. The most reliable sign of a head injury is _____.
   - **A.** pain
   - **B.** increased blood pressure
   - **C.** decreased LOC
   - **D.** tachypnea

6. What is the proper method for controlling bleeding from the scalp?
   - **A.** packing the wound
   - **B.** direct pressure
   - **C.** wet dressings
   - **D.** wrapping and elevating the head

Challenging Questions

7. What is the most fundamental part of the central nervous system and what does it control?

21

Soft-Tissue and Musculoskeletal Care

You are the Provider 1

You and your partner are sitting at a busy intersection waiting for the light to change when a large pickup truck runs the light and hits a motorcycle. The driver is thrown approximately 20' and slides across the asphalt to stop against a curb. His helmet is cracked on impact.

Your partner radios dispatch for assistance while you turn your lights on and block the intersection. Several other motorists get out of their cars to assist, including an off-duty fire fighter and a nurse.

Initial Assessment	Recording Time: 0 Minutes
Appearance	Multiple abrasions and possible fractures
Level of consciousness	Appears unresponsive
Airway	Snoring respirations
Breathing	Rapid and shallow
Circulation	Radials present

1. What should you do first?
2. Should the patient's helmet be removed or left in place?
3. How will you manage the airway?

◼ Introduction

The skin is the first line of defense against external forces, but it is still quite susceptible to injury. Injuries to soft tissues range from simple bruises and abrasions to serious lacerations and amputations and may involve exposure of deep structures such as blood vessels, nerves, and bones. Your priorities are to control bleeding, prevent further contamination, and protect the wound from further damage.

The musculoskeletal system serves to protect the internal organs and to give the body form, upright posture, and movement. The musculoskeletal system includes the bones and voluntary muscles of the body. Like the skin, bones and muscles are susceptible to external forces that can cause injury. Also at risk are the joints, tendons that attach muscles to bones, and ligaments that attach bones to one another.

This chapter begins with a review of the anatomy of the skin and the musculoskeletal system. Various types of soft-tissue and extremity injuries are reviewed, along with assessment techniques and emergency medical care for each type of injury. A detailed review of splinting is also included.

◼ The Anatomy and Functions of the Skin

The skin is the largest organ in the body. It varies in thickness, depending on age and its location. The skin of very young and very old people is thinner than the skin of a young adult. The skin covering your scalp, your back, and the soles of your feet is quite thick, whereas the skin of your eyelids, lips, and ears is very thin. Thin skin is more easily damaged than thick skin.

Technology

- Interactivities
- Vocabulary Explorer
- Anatomy Review
- Web Links
- Online Review Manual

Refresher.EMSzone.com

Anatomy of the Skin

The skin has two principal layers: the <u>epidermis</u> and the <u>dermis</u> Figure 21-1 ▶ . The epidermis is the tough, external layer that forms a watertight covering for the body. The epidermis is itself composed of several layers. The cells on the surface layer of the epidermis are constantly worn away. They are replaced by cells that are pushed to the surface when new cells form. Deeper cells contain pigment granules. Along with blood vessels in the dermis, these granules produce skin color.

The dermis is the inner layer of the skin. It lies below the epidermis. The dermis contains the structures that give the skin its characteristic appearance: hair follicles, sweat glands, and sebaceous glands. The sweat glands act to cool the body. They discharge sweat onto the surface of the skin through small pores, or ducts, that pass through the epidermis. Sebaceous glands produce sebum, the oily material that waterproofs the skin and keeps it supple. Sebum travels to the skin's surface along the shaft of adjacent hair follicles. Hair follicles are small organs that produce hair. There is one follicle for each hair, each connected with a sebaceous gland and a tiny muscle. This muscle pulls the hair erect whenever you are cold or frightened. Blood vessels in the dermis provide the skin with nutrients and oxygen. There are also specialized nerve endings within the dermis.

The skin covers all external surfaces of the body. The various openings in our body, including the mouth, nose, anus, and vagina, are not covered by skin. Instead, these openings are lined with <u>mucous membranes</u>. These membranes are similar to skin in that they provide a protective barrier against bacterial invasion, but mucous membranes differ in that they secrete a lubricating substance. Therefore, mucous membranes are moist, whereas skin is dry.

Functions of the Skin

The skin protects the body by keeping pathogens out and water in and assisting in body temperature regulation. The nerves in the skin report to the brain on the environment and on many sensations.

The skin is also the body's major organ for regulating temperature. In a cold environment, the blood vessels in the skin constrict, diverting blood away from the skin and decreasing the amount of heat that is radiated from the body's surface. In hot environments, the vessels in the skin dilate. The skin becomes flushed or red, and heat radiates from the body's surface. Also, sweat glands secrete sweat. As

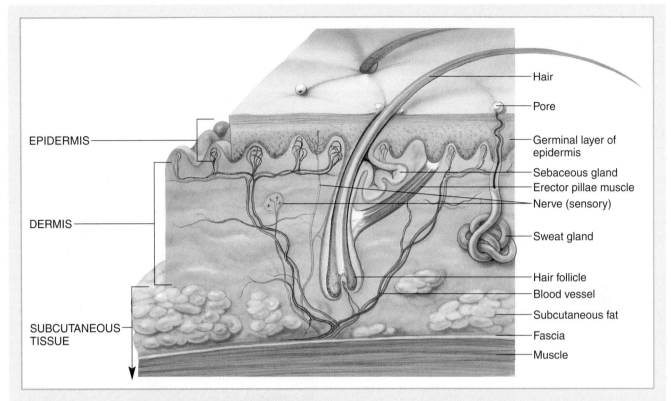

EPIDERMIS

DERMIS

SUBCUTANEOUS TISSUE

Hair

Pore

Germinal layer of epidermis

Sebaceous gland

Erector pillae muscle

Nerve (sensory)

Sweat gland

Hair follicle

Blood vessel

Subcutaneous fat

Fascia

Muscle

Figure 21-1 The skin is composed of a tough external layer called the epidermis and a vascular inner layer called the dermis.

the sweat evaporates from the skin's surface, your body temperature drops, and you begin to cool down.

Any break in the skin allows bacteria to enter and raises the possibilities of infection, fluid loss, and loss of temperature control.

■ Types of Soft-tissue Injuries

Soft tissues are often injured because they are exposed to the environment. There are three types of soft-tissue injuries:

- Closed injuries, in which soft-tissue damage occurs beneath the skin or mucous membrane but the surface remains intact
- Open injuries, in which there is a break in the surface of the skin or the mucous membrane, exposing deeper tissue to potential contamination
- Burns, in which the soft tissue receives more energy than it can absorb without injury. The source of this energy can be thermal heat, frictional heat, toxic chemicals, electricity, or nuclear radiation.

Closed Injuries

Closed soft-tissue injuries are characterized by a history of blunt trauma, pain at the site of injury, swelling beneath the skin, and discoloration. Such injuries can vary from mild to quite severe.

A contusion, or bruise, results from blunt force striking the body. The epidermis remains intact, but cells within the dermis are damaged, and small blood vessels are usually torn. The depth of the injury varies, depending on the amount of energy absorbed. As fluid and blood leak into the damaged area, the patient may have swelling and pain. The buildup of blood produces a characteristic blue or black discoloration called ecchymosis Figure 21-2 ▶ .

A hematoma is blood that has collected within damaged tissue or in a body cavity whenever a large blood vessel is damaged and bleeds rapidly Figure 21-3 ▶ . It is usually associated with extensive tissue damage. A hematoma can result from a soft-tissue injury, a fracture, or any injury to a large blood vessel. In severe cases, the hematoma may contain more than a liter of blood.

Figure 21-2 Contusions, more commonly known as bruises, occur as a result of a blunt force striking the body. The buildup of blood produces a characteristic blue or black discoloration (ecchymosis).

A crushing injury occurs when a great amount of force is applied to the body 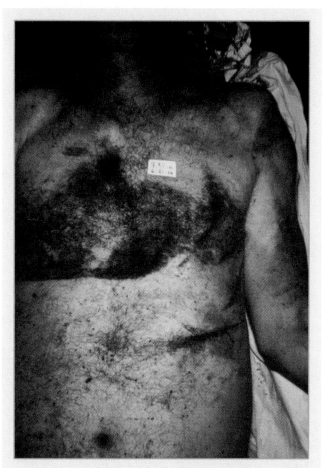. The extent of the damage depends on how much force is applied and the amount of time over which it is applied. In addition to causing some direct soft-tissue damage, continued compression of the soft tissues will cut off their circulation, producing further tissue destruction. For example, if a patient's legs are trapped under heavy debris, damage to the leg tissues will continue until the debris is removed.

Another form of compression can result from the swelling that occurs whenever tissues are injured. Ex-

Figure 21-4 The damage associated with a crush or compression injury varies depending on the direct damage to the soft tissues and on how long the circulation was cut off in the tissue.

cessive swelling often follows significant injury to the extremities. The cells that are injured leak watery fluid into the spaces between the cells. The pressure of the fluid may become great enough to compress the tissue and cause further damage. This is especially true if the blood vessels become compressed, cutting off blood flow to the tissue. This condition is called <u>compartment syndrome</u>.

Severe closed injuries can also damage internal organs. The greater the amount of energy absorbed from the blunt force, the greater the risk of injury to deeper structures. Therefore, you must assess all patients with closed injuries for more serious hidden injuries. Remain alert for signs of shock and internal bleeding.

Open Injuries

Open injuries differ from closed injuries in that the protective layer of skin is damaged, which produces more extensive bleeding. More important, however,

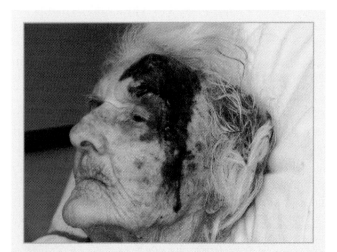

Figure 21-3 A hematoma develops whenever a large blood vessel is damaged and bleeds rapidly.

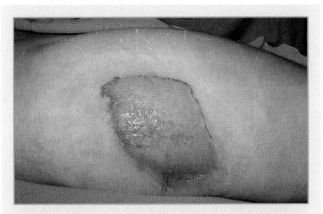

Figure 21-5 Abrasions usually do not penetrate completely through the dermis, but blood may ooze from the capillaries. These wounds are typically superficial and result from rubbing or scraping across a hard, rough surface.

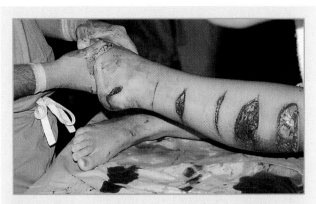

Figure 21-6 Lacerations vary in depth and can extend through the skin and subcutaneous tissue to the underlying muscles, nerves, and blood vessels. These wounds can be smooth or jagged as a result of a cut by a sharp object or a blunt force that tears the tissue.

a break in the protective skin layer or mucous membrane means that the wound is contaminated and may become infected. Contamination describes the presence of infectious organisms (pathogens) or foreign bodies, such as dirt, gravel, or metal. You must address these two problems in your treatment of open soft-tissue wounds. There are four types of open soft-tissue wounds that you must be prepared to manage: abrasions, lacerations, avulsions, and penetrating wounds.

An <u>abrasion</u> is a wound of the superficial layer of the skin caused by friction when a body part rubs or scrapes across a rough or hard surface. An abrasion usually does not penetrate completely through the dermis, but blood may ooze from the injured capillaries in the dermis. Known by a variety of names, including road rash, road burn, strawberry, and rug burn, abrasions can be extremely painful Figure 21-5 ▲ .

A <u>laceration</u> is a jagged cut caused by a sharp object or a blunt force that tears the tissue, an <u>incision</u> is a sharp, smooth cut. The depth of the injury can vary, extending through the skin and subcutaneous tissue, even into the underlying muscles and adjacent nerves and blood vessels Figure 21-6 ▶ . Lacerations and incisions may appear linear (regular) or stellate (irregular) and may occur along with other types of soft-tissue injury. Lacerations and incisions that involve arteries or large veins may result in severe bleeding.

An <u>avulsion</u> is an injury that separates various layers of soft tissue so that the skin is completely detached or hangs as a flap Figure 21-7 ▶ . Often there is significant bleeding. If the avulsed tissue is hanging from a small piece of skin, the circulation through the flap may be at risk. If you can, replace the avulsed flap

in its original position. If an avulsion is complete, you should wrap the separated tissue in sterile gauze and take it with you to the emergency department.

We usually think of amputations as involving the upper and lower extremities, but other body parts, such as the scalp, ear, nose, penis, or lips, may also be totally avulsed, or amputated. You can easily control the bleeding from some amputations, such as the fingers, with pressure dressings. But if an avulsion involves a large area of muscle mass, such as a thigh, there may be massive bleeding. In this situation, you need to treat the patient for shock. The use of pressure points may also be necessary to control the bleeding.

A <u>penetrating wound</u> is an injury resulting from a sharp, pointed object, such as a knife, ice pick, splinter, or bullet. Such objects leave relatively small

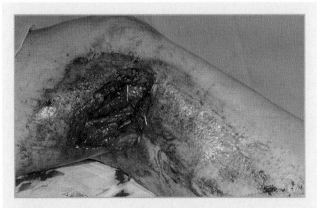

Figure 21-7 Avulsions are injuries characterized by complete separation of tissue or tissue hanging as a flap. Significant bleeding is common.

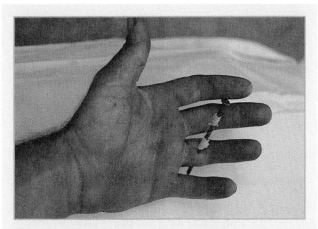

Figure 21-8 Penetrating wounds may cause very little external bleeding but can damage structures deep within the body.

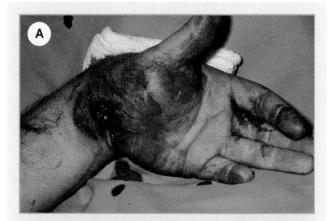

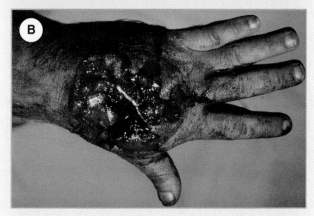

Figure 21-9 **A.** An entrance wound from a gunshot may have burns around the edges. **B.** An exit wound is often larger and associated with greater damage to soft tissues locally.

entrance wounds, so there may be little external bleeding ▸Figure 21-8▴. However, these objects can damage structures deep within the body and cause internal bleeding. If the wound is to the chest or abdomen, the injury can cause rapid, fatal bleeding.

Stabbings and shootings often result in multiple penetrating injuries. You must assess patients carefully to identify all wounds. Because a penetrating object can pass completely through the body, always count the number of penetrating injuries (or holes), especially with gunshot wounds. Entrance wounds and exit wounds may be difficult to tell apart in a prehospital setting, especially with the different types of ammunition available. Entrance wounds are usually smaller than exit wounds ▸Figure 21-9▸. Gunshot wounds have some unique characteristics that require special care. The amount of energy transmitted by a gunshot injury is directly related to the speed of the bullet. If possible, try to find out the type of gun that was used in the shooting. Shotgun wounds create multiple paths of missiles (shot) and create a larger surface area and volume of tissue damage.

Open wounds caused by crushing forces may involve damaged internal organs or broken bones, in addition to extensive soft-tissue damage ▸Figure 21-10▸. Although external bleeding may be minimal, internal bleeding may be severe, even life threatening. The crushing force damages soft tissues, vessels, and nerves.

■ Assessment of Closed and Open Injuries

Scene Size-up

Soft-tissue injuries can result in scenes where there is a lot of blood. Control of the blood and bloody con-

taminants can be difficult unless you are careful about what you touch and where. Using body substance isolation (BSI) precautions can minimize your direct exposure to body fluids. However, reaching into a medical kit for supplies with bloody gloves will extend the area of contamination and increase the risk

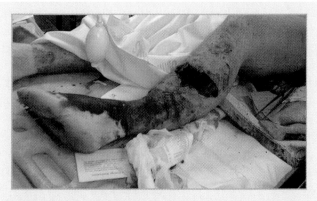

Figure 21-10 A crushing wound is characterized by extensive tissue damage and deformity that is often accompanied by swelling and extreme pain

of exposure to you or other rescuers. Place several pairs of gloves in your pocket for easy access in case you need another pair. If your gloves tear or there are multiple patients with bleeding, you may need more gloves immediately available.

Because of the color of blood and how well it soaks through clothing, you can often identify patients with bleeding as you approach the scene. However, bleeding can be hidden under thick clothing such as denim and leather. Eye exposures may occur from splashes and droplets at a busy scene. Eye protection should be required when managing open wounds.

As you put together information from dispatch and your observations of the scene, consider how the mechanism of injury (MOI) produced the injuries expected. This helps you develop an early index of suspicion for underlying injuries in the patient. The MOI may also provide indications of safety threats (shootings, assaults). Make sure the scene is safe, and consider requesting additional help early.

Initial Assessment

General Impression

As you approach the trauma patient, important indicators will alert you to the seriousness of the patient's condition. Is the patient awake and interacting with his or her surroundings or lying still, making no sounds? Does the patient have any apparent life threats such as significant bleeding? How is the patient's skin color? Is he or she responding to you appropriately or inappropriately? Observations such as bleeding and skin color and condition contribute to your general impression and help to determine your treatment priorities and the urgency of care needed. A good question to ask is, "How sick is my patient based on what I know right now?"

Airway and Breathing

Next, ensure that the patient has a clear and patent airway. Open soft-tissue injuries of the face and neck have a potential to interfere with the effectiveness of the airway and breathing. Because trauma was involved, protect the patient from further spinal injury as you manage the airway. If the patient is unresponsive or has a significantly altered level of consciousness, consider inserting an oropharyngeal airway or nasopharyngeal airway. You must also quickly assess for adequate breathing. Observe the rate and depth of respirations. Listen to breath sounds quickly on each side of the chest. Palpate the chest wall for DCAP-BTLS. Cover any open wounds to the chest with an occlusive dressing. Provide high-flow oxygen or assisted ventilations with a bag-mask device as needed.

Circulation

You must quickly assess the patient's pulse rate and quality; determine the skin condition, color, and temperature. Closed soft-tissue injuries do not have visible

You are the Provider 2

The helmet is removed and your partner is able to open the airway while stabilizing the cervical spine. You see a small amount of blood and note that two of his teeth are broken. You suction the airway, but do not see the broken teeth. You assess his airway, apply oxygen, and assess circulation.

You perform a rapid trauma assessment and note that he has an unstable pelvis, crepitus in the tibia/fibula area bilaterally, and an angulated ankle on the right.

Vital Signs	Recording Time: 3 Minutes
Skin	Pale, diaphoretic
Pulse	116 beats/min, irregular
Blood pressure	124/68 mm Hg
Respirations	12 breaths/min via bag-mask ventilations

4. What is the best option for packaging this patient?
5. How should his fractures be managed?
6. What do the vital signs indicate?

signs of bleeding. Because the bleeding is occurring inside the body, shock may be present. Your assessment of the pulse and skin will give you an indication as to how aggressively you need to treat for shock.

If visible significant bleeding is seen, you must begin the steps necessary to control bleeding. Significant bleeding is an immediate life threat and must be controlled quickly using appropriate methods. In dark environments, bleeding can be hidden because of its color. Thick clothing may also hide bleeding. Blood flowing freely from veins in a large gash can be as much of a threat as blood spurting from an artery. Life-threatening bleeding must be controlled in the initial assessment.

Transport Decision

During your initial assessment, determine whether your patient needs immediate transport or stabilization on scene. If your patient has an airway or breathing problem, signs of shock, or significant bleeding, you must consider rapid transport or requesting ALS support. The condition of patients who have visible significant bleeding or signs of significant internal bleeding may quickly become unstable. Although treatment in the initial assessment is directed at quickly addressing life threats, you should not delay transport of a trauma patient, particularly one in whom a closed soft-tissue injury may be a sign of a more serious deeper injury. Patients with a significant MOI may require a rapid physical exam to identify these injuries.

Focused History and Physical Exam

After the initial assessment is complete, determine which type of physical exam needs to be performed. A rapid physical exam is based on a significant MOI, whereas a focused physical exam is based on a nonsignificant MOI. In a responsive patient who has a simple open or closed injury and no significant MOI, consider a focused physical exam.

Patients with a significant MOI and those who are unconscious need a complete and rapid exam to iden-

tify all of the injuries and to prepare for packaging and rapid transport.

Focused Physical Exam

Focus your assessment on the isolated injury, the patient's complaint, and the body region affected. Ensure that control of the bleeding is maintained, and note the location of the injury. In an injured extremity, assess pulse and motor and sensory function. For injuries to the torso, assess respiratory, circulatory, and neurologic systems in the affected area.

Rapid Physical Exam

If significant trauma has likely affected multiple systems, start with a rapid trauma assessment, quickly looking from head to toe for DCAP-BTLS to identify all of the injuries.

You should not delay transport of a trauma patient, particularly a patient with significant bleeding, even if it is controlled. Identifying injuries during a rapid physical exam may help you prepare your patient for transport. For example, noting a hip or extremity injury in your patient during this exam would suggest log rolling the patient away from the injured extremity when possible. Spinal stabilization should be completed here, including application of a cervical spine stabilization device and securing the patient to a backboard, if not already done in the initial assessment.

Baseline Vital Signs

Remember you must be concerned with both visible bleeding and bleeding that is unseen. Patients with closed soft-tissue injuries may have internal bleeding, and their condition may rapidly become unstable. Determining a baseline set of vital signs will be important to identify how quickly the patient's condition is changing. Signs such as tachycardia, increased respiratory rate, low blood pressure, weak pulse, and cool, moist, and pale skin indicate hypoperfusion. Remember that soft-tissue injuries, even without a significant MOI, can cause shock.

SAMPLE History

Make every attempt to obtain a SAMPLE history from your patient. If the patient is not responsive, attempt to obtain the SAMPLE history from others, such as bystanders or family members. Medical identification jewelry and cards in wallets may also provide information about the patient's medical history. Using OPQRST may provide some background on isolated

EMT-B Safety

Amputations may involve splashing if an artery is severed. Use goggles or a face shield and a gown in conjunction with gloves when splashing is possible.

extremity injuries. Any information you receive will be valuable if the patient loses consciousness.

Interventions

For external bleeding, cover the wound and control the bleeding as quickly as possible. Provide complete spinal immobilization early if you suspect that your patient has spinal injuries. Providing high-flow oxygen to patients with soft-tissue injuries may help reduce the effects of shock and assist in perfusion of damaged tissues. If the patient has signs of hypoperfusion, treat aggressively for shock and provide rapid transport to the hospital. Do not delay transport of a seriously injured trauma patient to complete nonlifesaving treatments in the field, such as splinting extremity fractures; instead, complete these types of treatments en route to the hospital.

Detailed Physical Exam

If the patient's condition is stable and problems do not persist after the initial assessment, perform a thorough detailed physical exam. Many times, short transportation times and unstable patient conditions that require continuous monitoring and treatment make this assessment impractical.

Ongoing Assessment

Repeat the initial assessment. Is the airway still adequate? Is breathing still adequate? Is the pulse still adequate? Is perfusion adequate? Are the treatments you provided for problems with the ABCs still effective? How is the patient's condition improving with these interventions? Reassess vital signs. Assess these signs frequently, and note trends that indicate whether the patient's condition is getting better or worse.

Communication and Documentation

You should include a description of the MOI and the position in which you found the patient as you arrived on scene. In cases involving severe external bleeding, it is important to recognize, estimate, and report the amount of blood loss that has occurred and how rapidly or how much time has passed since the bleeding started. This is a challenge, especially if the surface is wet, absorbs fluids, or is dark. You should attempt to report blood loss using terms that you are comfortable with and that will easily be understood by other personnel. For example, you may say "approximately a liter was lost," or "the bleeding has soaked through three trauma dressings." It is not as important how you describe it, but that you describe it accurately. You must include the location and description of any soft-tissue injuries and other wounds you have located and treated. Describe the size and depth of the injury. Provide an accurate account of how you treated these injuries. All of this information is important to include in your verbal and written communication.

You are the Provider 3

You package the patient on a long backboard with the PASG in place. Once in the ambulance and en route, you continue with your assessment and interventions. You note multiple abrasions over his chest and arms. The upper part of his left arm has a large avulsion.

The PASG is inflated as a splint for the pelvis and lower extremities. A pillow is placed under his ankle and he is covered with a blanket. His airway is being maintained by a fire fighter who agrees to ride in to the hospital.

Reassessment	Recording Time: 7 Minutes
Pulse	126 beats/min, weak
Blood pressure	112/60 mm Hg
Respirations	Ventilating at 12 breaths/min
Breath sounds	Clear bilaterally
Level of consciousness	Deep pain responsive

7. What is the proper management for the avulsion?
8. What is the treatment for the abrasions?
9. If you were not using the PASG, would a traction splint be appropriate for this patient?

Emergency Medical Care

Small contusions require no special emergency medical care. More extensive closed injuries may involve significant swelling and bleeding beneath the skin, which could lead to hypovolemic shock. If life-threatening bleeding is observed, apply direct pressure to control the bleeding. If the wound is in the chest or upper abdomen, place an occlusive dressing on the wound.

Soft-tissue injuries may look rather dramatic. However, you must still focus on airway and breathing first. Always maintain the airway and provide oxygen in patients with potentially serious injuries. If the patient has inadequate breathing, you may have to assist breathing with bag-mask ventilation.

Treat a closed soft-tissue injury by applying the acronym RICES:

- **Rest**—keep the patient as quiet and as comfortable as possible.
- **Ice** (or a cold pack) slows bleeding by causing blood vessels to constrict and also reduces pain.
- **Compression** over the injury site slows bleeding by compressing the blood vessels.
- **Elevation** of the injured part just above the level of the patient's heart decreases swelling.
- **Splinting** decreases bleeding and also reduces pain by immobilizing a soft-tissue injury or an injured extremity.

For open soft-tissue injuries, follow the steps in Skill Drill 21-1 ▶:

1. **Apply a dry, sterile dressing** over the entire wound. Apply pressure to the dressing with your gloved hand (**Step ①**).
2. **Maintain the pressure,** and secure the dressing with a roller bandage (**Step ②**).
3. **If bleeding continues or recurs, leave the original dressing in place.** Apply a second dressing on top of the first, and secure it with another roller bandage (**Step ③**).
4. **Splint the extremity** to stabilize the injury, even if there is no suspected fracture, to help minimize movement, further control the bleeding, and keep the dressing in place (**Step ④**).

In addition to using these measures to control bleeding and swelling, you should be alert for signs of developing shock, including anxiety or agitation, changes in mental status, increased heart rate, increased respiratory rate, diaphoresis, cool or clammy skin, and decreased blood pressure. Any or all of these signs may indicate internal bleeding resulting from injuries to internal organs. If the patient appears to be in shock, you should place the patient in the shock position (supine with legs elevated 6" to 12"); or, if the patient is on a backboard or stretcher, use the Trendelenburg position (on a backboard or stretcher with the feet 6" to 12" higher than the head), provide supplemental high-flow oxygen, and transport promptly to the hospital.

Severe bleeding often accompanies significant trauma. When significant trauma exists, do not spend time on scene splinting the wound. Apply a pressure bandage, and splint during transport if time allows.

Keep in mind that a patient who is bleeding significantly from an open wound is at risk for hypovolemic shock. You must be alert for this possibility and provide treatment in all cases of significant trauma and for patients with moderate to severe bleeding.

■ Abdominal Wounds

An open wound in the abdominal cavity may expose internal organs. In some cases, the organs may even protrude through the wound, which is called an <u>evisceration</u> Figure 21-11 ▶. Do not touch or move the exposed organs. Cover the wound with sterile gauze compresses moistened with saline solution and secured with a sterile dressing. Because the open abdomen radiates body heat very effectively and because exposed organs lose fluid rapidly, you must

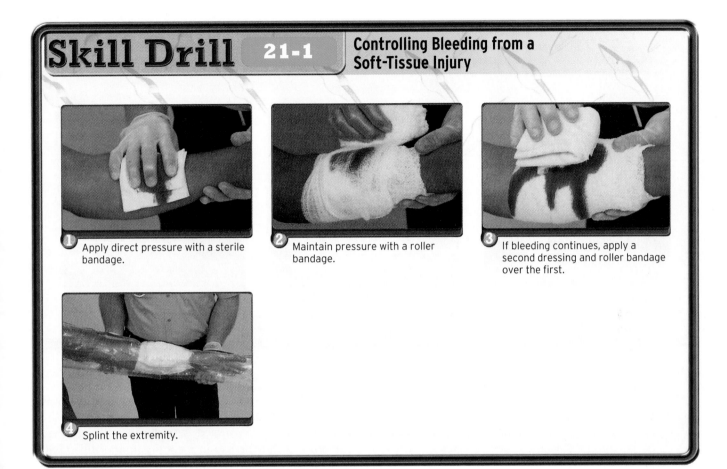

Skill Drill 21-1 Controlling Bleeding from a Soft-Tissue Injury

1. Apply direct pressure with a sterile bandage.

2. Maintain pressure with a roller bandage.

3. If bleeding continues, apply a second dressing and roller bandage over the first.

4. Splint the extremity.

keep the organs moist and warm. If you do not have gauze compresses, you may use moist sterile dressings, covered and secured in place with a bandage and tape. Do not use any material that is adherent or loses its substance when wet, such as toilet paper, facial tissue, paper towels, or absorbent cotton. If the patient's

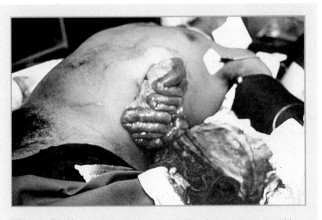

Figure 21-11 An abdominal evisceration is an open wound to the abdomen in which organs protrude through the wound.

legs and knees are uninjured, and spinal injury is *not* suspected, flex them to relieve pressure on the abdomen. Most patients with abdominal wounds require immediate transport to a trauma center, depending on the local protocol.

■ Impaled Objects

Occasionally, a patient will have an object, such as a knife, fishhook, wood splinter, or piece of glass, impaled in his or her body. To treat this, follow the steps in Skill Drill 21-2 :

1. **Do not attempt to move or remove the object** unless it is impaled through the cheek causing airway obstruction or if the object is in the chest and interferes with CPR. In most cases, a surgeon will have to remove the object. Removing it in the field may cause more bleeding or damaged nerves, blood vessels, or muscles within the wound (**Step ①**). Stabilize the impaled body part.

2. **Remove any clothing covering the injury. Control bleeding, and apply a bulky dressing** to stabilize the object. A combination of soft dressings,

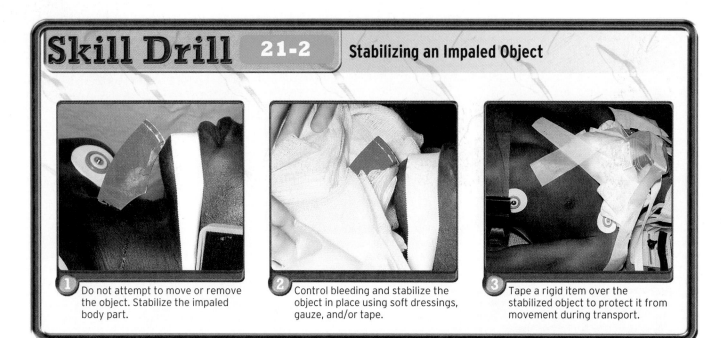

Skill Drill **21-2**   Stabilizing an Impaled Object

1. Do not attempt to move or remove the object. Stabilize the impaled body part.

2. Control bleeding and stabilize the object in place using soft dressings, gauze, and/or tape.

3. Tape a rigid item over the stabilized object to protect it from movement during transport.

gauze, and tape may be effective, depending on the location and size of the object. To prevent further injury, manually secure the object by incorporating it into the dressing (**Step 2**).

3. **Protect the impaled object** from being bumped or moved during transport by taping a rigid item such as a plastic cup, a section of a plastic water bottle, or a supply container over the stabilized object and its bandaging (**Step 3**).

The only exception to the rule of not removing an impaled object is an object in the cheek that obstructs breathing. In this situation, restoring the airway takes priority. If the object is very long, cut off (shorten) the exposed portion, first securing it to minimize motion and thus internal damage and pain. Once the object has been secured and the bleeding is under control, manage the airway and provide prompt transport.

■ Amputations

Surgeons today can occasionally reattach amputated parts. However, correct prehospital care of the amputated part is vital to successful reattachment. With partial amputations, make sure to immobilize the part with bulky compression dressings and a splint to prevent further injury. Do not sever any partial amputations; this may complicate later reattachment.

With a complete amputation, make sure to wrap the part in a sterile dressing and place it in a plastic bag. Follow your local protocols regarding how to preserve amputated parts. In some areas, dry sterile dressings are recommended for wrapping amputated parts; in other areas, dressings moistened with sterile saline are recommended. Put the bag in a cool container filled with ice. Lay the wrapped part on a bed of ice; do not pack it in ice. The goal is to keep the part cool without allowing it to freeze or develop frostbite. The amputated part should be transported with the patient. Remember that the wound needs to be cared for, including control of bleeding and appropriate bandaging.

■ Neck Injuries

An open neck injury can be life threatening. If the veins of the neck are open to the environment, they may suck in air **Figure 21-12 ▶**. If enough air is sucked into a blood vessel, it can actually block the flow of blood in the lungs, resulting in a life-threatening air embolism. To control bleeding and prevent the possibility of air embolism, cover the wound with an occlusive dressing. Apply manual pressure, but do not compress both carotid vessels at the same time; doing so may impair circulation to the brain and cause a stroke. Secure a pressure dressing over the wound by wrapping roller gauze loosely around the neck and then firmly under the arm.

■ Burns

Burns account for more than 10,000 deaths a year. Burns are also among the most serious and painful of all inju-

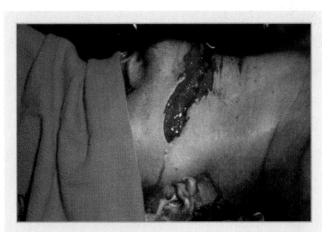

Figure 21-12 Open injuries to the neck can be very dangerous. If veins are open to the environment, they can suck in air, resulting in a potentially fatal condition called air embolism.

ries. A burn occurs when the body, or a body part, receives more radiant energy than it can absorb without injury. Potential sources of this energy include heat, toxic chemicals, and electricity. The proper emergency care of a burn may increase a patient's chances of survival and decrease the risk or duration of a long-term disability. Although a burn may be the patient's most obvious injury, you should always perform a complete assessment to determine whether there are other serious injuries.

Burn Severity

The severity of a burn may influence the choice of a treatment facility Table 21-1 ▼ .

Five factors will help you determine the severity of a burn:

- The depth of the burn
- The extent of the burn
- Critical areas (face, upper airway, hands, feet, genitalia) involved (also includes circumferential burns, which are burns that go completely around a body part such as an arm or foot).
- The presence of preexisting medical conditions or other injuries
- The patient is younger than 5 years or older than 55 years

Significant airway burns are also life threatening. You should suspect airway involvement if the patient has singeing of the hair within the nostrils, soot around the nose and mouth, hoarseness, or hypoxia.

Depth

Burns are first classified according to their depth Figure 21-13 ▶ :

- A superficial (first-degree) burn involves only the top layer of skin (epidermis). The skin turns red but does not blister or actually burn through. The burn site is painful. A sunburn is a good example of a superficial burn.
- A partial-thickness (second-degree) burn involves the epidermis and some portion of the dermis. These burns do not destroy the entire thickness of the skin, nor is the subcutaneous tissue injured. Typically, the skin is moist,

Table 21-1 Classification of Burns in Adults

Critical Burns

- Full-thickness burns involving the hands, feet, face, upper airway, genitalia, or circumferential burns of other areas
- Full-thickness burns covering more than 10% of the body's total surface area
- Partial-thickness burns covering more than 30% of the body's total surface area
- Burns associated with respiratory injury (smoke inhalation or inhalation injury)
- Burns complicated by fractures
- Burns on patients younger than 5 years or older than 55 years that would be classified as "moderate" on young adults

Moderate Burns

- Full-thickness burns involving 2% to 10% of the body's total surface area (excluding hands, feet, face, genitalia, or upper airway)
- Partial-thickness burns covering 15% to 30% of the body's total surface area
- Superficial burns covering more than 50% of the body's total surface area

Minor Burns

- Full-thickness burns covering less than 2% of the body's total surface area
- Partial-thickness burns covering less than 15% of the body's total surface area
- Superficial burns covering less than 50% of the body's total surface area

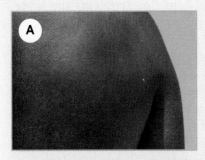
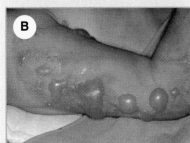
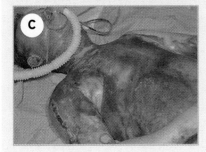

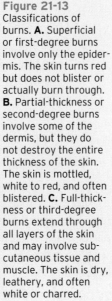

Figure 21-13 Classifications of burns. **A.** Superficial or first-degree burns involve only the epidermis. The skin turns red but does not blister or actually burn through. **B.** Partial-thickness or second-degree burns involve some of the dermis, but they do not destroy the entire thickness of the skin. The skin is mottled, white to red, and often blistered. **C.** Full-thickness or third-degree burns extend through all layers of the skin and may involve subcutaneous tissue and muscle. The skin is dry, leathery, and often white or charred.

Geriatric Needs

When treating geriatric patients with burns, it is important to be vigilant for the possibility of geriatric abuse. Geriatric patients who are institutionalized, disoriented, or incapable of clear communications are particularly susceptible to abuse.

Signs of abuse in the geriatric patient include evidence of multiple injuries in various stages of healing, injuries that do not seem to correspond to the history provided by caregivers, and burns associated with a suspicious history.

Burns that appear in a "pattern" are suspicious for intentional injuries. Multiple, small circular burns may be indicative of cigarette or cigar injuries. Other patterns may indicate irons, stovetops, or other hot surfaces not easily encountered accidentally. Scalding injuries to hands or feet may also be indicative of abuse. It is important to remember that these injuries are often inflicted in areas not readily seen. If the situation is suspicious for geriatric abuse, be sure to fully examine the patient under his or her clothing for signs of abuse. As always, appropriate support and transport of the patient in timely fashion remains a priority.

mottled, and white to red. Blisters are common. Partial-thickness burns cause intense pain.

- A <u>full-thickness (third-degree) burn</u> extends through all skin layers and may involve subcutaneous layers, muscle, bone, and internal organs. The burned area is dry and leathery and may appear white, dark brown, or even charred. Some full-thickness burns feel hard to the touch. Clotted blood vessels or subcutaneous tissue may be visible under the burned skin. If the nerve endings have been destroyed, a severely burned area may have no feeling. However, the surrounding, less severely burned areas may be extremely painful.

A pure full-thickness burn is unusual. Severe burns are typically a combination of superficial, partial-thickness, and full-thickness burns. Superficial burns heal well without scarring. Small partial-thickness burns also heal without scarring. However, deep partial-thickness burns and all full-thickness burns are best managed surgically.

Extent

One quick way to estimate the surface area that has been burned is to compare it with the size of the patient's palm, which is roughly equal to 1% of the patient's total body surface area. This technique is called "The Palmer Method." Another useful measurement system is the <u>Rule of Nines</u>, which divides the body into sections, each of which is approximately 9% of the total surface area `Figure 21-14 ▶`. Remember that the head of an infant or child is relatively larger than the head of an adult, and the legs are relatively smaller.

■ Assessment of Burns

Scene Size-up

Patients with burns can be very difficult to manage physically and emotionally. It is easy to become overwhelmed by the sight, sounds, and smells of burn injuries. As you prepare mentally to care for a burn

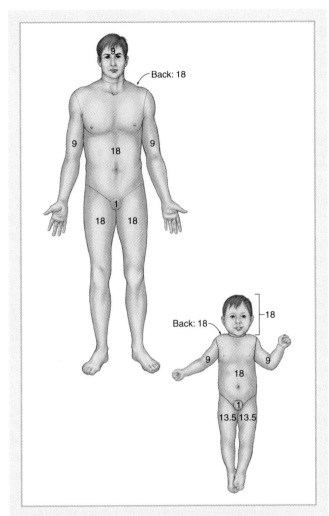

Figure 21-14 The Rule of Nines is a quick way to estimate the amount of surface area that has been burned. It divides the body into sections, each representing approximately 9% of the total body surface area.

Pediatric Needs

Burns to children are generally considered more serious than burns to adults. This is because infants and children have more surface area relative to total body mass, which means greater fluid and heat loss. In addition, children do not tolerate burns as well as adults do. Children are also more likely to go into shock, develop hypothermia, and experience airway problems because of the unique differences of their ages and anatomy.

Many burns in infants and children result from child abuse. The classic burn resulting from deliberate immersion involves the hands and wrists, as well as the feet, lower legs, and buttocks. Similarly, burns around the genitals and multiple cigarette burns should be viewed as possible abuse. You should report all suspected cases of abuse to the proper authorities.

units are needed, call for additional resources early. Anticipate using gloves and eye protection with any burn patient and gowns when serious injuries are expected. Remember, the burn patient is a trauma patient. Consider the potential for spinal injuries and other injuries.

Initial Assessment

General Impression

As you approach the burn trauma patient, simple clues can help identify how serious the injuries are and how quickly you need to assess and treat. Considerations for a significant MOI include a hoarse voice or your determination that the patient has been in an enclosed space with a fire or an intense heat source. Similarly, if the patient has singed facial hair, eyebrows, nasal hair, or moustache, your general impression would be that the patient has a potential airway and/or breathing problem.

Child abuse and elder abuse are unpleasant situations to handle. Unfortunately, they are often situations that involve burns. As you enter a scene where burns are involved, be suspicious of red flags that may indicate abuse.

The burned patient you encounter may have graphic injuries; however, you must not be distracted

patient, prepare yourself emotionally as well. Focus on your patient and immediate care. Do not get caught up in the issues surrounding child or elder abuse or dramatic-looking wounds. Focus on your goal: to quickly assess, treat, and transport your patient.

As you arrive on scene, observe the scene for hazards and threats to the safety of the crew, bystanders, and the patient. When responding to a burn injury, ensure that the factors that led to the patient's burn injury do not pose a hazard to you and your crew. Is the electricity turned off? Is the chemical leak secure? Has the fire been extinguished? At vehicle crashes, ensure that there are no energized electrical lines or leaking fuel in the area where you will be working. Begin with scene safety as the highest priority. If you determine that the power company, the fire department, or ALS

from the initial assessment. As you begin the initial assessment, always consider the need for manual spinal stabilization and determine responsiveness using the AVPU scale.

Airway and Breathing

Ensure that the patient has a clear and patent airway. If the patient is unresponsive or has a significantly altered level of consciousness, consider inserting an oral airway. Be alert to signs that the patient has inhaled hot gases or vapors, such as singed facial hair or soot present in or around the airway. Copious secretions and frequent coughing may also indicate a respiratory burn. You must also quickly assess for adequate breathing. Palpate the chest wall for DCAP-BTLS. Check for clear and equal breath sounds, and provide high-flow oxygen or assist breathing with bag-mask ventilation as needed. Burn patients are trauma patients. Evaluate and treat them for spinal injuries and airway problems concurrently.

Circulation

You must quickly assess the pulse rate and quality and determine perfusion based on the color, temperature, and condition of the skin. If you see significant bleeding, you must take the necessary steps to control it. Significant bleeding is an immediate life threat. If the patient has obvious life-threatening bleeding, it must be controlled quickly. Shock frequently develops in burn patients. Support their circulation by placing them in the shock position. Burn patients can become hypothermic owing to the damaged skin's limited ability to regulate body temperature.

Transport Decision

If the patient you are treating has an airway or breathing problem, significant burn injuries, significant external bleeding, or signs and symptoms of internal bleeding, you must consider rapid transport. Rendezvous with ALS providers may be appropriate for burn patients with moderate or severe burns and burns involving the airway. ALS providers can treat these pa-

tients with endotracheal intubation and intravenous fluids to support airway, breathing, and circulation (shock) problems. These problems can progress so rapidly that immediate ALS help can make the difference between life and death.

Focused History and Physical Exam
Rapid or Focused Physical Exam

After the initial assessment is complete, determine which assessment will be performed next, a rapid physical exam or a focused physical exam. In a responsive patient who has an isolated injury with a limited MOI, consider a focused physical exam. Focus your assessment on the isolated injury, the patient's complaint, and the body region affected. If the patient has a small burned area, focus on that injury. Dress the burn with the appropriate bandage, note the location, and estimate the size of the injury. Assess all underlying systems. In an extremity, assess pulse and motor and sensory function in the injured extremity.

If there is a significant amount of body surface burned or significant trauma that may affect multiple systems, start with a rapid trauma assessment, quickly assessing the patient from head to toe looking for DCAP-BTLS. Make a rough estimate, using the Rule of Nines, of the extent of the burned area. Package the patient for transport based on your findings. Remember to stabilize your patient for spinal injuries as appropriate. You should not delay transport of a seriously injured patient to complete a detailed physical exam.

Baseline Vital Signs and SAMPLE History

Determining an early set of baseline vital signs will help you know how your patient is tolerating his or her injuries. Vitals can be obtained en route, decreasing the delay to definitive care in a patient with moderate to severe burns.

Interventions

The goals of treating patients with burns are to stop the burning process, assess and treat airway and breath-

You are the Provider 4

En route to the hospital you note that the patient's abdomen is becoming distended and rigid. His mental status is not improving, and his vital signs are deteriorating slightly. The trauma team does a rapid assessment and he is rushed into surgery where they are able to stop the bleeding from his abdomen and stabilize his fractures. His other injuries are also addressed. He is placed in intensive care after surgery and then discharged to a rehabilitation center.

Teamwork Tips

Anticipate the need for early airway intervention. Call for an ALS unit as soon as you recognize the potential for airway edema as evidenced by singed facial hair, soot present in or around the airway, and/or copious secretions or frequent coughing.

ing, support circulation, and provide rapid transport. Because burn patients are also trauma patients, provide complete spinal stabilization if you suspect spinal injuries. Oxygen is mandatory for inhalation burns, but it is also helpful with smaller burns. If the patient has signs of hypoperfusion, treat aggressively for shock and provide rapid transport to the appropriate hospital. Cover all burns according to your local protocols. The risk of infection is very high and can be reduced if you cover large areas that are burned with sterile burn sheets or clean linen. Do not delay transport of a seriously injured patient to complete nonlifesaving treatments in the field, such as splinting extremity fractures.

Detailed Physical Exam

If the patient's condition is stable, perform a thorough detailed physical examination. Many times, short transportation times and unstable patient conditions make this assessment impractical.

Ongoing Assessment

Repeat the initial assessment and vital signs. Reevaluate interventions and treatment you have provided to the patient, particularly those used to treat airway and breathing problems and shock.

Communication and Documentation

Provide hospital personnel with a description of how the burn occurred. Many times they can determine

Documentation Tips

Report the extent of burns including:
- Amount of body surface area burned
- Depth of the burn
- Location of the burn

the appropriate treatment for chemical burns or calculate appropriate treatments for other types of burns with advanced notice. Your report and documentation should include the extent of the burns. This should include the amount of body surface area involved, the depth of the burn, and the location. For example, you may say 10% full-thickness burns, 15% partial-thickness burns, and 25% superficial burns to the chest, abdomen, and left lower extremity. If special areas are involved (genitalia, feet, hands, face, or circumferential), they should be specifically mentioned and documented.

Emergency Medical Care

Your first responsibility in caring for a burn patient is to stop the burning process and prevent additional injury. Follow these steps in caring for a burn patient Skill Drill 21-3 ▶ :

1. **Follow BSI precautions.** Because a burn destroys the patient's protective skin layer, always wear gloves and eye protection when treating a burn patient.

2. **Move the patient away from the burning area.** If any clothing is on fire, wrap the patient in a blanket. Remove any smoldering clothing and/or jewelry.

3. If allowed by local protocol, **immerse the area in cool, sterile water or saline solution,** or cover with a clean, wet, cool dressing if the skin or clothing is hot. Some EMS systems allow cooling with water only when 10% or less body surface area is burned. Water will not only stop the burning, but it also relieves pain. Prolonged immersion, however, may increase the risk of infection and hypothermia. As an alternative to immersion, the burned area can be irrigated until the burning stops, followed by the application of a sterile dressing (**Step ①**).

4. **Provide high-flow oxygen.** Remember that more fire victims die of smoke inhalation than of skin burns. A patient who has facial burns or has inhaled smoke or fumes may experience respiratory distress. Keep in mind that a patient who appears to be breathing well at first may suddenly experience severe respiratory distress. Continually assess the airway (**Step ②**).

5. **Rapidly estimate the severity of the burn.** Cover the burned area with a dry, sterile dressing to prevent further contamination. Sterile gauze is best if the area is not too large. You may cover

Skill Drill   21-3   Caring for Burns

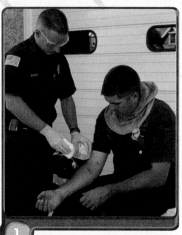

1 Follow BSI precautions to help prevent infection. If safe to do so, remove the patient from the burning area; extinguish or remove hot clothing and jewelry as necessary. If the wound(s) is still burning or hot, immerse the hot area in cool, sterile water, or cover with a wet, cool dressing.

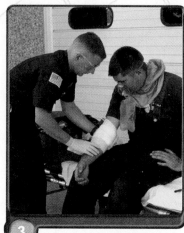

2 Provide high-flow oxygen and continue to assess the airway.

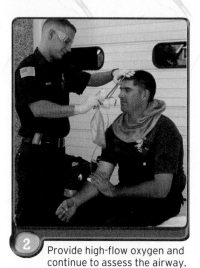

3 Estimate the severity of the burn, then cover the area with a dry, sterile dressing or clean sheet. Assess and treat the patient for any other injuries.

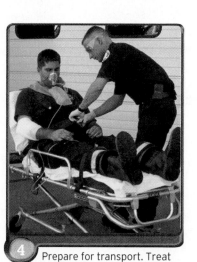

4 Prepare for transport. Treat for shock.

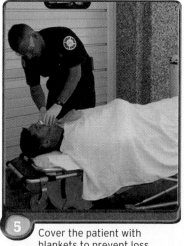

5 Cover the patient with blankets to prevent loss of body heat. Transport promptly.

larger areas with a clean, white sheet. Most important, do not put anything else on the burned area. Never use ointments, lotions, or antiseptics of any kind. In addition, do not intentionally break any blisters.

6. **Check for traumatic injuries or other medical conditions** that may be more immediately life threatening (**Step ③**).

7. **Treat the patient for shock** (**Step ④**).

8. An extensive burn can produce hypothermia (loss of body heat). **Prevent further heat loss by covering the patient with blankets.**

9. **Provide prompt transport.** Do not delay transport to perform a prolonged assessment or to apply dressings to burns in a patient in critical condition (**Step ⑤**).

■ Chemical Burns

A chemical burn can occur whenever a toxic substance contacts the body. Most chemical burns are caused by strong acids or strong alkalis. The eyes are particularly vulnerable to chemical burns. Sometimes the fumes alone from strong chemicals can cause respiratory tract burns.

To prevent exposure to hazardous materials, you must wear the appropriate chemical-resistant gloves and eye protection whenever you are caring for a patient with a chemical burn. Be particularly careful not to get any chemical, dry or liquid, on yourself or on your uniform. Remember that exposure risk is also present when you are cleaning up after a call. In cases of severe chemical burns or exposure, consider calling for assistance from the HazMat team.

The emergency care of a chemical burn is basically the same as treatment for a thermal burn. To stop the burning process, remove any chemical from the patient. A dry chemical that is activated by contact with water may damage the skin more when it is wet than when it is dry. Therefore, always brush dry chemicals off the skin and clothing before flushing the patient with water. Remove the patient's clothing, including shoes, socks, and gloves and any jewelry or glasses.

Immediately begin to flush the burned area with large amounts of water, taking care not to contaminate other areas or make the patient hypothermic. Never direct a forceful stream of water from a hose at the patient; the extreme water pressure may mechanically injure the burned skin. Continue flooding the area with gallons of water for 15 to 20 minutes after the patient says the burning pain has stopped. If an eye has been burned, hold the eyelid open while flooding the eye with a gentle stream of water. Continue flushing the contaminated area on the way to the hospital.

■ Musculoskeletal Injuries

A fracture is a broken bone. More precisely, it is a break in the continuity of the bone, often occurring as a result of an external force (Figure 21-15 ▶). The break can occur anywhere on the surface of the bone and in many different types of patterns.

A dislocation is a disruption of a joint in which the bone ends are no longer in contact. The supporting ligaments are often torn, usually completely, allowing the bone ends to separate completely from each other (Figure 21-16 ▶). A subluxation is similar to a dislocation except the disruption of the joints is not complete. A

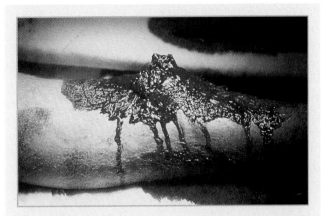

Figure 21-15 A fracture can occur anywhere on the surface of a bone and may or may not break the skin.

subluxation is an incomplete dislocation of a joint. A fracture-dislocation is a combination injury at the joint in which the joint is dislocated and there is a fracture of the end of one or more of the bones.

A sprain is a joint injury in which there is some partial or temporary dislocation of the bone ends and partial stretching or tearing of the supporting

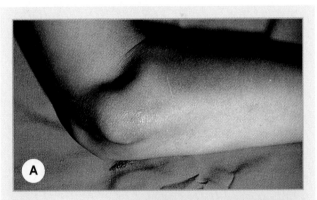

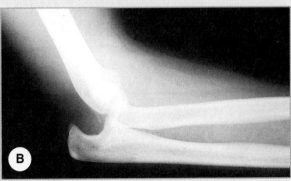

Figure 21-16 A dislocation is a disruption of a joint in which the bone ends are no longer in contact. **A.** The clinical appearance of an elbow dislocation. **B.** Radiographic appearance of the same elbow.

ligaments. After the injury, the joint surfaces generally fall back into alignment, so the joint is not significantly displaced. Sprains can range from mild to severe, depending on the amount of damage done to the supporting ligaments. The most severe sprains involve complete dislocation of the joint; mild sprains typically heal rather quickly.

A <u>strain</u>, or muscle pull, is a stretching or tearing of the muscle, causing pain, swelling, and bruising of the soft tissues in the area. Unlike a sprain, no ligament or joint damage typically occurs.

Injury to bones and joints is often associated with injury to the surrounding soft tissues, especially to the adjacent nerves and blood vessels. The entire area is known as the zone of injury (Figure 21-17 ▾). Depending on the amount of kinetic energy the tissues absorb from forces acting on the body, the zone may extend to a distant point. For this reason, you should not focus on a patient's obvious injury without first completing a rapid assessment to check for associated injuries, which may be even more serious. This is especially true in assessing damage from high-energy trauma or gunshots.

Mechanism of Injury

Significant force is generally required to cause fractures or dislocations. This force may be applied to the limb in any of the following ways:

- Direct blows
- Indirect forces
- Twisting forces
- High-energy injury

A direct blow fractures the bone at the point of impact. An example is the patella (kneecap) that fractures when it strikes the dashboard in an automobile crash.

Indirect force may cause a fracture or dislocation at a distant point, as when a person falls and lands on an outstretched hand. The direct impact may cause a wrist fracture, but the indirect force can cause dislocation of the elbow or a fracture of the forearm, humerus, or even clavicle. Therefore, when caring for patients who have fallen, you must identify the point of contact and the mechanism of injury so that you will not overlook associated injuries.

Twisting forces are a common cause of musculoskeletal injury, especially to the anterior cruciate ligament of the knee. Skiing injuries often happen this way.

High-energy injuries, such as those that occur in automobile crashes, falls from heights, gunshot wounds, and other extreme forces, produce severe damage to the skeleton, surrounding soft tissues, and vital internal organs. A patient may have multiple injuries to many body parts, including more than one fracture or dislocation in a single extremity.

A significant MOI is not necessary to fracture a bone. A slight force can easily fracture a bone that is weakened by a tumor or osteoporosis. In geriatric patients with osteoporosis, minor falls, simple twisting injuries, or even a muscle contraction can cause a fracture, most often of the wrist, spine, or hip. You should suspect the presence of a fracture in any older patient who has sustained even a mild injury.

Fractures

Fractures are classified as closed or open. In assessing and treating patients with possible fractures or dislocations, you should determine whether the overlying skin is damaged. If it is not, the patient has a <u>closed fracture</u>. With an <u>open fracture</u>, there is an external wound, caused by the same blow that fractured the bone or by

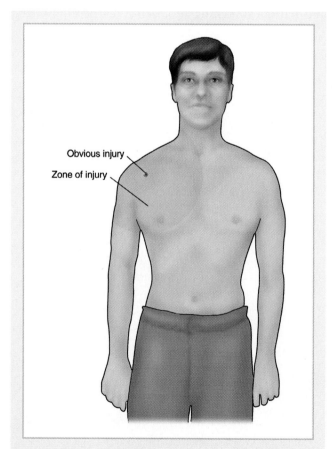

Figure 21-17 The zone of injury is the area of soft tissue, including the adjacent nerves and blood vessels, that surrounds the obvious injury of a bone or joint.

the broken bone ends lacerating the skin. The wound may vary in size from a very small puncture to a gaping tear that exposes bone and soft tissue. Regardless of the extent and severity of the damage to the skin, you should treat any injury that breaks the skin as a possible open fracture. Greater blood loss and a higher likelihood of infection are complications that you must try to limit.

Fractures are also described by whether the bone is moved from its normal position. A nondisplaced fracture (also known as a hairline fracture) is a simple crack of the bone that may be difficult to distinguish from a sprain or simple contusion. Radiographs are required for hospital personnel to diagnose a nondisplaced fracture. A displaced fracture produces actual deformity, or distortion, of the limb by shortening, rotating, or angulating it. Often, the deformity is obvious and can be associated with crepitus or free movement of a bone that is not normal for that region of the body. In some cases, the deformity is minimal. Be sure to look for differences between the injured limb and the opposite, uninjured limb in any patient with a suspected fracture of an extremity Figure 21-18 ▾ .

You should suspect a fracture if one or more of the following signs is present in any patient who has a history of injury and reports pain.

Deformity

The limb may appear to be shortened, rotated, or angulated at a point where there is no joint Figure 21-19 ▸ . Always use the opposite limb as a mirror image for comparison.

Tenderness

Point tenderness on palpation in the zone of injury is the most reliable indicator of an underlying fracture,

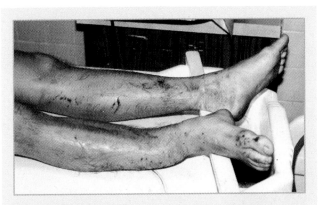

Figure 21-19 Obvious deformity, shortening, rotation, or angulation should increase your index of suspicion for a fracture. Remember to compare the injured limb with the opposite, uninjured limb.

although it does not tell you the type of fracture. Be sure to wear gloves if there are any open wounds.

Guarding

An inability to use the extremity is the patient's way of immobilizing it to minimize pain. The muscles around the fracture contract in an attempt to prevent movement of the broken bone. Guarding does not occur with all fractures; some patients may continue to use the injured part.

Swelling

Rapid swelling usually indicates bleeding from a fracture, and, typically, the patient complains of severe pain. Significant swelling may mask deformity of the extremity Figure 21-20 ▾ . Generalized swelling from fluid buildup may occur several hours after an injury.

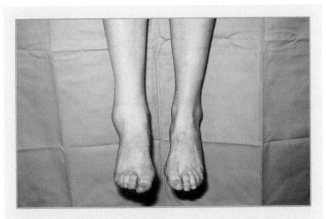

Figure 21-18 You should always compare the injured limb with the uninjured limb when checking for deformity.

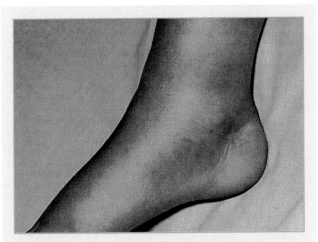

Figure 21-20 Swelling that occurs in association with a fracture can often mask deformity of the limb.

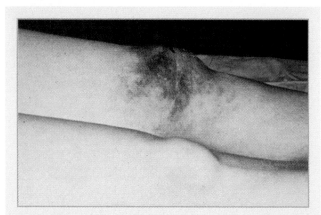

Figure 21-21 Fractures almost always have associated bruising of the surrounding soft tissue.

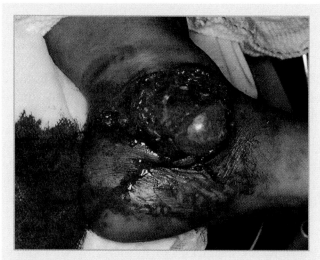

Figure 21-22 Bone ends may protrude through the skin or be visible within the wound of an open fracture.

Bruising

Fractures are almost always associated with ecchymosis (discoloration) of the surrounding soft tissues . Bruising may be present after almost any injury and may take hours to develop. The discoloration associated with acute injuries is usually a reddened area of the skin.

Crepitus

Crepitus is a grating or grinding sensation that can be felt and sometimes heard when fractured bone ends rub together.

False Motion

Also called free movement, this is motion at a point in the limb where there is no joint. It is a positive indication of a fracture.

Exposed Fragments

In open fractures, bone ends may protrude through the skin or be visible within the wound Figure 21-22 ▶ .

Locked Joint

A joint that is locked into position is difficult and painful to move. Keep in mind that crepitus and false motion appear only when a limb is moved or manipulated and are associated with injuries that are extremely painful. Do not manipulate the limb excessively in an effort to elicit these signs.

Dislocations

A dislocated joint sometimes will reduce spontaneously, or return to its normal position, before your as-

sessment. In this situation, you will be able to confirm the dislocation only by taking a patient history. Often, however, injury to the supporting ligaments and capsule is so severe that the joint surfaces remain completely separated from one another. A dislocation that does not spontaneously reduce is a serious problem. The ends of the bone can be locked in a displaced position, making any attempt at motion of the joint very difficult and painful. Commonly dislocated joints include the fingers, shoulders, elbows, and knees.

The signs and symptoms of a dislocated joint are similar to those of a fracture Figure 21-23 ▶ :

- Marked deformity
- Swelling
- Pain that is aggravated by any attempt at movement
- Tenderness on palpation
- Virtually complete loss of normal joint motion (locked joint)
- Numbness or impaired circulation to the limb or digit

Sprains

A sprain occurs when a joint is twisted or stretched beyond its normal range of motion. This results in the supporting capsule and ligaments being stretched or torn. A sprain should be considered a partial dislocation or subluxation. The alignment generally returns to a fairly normal position, although there may be some displacement. Note that severe deformity does not typically occur with a sprain. Sprains most often occur in the knee and the ankle, but a sprain

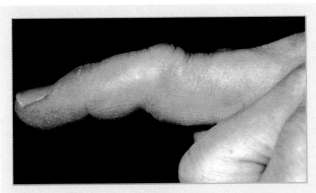

Figure 21-23 Joint dislocations, such as this finger, are characterized by deformity, swelling, pain with any movement, tenderness, locking, and impaired circulation.

can occur in any joint. The following signs and symptoms often indicate that the patient may have a sprain Figure 21-24 ▾ :

- Point tenderness can be elicited over the injured ligaments.
- Swelling and ecchymosis appear at the point of injury to the ligament as a result of torn blood vessels.
- Pain prevents the patient from moving or using the limb normally.
- Instability of the joint is indicated by increased motion, especially at the knee; however, this may be masked by severe swelling and guarding.

Compartment Syndrome

You should be aware of compartment syndrome, which most commonly occurs in a fractured tibia or forearm of children and is often overlooked, especially in patients with an altered level of consciousness.

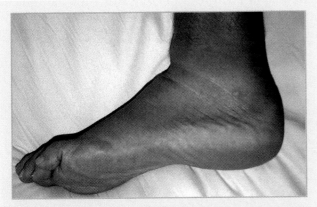

Figure 21-24 Sprains most often occur in the knee or ankle and are characterized by swelling, bruising, point tenderness, pain, and joint instability.

Compartment syndrome refers to elevated pressure within a fascial compartment. Fascia is the fibrous tissue that surrounds and supports the muscles and neurovascular structures.

Compartment syndrome typically develops within 6 to 12 hours after injury, usually as a result of excessive bleeding, a severely crushed extremity, or the rapid return of blood to an ischemic limb. This syndrome is characterized by pain that is out of proportion to the injury, pain on passive stretch of muscles within the compartment, pallor, decreased sensation, and decreased power (ranging from decreased strength and movement of the limb to complete paralysis).

If you suspect that a patient has compartment syndrome, splint the affected limb, keeping it at the level of the heart, and provide immediate transport, reassessing pulse and motor and sensory function frequently during transport. Compartment syndrome must be managed surgically.

■ Assessing Musculoskeletal Injuries

Always carefully assess the MOI to try to determine the amount of kinetic energy that an injured extremity may have absorbed, and maintain a high index of suspicion for associated injuries.

It is not important to distinguish between fractures, dislocations, sprains, and contusions. In most cases, your assessment will be reported as an "extremity injury." However, you must be able to distinguish mild injuries from severe injuries because some severe injuries may compromise neurovascular function.

Scene Size-up

Information from dispatch may indicate the MOI and the number of patients involved. Remember, the information given by the dispatcher is only as accurate as what the patient or bystanders report. In addition, the situation may change before your arrival at the scene. This information can still be used to help you consider whether spinal stabilization is needed, what equipment you may need, and whether hazards might be present.

As you arrive on scene, observe for hazards and threats to the safety of the crew, bystanders, and the patient. Try to identify the MOI: Could the forces involved produce injuries other than the musculoskeletal injuries reported by dispatch? BSI precautions may be as simple as gloves. Eye protection may also be indicated. Evaluate the need for law enforcement personnel, ALS, or additional ambulances, and request them early based on your initial scene assessment.

Initial Assessment

General Impression

Assess the patient's level of consciousness as you approach. Ask the patient his or her chief complaint and about the mechanism of injury. Was it a direct blow, indirect force, twisting force, or high-energy injury? In many of these situations, the musculoskeletal complaints will be simple and usually not life threatening; however, some situations, such as those with a significant MOI, will include multiple system trauma that includes musculoskeletal injuries. This initial interaction with your patient will provide you with a starting point and help you distinguish simple from complex injuries. If there was significant trauma and multiple body systems are affected, the musculoskeletal injuries are usually a lower priority. Scene time should not be wasted on prolonged musculoskeletal assessment or splinting.

Airway and Breathing

Fractures and sprains usually do not create airway and breathing problems. Other conditions, such as head injuries, intoxication, or other related illnesses and injuries may cause inadequate breathing. Evaluating the chief complaint and MOI will help you identify whether the patient has an open airway and whether breathing is present and adequate. Oxygen may be given to relieve anxiety and improve perfusion. Even though an injury to the arm or leg may be obvious, take the time to evaluate the adequacy of the airway and breathing. Little else matters if the patient's airway and breathing are inadequate.

Circulation

Your circulatory assessment should focus on determining whether the patient has a pulse, has adequate perfusion, or is bleeding. If your patient is conscious, as most patients with fractures and dislocations are, he or she will have a pulse. If the patient is unconscious, make sure there is a pulse and the patient is not in cardiac arrest. Hypoperfusion (shock) and bleeding will most likely be your primary concern. If the skin is pale, cool, or clammy and capillary refill time is slow, treat your patient for shock immediately. Maintain a normal body temperature, and improve perfusion with oxygen and by placing the patient in the shock position. If musculoskeletal injuries in the extremities are suspected, they at least must be initially stabilized, if not splinted, before moving.

Fractures can break through the skin and cause external bleeding. This may occur during the initial injury or during manipulation of the extremity while preparing for splinting or transport. Careful handling of the extremity will minimize this risk. If external bleeding is present, bandage the extremity quickly to control bleeding. The dressings that cover the wound and bone should be kept sterile to reduce the potential for bone infections. The bandage should be secure enough to control bleeding without restricting circulation distal to the injury. Monitor bandage tightness by assessing the circulation, sensation, and movement distal to the bandage. Swelling from fractures and internal bleeding may cause bandages to become too tight.

Transport Decision

If the patient you are treating has an airway or breathing problem or significant bleeding, you must consider rapid transport to the hospital for treatment. A patient who has a significant MOI but appears to be in otherwise stable condition should also be transported promptly to the closest appropriate hospital. Patients with bilateral fractures of the long bones (humerus, femur, or tibia) have been subjected to a high amount of kinetic energy. This should dramatically increase your index of suspicion for serious unseen injuries. When a decision for rapid transport is made, a backboard can be used as a splinting device to splint the whole body rather than splinting each extremity individually. Time taken to splint arms and legs individually delays prompt surgical intervention that may be needed for other injuries when a significant MOI has occurred. Individual splints should be applied en route if the ABCs are stable and time permits.

Patients with a simple MOI, such as twisting of an ankle or dislocating a shoulder, may be further assessed and their condition stabilized on scene before transport if no other problems are identified. Careful handling of fractures while preparing for transport is necessary to limit pain and prevent sharp bone ends from breaking through the skin or damaging nerves and blood vessels.

Focused History and Physical Exam

The focused history and physical exam is based on the MOI. The three parts of this step include a history from the patient, vital signs, and physical exam. Patients with musculoskeletal injuries may fall into a significant or nonsignificant MOI category.

During your assessment of musculoskeletal trauma, use the DCAP-BTLS approach. Identify any extremity deformities that likely represent significant musculoskeletal injury and stabilize appropriately.

Contusions and abrasions may overlie more subtle injuries and should prompt you to carefully evaluate the stability and neurovascular status of the limb. The presence of puncture wounds or other signs of penetrating injury should alert you to the possibility of an open fracture. Associated burns must be identified and treated appropriately. Palpate for tenderness, which, like contusions or abrasions, may be the only significant sign of an underlying musculoskeletal injury. When lacerations are present in an extremity, open fracture must be considered, bleeding controlled, and dressings applied. Careful inspection for swelling with comparison with the opposite limb may also reveal musculoskeletal injury.

Rapid Physical Exam for Significant Trauma

When significant trauma is involved, you should take a moment to rapidly check your patient from head to toe for any additional injury that may be present. Begin with the head and work systematically toward the feet, checking the head, chest, abdomen, extremities, and back. The goal is to identify hidden and potentially life-threatening injuries. This rapid exam will also help you prepare for packaging and rapid transport. Knowing whether an arm or leg is broken will be important when log rolling the patient onto a backboard and securing the patient to the board.

Focused Physical Exam for Nonsignificant Trauma

When the MOI is not significant and your patient has a simple strain, sprain, dislocation, or fracture, you can take the time to focus your exam on that particular injury. Look for DCAP-BTLS. Evaluate the circulation, motor function, and sensation distal to the injury. If the patient has two or more extremities injured, treat the patient as a significant trauma patient and provide rapid transport to the hospital. The likelihood of other more severe injuries is greater when two or more bones have been broken. Be sure to assess the entire zone of injury by removing clothing from the area and looking and palpating for injuries. In musculoskeletal injuries, this zone generally extends from the joint above (proximal) to the joint below (distal), front and back. Do not forget to check perfusion, motion, and sensation.

Many important blood vessels and nerves lie close to the bone, especially around the major joints. Therefore, any injury or deformity of the bone may be associated with vessel or nerve injury. For this reason, you must assess neurovascular function during the rapid or focused physical exam and repeat it in the detailed exam and every 5 to 10 minutes in the ongoing assessment, depending on the patient's condition. Always recheck the neurovascular function (pulse, motor function, and sensation) before and after you splint or otherwise manipulate the limb. Manipulation can cause a bone fragment to press against or impale a nerve or vessel. Failure to restore circulation in this situation can lead to death of the limb. Always give priority to patients with impaired circulation resulting from bone fragments.

Because many of the steps require patient cooperation, you will not be able to assess sensory and motor function in an unconscious patient, but you can still evaluate the limb for deformity, swelling, ecchymosis, false motion, and crepitus. If a patient is unconscious, perform an initial assessment first and then examine the extremities.

Baseline Vital Signs

Determine a baseline set of vital signs, including pulse rate, rhythm, and quality; respiratory rate, rhythm, and quality; blood pressure; skin condition; and pupil size and reaction to light. These baseline indicators need to be obtained as soon as possible. Trending these vital signs helps you understand whether your patient's condition is improving or getting worse over time, particularly during long transports. Shock or hypoperfusion is common in musculoskeletal injuries, and this baseline information will be important for ongoing assessment of your patient's condition.

SAMPLE History

A SAMPLE history should be obtained for all trauma patients. How much and in what detail you explore this history depends on the seriousness of the patient's condition and how quickly you need to transport the patient. Prehospital providers may have access to family members and others who have information about the patient's history. Make an attempt to obtain this history without delaying time to definitive care.

OPQRST can be of limited use in cases of severe injury and is usually too lengthy when life-threatening injuries require immediate attention. However, OPQRST may be useful in situations when the MOI is unclear, the patient's condition is stable, or details of the injury are uncertain.

Interventions

Because trauma patients often have multiple injuries, you must assess their overall condition, stabilize the ABCs, and control serious bleeding before further treating the injured extremity. In a critically injured patient, you should secure the patient to a long backboard to stabilize the spine, pelvis, and extremities and provide prompt transport to a trauma center. In this situation, extensive evaluation and splinting of limb injuries in the field is a waste of valuable time.

If the patient has no life-threatening injuries, you may take extra time at the scene to stabilize the patient and more completely evaluate the injured extremity. If possible, gently and carefully remove the patient's clothing to look for open fractures or dislocations, severe deformity, swelling, and ecchymosis. A good rule to follow is to check the patient's circulation, motor function, and sensation before and after splinting.

When you have finished assessing the extremity, apply a splint to stabilize the injury before transport. To minimize the potential for problems, the splint should be well padded. A comfortable and secure splint will reduce pain, improve shock, and minimize compromised circulation.

The main goal in providing care for musculoskeletal injuries is stabilization in the most comfortable position that allows for maintenance of good circulation distal to the injury. This should be done whether you are preparing the patient for rapid transport or have as much time as you need to assess and treat the patient.

Detailed Physical Exam

During the detailed physical exam, you can inspect and gently palpate the other extremities and the spine to identify areas of point tenderness that may indicate underlying fractures, dislocations, or sprains. Remember to compare the injured limb with the opposite, uninjured limb.

Ongoing Assessment

Repeat the initial assessment and vital signs. Assess the effectiveness of interventions and treatment you have provided to the patient. If a splint was applied, reassess the patient's distal neurovascular function and color of the injured extremity distal to the injury site. It is difficult to intervene when problems develop if you do not assess and reassess your patient's condition frequently.

Communication and Documentation

Your radio report to the hospital should include a description of injuries found during your assessment. In particular, you should report problems with the patient's ABCs, whether fractures are open, and whether circulation is compromised. How much you include in your radio report will depend on your local protocols.

Documentation Tips

Be sure to document the MOI along with a description of injuries. Note any loss of consciousness and PMS (pulse, motor, sensation) before and after splinting or movement.

Additional details can be given during your verbal report at the hospital when you transfer care.

Document complete descriptions of injuries and the MOIs associated with them. Hospital staff may later refer to these notes during confusing situations or when communication problems occur. It is important to assess and document the presence or absence of circulation, motor function, and sensation distal to the injury before you move an extremity, after manipulation or splinting of the injury, and on arrival at the hospital. Careful documentation provides a basis for ongoing care; in addition, it may prevent you from being included in legal action when patients are unhappy about outcomes from injuries. Do not rely on your memory to remember details from situations; it is unreliable and will not hold up in a court of law.

■ Emergency Medical Care

Your first steps in providing care for any patient are the initial assessment and stabilizing the patient's ABCs. Follow the steps in Skill Drill 21-4 ▶ when caring for patients with musculoskeletal injuries:

1. **Completely cover open wounds** with dry, sterile dressings, and apply direct pressure to control bleeding. Once you have applied a dressing, treat an open fracture in the same way as a closed fracture (**Step 1**).
2. **Apply the appropriate splint,** and elevate the extremity. Patients with lower extremity injuries should lie supine with the limb elevated about 6" to minimize swelling. For any patient, be sure to position the injured limb slightly above the level of the heart. Never allow the injured limb to flop about or dangle from the edge of the backboard. Always assess pulse and motor and sensory function before and after the application of splints (**Step 2**).
3. **If swelling is present, apply cold packs.** Avoid placing cold packs directly on the skin or other exposed tissues. Placing a cold pack on top of an air splint or other thick, insulating material will not help reduce swelling (**Step 3**).

Skill Drill 21-4   Caring for Musculoskeletal Injuries

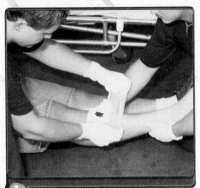

1 Cover open wounds with a dry, sterile dressing, and apply pressure to control bleeding.

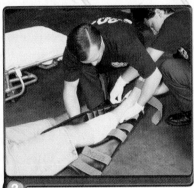

2 Apply a splint and elevate the extremity about 6" (slightly above the level of the heart).

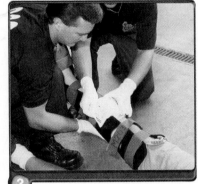

3 Apply cold packs if there is swelling, but do not place them directly on the skin.

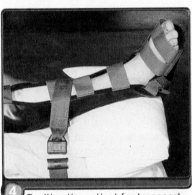

4 Position the patient for transport and secure the injured area.

4. **Prepare the patient for transport.** A patient with an isolated upper extremity injury will most likely be more comfortable in a semiseated position rather than lying flat (assuming there is no risk of spinal injury, either position is acceptable). Ensure that the extremity is elevated above the level of the heart and secured so that it does not dangle from the edge of the backboard (**Step ④**).

Splinting

A <u>splint</u> is a flexible or rigid device that is used to protect and maintain the position of an injured extremity. Unless the patient has life-threatening injuries, you should splint all injured extremities before moving the patient. By preventing movement of fracture fragments, bone ends, a dislocated joint, or damaged soft

tissues, splinting reduces pain and makes it easier to transfer and transport the patient. In addition, splinting helps to prevent the following:

- Further damage to muscles, the spinal cord, peripheral nerves, and blood vessels by broken bone ends
- Laceration of the skin by broken bone ends. One of the primary indications for splinting is to prevent a closed fracture from becoming an open fracture (conversion)
- Restriction of distal blood flow resulting from pressure of the bone ends on blood vessels
- Excessive bleeding of the tissues at the injury site caused by broken bone ends
- Increased pain from movement of bone ends
- Paralysis of extremities resulting from a damaged spine

General Principles of Splinting

The following principles of splinting apply to most situations:

1. **Expose the area** of any suspected fracture or dislocation so that you can inspect the extremity for DCAP-BTLS.
2. **Note and record the patient's neurovascular status** distal to the site of the injury, including pulse, sensation, and movement. Continue to monitor the neurovascular status until the patient reaches the hospital.
3. **Cover all wounds with a dry, sterile dressing** before splinting. Be sure to follow BSI precautions. Do not intentionally replace protruding bones. Notify the receiving hospital of all open wounds.
4. **Do not move the patient before splinting** an extremity unless there is an immediate hazard to the patient or yourself.
5. In a suspected fracture of the shaft of any bone, be sure to **stabilize the joints above and below the fracture.**
6. With injuries in and around the joint, be sure to **stabilize the bones above and below the injured joint.**
7. **Pad all rigid splints** to prevent local pressure and discomfort to the patient.
8. While applying the splint, **maintain manual stabilization** to minimize movement of the limb and to support the injury site.
9. If fracture of a long bone shaft has resulted in severe deformity, **use constant, gentle manual traction** to align the limb so that it can be splinted. This is especially important if the distal part of the extremity is cyanotic or pulseless.
10. **If you encounter resistance** to limb alignment, splint the limb in the position found.
11. **Stabilize all suspected spinal injuries** in a neutral in-line position on a backboard.
12. **If the patient has signs of shock** (hypoperfusion), align the limb in the normal anatomic position and provide transport (total body stabilization).
13. **When in doubt, splint.**

General Principles of In-line Traction Splinting

Application of in-line <u>traction</u> is the act of pulling on a body structure in the direction of its normal alignment. It is the most effective way to realign a fracture of the shaft of a long bone so that the limb can

be splinted more effectively. Excessive traction can be harmful to an injured limb. When applied correctly, however, traction stabilizes the bone fragments and improves the overall alignment of the limb. You should not attempt to reduce the fracture or force all the bone fragments back into alignment. In the field, the goals of in-line traction are as follows:

1. To stabilize the fracture fragments to prevent excessive movement
2. To align the limb sufficiently to allow it to be placed in a splint
3. To avoid potential neurovascular compromise

The amount of traction that is required to accomplish these objectives varies but often does not exceed 15 lb. You should use the least amount of force necessary. Grasp the foot or hand at the end of the injured limb firmly; once you start pulling, you should not stop until the limb is fully splinted. The direction of traction applied is always along the long axis of the limb. Imagine where the normal, uninjured limb would lie, and pull gently along the line of that imaginary limb until the injured limb is in approximately that position Figure 21-25 ▾ . Grasping the foot or hand and the initial pull of traction usually causes some discomfort as the bone fragments move. It helps if a second person can support the injured limb directly under the site of the fracture. This initial discomfort quickly subsides, and you can then apply further gentle traction. However, if the patient strongly resists the traction or if it causes more pain that persists, you must stop and splint the limb in the position it is in.

Remember that many different materials can be used as splints if necessary. When no splinting materials are available, the arm can be bound to the chest wall, and an injured leg can be bound to the uninjured leg to

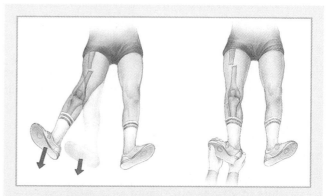

Figure 21-25 To apply traction, imagine the position where the normal uninjured limb would lie, then gently pull along that line until the injured limb is in that position. Do not release traction once you have applied it until a splint has been applied to the limb.

provide at least temporary stability. The three basic types of splints are rigid, formable, and traction splints.

Rigid Splints

Rigid (nonformable) splints are made from firm material and are applied to the sides, front, and/or back of an injured extremity to prevent motion at the injury site. Common examples of rigid splints include padded board splints, molded plastic and metal splints, padded wire ladder splints, and folded cardboard splints. As always, be sure to follow BSI precautions. Review the steps in Skill Drill 21-5 :

1. First EMT-B: **Gently support the limb** at the site of injury as others prepare and begin to position the equipment. Apply steady, in-line traction if necessary. Maintain this support until the splint is completely applied (**Step ①**).

2. Second EMT-B: **Place the rigid splint under or alongside the limb** (**Step ②**).

3. Second EMT-B: **Place padding between the limb and the splint** to make sure there is even pressure and even contact. Look for bony prominences, and pad them.

4. Second EMT-B: **Secure the splint** to the limb (**Step ③**).

5. Second EMT-B: **Check and record** the distal pulse, motor function, and sensation (**Step ④**).

Formable (Air) Splints

The most commonly used formable or soft splint is the precontoured, inflatable, clear plastic air splint. These are available in a variety of sizes and shapes, with or without a zipper that runs the length of the splint. Always inflate the splint after applying it. The

Skill Drill 21-5 — Applying a Rigid Splint

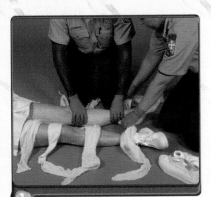
1. Provide gentle support and in-line traction for the limb.

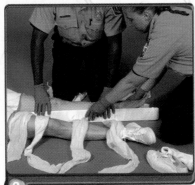
2. Second EMT places the splint alongside or under the limb. Pad between the limb and the splint as needed to ensure even pressure and contact.

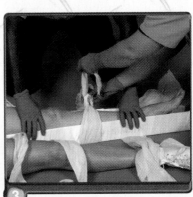
3. Secure the splint to the limb with bindings.

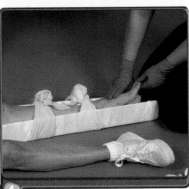
4. Assess and record distal neurovascular function.

air splint is comfortable, provides uniform contact, and has the added advantage of applying firm pressure to a bleeding wound. Air splints are used to stabilize injuries below the elbow or below the knee.

Air splints have some drawbacks, particularly in cold weather areas. The zipper can stick, clog with dirt, or freeze. Significant changes in the weather affect the pressure of the air in the splint, which decreases as the environment grows colder and increases as the environment grows warmer. The same thing happens when there are changes in altitude, which can be a problem with helicopter transport of patients. Therefore, you should carefully monitor the splint and let air out if the splint becomes overinflated.

The method of applying an air splint depends on whether it has a zipper. With either type, you must first cover all wounds with a dry, sterile dressing. For a splint that has a zipper, follow the steps in Skill Drill 21-6 ▼:

1. **Apply gentle traction and support** the site of injury. Have your partner place the open, deflated splint around the limb (**Step ①**).
2. **Zip the splint up and inflate it** by pump or by mouth. When this is done, test the pressure in the splint. With proper inflation, you should just be able to compress the walls of the splint together with a firm pinch between the thumb and index finger near the edge of the splint.
3. **Check and record pulse and motor and sensory functions,** and monitor them until the patient reaches the hospital (**Step ②**).

If you use an unzipped or partially zippered type of air splint, follow the steps in Skill Drill 21-7 ▶:

1. **Support the patient's injured extremity** until splinting is accomplished.
2. **Place your arm through the splint.** Extend your hand beyond the splint, and grasp the hand or foot of the injured extremity (**Step ①**).
3. **Apply gentle traction** to the hand or foot while sliding the splint onto the injured extremity. The hand or foot of the injured extremity should always be included in the splint (**Step ②**).
4. **Inflate the splint** by pump or by mouth (**Step ③**).
5. **Test the pressure** in the splint.
6. **Check and record pulse and motor and sensory functions,** and reassess en route.

Skill Drill 21-6 Applying a Zippered Air Splint

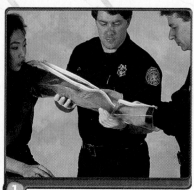

1 Support the injured limb and apply gentle traction as your partner applies the open, deflated splint.

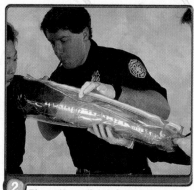

2 Zip up the splint, inflate it by pump or by mouth, and test the pressure. Check and record distal neurovascular function.

Skill Drill 21-7 — Applying an Unzipped Air Splint

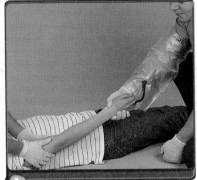

1 Support the injured limb. Have your partner place his or her arm through the splint to grasp the patient's hand or foot.

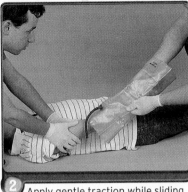

2 Apply gentle traction while sliding the splint onto the injured limb.

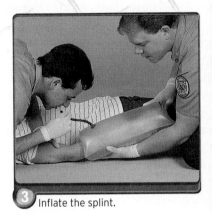

3 Inflate the splint.

Other formable splints include vacuum splints, pillow splints, SAM splints, sling and swathe, and a pneumatic antishock garment (PASG) for pelvic fractures. Just like an air splint, a vacuum splint can be easily shaped to fit around a deformed extremity. Instead of pumping air in, however, you can use a hand pump to pull the air out through a valve. Review the steps in Skill Drill 21-8 ▾ to apply a vacuum splint:

1. **Support and stabilize the injured extremity,** applying traction if needed, while your partner applies the splint (**Step ①**).
2. **Gently place the injured limb onto the vacuum splint** and wrap the splint around the extremity (**Step ②**).
3. **Draw the air out of the splint** through the suction valve, and then seal the valve. Once the valve is sealed, the vacuum splint becomes rigid,

Skill Drill 21-8 — Applying a Vacuum Splint

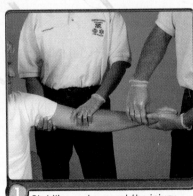

1 Stabilize and support the injury.

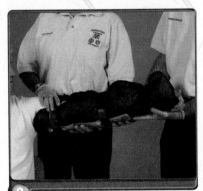

2 Place the splint and wrap it around the limb.

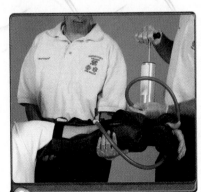

3 Draw the air out of the splint through the suction valve, and then seal the valve.

conforming to the shape of the deformed extremity and stabilizing it (**Step ③**). If the vacuum splint has straps, adjust them to secure the splint.

4. **Check and record pulse and motor and sensory functions,** and reassess en route.

Traction Splints

Traction splints are used primarily for fractures of the shaft of the femur, which are characterized by pain, swelling, and deformity of the midthigh. A traction splint should not be used if the patient has an obvious injury of the knee or ankle joint, foot, or lower leg. Several different types of lower extremity traction splints are commercially available, such as the Hare traction splint, the Sager splint, and the Kendrick splint, each with its own unique method of application with which you must be familiar. The Hare and Sager splints are reviewed in this chapter.

Do not use traction splints for any of the following conditions:

- Injuries of the upper extremity
- Injuries close to or involving the knee
- Injuries of the hip
- Injuries of the pelvis
- Partial amputations or avulsions with bone separation
- Lower leg, foot, or ankle injury

See **Skill Drill 21-9 ▶** to review the steps in applying a Hare traction splint:

1. **Expose the injury** by cutting open the patient's pant leg. Follow BSI precautions as needed. Be sure to assess and record the pulse, motor function, and sensation distal to the injury.

2. **Place the splint beside the patient's uninjured leg,** and adjust it to the proper length, with the ring at the ischial tuberosity and the splint extending 6" beyond the foot. Open and adjust the four Velcro support straps, which should be positioned at the midthigh, above the knee, below the knee, and above the ankle (**Step ①**).

3. First EMT-B: **Manually support and stabilize the injured leg** so that no motion will occur at the fracture site while the second EMT-B fastens the appropriately sized ankle hitch about the patient's ankle and foot. The patient's shoe should be removed (**Step ②**).

4. First EMT-B: **Support the leg at the site of the suspected injury** while the second EMT-B manually applies gentle longitudinal traction to the ankle hitch and foot. Use only enough force to align (reposition) the leg so that it will fit into the splint; do not attempt to align the fracture fragments anatomically (**Step ③**).

5. First EMT-B: **Slide the splint into position** under the patient's injured leg, making certain that the ring is seated well on the ischial tuberosity (**Step ④**).

6. **Pad the groin area,** and gently apply the ischial strap (**Step ⑤**).

7. First EMT-B: While the second EMT-B continues to maintain traction, **connect the loops of the ankle hitch** to the end of the splint. Then apply gentle traction to the connecting strap between the ankle hitch and the splint, just strongly enough to maintain alignment. Use caution. This splint comes with a ratchet mechanism to tighten the strap, which can overstretch the limb and further injure the patient. Adequate traction has been applied when the leg is the same length as the other leg or the patient feels relief (**Step ⑥**).

8. Once proper traction has been applied, **fasten the support straps** so that the leg is securely held in the splint. Check all proximal and distal support straps to make sure they are secure (**Step ⑦**).

9. **Reassess distal pulses,** motor function, and sensation.

10. **Place the patient securely on a long backboard** for transport. You may need to load the patient feet first into the ambulance so that you do not shut the door against the splint (**Step ⑧**).

Because this traction splint stabilizes the leg by producing countertraction on the ischium and in the groin, use care to pad these areas well. You must avoid excessive pressure on the external genitalia. Always use commercially available padded ankle hitches rather than pieces of rope, cord, or tape.

The Sager splint is lightweight and easy to store, applies a measurable amount of traction, and can be used with a PASG. Best of all, you can apply it by yourself when necessary. As with any splint, in addition to knowing the precise sequence of steps to apply the splint properly, you must practice the splinting technique frequently to maintain the necessary skills. Follow the steps below to apply a Sager splint **Skill Drill 21-10 ▶** :

1. **Expose the injured extremity.** Assess and record the pulse, motor function, and sensation distal to the injury.

2. **Estimate the proper splint length** by placing it alongside the injured limb, so that the wheel is at the level of the heel (**Step ①**).

Skill Drill 21-9 Applying a Hare Traction Splint

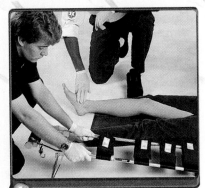

1 Expose the injured limb and check pulse, motor, and sensory function. Place the splint beside the uninjured limb, adjust the splint to proper length, and prepare the straps.

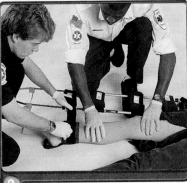

2 Support the injured limb as your partner fastens the ankle hitch about the foot and ankle.

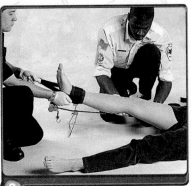

3 Continue to support the limb as your partner applies gentle in-line traction to the ankle hitch and foot.

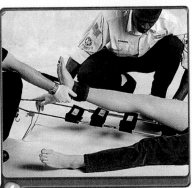

4 Slide the splint into position under the injured limb.

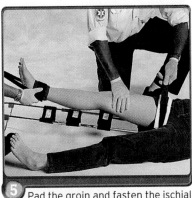

5 Pad the groin and fasten the ischial strap.

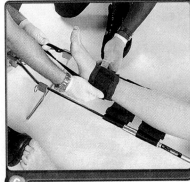

6 Connect the loops of the ankle hitch to the end of the splint as your partner continues to maintain traction. Carefully tighten the ratchet to the point that the splint holds adequate traction.

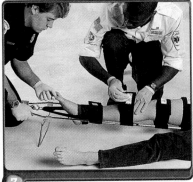

7 Secure and check support straps. Reassess pulse, motor, and sensory functions.

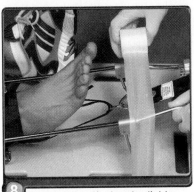

8 Secure the patient and splint to the backboard in a way that will prevent movement of the splint during patient movement and transport.

Skill Drill 21-10   Applying a Sager Traction Splint

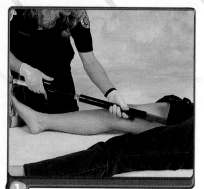

1 After exposing the injured area, assess pulse and motor and sensory function. Estimate the proper splint length by placing it alongside the injured limb.

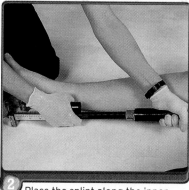

2 Place the splint along the inner aspect of the leg.

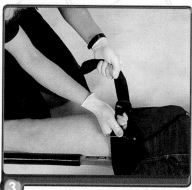

3 Apply the thigh strap at the upper thigh, and secure snugly.

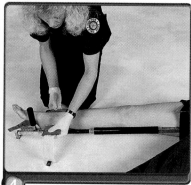

4 Fasten the ankle harness tightly around the patient's ankle just above the ankle bone. Snug the cable ring against the bottom of the foot.

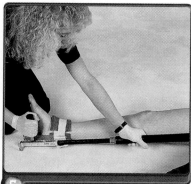

5 Extend the splint's inner shaft to apply traction to a maximum of 15 lb or approximately 10% of the patient's body weight. Stop when the injured leg is the same length as the uninjured leg or the patient feels relief.

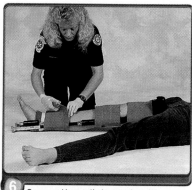

6 Secure the splint evenly with the elasticized straps. Place one over the fracture site, one over the knee, and the other midway between the knee and ankle.

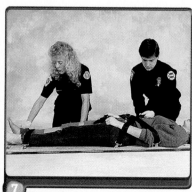

7 Reassess pulse, motor, and sensory function and then secure the patient to a long backboard.

3. **Place the splint along the inner aspect of the leg** (**Step** 2).
4. Slide the thigh strap around the upper thigh so that the perineal cushion is snug against the groin and the ischial tuberosity. **Tighten the thigh strap snugly** (**Step** 3).
5. **Secure the ankle harness** tightly around the patient's ankle just above the ankle bone. Pull the cable ring snugly up against the bottom of the foot (**Step** 4).
6. **Pull out the inner shaft** of the splint to apply traction of approximately 10% of body weight, using a maximum of 15 lb (**Step** 5).
7. **Secure the splint to the leg** using the elasticized straps (**Step** 6).
8. **Secure the patient to a long backboard,** and reassess pulse and motor and sensory function (**Step** 7).

You are the Provider Summary

Early recognition, care, and transport of the trauma patient ensure the best hope for survival in critical situations. There is no way to control internal bleeding in the field. Perform a rapid trauma assessment and only vital interventions on scene. All other assessments and care should be done en route to the closest appropriate facility.

1. **What should you do first?**
   - Ensure scene safety.
   - Recognize load-and-go based on the mechanism of injury.
   - Assume c-spine control.
   - Assess level of consciousness.
   - Assess ABCs.

2. **Should the patient's helmet be removed or left in place?**
   It should be removed so the airway can be opened with a jaw-thrust maneuver.

3. **How will you manage the airway?**
   Open the airway with a jaw-thrust maneuver. If it is patent, assess rate, quality, and degree of distress. Apply the appropriate oxygen therapy including airway adjunct if tolerated.

4. **What is the best option for packaging this patient?**
   Use PASG on long backboard. Remember that the primary indication for the use of the PASG is an unstable pelvis.

5. **How should his fractures be managed?**
   The PASG can be used to stabilize all of his lower extremity fractures. Individual splints would be time consuming and hinder use of the PASG for the unstable pelvis.

6. **What do the vital signs indicate?**
   They show signs of compensated shock.

7. **What is the proper management for the avulsion?**
   Rinse the avulsed part off if there is contamination. Move the avulsed part into its normal position. Cover with a dry dressing.

8. **What is the treatment for the abrasions?**
   Control any bleeding and cover with dry dressings.

9. **If you were not using the PASG, would a traction splint be appropriate for this patient?**
   No. The traction splint is for isolated femur fractures. It is contraindicated with an unstable pelvis and lower extremity fractures.

Assessment and Emergency Care

	Closed Injuries	Open Injuries	Burns
Scene Size-up	Body substance isolation precautions should include a minimum of gloves and eye protection. Ensure scene safety and determine NOI/MOI. Consider the number of patients, the need for additional help/ALS, and c-spine stabilization.	Body substance isolation precautions should include a minimum of gloves and eye protection. Ensure scene safety and determine NOI/MOI. Consider the number of patients, the need for additional help/ALS, and c-spine stabilization.	Body substance isolation precautions should include a minimum of gloves and eye protection. Ensure scene safety and determine NOI/MOI. Consider the number of patients, the need for additional help/ALS, and c-spine stabilization.
Initial Assessment			
■ General impression	Determine level of consciousness and treat any immediate threats to life. Determine priority of care based on environment and patient's chief complaint.	Determine level of consciousness and treat any immediate threats to life. Determine priority of care based on environment and patient's chief complaint.	Determine level of consciousness and treat any immediate threats to life. Determine priority of care based on environment and patient's chief complaint.
■ Airway	Ensure patent airway. Maintain spinal stabilization as necessary.	Ensure patent airway. Maintain spinal stabilization as necessary.	Ensure patent airway. Maintain spinal stabilization as necessary.
■ Breathing	Listen for abnormal breath sounds and evaluate depth and rate of respirations. Maintain ventilations as needed. Provide high-flow oxygen at 15 L/min and inspect the chest wall, assessing for DCAP-BTLS.	Listen for abnormal breath sounds and evaluate depth and rate of respirations. Maintain ventilations as needed. Provide high-flow oxygen at 15 L/min and inspect the chest wall, assessing for DCAP-BTLS.	Listen for abnormal breath sounds and evaluate depth and rate of respirations. Maintain ventilations as needed. Provide high-flow oxygen at 15 L/min and inspect the chest wall, assessing for DCAP-BTLS.
■ Circulation	Evaluate distal pulse rate and quality; observe skin color, temperature, and condition and treat accordingly.	Evaluate distal pulse rate and quality; observe skin color, temperature, and condition. Observe patient for shock and treat bleeding appropriately.	Evaluate distal pulse rate and quality; observe skin color, temperature, and condition and treat accordingly. Prevent heat loss.
■ Transport decision	Prompt transport	Prompt transport	Prompt transport
Focused History and Physical Exam	*NOTE: The order of the steps in the focused history and physical exam differs depending on whether or not the patient has a significant MOI. The order below is for a patient with a significant MOI. For a patient without a significant MOI, perform a focused trauma assessment, obtain vital signs, and obtain the history.*		
■ Rapid trauma assessment	Reevaluate the MOI(s). Perform a rapid trauma assessment, treating all life threats immediately. Log roll and secure patient to backboard for all patients with a significant MOI from the clavicles up.	Reevaluate the MOI(s). Perform a rapid trauma assessment, treating all life threats immediately. Log roll and secure patient to backboard for all patients with a significant MOI from the clavicles up.	Reevaluate the MOI(s). Perform a rapid trauma assessment, treating all life threats immediately. Estimate amount of body surface injured. Stabilize the patient for spinal injuries as appropriate.

	Closed Injuries	Open Injuries	Burns
■ Baseline vital signs	Take vital signs, noting skin color and temperature as well as patient's level of consciousness. Use pulse oximetry if available.	Take vital signs, noting skin color and temperature as well as patient's level of consciousness. Be alert to potential internal bleeding. Use pulse oximetry if available.	Take vital signs, noting skin color and temperature as well as patient's level of consciousness. Use pulse oximetry if available.
■ SAMPLE history	Obtain SAMPLE history. If the patient is not responsive, attempt to get history from family members, friends, or bystanders.	Obtain SAMPLE history. If the patient is not responsive, attempt to get history from family members, friends, or bystanders.	Obtain SAMPLE history. If the patient is not responsive, attempt to get history from family members, friends, or bystanders.
■ Interventions	Provide complete spinal stabilization early if you suspect that your patient has spinal injuries. Treat signs of hypoperfusion (shock) and consider ALS if available. Splint a painful, swollen, deformed extremity.	Provide complete spinal stabilization early if you suspect that your patient has spinal injuries. Treat signs of hypoperfusion (shock) and consider ALS if available. Splint a painful, swollen, deformed extremity.	Stop the burning process. Provide complete spinal stabilization if you suspect spinal injuries. Aggressively treat signs of hypoperfusion (shock) and consider ALS if available. Cover burns with dry, sterile dressings or per protocol.
Detailed Physical Exam	Complete a detailed physical exam.	Complete a detailed physical exam.	Complete a detailed physical exam.
Ongoing Assessment	Repeat the initial assessment, rapid or focused assessment, and reassess interventions performed. Reassess vital signs every 5 minutes for the unstable patient, every 15 minutes for the stable patient.	Repeat the initial assessment, rapid or focused assessment, and reassess interventions performed. Reassess vital signs every 5 minutes for the unstable patient, every 15 minutes for the stable patient.	Repeat the initial assessment, rapid or focused assessment, and reassess interventions performed. Reassess vital signs every 5 minutes for the unstable patient, every 15 minutes for the stable patient.
■ Communication and documentation	Contact medical control with a radio report. Relay any change in level of consciousness or difficulty breathing. Be sure to document physician's orders and changes in patient condition, and at what time they occurred.	Contact medical control with a radio report. Relay any change in level of consciousness or difficulty breathing. Document the MOI and the position in which the patient was found. Report location and description of injury, significant blood losses, and how you treated the injury. Document physician's orders and changes in patient condition, and at what time they occurred.	Contact medical control with a radio report. Describe how the burn occurred, and the extent of the burn(s). Relay any change in level of consciousness or difficulty breathing. Be sure to document physician's orders and changes in patient condition, and at what time they occurred.

Assessment and Emergency Care

Assessment and Emergency Care

NOTE: While the steps below are widely accepted, be sure to consult and follow your local protocol.

Closed Injuries

1. Keep the patient as quiet and comfortable as possible.
2. Apply ice (or cold packs).
3. Apply direct pressure.
4. Elevate the injured part just above the level of the patient's heart.
5. Splint the injured area.

Open Injuries

1. Apply direct pressure with a sterile bandage.
2. Maintain pressure with a roller bandage.
3. If bleeding continues, apply a second dressing and roller bandage over the first.
4. Splint the extremity.

Burns

1. Follow BSI precautions.
2. Move the patient away from the burning area.
3. Immerse the burned skin in cool, sterile water.
4. Provide high-flow oxygen.
5. Cover the patient with a clean blanket.
6. Rapidly estimate the burn's severity.
7. Check for traumatic injuries.
8. Treat the patient for shock.
9. Provide prompt transport.

Abdominal Injuries

1. Do not touch or move exposed organs.
2. Keep organs moist. Use moist sterile dressings, cover and secure in place.
3. If the patient's legs and knees are uninjured, flex them to relieve pressure on the abdomen.

Impaled Objects

1. Do not attempt to move or remove the object.
2. Control bleeding and stabilize the object in place using soft dressings, gauze, and/or tape.
3. Tape a rigid item over the stabilized object to protect it from movement during transport.

Neck Wounds

1. Cover wound with occlusive dressing.
2. Apply manual pressure, but do not compress both carotid vessels at the same time.
3. Secure dressing over the wound.

Chemical Burns

1. Stop the burning process; safely remove any chemical from the patient, always brushing off a dry chemical.
2. Remove all of the patient's clothing.
3. Flush the burn area with large amounts of water for 15 to 20 minutes after the patient says the burning has stopped.

Musculoskeletal Injuries

Scene Size-up	Body substance isolation precautions should include a minimum of gloves and eye protection. Ensure scene safety and determine NOI/MOI. Consider the number of patients, the need for additional help/ALS, and c-spine stabilization.
Initial Assessment	
■ General impression	Determine level of consciousness and treat any immediate threats to life. Determine priority of care based on environment and patient's chief complaint.
■ Airway	Ensure patent airway.
■ Breathing	Listen for abnormal breath sounds and evaluate depth and rate of the respirations. Look for symmetric chest rise and fall. Maintain ventilations as needed. Provide high-flow oxygen at 15 L/min and inspect the chest wall, assessing for DCAP-BTLS.
■ Circulation	Evaluate pulse rate and quality; observe skin color, temperature, and condition, and treat accordingly.
■ Transport decision	Prompt transport
Focused History and Physical Exam	NOTE: The order of the steps in the focused history and physical exam differs depending on whether or not the patient has a significant MOI. The order below is for a patient with a significant MOI. For a patient without a significant MOI, perform a focused trauma assessment, obtain vital signs, and obtain the history.
■ Rapid trauma assessment	Reevaluate the mechanism of injury. Perform a rapid trauma assessment, treating all life-threats immediately. Log roll and secure patient to backboard for all patients with a suspected spinal injury.
■ Baseline vital signs	Take vital signs, noting skin color and temperature as well as patient's level of consciousness. Use pulse oximetry if available.
■ SAMPLE history	Obtain SAMPLE history. If the patient is unresponsive, attempt to obtain information from family members, friends, or bystanders. Consider obtaining pertinent OPQRST information for patients with minor injuries.
■ Interventions	Provide complete spinal immobilization early if you suspect that your patient has spinal injuries. Maintain an open airway and suction as needed. Immobilize musculoskeletal injuries as per protocol; treat signs of shock and any other life threats.
Detailed Physical Exam	Complete a detailed physical exam.
Ongoing Assessment	Repeat the initial assessment, rapid/focused assessment, and reassess interventions performed. Reassess vital signs every 5 minutes for the unstable patient, every 15 minutes for the stable patient.
■ Communication and documentation	Contact medical control with a radio report. Relay any change in level of consciousness or difficulty breathing. Describe the MOI and any interventions you performed. Be sure to document any physician's orders and changes in the patient's condition and at what time they occurred.

Assessment and Emergency Care

Assessment and Emergency Care

NOTE: While the steps below are widely accepted, be sure to consult and follow your local protocol.

Musculoskeletal Injuries

Caring for Musculoskeletal Injuries

1. Cover open wounds with a dry, sterile dressing, and apply pressure to control bleeding.
2. Assess pulse, motor function, and sensory function prior to splinting.
3. Apply a splint and elevate the extremity about 6" (slightly above the level of the heart).
4. Assess pulse, motor function, and sensory function immediately after splinting and frequently in transit.
5. Apply cold packs if there is swelling, but do not place them directly on the skin.
6. Position the patient for transport and secure the injured area.

Applying a Rigid Splint

1. Provide gentle support and in-line traction for the limb.
2. Second EMT places the splint alongside or under the limb. Pad between the limb and the splint as needed to ensure even pressure and contact.
3. Secure the splint to the limb with bindings.
4. Assess and record distal neurovascular function.

Applying a Zippered Air Splint

1. Support the injured limb and apply gentle traction as your partner applies the open, deflated splint.
2. Zip up the splint, inflate it by pump or by mouth, and test the pressure. Check and record distal neurovascular function.

Applying an Unzippered Air Splint

1. Support the injured limb. Have your partner place his or her arm through the splint to grasp the patient's hand or foot.
2. Apply gentle traction while sliding the splint onto the injured limb.
3. Inflate the splint.

Applying a Vacuum Splint

1. Stabilize and support the injury.
2. Place the splint and wrap it around the limb.
3. Draw the air out of the splint and seal the valve.

Applying a Hare Traction Splint

1. Expose the injured limb and check pulse, motor, and sensory function. Place the splint beside the uninjured limb, adjust the splint to proper length, and prepare the straps.
2. Support the injured limb as your partner fastens the ankle hitch about the foot and ankle.
3. Continue to support the limb as your partner applies gentle in-line traction to the ankle hitch and foot.
4. Slide the splint into position under the injured limb.
5. Pad the groin and fasten the ischial strap.
6. Connect the loops of the ankle hitch to the end of the splint as your partner continues to maintain traction. Carefully tighten the ratchet to the point that the splint holds adequate traction.
7. Secure and check support straps. Assess pulse, motor, and sensory functions.
8. Secure the patient and splint to the backboard in a way that will prevent movement of the splint during patient movement and transport.

Applying a Sager Traction Splint

1. After exposing the injured area, check the patient's pulse and motor and sensory function. Adjust the thigh strap so that it lies anteriorly when secured.
2. Estimate the proper length of the splint by placing it next to the injured limb. Fit the ankle pads to the ankle.
3. Place the splint at the inner thigh, apply the thigh strap at the upper thigh, and secure snugly.
4. Tighten the ankle harness just above the malleoli. Snug the cable ring against the bottom of the foot.
5. Extend the splint's inner shaft to apply traction of about 10% of body weight.
6. Secure the splint with elasticized cravats.
7. Secure the patient to a long backboard. Check pulse, motor, and sensory functions.

Prep Kit

Ready for Review

- The skin has three layers: the epidermis (tough outer layer), the dermis (inner layer containing hair follicles, sweat glands, and sebaceous glands), and the subcutaneous (containing fat and muscle layers).
- The main functions of the skin are to keep pathogens out and fluid in, maintain body temperature, and provide environmental information to the brain.
- Soft-tissue injuries are classified into three groups: closed injuries, open injuries, and burns.
- Closed injuries include hematomas and crushing injuries. Treatment includes RICES (rest, ice, compression, elevation, and splinting).
- Open injuries produce more extensive bleeding and increase the risk for infection. There are five types of open injuries: abrasions, lacerations, incisions, avulsions, and penetrating.
- To treat open injuries, control bleeding and apply sterile dressings; avoid cleaning an open wound because this may aggravate bleeding.
- Burns are serious and painful soft-tissue injuries caused by heat (thermal), chemicals, electricity, and radiation.
- Burns are classified primarily by the depth and extent of the burn injury and the body area involved. Burns are considered superficial, partial thickness, or full thickness based on the depth involved.
- Emergency care for burns includes the following:
  - Use BSI precautions to protect yourself from potentially contaminated body fluid and to protect the patient from potential infection.
  - Cool the burned area to prevent further cellular damage.
  - Remove jewelry or constrictive clothing; never attempt to remove synthetic material that may have melted into the burned skin.
  - Ensure an open and clear airway, provide high-flow oxygen, and be alert to signs and symptoms of inhalation injury such as difficulty breathing, stridor, and wheezing.
  - Place sterile dressings over the burned area(s); prevent hypothermia by covering the patient with a clean blanket. Provide prompt transport.
- Dressings and bandages are designed to control bleeding, protect the wound from further damage, prevent further contamination, and prevent infection.
- There are 206 bones in the human body. When this living tissue is fractured, it can produce bleeding and significant pain.
- A joint is a junction where two bones come into contact. Joints are stabilized by ligaments.
- A fracture is a broken bone, a dislocation is a disruption of a joint, a sprain is a stretching injury to the ligaments around a joint, and strain is stretching of muscle.

- Depending on the amount of kinetic energy absorbed by tissues, the zone of injury may extend beyond the point of contact. Always maintain a high index of suspicion for associated injuries.
- Fractures of the bones are classified as open or closed. Both are splinted in a similar manner, but remember to control bleeding and apply a sterile dressing to an open extremity injury before splinting.
- Fractures and dislocations are often difficult to diagnose without radiographs. Stabilize the injury with a splint, and transport the patient.
- Signs of fractures and dislocations include pain, deformity, point tenderness, false movement, crepitus, swelling, and bruising.
- Always assess the trauma patient with the same technique: address the initial assessment and correct problems, determine whether you will use the rapid trauma exam or focused trauma exam, obtain the SAMPLE history, and obtain baseline vital signs. When treating musculoskeletal injuries, always assess for pulse and motor and sensory function before and after applying a splint. Reassess these functions during the ongoing assessment.
- Compare the unaffected extremity with the injured extremity for differences whenever possible.
- There are three main types of splints used by EMS: rigid splints, traction splints, and air splints.
- Remember to splint the injured extremity from the joint above to the joint below the injury site for complete stabilization.

Vital Vocabulary

abrasion Loss or damage of the superficial layer of skin as a result of a body part rubbing or scraping across a rough or hard surface.

avulsion An injury in which soft tissue is torn completely loose or is hanging as a flap.

burns Injuries in which the soft tissue receives more energy from thermal heat, frictional heat, toxic chemicals, electricity, or nuclear radiation than it can absorb without injury.

Technology

- Interactivities
- Vocabulary Explorer
- Anatomy Review
- Web Links
- Online Review Manual

closed fracture A fracture in which the skin is not broken.

closed injuries Injuries in which damage occurs beneath the skin or mucous membrane but the surface remains intact.

compartment syndrome Swelling in a confined space that produces dangerous pressure; may cut off blood flow and damage sensitive tissue.

contusion A bruise without a break in the skin.

crepitus A grating or grinding sensation or sound caused by fractured bone ends or joints rubbing together.

dermis The inner layer of the skin, containing hair follicles, sweat glands, nerve endings, and blood vessels.

dislocation Disruption of a joint in which ligaments are damaged and the bone ends are completely displaced.

ecchymosis Discoloration associated with a closed wound; signifies bleeding.

epidermis The outer layer of skin that acts as a watertight protective covering.

evisceration The displacement of organs outside the body.

fracture A break in the continuity of a bone.

full-thickness (third-degree) burn A burn that affects all skin layers and may affect the subcutaneous layers, muscle, bone, and internal organs, leaving the area dry, leathery, and white, dark brown, or charred.

hematoma Blood collected within the body's tissues or in a body cavity.

incision A sharp or smooth cut.

laceration A jagged open wound.

mucous membranes The linings of body cavities and passages that are in direct contact with the outside environment.

occlusive dressing A dressing made of Vaseline gauze, aluminum foil, or plastic that prevents air and liquids from entering or exiting a wound.

open fracture Any break in a bone in which the overlying skin has been damaged.

open injuries Injuries in which there is a break in the surface of the skin or the mucous membrane, exposing deeper tissue to potential contamination.

partial-thickness (second-degree) burn A burn affecting the epidermis and some portion of the dermis but not the subcutaneous tissue, characterized by blisters and skin that is white to red, moist, and mottled.

penetrating wound An injury resulting from a sharp, pointed object.

Rule of Nines A system that assigns percentages to sections of the body, allowing calculation of the amount of skin surface involved in the burned area.

splint A flexible or rigid appliance used to protect and maintain the position of an injured extremity.

sprain A joint injury involving damage to supporting ligaments and sometimes partial or temporary dislocation of bone ends.

strain Stretching or tearing of a muscle; also called a muscle pull.

superficial (first-degree) burn A burn affecting only the epidermis, characterized by skin that is red but not blistered or actually burned through.

traction Longitudinal force applied to a structure.

Assessment in Action

Burns account for over 10,000 deaths a year. You and your partner are called to a patient burned at a factory. While en route to the location, you discuss the procedures for assessment and treatment of burns.

1. Respiratory burns may be indicated by _____.
   - **A.** eupnea
   - **B.** singed facial hair
   - **C.** hiccups
   - **D.** lack of secretions

2. Documentation of a burn patient should include:
   - **A.** the location of the burn.
   - **B.** the amount of BSA involved.
   - **C.** the depth of the burn.
   - **D.** all of the above.

3. A sunburn is an example of what degree of burn?
   - **A.** first degree
   - **B.** second degree
   - **C.** third degree
   - **D.** fourth degree

4. Potential sources of burns include _____.
   - **A.** heat
   - **B.** toxic chemicals
   - **C.** electricity
   - **D.** all of the above

5. What is the correct procedure for treating a patient who has been burned by a dry chemical?
   - **A.** remove by flushing with water
   - **B.** apply wet dressing to the burned area
   - **C.** brush excess chemical from skin
   - **D.** rapid transport to emergency department for decontamination

6. Critical areas of the body include the face, hands, feet, and _____?
   - **A.** chest
   - **B.** genitalia
   - **C.** knees
   - **D.** back

Challenging Questions

7. Explain "The Palmer Method."

22

Chest and Abdominal Injuries

You are on scene with a 41-year-old man with a gunshot wound to the chest. The entrance wound is on the right side, midclavicular, between the fourth and fifth intercostal spaces. The blood is bubbling around the site and you hear a sucking sound as he breathes. A fire fighter is providing cervical spine control while your partner gathers supplies.

Initial Assessment	Recording Time: 0 Minutes
Appearance	Pale, diaphoretic
Level of consciousness	Responsive to painful stimuli
Airway	Open and clear
Breathing	A little fast and shallow
Circulation	Radial pulses present

1. What is the first step in treating this patient?
2. What structures may have been affected by the gunshot wound?
3. How is this injury classified?
4. What type of oxygen should this patient receive?

Introduction

Trauma situations often result in injuries to the chest and abdomen. Given the location of the heart, lungs, and great blood vessels within the chest cavity, potentially serious injuries may occur. Any injury that interferes with the body's mechanics of normal breathing must be treated without delay to minimize or prevent permanent damage to tissues that depend on a continuous supply of oxygen. Blood from the thoracic organs or major vessels can collect in the chest cavity, compressing the lungs. Air can collect in the chest as well. Serious injuries and significant blood loss may also occur to the organs in the abdominal cavity. Quick action when caring for patients with these injuries is crucial to a successful outcome. This chapter reviews the anatomy and physiology of the chest and abdomen. It then describes common signs, symptoms, and assessment for specific chest and abdominal injuries. The chapter concludes with a review of the emergency medical care for patients with chest and abdominal injuries.

Anatomy and Physiology of the Chest

A review of the anatomy of the chest and the mechanism by which gases are exchanged during breathing will help you understand the reasoning behind the emergency medical care of chest injuries.

A key point to remember is the difference between the concepts of ventilation and respiration. Ventilation is the body's ability to move air in and out of the chest and lung tissue. Any injury that affects the patient's ability to move air in and out of the chest is significant and may be life threatening. Respiration is the exchange of gases in the alveoli—the terminal point of the pulmonary system. Oxygen must be delivered to the cells, and carbon dioxide (a waste product of cell function) must be removed from the body for proper organ system function.

The chest (thoracic cage) extends from the lower end of the neck to the diaphragm (Figure 22-1). In a person who is lying down or who has just completed exhalation, the diaphragm may rise as high as the nipple line. A penetrating injury to the chest, such as a gunshot or stab wound, not only may damage the lung and diaphragm, but also may injure the liver or stomach.

Each side of the chest contains a lung that is separated into lobes. The right lung has three lobes, and the left lung has two lobes. A thin membrane (pleura) covers the lungs. The lining on the inner chest wall is called the parietal pleura. The lung itself is covered by a lining called the visceral pleura. Between these

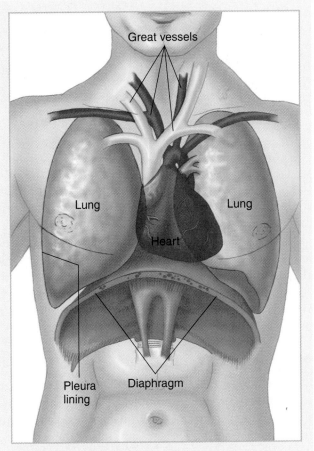

Figure 22-1 A view of the anterior aspect of the chest shows the major organs beneath the surface.

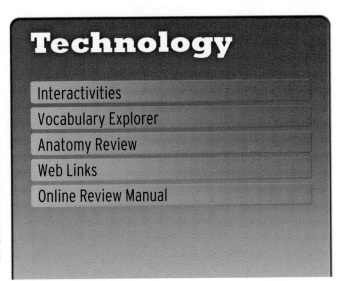

Refresher.EMSzone.com

Technology

Interactivities

Vocabulary Explorer

Anatomy Review

Web Links

Online Review Manual

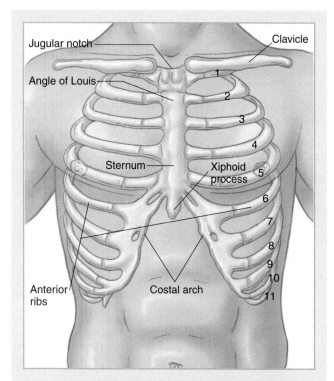

Figure 22-2 The organs within the chest are protected by the ribs, which are connected in back to the vertebrae and in the front, through the costal cartilages, to the sternum.

linings is a small amount of fluid that allows the lungs to move freely against the inner chest wall as breathing occurs.

The contents of the chest are partially protected by the ribs, which are connected in the back to the vertebrae and in the front, through the costal cartilages, to the sternum (Figure 22-2 ▲). The trachea divides into the left and right mainstem bronchi, which supply air to the lungs. The thoracic cage also contains the heart and the great vessels: the aorta, the right and left subclavian arteries and their branches, and the superior and inferior vena cava. The esophagus runs through the back of the chest, connecting the pharynx with the stomach and the abdomen below. The diaphragm is a muscle that separates the thoracic cavity from the abdominal cavity.

Mechanics of Ventilation

On inhalation, the intercostal muscles between the ribs contract, elevating the rib cage. At the same time, the diaphragm contracts and pushes the contents of the abdomen down. The pressure inside the chest decreases, and air enters the lungs through the nose and mouth. On exhalation, the intercostal muscles and diaphragm relax, and the organs and tissues move back

to their normal positions, allowing air to be exhaled. Note that the nerves supplying the diaphragm (the phrenic nerves) exit the spinal cord at C3, C4, and C5. A patient whose spinal cord is injured below the C5 level will lose the power to move his or her intercostal muscles, but the diaphragm will still contract. The patient will still be able to breathe because the phrenic nerves remain intact. Patients with spinal cord injuries at C3 or above can lose their ability to breathe entirely.

■ Injuries of the Chest

Chest injuries can be open or closed. A closed chest injury is one in which the skin is not broken. This type of injury is generally caused by blunt trauma, such as when a driver strikes a steering wheel in a motor vehicle crash or a person is struck by a falling object or is struck in the chest by an object during a fight or physical assault (Figure 22-3 ▼). In an open chest injury, the chest wall itself is penetrated by an object such as a knife, a bullet, a piece of metal, or the broken end of a fractured rib.

In blunt trauma, a blow to the chest may fracture the ribs, the sternum, or whole areas of the chest wall; bruise the lungs and the heart; and even damage the aorta. Almost one third of people who are killed immediately in car crashes die as a result of traumatic rupture of the aorta. Closed chest injuries can result in significant internal bleeding when broken ribs lacerate the organs or blood vessels. Damage to the chest wall structures may result in decreased ability of patients to ventilate on their own. Also, vital organs can actually be torn from their attachment in the chest cavity with-

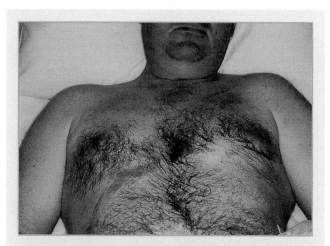

Figure 22-3 Closed injuries usually result from blunt trauma, such as when a person strikes the steering wheel in a motor vehicle crash or is struck by a falling object.

out any break in the skin. This condition can cause serious and life-threatening internal bleeding.

Signs and Symptoms

Signs and symptoms of chest injury include the following:

- Pain at the site of injury
- Pain localized at the site of injury that is aggravated by or increased with breathing
- Bruising of the chest wall
- Crepitus with palpation of the chest
- Any penetrating injury to the chest
- Dyspnea (difficulty breathing, shortness of breath)
- <u>Hemoptysis</u> (coughing up blood)
- Failure of one or both sides of the chest to expand normally with inspiration
- Rapid, weak pulse and low blood pressure after experiencing trauma to the chest
- Cyanosis around the lips or fingernails

After a chest injury, any change in normal breathing (rate, depth, quality, and effort) indicates a potentially life-threatening injury. Respirations less than 12 breaths/min or more than 20 breaths/min may indicate inadequate breathing. Patients with chest injuries often have rapid and shallow respirations because it hurts to take a deep breath. Remember that the patient may be making breathing attempts but may not actually be moving air. Chest wall trauma such as a sucking chest wound or flail chest may interfere with the ability to actually move air.

As with any other injury, pain and tenderness are common at the point of impact as a result of a bruise or fracture. Pain is usually aggravated by the normal process of breathing. Irritation of or damage to the pleural surfaces causes a characteristic sharp or sticking pain with each breath when these normally smooth surfaces slide on one another. This sharp pain is called *pleuritic pain.*

In trauma patients, <u>dyspnea</u> has many causes, including airway obstruction, damage to the chest wall, improper chest expansion due to the loss of normal control of breathing, or lung compression because of accumulated blood or air in the chest cavity. Dyspnea in an injured patient indicates potential compromise of lung function. Prompt, aggressive support of oxygenation and ventilation with rapid transport is required.

Hemoptysis, the spitting or coughing up of blood, usually indicates that the lung itself or the air passages have been damaged. With a laceration of the lung tis-sue, blood can enter the bronchial passages and is coughed up as the patient tries to clear the airway.

A rapid, weak pulse and low blood pressure are the principal signs of hypovolemic shock, which can result from extensive bleeding from lacerated structures within the chest cavity. Shock following a chest injury may also result from insufficient oxygenation of the blood by the poorly functioning lungs.

Cyanosis in a patient with a chest injury is a sign of inadequate respiration. The classic blue or ashen gray appearance indicates that blood is not being oxygenated sufficiently. Patients with cyanosis are unable to provide a sufficient supply of oxygen to the blood through the lungs and require immediate ventilation and oxygenation.

■ Complications of Chest Injuries

Pneumothorax

In any chest injury, damage to the heart, lungs, and great vessels can be complicated by the accumulation of air in the pleural space (a <u>pneumothorax</u>, or collapsed lung). In this condition, air enters through a hole in the chest wall or the surface of the lung as the patient attempts to breathe, causing the affected lung to collapse `Figure 22-4 ▼`. As a result, any blood that passes through the collapsed portion of the lung is not oxygenated, resulting in hypoxia. Depending on the size of the hole and the rate at which air fills the cavity, the lung may collapse in a few seconds or a

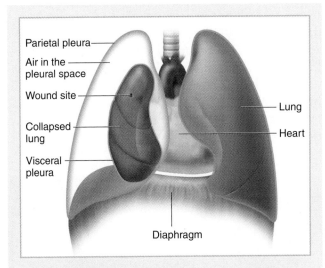

Figure 22-4 Pneumothorax occurs when air leaks into the space between the pleural surfaces from an opening in the chest wall or the surface of the lung. The lung collapses as air fills the pleural space.

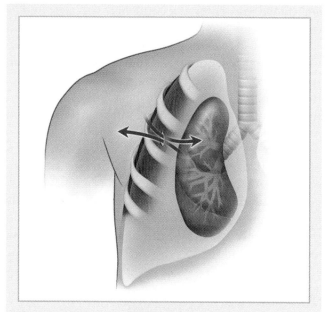

Figure 22-5 With a sucking chest wound, air passes from the outside into the pleural space and back out with each breath, creating a sucking sound.

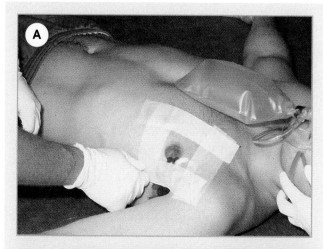

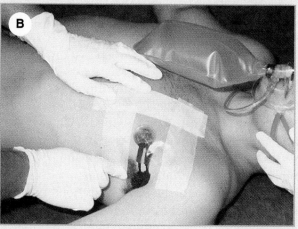

Figure 22-6 A sucking chest wound can be sealed with a large, airtight dressing that seals all four sides, **A,** or seals three sides with the fourth left open as a flutter valve, **B.** Your local protocol will dictate the way you are to care for this injury.

few hours. In the uncommon situation when the hole is in the chest wall, you can actually hear a sucking sound as the patient inhales and the sound of rushing air as he or she exhales. For this reason, an open or penetrating wound to the chest wall is often called a sucking chest wound (Figure 22-5 ▲).

This type of open pneumothorax is a true emergency requiring immediate emergency medical care and transport. Initial emergency care, after clearing and maintaining the airway and providing oxygen, is to rapidly seal the open wound with a sterile occlusive dressing (Figure 22-6 ▶). The occlusive dressing will seal the wound and prevent air from being sucked into the chest through the wound. Several sterile materials, including Vaseline gauze and aluminum foil, may be used to seal the wound. Use a dressing that is large enough so that it is not pulled or sucked into the chest cavity. Depending on your local protocol,

Teamwork Tips

Immediately cover a sucking chest wound with your gloved hand while your partner secures an occlusive dressing. A sucking chest wound is a part of "airway" and should be corrected as soon as it is found.

you may tape the dressing down on all four sides or only three sides so that air can exit but not enter the wound.

Spontaneous Pneumothorax

Some people are born with or develop weak areas on the surface of the lungs. This weakened area of the lung is called a *bleb*. Occasionally, such a weak area will rupture spontaneously, allowing air to leak into the pleural space. Unrelated to trauma, a spontaneous pneumothorax simply happens with normal breathing or may occur during physical activity or a coughing episode. The patient experiences sudden, sharp chest pain and increasing difficulty breathing. A portion of the affected lung collapses, losing its ability to ventilate normally. The amount of pneumothorax that develops varies, as does the amount of respiratory distress the patient experiences.

You should suspect a spontaneous pneumothorax in a patient who experiences sudden chest pain and shortness of breath without a specific known cause. Treatment includes the administration of oxygen and transport.

Tension Pneumothorax

A potential complication that may develop following a chest injury with pneumothorax is a <u>tension pneumothorax</u> (Figure 22-7 ▾). This occurs when there is significant ongoing air accumulation in the pleural space. The air gradually increases the pressure in the chest, first causing the complete collapse of the affected lung and then pushing the mediastinum (the central part of the chest containing the heart and great vessels) into the opposite side of the chest. This prevents blood from returning through the vena cava to the heart and can cause shock and cardiac arrest.

If signs and symptoms of a tension pneumothorax develop after sealing an open chest wound, you should partly remove the dressing to relieve the tension. You may hear a rush of air out of the chest cavity, although this does not occur in all cases.

Tension pneumothorax occurs more commonly as a result of closed, blunt injury to the chest in which a fractured rib lacerates a lung or bronchus. Only very rarely does a tension pneumothorax arise spontaneously.

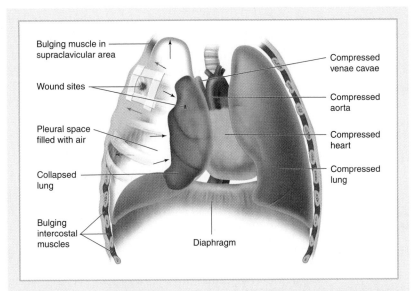

Figure 22-7 A tension pneumothorax can develop if a penetrating chest wound is bandaged tightly and air from a damaged lung cannot escape. The air then accumulates in the pleural space, eventually causing compression of the heart and great vessels.

Labels: Bulging muscle in supraclavicular area; Wound sites; Pleural space filled with air; Collapsed lung; Bulging intercostal muscles; Diaphragm; Compressed venae cavae; Compressed aorta; Compressed heart; Compressed lung

The common signs and symptoms of tension pneumothorax include increasing respiratory distress, distended neck veins, deviation of the trachea to the side of the chest opposite the tension pneumothorax, tachycardia, low blood pressure, cyanosis, and decreased breath sounds on the side of the pneumothorax. A tension pneumothorax is a life-threatening condition. Support ventilation with high-flow oxygen and request ALS support or transport immediately to the closest hospital.

Hemothorax

In blunt and penetrating chest injuries, blood can collect in the pleural space from bleeding around the rib cage or from a lung or great vessel. This condition is called a <u>hemothorax</u>. You should suspect a hemothorax if the patient has signs and symptoms of shock or decreased breath sounds on the affected side. The presence of air and blood in the pleural space is known as a hemopneumothorax.

Rib Fractures

Rib fractures are common, particularly in older patients. Because the upper four ribs are well protected by the bony girdle of the clavicle and scapula, a fracture of one of these ribs is a sign of a very significant mechanism of injury (MOI).

Remember that a fractured rib that penetrates the pleural space may lacerate the surface of the lung, causing a pneumothorax, a tension pneumothorax, a hemothorax, or a hemopneumothorax. One sign of this development can be a crackly feeling to the skin in the area (also called crepitus or subcutaneous emphysema), which indicates that air escaping from a lacerated lung is leaking into the chest wall.

Patients with one or more cracked ribs usually complain of localized tenderness and pain when breathing. The pain is the result of broken ends of the fracture rubbing against each other with each inspiration and expiration. Patients will tend to avoid taking deep breaths, and their respirations are usually rapid and shallow. They will often hold the affected portion of the rib cage in an effort to minimize the discomfort. Patients should receive supplemental oxygen during assessment and transport.

Flail Chest

Ribs may be fractured in more than one place. A flail chest is when two or more ribs are fractured in two or more places or if the sternum is fractured along with several ribs and a segment of chest wall is detached from the rest of the thoracic cage   Figure 22-8 ▼ . With this paradoxical motion, the detached portion of the chest wall moves opposite the rest of the chest wall. This occurs because of negative pressure that has built up in the thorax. Breathing with a flail chest can be painful and ineffective, and hypoxemia easily results.

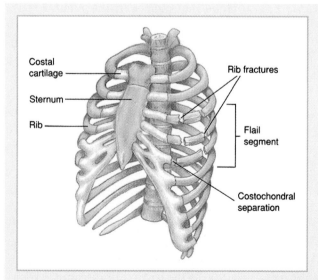

Figure 22-8 When three or more adjacent ribs are fractured in two or more places, a flail chest results. A flail segment will move paradoxically when the patient breathes.

A flail segment seriously interferes with the body's normal mechanics of ventilation and must be addressed quickly.

Your treatment of a patient with a flail chest should include maintaining the airway, providing respiratory support if necessary, giving supplemental oxygen, and performing ongoing assessments for possible pneumothorax or other respiratory complications. Treatment may also include positive-pressure ventilation with a bag-mask device.

The patient may find it easier and less painful to breathe if the flail segment is immobilized. You can tape a bulky pad against that segment of the chest for this purpose, but don't tape it so tightly that the dressing prevents adequate ventilation. You can also immobilize a flail chest by splinting the chest with the patient's arm, placing a sling and swathe on the arm, and securing it to the chest wall snugly. Keep in mind that although flail chest itself is a serious condition, it suggests an injury that was forceful enough to cause other serious internal damage and possible spinal injury as well. Often the flail chest contributes less to the patient's ventilation difficulties than does the underlying pulmonary contusion (bruised lung segment).

Pulmonary Contusion

In addition to fracturing ribs, any severe blunt trauma to the chest can also injure the lung. The alveoli may become filled with blood, and fluid accumulates in the injured area, leaving the patient hypoxic. Severe pulmonary contusion, bruising of the lung, should always be suspected in patients with a flail chest and usually develops during a period of hours. If you believe that a patient may have a pulmonary contusion, you should provide respiratory support and supplemental oxygen to ensure adequate ventilation.

Traumatic Asphyxia

Sometimes a patient will experience a sudden, severe compression of the chest, which produces a rapid increase in pressure within the chest. This may occur in an unrestrained driver who hits a steering wheel or a pedestrian who is compressed between a vehicle and a wall. The sudden increase in intrathoracic pressure results in a characteristic appearance, including distended neck veins, cyanosis in the face and neck, and hemorrhage into the sclera of the eye, signaling the bursting of small blood vessels. This is called traumatic asphyxia. These findings suggest an underlying injury to the heart and possibly a pulmonary contusion. You should provide ventilatory support with supplemental oxygen and monitor the patient's vital signs, as you provide immediate transport.

Blunt Myocardial Injury

A myocardial contusion (bruising of the heart muscle) can occur with blunt trauma to the chest. If the bruising is significant, the heart may not pump efficiently or be able to maintain adequate blood pressure. Often the pulse rate is irregular. There is no specific diagnostic test at this time, and there is no prehospital treatment for the condition. Still, you should suspect myocardial contusion in all cases of severe blunt injury to the chest. Check the patient's pulse carefully, and note any irregularities. Provide supplemental oxygen, and transport immediately.

Pericardial Tamponade

In pericardial tamponade, blood or other fluid collects in the pericardium, the fibrous sac surrounding the heart Figure 22-9 ▼. This prevents the heart from filling during the diastolic phase, causing a decrease in the amount of blood pumped to the body and decreased blood pressure. Ultimately, as the blood accumulates in the pericardial sac, it compresses the heart until it can no longer function and the patient may go into cardiac arrest. Signs and symptoms of pericardial tamponade include very soft and faint heart tones (muffled heart

sounds), a weak pulse, low blood pressure, a decrease in the difference between the systolic and diastolic blood pressures, and jugular vein distention.

In trauma, even a small amount of fluid in the pericardial sac is enough to cause fatal pericardial tamponade. (Occasionally, fluid in surprisingly large amounts may collect in the pericardial sac as a chronic condition.) Pericardial tamponade is relatively uncommon, seen more often with penetrating injuries to the heart itself than with blunt trauma to the chest. If you suspect this life-threatening condition, provide appropriate respiratory support, supplemental oxygen, and prompt transport. Be sure to notify hospital staff of your suspicions so that preparations can be made for immediate treatment.

Laceration of the Great Vessels

The chest contains several large blood vessels: the superior vena cava, the inferior vena cava, the pulmonary arteries, four main pulmonary veins, and the aorta, with its major branches distributing blood throughout the body. Injury to any of these vessels may be accompanied by massive, rapidly fatal hemorrhage. Any patient with a chest wound who shows signs of shock may have an injury of these vessels. Frequently, there is significant internal blood loss within the chest cavity. You must remain alert to signs

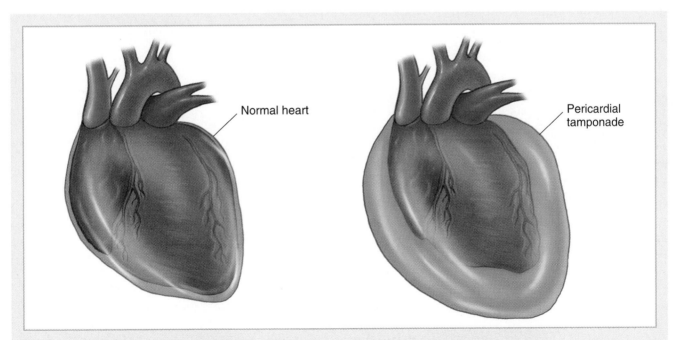

Figure 22-9 Pericardial tamponade is a potentially fatal condition in which fluid builds up within the pericardial sac, causing compression of the heart's chambers and dramatically impairing its ability to pump blood to the body.

and symptoms of shock and to changes in the baseline vital signs, such as tachycardia and hypotension.

Emergency treatment for these patients includes CPR, if appropriate, ventilatory support, and supplemental oxygen. Here, particularly, immediate transport to the hospital may be critical. The overwhelming majority of injuries to the great vessels in the chest are rapidly fatal.

■ Assessment of Chest Injuries

Scene Size-up

As you arrive on the scene, observe for hazards and threats to the safety of the crew, bystanders, and patient. Consider the possibility that the area where the patient is located may be a crime scene. Ensure that you and your crew use proper body substance isolation (BSI) precautions, and use a minimum of gloves and eye protection. Because of the color of blood and how well it soaks through clothing, you can often identify patients with bleeding as you approach the scene. As you observe the scene, look for indicators of and the significance of the MOI. Chest injuries are common in motor vehicle crashes, falls, and assaults. Dispatch information and visual inspection of the scene will often increase your suspicion of chest injury. Consider spinal immobilization based on the MOI. Ensure that the police are on scene at incidents involving violence, such as assaults and gunshot wounds. If you determine that the power company, fire department, or ALS units are needed, call for them early.

Initial Assessment

General Impression

During your initial assessment, you must quickly evaluate the patient's ABCs and treat potential life-threats. A responsive patient will usually tell you what is wrong (chief complaint). Note not only what the patient says, but also how he or she says it. Difficulty speaking may indicate several conditions, including chest trauma. Obvious injuries and the appearance of blood or difficulty breathing may be observed in an unresponsive patient. Look for cyanosis, irregular breathing, or chest rise and fall on only one side to indicate chest injuries. If no obvious problems present themselves, begin your assessment by focusing on the ABCs. The general impression will help you develop an index of suspicion for serious injuries and determine your sense of urgency for medical intervention. A good question to ask yourself is "How sick is this patient?" Patients with significant chest injuries will look sick and are often frightened or anxious.

Airway and Breathing

Next, ensure that the patient has a clear and patent airway. How you assess and manage the airway depends a great deal on whether you suspect a spinal injury. A significant number of patients with traumatic chest injuries also have spinal injuries, and proper precautions should be taken. Be suspicious, and protect the spine early in your care, even if your assessment later confirms that there is no spinal injury. Once you have

You are the Provider 2

A second fire fighter begins providing bag-mask ventilation and 100% oxygen. There are no other obvious injuries and no bleeding. When the patient is rolled over so you can check his posterior, you note an exit wound just below his right scapula in line with the entrance wound.

Vital Signs	Recording Time: 2 Minutes
Skin	Pale, diaphoretic
Pulse	114 beats/min, regular
Blood pressure	128/72 mm Hg
Respirations	Bag-mask ventilation

5. How should the exit wound be treated?
6. Should this patient be immobilized on a long backboard?

determined the patient has a patent airway, determine whether breathing is present and adequate.

With chest injuries, begin by inspecting for DCAP-BTLS. Listen to breath sounds. Absent or decreased breath sounds on one side usually indicate significant damage to a lung, preventing it from expanding properly. Assess for equal chest rise and fall. Check for paradoxical motion. If the patient has paradoxical movement of the chest wall or penetrating chest trauma, address this life threat at once. These conditions may interfere with the normal mechanics of breathing and can cause the patient's condition to deteriorate quickly. Apply an occlusive dressing to all open chest wounds, and stabilize paradoxical motion with a large bulky dressing and 2" tape. Apply oxygen with a nonrebreathing mask at 15 L/min. Provide positive pressure ventilation with 100% oxygen if breathing is inadequate and the patient has a decreased level of consciousness.

Circulation

Assess the patient's pulse to determine whether it is present and adequate. If it is too fast or too slow or if the skin is pale, cool, or clammy, consider your patient to be in shock and treat aggressively. Support the patient's circulatory system. External bleeding may not be obvious. However, internal bleeding in the chest can be significant and can be a quick cause of death. Control external bleeding with direct pressure and a bulky trauma dressing.

Transport Decision

Patients with compromised ABCs are considered priority patients. Sometimes the priority is obvious and the decision to transport quickly is easy. At other times, what is happening outside may not provide obvious clues to the seriousness of what is happening inside. Pay attention to clues such as skin color, temperature, and condition and level of consciousness. These symptoms may not be as dramatic as a large gash across the chest or a sucking chest wound, but they are equally important indicators of a life-threatening condition. When you find signs of poor perfusion or inadequate breathing, provide rapid transport. A delay on the scene to perform a lengthy assessment will reduce the chances of survival for your patient.

Focused History and Physical Exam
Rapid Physical Exam Versus Focused Physical Exam

After the initial assessment is complete, determine which physical exam will be performed: a rapid phys-

ical exam or a focused physical exam. For a patient who has an isolated injury to the chest with limited MOI, such as in a stabbing, consider a focused physical exam. Focus your assessment on the isolated injury, the patient's complaint, and the body region affected. Ensure that wounds are identified and bleeding is controlled. Note the location and extent of the injury. Assess all underlying systems. Examine the anterior and posterior aspects of the chest wall, and be alert to changes in the patient's ability to maintain adequate respirations.

If there is significant trauma (such as a blunt trauma or gunshot wound) likely affecting multiple systems, start with a rapid physical assessment looking for DCAP-BTLS to determine the nature and extent of thoracic injury. Using a systematic approach to patient assessment minimizes the chance of missing a significant injury. With chest trauma, it is important to not focus just on the chest wound. With significant trauma, you should quickly assess the entire patient from head to toe.

Baseline Vital Signs

Once you have stabilized the ABCs and have checked the patient from head to toe to identify injuries, obtain a baseline set of vital signs. This should include assessment of pulse, respirations, blood pressure, skin condition, and pupils. Each of these is a sign indicating how your patient is tolerating the injuries. Baseline vital signs are used to evaluate changes in the patient's condition.

SAMPLE History

Many chest trauma patients may be considered high priority and be rapidly transported to a hospital. A basic evaluation of allergies, medications, pertinent medical problems, and last oral intake should be completed. Most signs and symptoms have been identified in the initial assessment and the rapid or focused physical exam. The events leading to the incident are usually identified in the scene size-up and initial assessment. A SAMPLE history can be obtained quickly in most situations and can usually be obtained while accomplishing other tasks.

Interventions

Provide spinal immobilization based on the MOI. You should suspect spinal injuries in patients with penetrating and blunt trauma to the chest. Maintain an open airway, be prepared to suction the patient, and provide high-flow oxygen. If needed, provide assisted ventilation using a bag-mask device with high-flow oxygen. Control any significant external bleeding. Place an occlusive dressing over all open chest wounds, and stabilize flail segments with a bulky dressing. If the patient has signs of hypoperfusion, treat aggressively for shock and provide rapid transport to the appropriate hospital. Do not delay transport of a seriously injured trauma patient to complete nonlifesaving treatments such as splinting extremity fractures.

Detailed Physical Exam

Patients with a significant MOI to the chest have a high likelihood of other injuries. If time allows, perform a detailed physical exam en route. Your rapid physical exam identified injuries that needed immediate attention and helped you prepare for packaging and transportation. The detailed physical exam can now help determine all injuries and their extent. If there is no major trauma and no persistent problems are present after the initial assessment, a detailed physical exam may not be necessary. Many times, short transportation times and unstable patient conditions may make this assessment impractical.

Ongoing Assessment

The ongoing assessment identifies how your patient's condition is changing. It should focus on reassessing the patient's airway, breathing, pulse, perfusion, and bleeding. Has breathing improved now that the sucking chest wound is sealed? Or has it become more

Documentation Tips

Document a complete set of vitals signs:

- Blood pressure
- Pulse
- Respirations
- Skin color, temperature, moisture
- Pupillary response

Record vital signs every 5 minutes for a patient in unstable condition, and every 15 minutes for a patient in stable condition.

difficult? Do you need to release one side of the occlusive dressing? Other interventions should also be assessed to determine whether they are effective. For example, are pulse oximeter values rising now that the patient is receiving oxygen? Vital signs need to be reassessed and compared with the baseline vital signs. The condition of patients with chest trauma may deteriorate during transport to the hospital because of the seriousness of the injuries. Your reassessment will help identify conditions in a timely manner so that they can be addressed immediately.

Communication and Documentation

Communicating with hospital staff early when your patient has a significant MOI to the chest can help

You are the Provider 3

The patient is rolled back onto a long backboard and packaged for transport. Once he is loaded into the ambulance the fire fighter who is providing bag-mask ventilation tells you that the bag is getting difficult to squeeze. You note that the patient is very pale and radial pulses are rapid and extremely weak.

Reassessment	Recording Time: 5 Minutes
Pulse	126 beats/min, weak
Blood pressure	114/98 mm Hg
Respirations	Bag-mask ventilation
Breath sounds	Diminished on the right side
Pulse oximetry	93% with oxygen via bag-mask ventilation

7. Why do you think it is getting difficult to ventilate the patient?
8. What signs and symptoms are associated with this condition?
9. What is the treatment?

them be prepared with appropriate equipment and personnel when you arrive. If a penetrating injury is present, describe it in your report, along with the treatment you have provided. Your documentation should be complete and thorough. Remember, your documentation provides a basis for ongoing care and is your legal record of what happened.

■ The Anatomy of the Abdomen

The abdomen contains hollow and solid organs, any of which may be damaged. Hollow organs, including the stomach, intestines, ureters, and bladder, are actually structures through which materials pass Figure 22-10 ▾ . They usually contain food that is in the process of being digested, urine that is being passed to the bladder for release, or bile. When ruptured or lacerated, these organs spill their contents into the abdominal cavity (peritoneal cavity), causing an intense inflammatory reaction and possible infection. Peritonitis is an inflammation of the peritoneum that may be caused by this type of infection. The intestines and stomach contain acidlike substances that aid in the digestive process. When they spill or leak into the peritoneal cavity, pain and irritation to the peritoneum often follow. The first signs of peritonitis are severe abdominal pain, tenderness, and

muscular spasm. Later, bowel sounds diminish or disappear as the bowel stops functioning. A patient may feel nauseous and may vomit; the abdomen may become distended and firm to touch, and infection may occur. Peritonitis is serious and may become life threatening.

The liver, spleen, pancreas, and kidneys are solid organs Figure 22-11 ▾ . These organs function to produce enzymes, cleanse the blood, and produce energy. Solid organs have a rich blood supply, so injury can cause severe and unseen hemorrhage. The same is true of the aorta and inferior vena cava, whether the injury is open or closed. Blood may irritate the peritoneal cavity and cause the patient to complain of abdominal pain. However, the patient does not always complain of pain. The absence of pain and tenderness does not necessarily mean the absence of major bleeding in the abdomen.

The bony landmarks in the abdomen include the pubic symphysis, the costal arch, the iliac crests, and the anterior superior iliac spines. The major soft-tissue landmark is the umbilicus, which overlies the fourth lumbar vertebra. The abdomen is divided into four quadrants by two perpendicular lines that intersect at the umbilicus Figure 22-12 ▶ . These quadrants provide a frame of reference for identifying and reporting abdominal signs and symptoms.

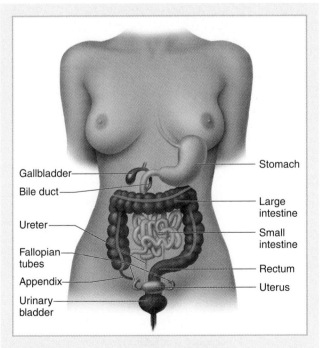

Figure 22-10 The hollow organs in the abdominal cavity are structures through which materials pass.

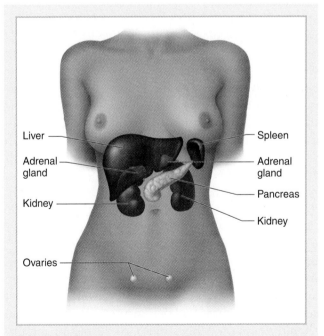

Figure 22-11 The solid organs are solid masses of tissue that do much of the chemical work in the body and receive a large, rich supply of blood.

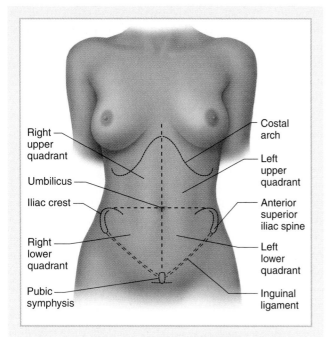

Figure 22-12 The abdominal cavity is divided into four quadrants, which serve as your means of identifying and reporting problems in the abdomen.

■ Injuries to the Abdomen

Abdominal injuries may be as obvious as loops of intestines protruding from a penetrating injury or hidden and internal such as a laceration to the liver or spleen. Traumatic injuries to the abdomen are considered open or closed and can involve hollow and/or solid organs. A closed abdominal injury is one in which blunt force trauma, some type of impact to the body, results in injury to the abdomen without breaking the skin. Examples include the patient striking the handlebar of a bicycle or the steering wheel of a car or when the patient is struck by an item such as a board or baseball bat during a fight or assault **Figure 22-13 ▶**. An open abdominal injury results from penetrating trauma in which an object enters the abdomen and opens the peritoneal cavity to the outside **Figure 22-14 ▶**. Stab wounds and gunshot wounds are examples of open injuries. Open wounds might not be deeper than the muscular wall of the abdomen. As an EMS provider, you cannot determine how deep an abdominal wound is. These injuries must be assessed and evaluated at the hospital. Therefore, you should maintain a high index of suspicion for unseen injuries, internal damage to organs, and potential life-threatening injuries and provide prompt transport.

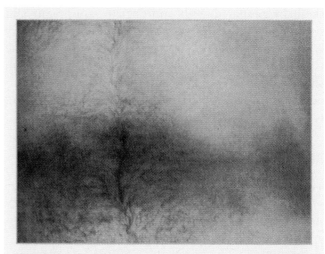

Figure 22-13 Blunt trauma to the abdomen can occur when a patient strikes the steering wheel of an automobile as a result of a crash.

Signs and Symptoms

Patients with abdominal injuries generally have one principal complaint—pain. Other significant injuries may mask the pain at first, and some patients may not be able to tell you about pain because they are uncon-

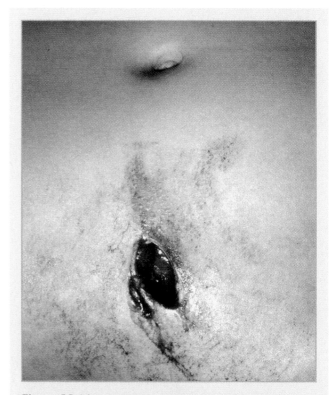

Figure 22-14 Because it is difficult to know how deep a penetrating injury is, assume organ damage and transport promptly.

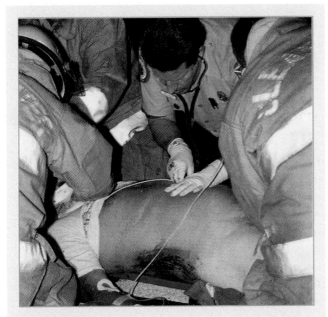

Figure 22-15 Bruising on the abdomen can provide clues to the possible injury of underlying organs.

scious or unresponsive. A very common sign of significant abdominal injury is tachycardia as the heart increases its pumping action to compensate for blood loss. This is an early indication of compensated shock. Later signs include evidence of shock such as decreased blood pressure and pale, cool, moist skin or changes in the patient's mental status, combined with trauma to the abdomen. In some cases, the abdomen may become distended from the accumulation of blood and fluid. As an EMT-B, you must look for other signs and symptoms of potential problems and injuries to the abdomen. Blunt injuries include bruises (often indicated by red areas of skin at this early stage) or other visible marks, whose location should guide your attention to underlying structures (Figure 22-15). For example, bruises in the right upper quadrant, left upper quadrant, or flank (the region of the lower rib cage) might suggest an injury to the liver, spleen, or kidney, respectively.

The signs of abdominal injury are usually more definite than the symptoms, including firmness on palpation of the abdomen, obvious penetrating wounds, bruises, and vital signs such as increased pulse rate, increased respiratory rate, decreased blood pressure, and shallow respirations (although these might not appear until later). Common symptoms include abdominal tenderness, particularly localized tenderness, difficulty with movement because of pain, or inability to get comfortable—patients are often restless and may want to pull their knees up.

Types of Abdominal Injuries

Blunt Abdominal Wounds

A patient with a blunt abdominal wound may have one or more of the following:

- Severe bruising of the abdominal wall
- Laceration of the liver and/or spleen
- Rupture of the intestine
- Tears in the mesentery, membranous folds that attach the intestines to the walls of the body, and injury to blood vessels within them
- Rupture of the kidneys, or avulsion of the kidneys from their arteries and veins
- Rupture of the bladder, especially in a patient who had a full and distended bladder at the time of the crash
- Severe intra-abdominal hemorrhage
- Peritoneal irritation and inflammation in response to the rupture of hollow organs

A patient who has sustained a blunt abdominal injury should be log rolled onto a backboard. If the patient vomits, turn him or her to one side and clear the mouth and throat of vomitus. Monitor the patient's vital signs for any indication of shock such as pallor; cold sweat; rapid, thready pulse; or low blood pressure. Administer high-flow supplemental oxygen via nonrebreathing mask early, and treat for shock. Keep the patient warm with blankets, and provide prompt transport to the emergency department.

You are the Provider 4

You "burp" the dressing on the patient's chest by lifting one corner to allow the air to escape from the thorax. He is immediately easier to ventilate and his radial pulses improve. On arrival at the hospital, he is treated by the trauma team and taken into surgery. There were no injuries other than the punctured lung, and the patient makes a complete recovery.

10. What is significant about a pneumothorax developing tension?

Injuries From Seat Belts and Airbags

Seat belts have prevented many thousands of injuries and saved many lives, including those of people who otherwise would have been ejected. However, seat belts occasionally cause blunt injuries of the abdominal organs. When worn properly, a seat belt lies below the anterior superior iliac spines of the pelvis and against the hip joints. If the belt lies too high, it can squeeze abdominal organs or great vessels against the spine when the car suddenly decelerates or stops Figure 22-16 ▾ . Occasionally, fractures of the lumbar spine have been reported. Remember that the use of seat belts in many cases turns what could have been a fatal injury into a manageable one.

In all current-model automobiles, the lap and shoulder safety belts are combined into one so that

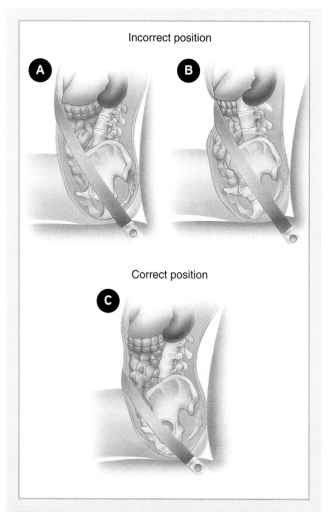

Figure 22-16 The proper position for a seat belt is below the anterior superior iliac spines of the pelvis and against the hip joints, as shown in diagram **C.** Diagrams **A** and **B** show improper positioning of seat belts.

they may not be used independently. Of course, people can still place the diagonal portion of the belt behind the back, significantly reducing the effectiveness of this design. In some older cars, only lap belts or two separate belts are provided. Used alone, diagonal shoulder safety belts can cause injuries of the upper part of the trunk, such as a bruised chest, fractured ribs, lacerated liver, or even decapitation. Far fewer head and neck injuries are seen when this belt is used in combination with a lap belt and a headrest.

The airbag, which is standard in today's vehicles, represents a great advance in automotive safety. In head-on collisions, it can be a genuine lifesaver. However, because frontal airbags provide no protection in a side impact or rollover, they must be used in combination with safety belts. Small children and short stature individuals who are in the front seat of the automobile are at risk of injury if an airbag is deployed. Special attention should be used in evaluating these patients when a deployed airbag is noted. Remember to inspect beneath the airbag for signs of damage to the steering column.

Penetrating Abdominal Injuries

Patients with penetrating injuries generally have obvious wounds and external bleeding. However, the patient could also have significant internal bleeding that you cannot see. A large wound may have protrusions of bowel, fat, or other structures. In addition to pain, patients with these injuries often report nausea and vomiting. Patients with peritonitis generally prefer to lie very still with their legs drawn up because it hurts to move or straighten their legs.

Some penetrating injuries go no deeper than the abdominal wall, but the severity of the injury often cannot be determined in the prehospital setting. Only a surgeon can accurately assess the damage. You should assume that the object has penetrated into the abdominal cavity and has possibly injured one or more organs, even if there are no immediate obvious signs.

If major blood vessels are cut or solid organs are lacerated, bleeding may be rapid and severe. Other signs of abdominal trauma may develop slowly, particularly in penetrating wounds to hollow organs. Once such an organ is punctured and its contents are spilled into the abdominal cavity, peritonitis may develop, but this may take several hours.

In caring for a patient with a penetrating wound to the abdomen, administer oxygen and treat for shock. Inspect the patient's back and sides for exit wounds, and apply a dry, sterile dressing to all open wounds. If the penetrating object is still in place, apply a stabilizing bandage around it to control external bleeding and minimize movement of the object.

Abdominal Evisceration

Severe trauma to the abdominal wall may result in an <u>evisceration</u>, in which internal organs or fat protrude through the wound `Figure 22-17 ▼`. Never try to replace an organ that is protruding from an abdominal wound, whether it is a small fold of tissue or nearly all of the intestines. Instead, cover it with sterile gauze compresses moistened with sterile saline solution and secure with a sterile dressing. (Protocols in some EMS systems call for an occlusive dressing over the organs, secured by trauma dressings.) Because the open abdomen radiates body heat very effectively and because exposed organs lose fluid rapidly, you must keep the organs moist and warm. If you do not have gauze compresses, you may use moist, sterile dressings, covered and secured in place with a bandage and tape. Do not use any material that is adherent or loses its substance when wet, such as toilet paper, facial tissue, paper towels, or absorbent cotton.

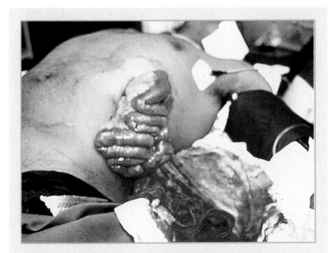

Figure 22-17 An abdominal evisceration is an open abdominal wound from which internal organs or fat protrude.

■ Assessment of Abdominal Injuries

Scene Size-up

Your scene size-up begins with the information reported from dispatch, which can help you prepare for the call. Sometimes this information is sketchy or inaccurate, but it will still provide some information to consider as you respond to the call. BSI precautions should be taken before arrival on scene.

As you arrive on scene, continue to gather information that will help manage the incident. Observe the scene for hazards and threats to your safety. If dispatch information indicates a possible assault, domestic dispute, or shooting, all of which commonly lead to abdominal injuries, be sure that law enforcement personnel have controlled the scene. As you observe the scene, determine the MOI and consider early spinal precautions. How many victims might be involved in the incident? If you determine additional resources are needed, call for them early in your assessment.

Initial Assessment
General Impression

Your goal in the initial assessment is to evaluate the patient's ABCs and then immediately care for any life-threats. The general impression, including an evaluation of the patient's age, chief complaint, and level of consciousness, will help you establish the seriousness of the patient's condition. Some abdominal injuries will be obvious and graphic. Most will be subtle and may go unnoticed. The MOI together with the chief complaint will help you focus on the immediate problem. Remember, the trauma or blow to the abdomen may have been hours or even days earlier, and the pain is just now bad enough for the person to seek help. Ask about previous injuries associated with a chief complaint of abdominal pain.

Quickly assess the patient's chief complaint, noting the position the patient is in. If the chief complaint involves sexual or physical assault, the patient may be hesitant to discuss what happened. Bleeding from the reproductive or genitourinary organs is common after sexual assault, but again, patients may be hesitant to discuss this or to be examined to determine severity. Movement of the body or the abdominal organs irritates the inflamed peritoneum, causing additional pain. To minimize this pain, patients will lie still, usually with the knees drawn up, and their breathing will be rapid and shallow. For the same reason, they will contract their abdominal muscles, a sign called <u>guarding</u>.

Airway and Breathing

Next, ensure that the patient has a clear and patent airway. If a spinal injury is suspected, prevent the patient from moving by having a team member hold the patient's head still and verbally reminding the patient not to move. Patients may report that they feel nauseous, and they may vomit. Remember to keep the airway clear of vomitus so that it is not aspirated into the lungs, especially in a patient who is unconscious or has an altered level of consciousness. Turn the patient to one side, using spinal precautions if necessary, and try to clear any material from the airway.

You must also quickly assess the patient for adequate breathing. A distended abdomen or pain may prevent adequate inhalation. When these guarded respirations decrease breathing effectiveness, providing supplemental oxygen with a nonrebreathing mask will help improve oxygenation. If the patient's level of consciousness is decreased and respirations are shallow, consider assisting ventilation with a bag-mask device.

Circulation

Superficial abdominal or genitalia injuries usually do not produce significant external bleeding. Internal bleeding from open or closed abdominal injuries can be profound. Trauma to the kidneys, liver, and spleen can cause significant internal bleeding. Evaluate the patient's pulse and skin color, temperature, and condition. If you suspect shock, treat the patient aggressively by providing oxygen, positioning the patient in the shock position, and keeping the patient warm. Wounds should be covered and bleeding controlled as quickly as possible.

Transport Decision

Due to the nature of abdominal injuries, a short on-scene time and rapid transport are generally indicated. Abdominal pain together with an MOI that suggests injury to the abdomen or flank is a good indication for rapid transport. In the prehospital environment, it is difficult to determine whether the liver, spleen, or kidney has been injured. Hollow organs that have ruptured are also difficult to identify without more advanced diagnostic equipment. The condition of patients who have visible significant bleeding or signs of significant internal bleeding may quickly become unstable. Treatment is directed at quickly addressing

EMT-B Safety

When there is the potential for violence, be sure law enforcement has secured the scene before approaching.

life-threats and providing rapid transportation to the closest appropriate hospital.

Focused History and Physical Exam

Remove or loosen clothes to expose the injured areas of the body for the physical assessment. Provide privacy as needed, or wait until you are in the back of the ambulance. A patient without a suspected spinal injury should be allowed to stay in the position of comfort—with legs pulled up toward the abdomen. A patient without a suspected spinal injury should not be forced to lie flat for the physical exam or transport. Determine which physical assessment process you will use—rapid physical exam or focused physical exam.

Use DCAP-BTLS to help identify specific signs and symptoms of injury. Inspect and palpate the abdomen for the presence of deformity, which may be subtle in abdominal injuries. Look for the presence of contusions and abrasions, which can help localize focal points of impact and may indicate significant internal injury. Puncture wounds and other penetrating injuries must not be overlooked because the intra-abdominal extent of these injuries may be life threatening. The presence of burns must be noted and managed appropriately. Palpate for tenderness, and attempt to localize it to a specific quadrant of the abdomen. Identify and treat any lacerations with appropriate dressings. Swelling may involve the abdomen globally and indicate significant intra-abdominal injury. In pediatric patients, the liver and spleen are very large in the abdomen and are more easily injured. The soft, flexible ribs of infants and young children do not protect these organs very well.

Rapid Physical Exam for Significant MOI

If there is a significant MOI, a rapid physical exam will help you quickly identify any injuries your patient may have, not just abdominal injuries. Begin with the head and finish with the lower extremities, moving in a systematic manner. Your goal is not to identify the extent of all the injuries but to determine whether injuries are present. If you find a life threat, stop and treat it immediately. The injuries you find will help you in packaging your patient for transport.

Focused Physical Exam for Nonsignificant MOI

If the MOI suggests an isolated injury to the abdomen, a focused exam of the injured area only may be sufficient. Assess the abdomen for wounds through which bullets, knives, or other missile-type foreign bodies may have passed. Keep in mind that the size of the wound does not necessarily indicate the extent of the underlying injuries. If you find an entry wound, you must always check for a corresponding exit wound in the patient's back or sides. If the injury was caused by a high-velocity missile from a rifle, you may see a small, harmless-looking entrance wound with a large, gaping exit wound. Bruises or other visible marks are important clues to the cause and severity of any blunt injury. Steering wheels and seat belts produce characteristic patterns of bruising on the abdomen or chest.

The kidneys are located in the flank region of the back. Inspect and palpate this area for tenderness, bruising, swelling, and other signs of trauma. Genital injuries can be awkward to evaluate and can be even more awkward to treat. Privacy is a genuine concern. Expose only what is needed, and cover what has been exposed. Being professional will help reduce anxiety for you and your patient.

Baseline Vital Signs

Quickly obtain the patient's baseline vital signs. Many abdominal emergencies, in addition to those that cause severe bleeding, can cause a rapid pulse and low blood pressure. Your record of vital signs, made as early as possible and periodically thereafter (every 5 minutes in a patient whom you suspect to have a serious injury), will help you identify changes in the patient's condition and be alert to signs of decompensation from blood loss.

SAMPLE History

Next, obtain a SAMPLE history from your patient. Using OPQRST (Onset of the pain, Provoking or palliating factors, Quality of the pain, Region of the pain [primary location and areas of radiating or referred pain], Severity of the pain, and Time (duration) the patient has been experiencing pain) to assess for pain may provide helpful information. If the patient is not responsive, attempt to get the SAMPLE history from friends or family members.

Interventions

Manage airway and breathing problems based on signs and symptoms found in your initial assessment. Provide complete spinal stabilization to patients with suspected spinal injuries. If the patient has signs of hypoperfusion, provide aggressive treatment for shock and rapid transport to the appropriate hospital. If there is an evisceration, place a moist, sterile dressing over the wound, apply a bandage, and transport. Cover bleeding injuries to the genitalia with a moist dressing. Do not delay transport of a seriously injured trauma patient to complete nonlifesaving treatments.

Detailed Physical Exam

As time permits, conduct a detailed physical exam. Thoroughly examine the patient from head to toe to identify injuries and determine their severity. You may identify new injuries not found in the initial assessment or the focused history and physical exam. Provide additional treatments as necessary. Short transport times or continuous problems with the ABCs may prevent you from performing a detailed physical exam. Every effort should be made to thoroughly examine the patient before arrival at the hospital.

Ongoing Assessment

Recheck the areas of the initial assessment and vital signs. Reassess the effectiveness of the interventions and treatment you have provided to the patient. Identifying trends in pain, vital signs, and the progress of treatments will help determine whether the patient's condition is improving or getting worse. Adjustments in care can be based on these findings.

Communication and Documentation

Communicate the MOI and the injuries found during your assessment. Use of appropriate medical and anatomic terminology is important; however, when in doubt, just describe what you see. The information you provide will help hospital staff prepare for the patient. Documentation of your assessment and trends in vital signs is a tremendous help to physicians when evaluating the problem when the patient arrives in the emergency department. Continuity of care is maintained when the emergency department has an accurate record of your findings on scene and the treatments you have provided.

You are the Provider | Summary

Treating an open wound to the chest is considered part of your airway assessment/treatment. It should be covered as soon as found to slow the development of tension. Once the presence of tension is detected, it must be treated immediately in order for the patient to survive.

1. **What is the first step in treating this patient?**
   Immediately cover the entrance wound with a gloved hand. Have another rescuer cover the wound with an occlusive dressing taped on three sides and continue with your assessment of the ABCs.

2. **What structures may have been affected by the gunshot wound?**
   Lungs, trachea, diaphragm, vessels, muscles, bones, and if the bullet did not go straight through, any structure in the pathway.

3. **How is this injury classified?**
   Open or penetrating trauma.

4. **What type of oxygen should this patient receive?**
   His breathing is shallow, so he should be receive bag-mask ventilation and 100% oxygen.

5. **How should the exit wound be treated?**
   It should be covered with an occlusive dressing sealed on all four sides.

6. **Should this patient be immobilized on a long backboard?**
   Yes. The bullet could have struck the spine or it could have fragmented a bone that was struck causing fragments to strike or lodge in the spine. Also, the patient may have fallen when he was shot.

7. **Why do you think it is getting difficult to ventilate the patient?**
   The patient has a pneumothorax that is developing tension. As pressure builds up in the thorax, ventilation becomes more difficult.

8. **What signs and symptoms are associated with this condition?**
   The common signs and symptoms of a tension pneumothorax include increasing respiratory distress, distended neck veins, deviation of the trachea to the side of the chest opposite the tension pneumothorax, tachycardia, low blood pressure, cyanosis, and decreased breath sounds on the side of the pneumothorax.

9. **What is the treatment?**
   Burp the dressing. Simply lift one corner of the dressing to allow air to escape.

10. **What is significant about a pneumothorax developing tension?**
    The air gradually increases the pressure in the chest, first causing complete collapse of the affected lung and then pushing the mediastinum to the opposite side of the chest. This prevents blood from returning through the vena cava to the heart and can cause shock and cardiac arrest.

Chest Injuries

Scene Size-up	Body substance isolation precautions should include a minimum of gloves and eye protection. Ensure scene safety and determine NOI/MOI. Consider the number of patients, the need for additional help/ALS, and c-spine stabilization.

Initial Assessment

■ General impression	Determine level of consciousness and treat any immediate threats to life. Determine priority of care based on environment and patient's chief complaint.
■ Airway	Ensure patent airway. Maintain spinal immobilization as necessary.
■ Breathing	Listen for abnormal breath sounds and evaluate depth and rate of the respirations. Look for symmetric chest rise and fall. Maintain ventilations as needed. Provide high-flow oxygen at 15 L/min and inspect the chest wall assessing for DCAP-BTLS.
■ Circulation	Evaluate pulse rate and quality; observe skin color, temperature, and condition, and treat accordingly. Control bleeding and cover sucking chest wounds with an occlusive dressing.
■ Transport decision	Prompt transport

Focused History and Physical Exam	*NOTE: The order of the steps in the focused history and physical exam differs depending on whether or not the patient has a significant MOI. The order below is for a patient with a significant MOI. For a patient without a significant MOI, perform a focused trauma assessment, obtain vital signs, and obtain the history.*
■ Rapid trauma assessment	Reevaluate the mechanism of injury(s). Perform a rapid trauma assessment, treating all life-threats immediately. Log roll and secure patient to backboard for all patients with a suspected spinal injury.
■ Baseline vital signs	Take vital signs, noting skin color and temperature as well as patient's level of consciousness. Use pulse oximetry if available.
■ SAMPLE history	Obtain SAMPLE history. If the patient is unresponsive, attempt to obtain information from family members, friends, or bystanders.
■ Interventions	Provide complete spinal immobilization early if you suspect that your patient has spinal injuries. Maintain an open airway and suction as needed. Treat signs of shock and any other life threats.
Detailed Physical Exam	Complete a detailed physical exam if time allows.
Ongoing Assessment	Repeat the initial assessment, rapid/focused assessment, and reassess interventions performed. Reassess vital signs every 5 minutes for the unstable patient, every 15 minutes for the stable patient.
■ Communication and documentation	Contact medical control with a radio report. Relay any change in level of consciousness or difficulty breathing. Describe the MOI and any interventions you performed. Be sure to document any physician's orders or changes in the patient's condition and at what time they occurred.

NOTE: While the steps below are widely accepted, be sure to consult and follow your local protocol.

Pneumothorax	Hemothorax	Rib Fractures	Flail Chest
1. Clear and maintain an open airway.	1. Clear and maintain an open airway.	1. Clear and maintain an open airway.	1. Clear and maintain an open airway.
2. Provide high-flow oxygen.	2. Provide high-flow oxygen. Cover the patient with a blanket.	2. Provide high-flow oxygen. Cover the patient with a blanket.	2. Provide respiratory support if necessary.
3. Seal the wound with an occlusive dressing, using a large enough dressing so that it is not pulled or sucked into the chest cavity.	3. Treat the patient for shock.	3. Place in a position of comfort to support breathing, unless a spinal injury is suspected.	3. Provide high-flow oxygen.
4. Depending on your local protocol, you may tape the dressing down on all four sides, or create a flutter valve by taping only three sides of the dressing.			4. Stabilize flail segment by securing (or having the patient hold) a pillow firmly against the chest wall.

Abdomen and Genitalia Injuries

Scene Size-up	Body substance isolation precautions should include a minimum of gloves and eye protection. Ensure scene safety and determine NOI/MOI. Consider the number of patients, the need for additional help/ALS, and c-spine stabilization.
Initial Assessment	
■ General impression	Determine level of consciousness and treat any immediate threats to life. Determine priority of care based on environment and patient's chief complaint.
■ Airway	Ensure patent airway.
■ Breathing	Listen for abnormal breath sounds and evaluate depth and rate of the respirations. Look for symmetric chest rise and fall. Maintain ventilations as needed. Provide high-flow oxygen at 15 L/min and inspect the chest wall, assessing for DCAP-BTLS.
■ Circulation	Evaluate pulse rate and quality; observe skin color, temperature, and condition, and treat accordingly.
■ Transport decision	Prompt transport
Focused History and Physical Exam	NOTE: The order of the steps in the focused history and physical exam differs depending on whether or not the patient has a significant MOI. The order below is for a patient with a significant MOI. For a patient without a significant MOI, perform a focused trauma assessment, obtain vital signs, and obtain the history.
■ Rapid trauma assessment	Reevaluate the mechanism of injury. Perform a rapid trauma assessment, treating all life threats immediately. Log roll and secure patient to backboard if a spinal injury is suspected.
■ Baseline vital signs	Take vital signs, noting skin color and temperature as well as patient's level of consciousness. Use pulse oximetry if available.
■ SAMPLE history	Obtain SAMPLE history. If the patient is unresponsive, attempt to get it from family members, friends, or bystanders.
■ Interventions	Provide complete spinal immobilization early if you suspect that your patient has spinal injuries. Maintain an open airway and suction as needed. If an evisceration is present, place a moist, sterile dressing over the wound and bandage. Cover bleeding injuries to the genitalia with a moist dressing. Treat signs of shock and any other life threats.
Detailed Physical Exam	Complete a detailed physical exam if time allows.
Ongoing Assessment	Repeat the initial assessment, rapid/focused assessment, and reassess interventions performed. Reassess vital signs every 5 minutes for the unstable patient, every 15 minutes for the stable patient.
■ Communication and documentation	Contact medical control with a radio report. Relay any changes in the patient's condition. Describe the MOI and any interventions you performed. Be sure to document any changes in the patient's condition and at what time they occurred.

Prep Kit

Ready for Review

- Chest injuries are classified as closed or open. Closed injuries are often the result of blunt force trauma, and open injuries are the result of some object penetrating the skin and/or chest wall.
- Blunt trauma may result in fractures to the ribs and the sternum.
- A flail chest segment is two or more ribs broken in two or more places.
- A flail chest segment should be secured with a large, bulky dressing and 2" tape.
- Any penetrating injury to the chest may result in air entering the pleural space and may cause a pneumothorax. An occlusive dressing should be placed on all open wounds to the chest.
- A spontaneous pneumothorax may be the result of rupture of a weak spot on the lung allowing air to enter the pleural space and accumulate. This often is not a result of trauma and may occur during times of physical activity or a coughing episode.
- A pneumothorax may progress to a tension pneumothorax and cause cardiac arrest.
- Hemothorax is the result of blood accumulating in the pleural space after a traumatic injury when the vessels of the lung are lacerated and bleed.
- All patients with chest injuries should receive high-flow oxygen or bag-mask ventilation.
- Pulmonary contusion (bruised lung) may interfere with oxygen exchange in the lung tissue.
- A cardiac contusion is bruising of the heart muscle after traumatic injury. This condition may have the same signs and symptoms as a heart attack, including an irregular pulse. Remember that this is an injury to heart muscle from trauma, not from a heart attack.
- Pericardial tamponade is when blood collects in the space between the pericardial sac and the heart. This condition results in pressure building up inside the pericardial sac until the heart cannot pump effectively; cardiac arrest may occur quickly.
- The great vessels in the chest may be lacerated or torn and cause significant internal bleeding inside the patient's chest cavity.
- Abdominal injuries are categorized as open (penetrating trauma) or closed (blunt force trauma).
- Either classification of injury can result in injury to the hollow or solid organs of the abdomen and cause significant life-threatening bleeding.
- Blunt force trauma that causes closed injuries results from an object striking the body without breaking the skin.
- Penetrating trauma is often a result of a gunshot wound or stab wound. Other mechanisms of injury such as a fall on an object can also cause penetrating trauma to the chest or abdomen.
- Injury to the solid internal organs often causes significant unseen bleeding that can be life threatening.
- Injury to the hollow organs of the abdomen may cause irritation and inflammation to the peritoneum as caustic digestive juices leak into the peritoneum. A serious infection may also occur after several hours.
- Always maintain a high index of suspicion for serious intra-abdominal injury in trauma patients, particularly in a patient with signs of shock.
- Assess the abdomen for signs of bruising, rigidity, penetrating injuries, and complaints of pain.
- Never remove an impaled object from the abdominal region. Secure it in place with a large, bulky dressing and provide prompt transport.
- Be prepared to treat the patient for shock. Place the patient in the shock position, keep the patient warm, and provide high-flow oxygen.
- Never replace an organ that protrudes from an open injury to the abdomen (evisceration). Keep the tissues moist and warm. Cover the injury site with a large, sterile, moist, bulky dressing.
- Injuries to the kidneys may be difficult to detect due to the well-protected region of the body where they are located. Be alert to bruising or hematoma in the flank region.

Vital Vocabulary

closed abdominal injury Any injury of the abdomen caused by a nonpenetrating instrument or force, in which the skin remains intact; also called blunt abdominal injury.

closed chest injury An injury to the chest in which the skin is not broken, usually due to blunt trauma.

dyspnea Difficulty breathing.

evisceration The displacement of organs outside of the body.

flail chest A condition in which two or more ribs are fractured in two or more places or in association with a fracture of the sternum so that a segment of chest wall is effectively detached from the rest of the thoracic cage.

Technology

- Interactivities
- Vocabulary Explorer
- Anatomy Review
- Web Links
- Online Review Manual

Refresher.EMSzone.com

guarding Contracting the stomach muscles to minimize the pain of abdominal movement; a sign of peritonitis.

hemoptysis The spitting or coughing up of blood.

hemothorax A collection of blood in the pleural cavity.

hollow organs Structures through which materials pass, such as the stomach, small intestines, large intestines, ureters, and bladder.

myocardial contusion A bruise of the heart muscle.

occlusive dressing A dressing made of Vaseline gauze, aluminum foil, or plastic that prevents air and liquids from entering or exiting a wound.

open abdominal injury An injury of the abdomen caused by a penetrating or piercing instrument or force, in which the skin is lacerated or perforated and the cavity is opened to the atmosphere; also called penetrating injury.

open chest injury An injury to the chest in which the chest wall itself is penetrated by a fractured rib or, more frequently, by an external object such as a bullet or knife.

paradoxical motion The motion of the portion of the chest wall that is detached in a flail chest; the injured segment moves in during inhalation and out during exhalation, the opposite of normal chest wall motion during breathing.

pericardial tamponade Compression of the heart due to a buildup of blood or other fluid in the pericardial sac.

pericardium The fibrous sac that surrounds the heart.

pneumothorax An accumulation of air or gas in the pleural cavity.

pulmonary contusion A bruise of the lung.

solid organs Solid masses of tissue where much of the chemical work of the body takes place (such as the liver, spleen, pancreas, and kidneys).

spontaneous pneumothorax A pneumothorax that occurs when a weak area on the lung ruptures in the absence of major injury, allowing air to leak into the pleural space.

sucking chest wound An open or penetrating chest wall wound through which air passes during inspiration and expiration, creating a sucking sound.

tension pneumothorax An accumulation of air or gas in the pleural cavity that progressively increases the pressure in the chest with potentially fatal results.

Assessment in Action

Given the location of the heart, lungs, and great vessels within the chest cavity, potentially serious injuries may occur. Serious injuries and significant blood loss may also occur to the organs in the abdominal cavity. Quick action when caring for these patients is crucial to a successful outcome.

1. A weak area on the surface of the lungs is known as a(n):
   A. pneumothorax.
   B. bleb.
   C. aneurysm.
   D. evisceration.

2. Signs and symptoms of a tension pneumothorax include(s):
   A. distended neck veins.
   B. tachycardia.
   C. hypotension.
   D. All of the above.

3. What occurs during ventilation?
   A. The intercostal muscles and diaphragm relax.
   B. The intercostal muscles relax and the diaphragm contracts.
   C. The intercostal muscles and diaphragm contract.
   D. The intercostal muscles contract and the diaphragm relaxes.

4. Internal organs protruding through a wound is known as a(n):
   A. hemothorax.
   B. aneurysm.
   C. pneumothorax.
   D. evisceration.

5. _____ is a potentially fatal condition in which fluid builds up in the fibrous sac around the heart.
   A. Congestive heart failure
   B. Tension pneumothorax
   C. Pericardial tamponade
   D. Hemothorax

6. Two or more ribs fractured in two or more places is the definition of:
   A. a pneumothorax.
   B. a flail segment.
   C. a hemothorax.
   D. crepitice.

Challenging Questions

7. What is the treatment for a flail segment?

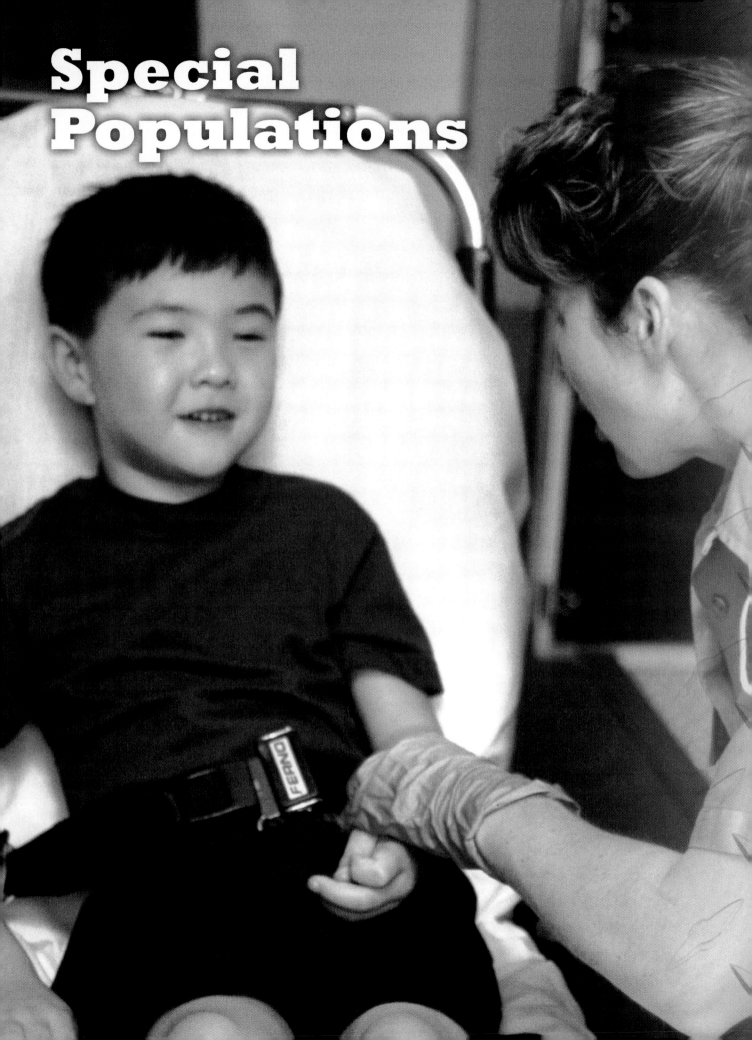

Special Populations

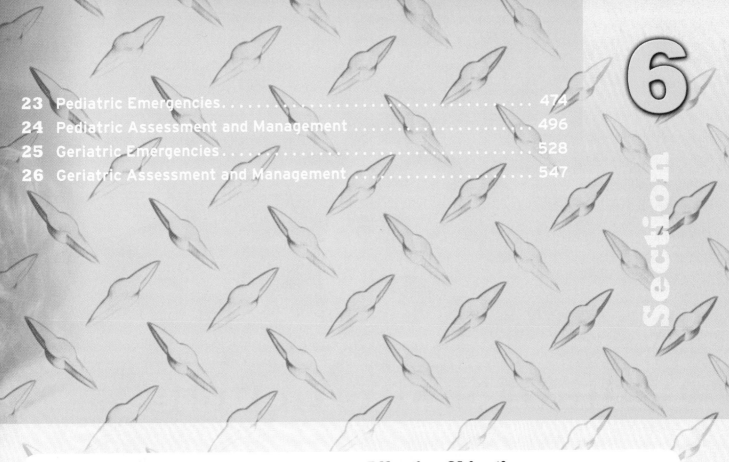

6

Section

Cognitive Objectives

1. Assess and provide care to the obstetric patient. (Chapter 17, p 313)
2. Assist with the delivery of an infant. (Chapter 17, p 315)
3. Assess and provide care to the newborn. (Chapter 17, p 319)
4. Assess and provide care to the mother immediately following delivery of a newborn. (Chapter 17, p 320)
   - Identify predelivery emergencies.
   - State the steps to assist in the delivery.
   - Discuss the steps in the delivery of the placenta.
   - List the steps in the emergency medical care of the mother postdelivery.
   - Summarize neonatal resuscitation procedures.
   - Describe the procedures for the following abnormal deliveries.
5. Assess and provide care to an ill or injured infant or child with: (Chapters 23 and 24)
   - Respiratory distress
   - Shock (hypoperfusion)
   - Cardiac arrest
   - Seizures
   - Trauma

Affective Objectives

1. Explain the rationale for having knowledge and skills appropriate for managing infant and child patients. (Chapter 23, p 475)
2. Understand the provider's own response (emotional) to caring for infants and children. (Chapter 23, p 475)

Psychomotor Objectives

1. Demonstrate steps to assist in the normal cephalic delivery. (Chapter 17, p 315)
2. Demonstrate postdelivery care of the infant. (Chapter 17, p 319)
3. Demonstrate postdelivery care of the mother. (Chapter 17, p 320)

23

Pediatric Emergencies

You are the Provider 1

You are called to a residence for a 2-year-old girl who was having a seizure before EMS arrival. The frantic mother meets you at the door with the distraught toddler wrapped in a blanket. She tells you this has never happened before.

Initial Assessment	Recording Time: 0 Minutes
Appearance	Flushed
Level of consciousness	Appears to be alert
Airway	Open and clear
Breathing	A little fast
Circulation	Tachycardic

1. What questions should you ask the mother?
2. How should you approach the patient?
3. How do you expect the patient to respond to you?

■ Introduction

Pediatrics is the specialized medical practice devoted to the care of young people. Many problems that are common in adults do not occur in children, and not everyone is comfortable caring for children. In most situations, handling an infant or child means that you must manage the parents as well. As you already know, it is vital that you remain calm and professional and keep your personal feelings in check as you work with infants, children, and their families throughout the emergency. Once you learn how to approach children of different ages and what to expect while caring for them, you will find that treating children also offers some very special rewards.

■ Anatomy and Physiology

Children grow and change rapidly. Understanding the anatomy of the pediatric patient and how their bodies work differently from adult bodies will help you immensely when you are assessing and treating them.

To manage the pediatric airway effectively, you should understand the anatomic differences between adults and children. To start with, the heart is higher in a child's chest, and the lungs are smaller. The opening to the trachea is higher in the neck, and the neck itself is shorter.

The anatomy of a child's airway differs from that of the adult airway. These differences will influence the treatment decisions that you make about pediatric patients, including whether intervention is needed and, if so, what procedure to use. Anatomic differences between a child and an adult that affect pediatric airway management techniques include the following Figure 23-1▾ :

- A larger, rounder occiput, or back of the head, which requires more careful positioning of the airway
- A proportionately larger tongue relative to the size of the mouth and a more anterior location in the mouth. The child's tongue is also larger relative to the small mandible and can easily block the airway.
- A floppy, U-shaped epiglottis that is larger than an adult's, relative to the size of the airway
- Less well-developed rings of cartilage in the trachea that may easily collapse if the neck is flexed or hyperextended
- A narrower, lower airway

Because of the smaller diameter of the trachea in infants (about the same as a drinking straw), their airway is easily obstructed by secretions, blood, and swelling.

An infant needs to breathe faster than an older child Table 23-1 ▶ . Children's lungs grow and develop an increased ability to handle exchange of oxygen as they become older. A respiratory rate of 30 to 60 breaths/min is normal for neonates, whereas teenagers

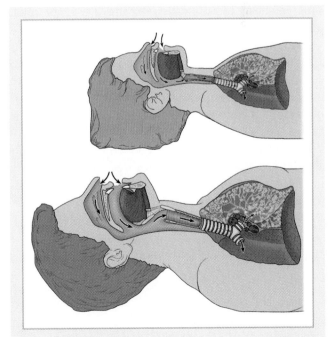

Figure 23-1 The anatomy of a child's airway differs from that of an adult in several ways. The back of the head is larger in a child, so head positioning requires more care. The tongue is proportionately larger and more anterior in the mouth. The trachea is lower and narrower.

Table 23-1 Pediatric Respiratory Rates

Age	Respirations (breaths/min)
Neonate: 0 to 1 month	30 to 60
Infant: 1 month to 1 year	25 to 50
Toddler: 1 to 3 years	20 to 30
Preschool age: 3 to 6 years	20 to 25
School age: 6 to 12 years	15 to 20
Adolescent: 12 to 18 years	12 to 16
Older than 18 years	12 to 20

have rates closer to the adult range (12 to 20 breaths/min). Breathing also requires the use of the chest muscles and diaphragm. Because intercostal muscles are not well developed in children, movement of the diaphragm, their major muscle of respiration, dictates the amount of air that they inspire. Anything that puts pressure on the abdomen of a young child can block the movement of the diaphragm and cause respiratory compromise. Gastric distention can interfere with movement of the diaphragm and lead to hypoventilation. Young children also experience muscle fatigue much more quickly than do older children. This can lead to respiratory failure if a child must physically fight to breathe for long periods.

An infant's heart rate can become as high as 200 beats or more per minute if the infant needs to compensate for injury or illness. This is the primary method the body uses to compensate for decreased perfusion. It is important to know the normal heart rate ranges when evaluating children (Table 23-2 ▼).

The ability in children to constrict blood vessels also helps them compensate for decreased perfusion. Pale skin is an early sign that a child may be compen-

Table 23-2 Pediatric Heart Rate

Age	Heart Rate (beats/min)
Infant	100 to 160
Toddler	90 to 150
Preschooler	80 to 140
School-age child	70 to 120
Adolescent	60 to 100

sating for decreased perfusion. Vessel constriction can be so profound that blood flow to the extremities can be diminished. Signs of vasoconstriction can include weak distal (for example, radial or pedal) pulses, delayed capillary refill, and cool hands or feet.

The skeletal system contains growth plates at the ends of long bones, which enable these bones to grow during childhood. As a result of the active growth plates, children's bones are weaker and more flexible, making them prone to fracture with stress. The bones of the skull also grow during infancy. Infants have two soft openings within the skull called fontanels. These will usually close completely by about 18 months of age.

■ Growth and Development

Between birth and adulthood, many physical and emotional changes occur in children. Although each child is unique, the thoughts and behaviors of children as a whole are often grouped into stages: infancy, the toddler years, preschool age, school age, and adolescence. Children in each stage struggle with developmental issues. Even though there are specific issues that are important to different age groups, there are also general rules that apply when you care for children of any age.

The Infant

Infancy is usually defined as the first year of life; the first month after birth is called the neonatal, or newborn, period. At first, infants respond mainly to physical stimuli such as light, warmth, hunger, and sound. Crying is one of their main avenues of expression. After the first few months, they learn to coo, smile, roll over, and recognize their parents or caregivers. Infants are usually not afraid of strangers because they are used to being the center of attention. By the end of their first year, they may show signs of separation anxiety (cry when separated) and prefer to be with their caregivers (Figure 23-2 ▶).

Begin your assessment by observing the infant from a distance as you approach. Older infants, from 6 months to a year, may begin to cry when touched or picked up by a stranger, so let the caregiver continue to hold the baby as you start your examination. Provide as much sensory comfort as you can. Warm your hands and the end of the stethoscope and offer a pacifier if the caregiver allows it. Have a caregiver hold the infant, if possible, during procedures. Plan to complete any painful procedure in an efficient manner,

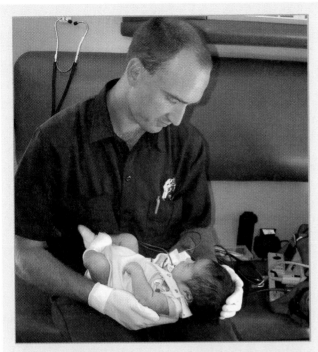

Figure 23-2 Infants are usually not afraid of strangers, but as they reach 6 months to 1 year, they may show signs that they prefer to be with their caregivers.

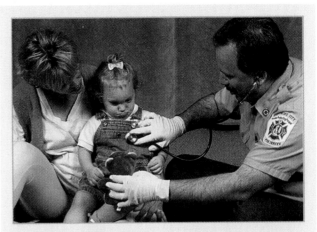

Figure 23-3 Leave a toddler on the caregiver's lap during your assessment, and use a toy to distract him or her.

and, if possible, plan to do any painful procedures at the end of the assessment process, so that if the child becomes agitated, it will not interfere with assessment. When splinting a suspected fracture, have all of the equipment you will need ready to avoid making the procedure take longer than necessary.

Toddlers

From 1 to about 3 years, a child is called a <u>toddler</u>. During this period, children begin to walk and explore the environment. They are able to open doors, drawers, boxes, and bottles. Because they are explorers by nature and are not afraid, injuries increase in this age group.

Stranger anxiety develops early in this period. Toddlers may resist separation from caregivers and be afraid to let others come near them. Because of their newly found independence, they may also be very unhappy about being restrained or held for procedures. Two-year-olds in particular have a well-deserved reputation for having their own ideas about almost everything, the "terrible twos." Toddlers have a hard time describing or localizing pain. Pain in the abdomen may be expressed as, "My tummy hurts," and examination may reveal tenderness throughout the body.

This is not because the child is trying to be difficult; the child does not have the verbal ability to be exact.

Toddlers can be curious and adventuresome, so you may be able to distract them Figure 23-3 . For example, you might allow the child to play with a tongue depressor while assessing his or her vital signs. Restrain the child for as short a time as possible, and allow him or her to be comforted by the caregiver immediately after a painful procedure. Begin your assessment at the hands or feet to keep from upsetting the child whenever possible.

The Preschool-Age Child

During <u>preschool age</u>, children (ages 3 to 6 years) are able to use simple language quite effectively and have lively imaginations. They can understand directions, be much more specific in describing their sensations, and identify painful areas when questioned. Much of their history must still be obtained from caregivers. Preschool-age children have a rich fantasy life, which can make them particularly fearful about pain and change involving their bodies. At this age, they often believe that their thoughts or wishes can cause injury or harm to themselves or others. They can believe that an injury was due to their bad deed earlier in the day.

Tell the child what you are going to do immediately before you do it so the child will not have time to develop frightening fantasies. At this age, children are easily distracted with counting games, small toys, and conversation Figure 23-4 . Be sure to adjust the level of game to the developmental level of the child; health care providers often assume that preschool children understand more than they actually do. Begin your

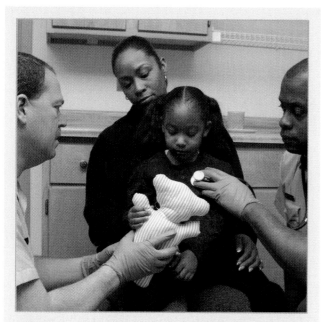

Figure 23-4 A preschool-age child can be easily distracted by games or conversation.

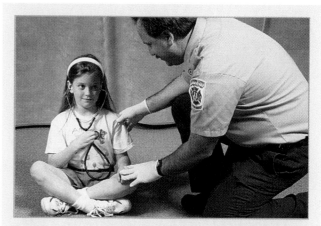

Figure 23-5 School-age children are more like adults because they can answer your questions and can help take care of themselves.

assessment with the feet and move toward the head, similar to assessing a toddler. Use adhesive bandages to cover any injuries because the child might be worried about keeping his or her body together in one piece.

The School-Age Child

During <u>school age</u>, children (ages 6 to 12 years) are beginning to act more like adults. They can think in concrete terms, respond sensibly to direct questions, and help take care of themselves. Your assessment should be more like that for an adult. You should talk to the child, not just the caregiver, while asking questions and performing your assessment.

School-age children are usually familiar with the process of physical examination. They have been to the doctor for childhood checkups and immunizations. You may begin at the head and move to the feet, similar to assessing adolescents and adults. Whenever possible, give the child appropriate choices: Would you like to sit up or lie down? Ask only questions for which you can control the answer. If you ask "Can I take your blood pressure?" and the answer is no, you will not be able to take it without upsetting the child. Instead, ask if you may find out their blood pressure on their right or left arm. (Asking if you may "take" the blood pressure may make younger patients think you will not give it back.) Giving them a choice that allows you to still obtain assessment information

allows the child some control. Encourage cooperation by allowing the child to listen to his or her own heartbeat through the stethoscope (Figure 23-5 ▲).

School-age children can understand the difference between emotional and physical pain and have concerns about what pain means. Give them simple explanations about what is causing their pain and what will be done about it. Games and conversation may distract them. Ask them to describe their favorite place, their pets, or their toys. Ask the caregiver's advice in choosing the right distraction. Rewarding a school-age child after a procedure can be very helpful in his or her future cooperation and recovery.

Adolescents

Most <u>adolescents</u> (ages 12 to 18 years) are able to think abstractly and can participate in decision making. This is when the focus of their strength has moved from parents to peers. They are very concerned about body image and how they appear to their peers and others their age. They may have very strong feelings against being observed during procedures.

Respect the adolescent's privacy at all times. Remember that adolescents can often understand very complex concepts and treatment options; you should provide them with information when they request it. You will find them more helpful and understanding of necessary procedures than younger patients.

Adolescents have a clear understanding of the purpose and meaning of pain. Whenever possible, explain any necessary procedures well in advance. Assess their pain by facial and body expression and by asking questions. To distract them, find out what they

Teamwork Tips

One rescuer should talk with the patient in an area *away* from the parents or caregivers while the second rescuer talks to the parents or caregivers.

are interested in, such as sports, books, movies, or friends, and get them talking.

Family Matters

It is important to remember that when children are ill or injured, especially children with chronic illnesses, you may have several patients to treat. Family members, especially the parent or primary caregiver, often need help or support when the child is sick or injured. A calm parent usually helps contribute to calmness in the child. An agitated parent usually means that the child will act the same way. Make sure that you are calm, efficient, professional, and sensitive as you deal with children and their families.

■ Pediatric Emergencies

Dehydration

Dehydration occurs when fluid losses are greater than fluid intake. The most common cause of dehy-

dration in children is vomiting and diarrhea. If left untreated, dehydration can lead to shock and, eventually, death. Infants and children are at greater risk than adults for dehydration because their fluid reserves are smaller than those in adults. Life-threatening dehydration can overcome an infant in a matter of hours.

Fever

Fever is a common reason that parents call 9-1-1. Simply defined, fever is an increase in body temperature, usually in response to an infection. Body temperatures of 100.4°F (38°C) or higher are considered abnormal. Fevers have many causes and are rarely life-threatening events. You should not underestimate the potential seriousness of fevers, such as those that occur in conjunction with a rash. You should be suspicious of whether the fever is a sign of serious illness, such as meningitis. Common causes of a high temperature in a child include infection (ear infection, pneumonia, meningitis, or urinary tract infection), drug ingestion, and high environmental temperatures.

Fever is due to an internal body mechanism in which heat generation is increased and heat loss is decreased. Hyperthermia differs from fever in that it is an increase in body temperature caused by an inability of the body to cool itself. Hyperthermia is typically seen in warm environments, such as a closed car on a hot day.

You are the Provider 2

The child is very apprehensive, but will allow you to touch her with her mother holding her. You note that she is very hot to the touch. Her mother tells you that she woke up vomiting and then started having a seizure. The seizure activity lasted about 3 minutes.

Vital Signs	Recording Time: 2 Minutes
Skin	Flushed, hot to touch
Pulse	136 beats/min
Temperature	103.2°F
Respirations	32 breaths/min

4. What might you do to distract the patient?
5. How should you perform your assessment?
6. What is the proper treatment for this patient?

Meningitis

Meningitis is an inflammation of the meninges, the tissue that covers the spinal cord and brain. It is an infection caused by bacteria, viruses, fungi, or parasites. If left untreated, meningitis can lead to permanent brain damage or death. Meningitis can occur in children and adults. Those at greater risk for meningitis include the following:

- Males
- Newborn infants
- Older people
- People whose immune systems have been weakened by AIDS or cancer
- People who have any history of brain, spinal cord, or back surgery
- Children who have had head trauma
- Children with shunts, pins, or other foreign bodies within the brain or spinal cord

At especially high risk are children with a ventriculoperitoneal (VP) shunt. Ventriculoperitoneal shunts drain excess fluids from around the brain into the abdomen. These special-needs children have tubing that can usually be seen and felt just under the scalp.

The signs and symptoms of meningitis vary, depending on the age of the patient. Fever and altered level of consciousness are common symptoms of meningitis in patients of all ages. Changes in level of consciousness can range from a mild or severe headache to confusion, lethargy, and/or an inability to understand commands or interact appropriately. The child may also experience a seizure, which may be a first sign of meningitis.

In describing children with meningitis, physicians often use the term "meningeal irritation" or "meningeal signs" to describe pain that accompanies movement. Bending the neck forward or back increases the tension within the spinal canal and stretches the meninges, causing a great deal of pain. Children with this characteristic stiff neck will often refuse to move their neck or lift their legs. One sign of meningitis in an infant is increasing irritability, especially when being handled. Infants with meningitis may also have a bulging fontanel.

One form of meningitis deserves special attention. *Neisseria meningitidis* is a bacterium that causes a rapid onset of meningitis symptoms, often leading to shock and death. Children with this bacterial meningitis typically have small, pinpoint, cherry-red spots or a larger purple-black rash Figure 23-6 ▶. This rash may be on part of the face or body. Children with this type of meningitis are at serious risk of sepsis, shock, and death.

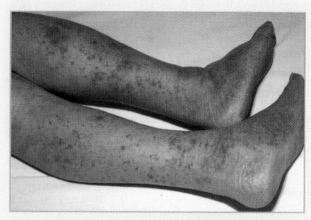

Figure 23-6 Children with *N meningitidis* typically have small, pinpoint, cherry-red spots or a larger purple-black rash.

All patients with possible meningitis should be considered highly contagious and infectious. You should use body substance isolation (BSI) precautions whenever you suspect meningitis and follow up with the hospital to learn the patient's final diagnosis. If you have been exposed to a child with bacterial meningitis, you should follow your department's infectious disease policy for medical review and treatment.

Seizures

A seizure is the result of disorganized electrical activity in the brain. Common causes of seizures are listed in Table 23-3 ▶. As you know, it can be frightening to see someone have a seizure, especially if the patient is an infant or young child. Remember to reassure the family and to approach assessment and management in a calm, step-by-step manner.

Febrile Seizures

Febrile seizures are common in children between the ages of 6 months and 6 years. Most pediatric seizures are due to fever alone, which is why they are called febrile seizures. These seizures typically occur on the first day of an illness that is accompanied by a high

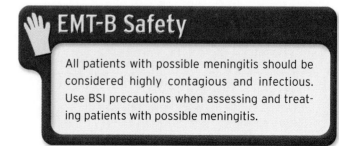

EMT-B Safety

All patients with possible meningitis should be considered highly contagious and infectious. Use BSI precautions when assessing and treating patients with possible meningitis.

Table 23-3 Common Causes of Seizures

- Fever
- Hypoglycemia (low blood glucose level)
- Idiopathic (no cause can be found)
- Lack of oxygen
- Poisoning
- Infection
- Child abuse
- Electrolyte imbalance
- Medications
- Previous seizure disorder
- Recreational drug use
- Head trauma

temperature. A common cause of a fever that causes a seizure is a middle ear infection. The seizures are characterized by generalized tonic-clonic activity, last fewer than 15 minutes, and have a short postictal phase or none at all. A seizure also may be a sign of a more serious problem, such as meningitis. Obtain a history from the caregivers because the child may have had a previous febrile seizure.

If you are called to care for a child who has had a febrile seizure, you often will find that the patient is awake, alert, and fully interactive when you arrive. Remember that a persistent fever can lead to another seizure.

Poisoning

Poisoning is common among children Table 23-4 ▼. The signs and symptoms of poisoning vary widely, depending on the substance, the route, and the age and

Table 23-4 Common Sources of Poisoning in Children

- Alcohol
- Aspirin and acetaminophen
- Household cleaning products such as bleach and furniture polish
- Houseplants
- Iron
- Prescription medications of family members
- Street drugs
- Vitamins

weight of the child. The child may appear normal at first, even in serious cases, or he or she may be confused, sleepy, or unconscious.

Infants may be poisoned as a result of being fed a harmful substance by a sibling or a caregiver or as a result of child abuse. Infants can be exposed to drugs and poisons left on floors and carpeting. They can also be exposed in a room or automobile in which harmful drugs, such as crack, cocaine, or PCP (phencyclidine hydrochloride), are being smoked. Toddlers are curious and often ingest poisons when they find them in the home or garage Figure 23-7 ▼. For example, many cleaning supplies are colored liquids. Toddlers may think the substance is juice or soda. Adolescents are more likely to have ingested alcohol and street drugs while partying or in a suicide attempt.

After you have completed your initial assessment, try to determine the following:

- What is the substance(s) involved?
- Approximately how much of the substance was ingested or involved in the exposure (for example, number of pills, amount of liquid)?

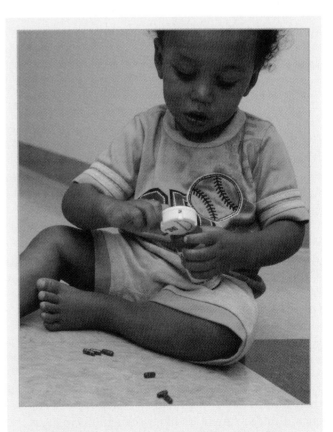

Figure 23-7 A curious child will try to taste or swallow almost any substance. A common victim of accidental ingestion of dangerous compounds is the unwatched toddler.

- What time did the incident occur?
- Are there changes in behavior or level of consciousness?
- Was there choking or coughing after the exposure?

■ Pediatric Trauma

Injuries are the number one killer of children in the United States. More children die of injuries in 1 year than of all other causes combined. As an EMT-B, you frequently treat injured children. The quality of care during the first few minutes after a child has been injured can have an enormous impact on that child's chances for complete recovery.

Infants and toddlers are most commonly hurt as a result of falls or abuse. Older children and adolescents are usually injured as a result of mishaps involving automobiles. According to information collected by the National Pediatric Trauma Registry, automobile accidents, including those involving bicycles and pedestrians, are the most significant threat to the well-being of children. Other common causes of traumatic injury and death include falls, gunshot wounds, blunt injuries, and sports activities. Another extremely serious and troublesome cause of injury is child abuse.

Physical Differences

Children are smaller than adults; therefore, when they are hurt in the same type of accident as an adult, the location of their injuries may differ. For example, the bumper of a car will strike an adult in the lower leg, whereas it will strike a child in the pelvis. In a crash involving sudden deceleration, an adult might injure a ligament in the knee; in that same accident, a child might injure the bones in the leg.

Children's bones and soft tissues are less well developed than those of adults. The force of an injury affects these structures differently than it does in an adult. Because a child's head is proportionately larger than an adult's, it exerts greater stress on the neck structures during a deceleration injury.

Psychological Differences

Children are also less mature psychologically than adults; therefore, they are often injured because of their undeveloped judgment and their lack of experience. Children are more likely than adults to cross the street without looking for oncoming traffic. As a result, children are more likely than adults to be struck by cars. Children and adolescents are also more likely to sustain injuries from diving into shallow water because they forget to check the depth of the water before they dive.

Injury Patterns

Although you are not responsible for diagnosing injuries in children, your ability to recognize and treat serious injuries in children has a tremendous impact on the outcome for the child. For this reason, it is important for you to understand what makes children more likely to have certain kinds of injuries.

Automobile Collisions

Children playing or riding a bicycle can dart in front of motor vehicles without looking. In such a situation, the driver may have little time to slow down or stop to prevent hitting the child. The area of greatest injury varies, depending on the size of the child and the height of the bumper at the time of impact. When vehicles slow down at the moment of impact, the bumper dips slightly, causing the point of impact with the child to be lowered. The exact area that is struck depends on the child's height and the final position of the bumper at the time of impact. Children who are injured in these situations often sustain high-energy injuries to the head, spine, abdomen, pelvis, or legs.

Sports Activities

Children, especially those who are older or adolescents, are often injured in organized sports activities. Head and neck injuries can occur after high-speed collisions in contact sports such as football, wrestling, ice hockey, field hockey, soccer, and lacrosse. Remember to stabilize the cervical spine when caring for children with sports-related injuries. You should be familiar with your local protocols related to helmet removal.

■ Injuries to Specific Body Systems

Head Injuries

Head injuries are common in children because the size of a child's head, in relation to the body, is larger than that of an adult. The signs and symptoms of head injury in a child are similar to those in an adult, but there are some important differences. Nausea and vomiting are common signs and symptoms of head injury in children. You should suspect a serious head injury in any child who experiences nausea and vomiting in conjunction with the mechanism of injury.

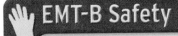

Chest Injuries

Chest injuries in children are usually the result of blunt trauma rather than penetrating objects. Remember that children have very soft, flexible ribs that can be compressed a great deal without breaking. Keep this in mind as you assess a child who has sustained blunt trauma to the chest. Even though there may be no external sign of injury, such as broken ribs, contusions, or bleeding, there may be significant injuries within the chest.

Abdominal Injuries

Abdominal injuries are common in children. Remember that children can compensate for significant blood loss better than adults without signs or symptoms of shock. They can also have a serious injury without early external evidence of a problem. All children with abdominal injuries should be monitored for signs and symptoms of shock, including a weak, rapid pulse; cold, clammy skin; decreased capillary refill (an early sign); confusion; and decreased systolic blood pressure (a late sign). Even in the absence of signs and symptoms of shock or with only a few signs and symptoms, you should remain cautious about the possibility of internal injuries.

Extremity Injuries

Children have immature bones with active growth centers. Growth of long bones occurs from the ends at specialized growth plates. These growth plates are potential weak spots in the bone and are often injured as a result of trauma. In general, children's bones bend more easily than do adults' bones. As a result, incomplete or greenstick fractures can occur.

Extremity injuries in children are generally managed in the same manner as those in adults. Painful, deformed limbs should be splinted. Specialized splinting equipment, such as a traction splint for fractures of the femur, should be used only if it fits the child. You should not attempt to use adult immobilization devices on a child unless the child is large enough to properly fit in the device.

Other Considerations

Pneumatic Antishock Garments

A pneumatic antishock garment (PASG) is rarely used on a pediatric patient. The problem with the use of a PASG on a child is that it rarely fits the child appropriately. The PASG should be used on children only if it fits properly. Techniques such as placing the child in one leg of the garment are absolutely contraindicated and should never be used. The abdominal compartment of the garment should be inflated on children with caution because excessive pressure on the abdomen will cause pressure on the diaphragm and compromise breathing.

Burns

Children can be burned in a variety of ways. The most common involve exposure to hot substances such as scalding water in a bathtub, hot items on a stove, or exposure to caustic substances such as cleaning solvents or paint thinners. You should suspect possible internal injuries from chemical ingestion when you see a child who has burns around the face and mouth.

A common problem following burn injuries in children is infection. Burned skin cannot resist infection as effectively as normal skin can. For this reason, sterile technique should be used in treating pediatric burn patients.

Table 23-5 provides general guidelines on classifying the severity of a burn to a child. These guidelines may help you determine which children should

Table 23-5 Severity of Burns in Children

Severity of Burn	Body Area Involved
Minor	Partial-thickness burns involving less than 10% of the body surface
Moderate	Partial-thickness burns involving 10% to 20% of the body surface
Critical	Any full-thickness burn
	Any partial-thickness burn involving more than 20% of the body surface
	Any burn involving the hands, feet, face, airway, or genitalia

be treated at a specialized burn center or a trauma center. Remember that you should consider the possibility of child abuse in any burn situation. Make sure you report any information about your suspicions to the appropriate authorities.

Submersion Injury

Submersion injuries include near drowning and drowning. In submersion situations, you must always take steps to ensure your own safety.

Drowning is the second most common cause of unintentional death among children in the United States; children younger than 5 years are at particular risk. At this age, children often fall into swimming pools and lakes, but many drown in bathtubs and even buckets. Older adolescents, who account for the most drownings after toddlers, drown when swimming or boating, and alcohol use is frequently a factor.

The principal injury from submersion is lack of oxygen. Even a few minutes (or less) without oxygen will affect the heart, lungs, and brain. This can lead to life-threatening problems such as cardiac arrest, respiratory difficulty, and coma. Submersion in icy water can rob the body of heat, resulting in hypothermia. While a very few, very cold victims of submersion hypothermia have survived long periods in cardiac arrest in icy water, most people in this situation die. Diving into the water increases the risk of neck and spinal cord injuries.

■ Child Abuse

The term <u>child abuse</u> means any improper or excessive action that injures or otherwise harms a child or infant. Child abuse includes physical abuse, sexual abuse, neglect, and emotional abuse. The intentional injury of a child, whether physical or emotional, is not rare in our society. More than 2 million cases of child abuse are reported to child protection agencies annually. Many of these children sustain life-threatening injuries, and some die. If suspected child abuse is not reported, the child is likely to be abused again and again, perhaps sustaining permanent injuries or death. You must be aware of the signs of child abuse and neglect and of your responsibility to report suspected abuse to law enforcement or child protection agencies.

Signs of Abuse

If you suspect that physical or sexual abuse is involved, you should ask yourself the following questions:

- Is the injury typical for the developmental level of the child?
- Is the method of injury reported by the parent or caregiver consistent with the child's injuries?
- Is the caregiver behaving appropriately (concerned about the child's well-being)?
- Is there evidence of drinking or drug use at the scene?

You are the Provider 3

You give the patient a penlight to hold and ask Mom to help by removing the child's clothing down to her diaper. Your partner begins sponging the patient with tepid water. Your assessment reveals nothing significant and she appears to be in no distress. Her mother tells you that she has been pulling at her ears since last night and she may have an ear infection.

Reassessment	Recording Time: 5 Minutes
Pulse	142 beats/min
Temperature	102.6°F
Respirations	32 breaths/min
Breath sounds	Clear bilaterally
Pulse oximetry	97% while breathing room air

7. What are some of the common causes of seizures?

8. If you are able to lower the patient's temperature, should she be transported? Why or why not?

- Was there a delay in seeking care for the child?
- Is there a good relationship between the child and the caregiver?
- Does the child have multiple injuries at different stages of healing?
- Does the child have any unusual marks or bruises that may have been caused by cigarettes, grids, or branding injuries?
- Does the child have several types of injuries, such as burns, fractures, and bruises?
- Does the child have any burns on the hands or feet that involve a glove distribution (marks that encircle a hand or foot in a pattern that looks like a glove)?
- Is there an unexplained decreased level of consciousness?
- Is the child clean and an appropriate weight for his or her age?
- Is there any rectal or vaginal bleeding?
- What does the home look like? Clean or dirty? Is it warm or cold? Is there age-appropriate food?

Your assessment in the field is critical to the overall care of the child. An easy way to remember what to look for is the mnemonic CHILD ABUSE shown in Table 23-6. As you assess the child, look for and pay particular attention to the following signs Figure 23-8 :

Bruises

Observe the color and location of any bruises. New bruises are pink or red. Over time, bruises turn blue,

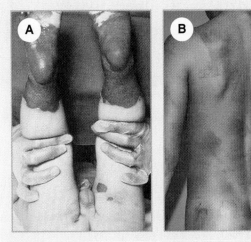

Figure 23-8 Signs of child abuse. **A.** Scald. **B.** Multiple injuries at different stages of healing.

then green, then yellow-brown and faded. Note the location. Bruises to the back, buttocks, or face are suspicious and are usually inflicted by a person.

Burns

Burns to the penis, testicles, vagina, or buttocks are usually inflicted by someone else, as are burns that encircle a hand or foot to look like a glove. You should suspect abuse if the child has cigarette burns or burns in a grid pattern.

Fractures

Fractures of the humerus or femur do not normally occur unless there was major trauma, such as a fall from a high place or a motor vehicle crash. Falls from bed are not usually associated with fractures.

Shaken Baby Syndrome

Infants may sustain life-threatening head trauma by being shaken or struck on the head, a life-threatening condition called shaken baby syndrome. With this condition, there is bleeding within the head and damage to the cervical spine as a result of intentional, forceful shaking. The infant will be found unconscious, often without evidence of external trauma. The call for help may be for an infant who has stopped breathing or is unresponsive. The infant may appear to be in cardiopulmonary arrest, but what has likely occurred is that the shaking tore blood vessels in the brain, resulting in bleeding around the brain. The pressure from the blood results in a coma.

Table 23-6 Child Abuse

Mnemonic for Assessing Possible Child Abuse

Consistency of the injury with the child's developmental age

History inconsistent with injury

Inappropriate parental concerns

Lack of supervision

Delay in seeking care

Affect

Bruises of varying ages

Unusual injury patterns

Suspicious circumstances

Environmental clues

Documentation Tips

Document all findings and make special note of any unusual injury patterns that may indicate child abuse.

Neglect

Children who are neglected are often dirty or too thin or appear developmentally delayed because of lack of stimulation. You may observe such children when you are making calls for unrelated problems. Report all cases of suspicious neglect.

Symptoms and Other Indicators of Abuse

An abused child may appear withdrawn, fearful, or hostile. You should be particularly concerned if the child refuses to discuss how an injury occurred. Occasionally, the parent or caregiver will reveal a history of several "accidents." Be alert for conflicting stories or a marked lack of concern from the parents or caregiver. Remember, the abuser may be a parent, caregiver, relative, or friend of the family. Sometimes the abuser is an acquaintance of a single parent.

EMT-Bs in all states must report all cases of suspected abuse, even if the emergency department fails to do so. Most states have special forms for reporting. Supervisors are generally forbidden to interfere with the reporting of suspected abuse, even if they disagree with the assessment. You do not have to prove that there has been abuse. Law enforcement and child protection agencies are mandated to investigate all reported cases.

Sexual Abuse

Children of any age and either sex can be victims of sexual abuse. Most victims of rape are older than 10 years, although younger children may be victims as well. This type of sexual abuse is often the result of longstanding abuse by relatives.

Your assessment of a child who has been sexually abused is usually limited. Sometimes, a sexually abused child is also beaten. Therefore, you should treat any bruises or fractures as well. Do not examine the genitalia of a young child unless there is evidence of bleeding or there is an injury that must be treated.

In addition, if you suspect that a child is a victim of sexual abuse, do not allow the child to wash, urinate, or defecate before a physician completes an exam. Although this step is difficult, it is important to preserve evidence. If the molested child is a girl, ensure that a female EMT-B or police officer remains with the child unless locating one will delay transport.

You must maintain professional composure the entire time you are assessing and caring for a sexually abused child. Assume a concerned, caring approach, and shield the child from onlookers and curious bystanders. Obtain as much information as possible from the child and any witnesses. The child may be hysterical or unwilling to say anything at all, especially if the abuser is a relative or family friend. You are in the best position to obtain the most accurate firsthand information about the incident. Therefore, you should record any information carefully and completely on the patient care report.

Transport all children who are victims of sexual assault. Sexual abuse of a child is a crime. Cooperate with law enforcement officials in their investigations.

■ Sudden Infant Death Syndrome

The death of an infant or a young child is called sudden infant death syndrome (SIDS) when, after a complete autopsy, the cause of death remains unexplained. SIDS is the leading cause of death in infants younger than 1 year, and most cases occur in infants younger than 6 months.

You are the Provider 4

You continue to cool her with tepid water en route to the hospital. On arrival, her temperature is down to 101.8° F. She is seen by the pediatrician on call and given antibiotics for her ear infection and an antipyretic for the fever. She is allowed to go home with an appointment to return to the doctor's office in 3 days for a checkup.

Although it is impossible to predict SIDS, there are several known risk factors:

- Mother younger than 20 years old
- Mother smoked during pregnancy
- Low birth weight

Deaths due to SIDS can occur at any time of the day. Most SIDS patients are discovered in the morning when the parents go in to check on the infant. If you are the first provider at the scene of suspected SIDS, you will face three tasks: assessment and management of the patient, communication with and support of the family, and assessment of the scene.

Assessment and Management

SIDS is a diagnosis of exclusion. All other potential causes must first be ruled out, a process that may take physicians quite a while. An infant who has been a victim of SIDS will be pale or blue, not breathing, and unresponsive.

Regardless of the cause, assessment and management of the infant remain the same. Remember that what you find in assessing the infant and the scene may provide important diagnostic information.

Begin with an assessment of the ABCs, and provide interventions as necessary. Depending on how much time has passed since the child was discovered, he or she may show signs of postmortem changes. These include stiffening of the body, called <u>rigor mortis</u>, and <u>dependent lividity</u>, which is the pooling of blood in the lower parts of the body or those that are in contact with the floor or bed.

If the child shows such signs, follow your local protocol, which may include calling medical control. In some EMS systems, a victim of SIDS may be declared dead on the scene. Deciding whether to start CPR on a child who shows clear signs of rigor mortis or dependent lividity can be very difficult. Family members may consider anything less as withholding critical care. In this situation, the best course of action may be to initiate CPR and transport the patient and the family to the nearest emergency department, where the family can receive more extensive support (follow local protocols). If there is no evidence of postmortem changes, begin CPR immediately.

As you assess the infant, pay special attention to any marks or bruises on the child before performing any procedures, including CPR. Also note any intervention such as CPR that was done by the parents before you arrived.

Communication With and Support of the Family

The death of a child is a stressful event for a family; it also tends to evoke strong emotional responses among health care providers, including EMS personnel Table 23-7. Part of your job at this point is to allow the family members to express their grief in ways that

TABLE 23-7 How You Can Help the Family of a Deceased Child

When Arriving on Site
- Introduce yourself quickly.
- Obtain a brief history.
- When possible, one provider should stay with the family.

If Resuscitation Is Attempted
- Give brief, frequent updates and explanations.
- Allow family members to stay within viewing distance if they wish.
- Allow family members to accompany child to the hospital when possible.

If No Resuscitation Is Performed
- Sit down with the family.
- Inform the family immediately.
- Explain why no resuscitation will be attempted.
- Offer to arrange for religious support, including baptism or last rites.

Beginning the Grieving Process
- Learn and use the child's name.
- Allow family to express emotions; be nonjudgmental.
- Give brief explanations and answers.
- Explain to the family that the cause of death is still unknown.
- Allow time for questions.

DO
- Tell the family how sorry you are.
- Tell the family whom they can call if they have questions later.
- Give written instructions and referrals.

DON'T
- Say, "I know how you feel."
- Say, "You have other children" or "You can have other children."
- Attempt to answer the question "Why did this happen?"
- Try to tell family that they will be feeling better in time.

Table 23-8 Common Questions Following Death of a Child

Q Was there pain?

A This often can be answered by a simple "No." If you are uncertain, you may give an indirect answer such as "We really don't know what patients feel in these circumstances."

Q What did he/she die of?

A Do not answer this question; you would probably be guessing at this point.

Q Why did this happen?

A Do not attempt to answer this question either, as the answer depends on one's own individual philosophy, or religion. "I wish I had an answer for you" is usually the most appropriate response.

Q What happens now?

A This question usually concerns the next few minutes or the next hour. If you know, you should give the family a general idea of what will happen. For example, if there is no history of illness, you can say that "a medical examination will be done, and then [child's name] will be taken to the mortuary."

may differ from your own cultural, religious, and personal practices. Provide support in whatever ways you can.

Many times, family members will ask specific questions about the event: Why did this happen? How did this happen? Let them know that their concerns will be addressed but that answers are not immediately available Table 23-8 ▲. Always use the infant's name when speaking to family members. If possible, allow the family to spend time with the infant and to ride in the ambulance to the hospital.

Scene Assessment

Carefully inspect the environment, noting the condition of the scene where the caregivers found the infant. Your assessment of the scene should concentrate on the following:

- Signs of illness, including medications, humidifiers, or thermometers
- The general condition of the house (Note any signs of poor hygiene.)
- Family interaction. Do not allow yourself to be judgmental about family interactions at this time. Do note and report any behavior that is clearly not within the acceptable range, such as physical and verbal abuse.

- The site where the infant was discovered
- Note all items in the infant's crib or bed, including pillows, stuffed animals, toys, and small objects.

The death of a child is difficult for everyone involved: parents, relatives, friends, and health care professionals. You should arrange for a proper debriefing after your involvement with the run comes to a close. This can be a session with a trained counselor or a group discussion with your colleagues or the entire health care team.

Apparent Life-threatening Event

Infants who are not breathing and are cyanotic and unresponsive when found by their families sometimes resume breathing and color with stimulation. These children have had what is called an apparent life-threatening event (ALTE), called "near-miss SIDS" in the past. In addition to cyanosis and apnea, a classic ALTE is characterized by a distinct change in muscle tone (limpness) and choking or gagging. After the event, a child may appear healthy and show no signs of illness or distress. You still should complete a careful assessment and provide immediate transport.

Pay strict attention to management of the airway. Assess the infant's history and, if possible, the environment. Allow caregivers to ride in the ambulance. If asked, explain that you cannot say what caused the event and that this is something that doctors will have to determine at the hospital.

Death of a Child

As with SIDS, the death of a child from any cause poses special challenges for EMS personnel. In addition to any medical treatment the child may require, you must be prepared to offer the family a high level of support and understanding as they begin the grieving process. First, the family may want you to initiate resuscitation efforts, which may or may not conflict with your EMS protocols. If the child is clearly deceased and, under protocol, can be declared dead in the field, but the family is so distraught that they insist that resuscitation efforts be made, initiate CPR and transport the child.

The extent of your interaction with the family will depend, to some degree, on the number of providers available at the scene. Always introduce yourself to the child's caregivers, and ask about the child's date of birth and medical history. If and when the decision is made to start or stop resuscitation efforts, inform the family immediately. Find a place for family members where they can watch the resuscitation without being in the way. Do not, in any case, speculate on the cause of the child's death. The family will want to see the child and should be asked whether they want to hold the child. Parents may be experiencing strong feelings of denial.

The following interventions are helpful in caring for the family at this time:

- Learn and use the child's name rather than the impersonal "your child."
- Speak to family members at eye level, maintaining good eye contact with them.
- Use the word "dead" or "died" when informing the family of the child's death; euphemisms such as "passed away" and "gone" are not effective.
- Acknowledge the family's feelings ("I know this is devastating for you"), but never say "I know how you feel," even if you have experienced a similar event; the statement will anger many people.
- Offer to call other family members or clergy if the family wants.
- Keep any instructions short, simple, and basic. Emotional distress may limit their ability to process information.
- Ask each adult family member individually whether he or she wants to hold the child.
- Wrap the dead child in a blanket, as you would if he or she were alive, and stay with the family while they hold the child.

Remember that each individual and each culture express grief in a different way, some more visibly than others. Some will require intervention; others will not. Most caregivers feel directly or indirectly responsible for the death of a child and may express this immediately; this does not mean that they actually are responsible. Parents often have questions that you should be prepared to answer. Although you should keep the possibility of abuse or neglect in mind, your role is not that of investigator. Any further inquiry is the responsibility of law enforcement personnel.

Again, coping with the death of a child can be stressful for health care professionals. You may find yourself with unexpected feelings of pain and loss. It is helpful to take some time before going back on the job to work through your feelings and talk about the event with your EMS colleagues. Be alert for signs of posttraumatic stress in yourself and oth-

Documentation Tips

When documenting a death, include lack of vital signs (pulseless and apneic) as well as your reason for not initiating BLS (for example, rigor mortis or dependent lividity).

ers: nightmares, restlessness, difficulty sleeping, lack of appetite, a constant need for food, and the like. Consider the need for professional help if these signs or symptoms continue. All EMS programs should have critical incident stress management protocols and debriefing teams available for traumatic incidents.

Although you may consider the death of a child to be a failure, your skill at coping with this kind of emotional event can be a great comfort to the family, helping them to accept their loss and begin the long process of grieving.

Infants and Children With Special Needs

The approach to health care in our society continues to focus on decreasing lengths of hospitalization, and technology continues to improve. As a result of these two factors, the number of infants and children with chronic diseases who are living at home or in other environments outside of the hospital continues to grow. You should be familiar with some of the special needs created by chronic diseases and conditions, particularly as they relate to the potential need for emergency medical care.

Some examples of infants and children with special needs include the following:

- Children who were born prematurely and have associated lung disease problems
- Small children or infants with congenital heart disease
- Children with neurologic disease (occasionally caused by hypoxemia at the time of birth, as with cerebral palsy)
- Children with congenital or acquired diseases resulting in altered body functions such as breathing, eating, urination, and bowel function

The parent or caregiver of a special-needs child will be an important part of your assessment. You must first determine the child's normal baseline status before an assessment of the current condition can be made. It is often helpful to ask, "What is different today?" The parents or guardians often know their child's history and condition better than some skilled health care workers might.

Occasionally, the children live at home but depend on artificial ventilators or other devices to maintain life. You assess and care for special-needs children the same as for all other patients. Your focus on the ABCs remains the priority.

Tracheostomy Tubes

Children who depend on home artificial ventilators or those who have chronic pulmonary medical conditions may breathe through a tracheostomy tube
Figure 23-9 ▾ . A tracheostomy tube is a tube placed in the neck that passes directly into the trachea. Because this tube bypasses the nose and mouth, the body can build up secretions in or around the tube. These tubes are prone to become obstructed by mucous plugs or foreign bodies. There may be bleeding or air leaking around the tube, which usually happens with new tracheostomies, and the tube can become loose or

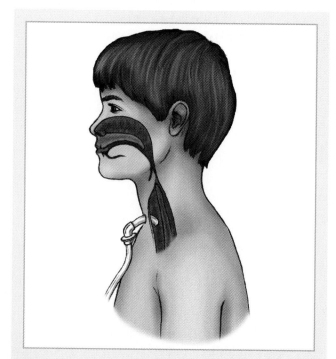

Figure 23-9 Some children require a tracheostomy tube to breathe.

dislodged. Occasionally, the opening around the tube may become infected. Your care of a patient with a tracheostomy tube includes maintaining an open airway. This can include suctioning the tube if necessary to clear a mucous plug, maintaining the patient in a position of comfort, and providing transport to the hospital. Call for ALS backup.

Artificial Ventilators

Children who use a ventilator at home cannot breathe without help. If the ventilator malfunctions, remove the child from the ventilator and begin bag-mask ventilation. To do this, remove the mask from a bag-mask device and directly attach the bag and valve to the tracheostomy tube.

Children using home ventilators will need artificial ventilation throughout transport. Artificial ventilation is provided through the tracheostomy tube. Remember that the patient's caregivers will know how the ventilator works and will be of great help to you in attaching the bag-mask device to the tube in preparation for transport.

Central Intravenous Lines

Children with chronic medical conditions such as gastrointestinal disturbances that require prolonged intravenous (IV) feeding or those with infections that require prolonged IV antibiotics will have indwelling IV catheters placed near the heart for long-term use. These catheters can be in the chest or the arm   Figure 23-10 ▸ . Problems associated with these devices may include broken lines, infections around the lines, clotted lines, and bleeding around the line or from the tubing attached to the line. If bleeding occurs, you should apply direct pressure to the tubing and provide transport to the hospital.

Gastrostomy Tubes

A gastrostomy tube, sometimes referred to as a G-tube, is a tube placed through the wall of the abdomen directly into the stomach for feeding a child who cannot be fed by mouth   Figure 23-11 ▸ . Because food is pumped into the stomach, it can back up the esophagus and into the lungs. Breathing problems may be complicated by aspiration of the tube contents into the lungs. You should always have suction readily available to clear any materials from the mouth and to prevent airway problems. Patients with gas-

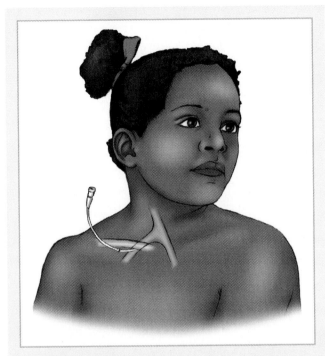

Figure 23-10 Children who require frequent IV medications may have a central line in place.

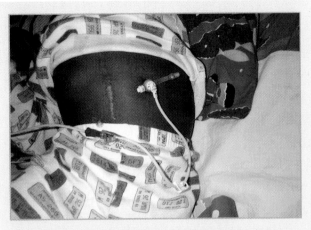

Figure 23-11 Gastrostomy tubes are placed through the skin into the stomach for children who cannot be fed by mouth.

Shunts

Some children with chronic neurologic conditions may have shunts in place. A <u>shunt</u> is a tube that extends from the brain to the abdomen to drain excess cerebrospinal fluid that may accumulate near the brain. Shunts keep pressures in the head from building up. If a shunt becomes clogged due to infection, changes in mental status and respiratory arrest may occur. Emergency medical care includes airway management and artificial ventilation during transport. During assessment, you will likely feel a device on the side of the head, behind the ear, beneath the skin. This device is a fluid reservoir, and the presence of this device should alert you to the possibility that the child has an underlying shunt. Should the shunt become dysfunctional, the child could be predisposed to respiratory arrest.

trostomy tubes who have difficulty breathing should be transported sitting or lying on the right side with the head elevated to prevent the contents of the stomach from passing into the lungs. Give supplemental oxygen if the patient has difficulty breathing. Children with diabetes who receive insulin and tube feedings may become hypoglycemic quickly if tube feedings are discontinued. Be alert for altered mental status.

You are the Provider Summary

Even though febrile seizures are rarely life-threatening, it is vital to cool the patient and transport for further evaluation and treatment for the cause of the fever. Remember to protect the airway and never cool the patient to the point of shivering, which may increase the temperature.

1. **What questions should you ask the mother?**
   - Does the child have any medical history?
   - What was going on prior to the seizure?
   - Does the child have a fever?
   - Has she given the child any medication?
   - Does she take any medications on a daily basis?
   - Is she allergic to any medications?
   - Has she fallen or hit her head?
   - Did she vomit?

2. **How should you approach the patient?**
   Form a general impression before approaching the patient. Talk softly and avoid sudden movements.

3. **How do you expect the patient to respond to you?**
   Toddlers are known for having stranger anxiety. If she is alert she may cling to her mother and cry.

4. **What might you do to distract the patient?**
   Give her something to hold or play with, like a tongue depressor or a penlight.

5. **How should you perform your assessment?**
   Unless the child appears to be in distress, start at the feet and work up.

6. **What is the proper treatment for this patient?**
   Cooling her down, but not to the point of shivering that could cause a reflex hyperthermia.

7. **What are some of the common causes of seizures?**
   - Fever
   - Hypoglycemia
   - Idiopathic
   - Hypoxia
   - Poisoning
   - Infection
   - Child abuse
   - Electrolyte imbalances
   - Medications
   - Previous seizure disorder
   - Recreational drug use
   - Head trauma

8. **If you are able to lower the temperature, should the patient be transported? Why or why not?**
   Yes. Unless the cause of the fever is treated, it is likely to recur and the patient may have another seizure.

Prep Kit

Ready for Review

- Children are not only smaller than adults and more vulnerable, they are also anatomically, physiologically, and psychologically different from adults in some important ways.
- Child anatomy contributes to some special challenges.
- The tongue is large relative to other structures, so it poses a higher risk of airway obstruction than in an adult.
- Head size and shape also make airway positioning a specialized task in children. Neonates and infants have high respiratory rates and breathe primarily with their abdomens.
- Vasoconstriction in the skin and increased heart rate are the major means of compensating for decreased perfusion of vital organs.
- The airway in a child has a smaller diameter than the airway in an adult and is, therefore, more easily obstructed.
- Because the diaphragm is the principal muscle of respiration in children and infants, gastric distention can create breathing difficulties.
- There are five developmental stages in childhood: infancy, the toddler years, preschool age, school age, and adolescence.
- General rules for dealing with children of all ages include appearing confident, being honest, and keeping caregivers together with the patient as much as possible.
- You should remember that children's bones are more flexible and bend more with injury and that the ends of the long bones, where growth occurs, are weaker and may be injured more easily.
- Children's internal organs are not as insulated by fat and may be injured more severely, and children have less circulating blood, so that, although children exhibit the signs of shock more slowly, they go into shock more quickly, with less blood loss.
- Children are not always as cautious as adults and tend to have more accidental poisoning, diving, and bicycle injuries.
- The most common cause of dehydration in children is vomiting and diarrhea. Life-threatening diarrhea can develop in an infant in hours.
- Febrile seizures may be a sign of a more serious problem such as meningitis.
- A victim of sudden infant death syndrome (SIDS) will be pale or blue, not breathing, and unresponsive. He or she may show signs of postmortem changes, including rigor mortis and dependent lividity.
- If family members insist or protocols mandate, you should initiate CPR and transport the infant and family to the emergency department, where the family can receive more extensive support. If the child does not

have any evidence of postmortem changes, begin CPR immediately.
- Carefully inspect the environment where a SIDS victim was found, looking for signs of illness, abusive family interactions, and objects in the child's crib.
- Provide support for the family in whatever way you can, but do not make judgmental statements. Allow them to spend time with the child and ride in the ambulance to the hospital.
- Any death of a child is stressful for family members and for health care providers. In dealing with the family, acknowledge their feelings, keep instructions short and simple, use the child's name, and maintain eye contact.
- Be prepared to respond to philosophical and medical questions, in most cases by indicating concern and understanding; do not be specific about the cause of death.
- Be alert for signs of posttraumatic stress in yourself and others after dealing with the death of a child. It can help to talk about the event and your feelings with your EMS colleagues.
- The number of children living at home who have chronic diseases and special needs is increasing.
- These patients will test your knowledge of special equipment and care procedures, your skills in obtaining pertinent history from family and caregivers, and your ability to detect urgent problems when you may not be completely familiar with the technical details involved. Learning everything you can from each special situation will help prepare you for similar responses in the future.

Vital Vocabulary

adolescents Children between 12 and 18 years of age.
apparent life-threatening event (ALTE) An event that causes unresponsiveness, cyanosis, and apnea in an infant, who then resumes breathing with stimulation.
child abuse Any improper or excessive action that injures or otherwise harms a child or infant; includes neglect and physical, sexual, and emotional abuse.

Technology

- Interactivities
- Vocabulary Explorer
- Anatomy Review
- Web Links
- Online Review Manual

Refresher.EMSzone.com

dehydration   A state in which fluid losses are greater than fluid intake into the body, leading to shock and death if untreated.

dependent lividity   Pooling of the blood in the lower parts of the body after death.

febrile seizures   Seizures relating to a fever.

gastrostomy tube   A feeding tube placed directly through the wall of the abdomen; used in patients who cannot ingest liquids or solids.

hypoventilation   Reduced minute volume, either from reduced rate and/or depth of breathing.

infancy   The first year of life.

meningitis   Inflammation of the meninges that cover the spinal cord and the brain.

neonatal   The first month after birth.

occiput   The back of the head.

pediatrics   The specialized medical practice devoted to the care of young people.

pneumatic antishock garment (PASG)   An inflatable device that covers the legs and abdomen; used to splint the lower extremities or pelvis or to control bleeding in the lower extremities, pelvis, or abdominal cavity.

preschool age   Between 3 and 6 years of age.

rigor mortis   Stiffening of the body after death.

school age   Between 6 to 12 years of age.

shaken baby syndrome   Bleeding within the head and damage to the cervical spine of an infant who has been intentionally and forcibly shaken; a form of child abuse.

shunt   A tube that diverts excess cerebrospinal fluid from the brain to the abdomen.

sudden infant death syndrome (SIDS)   Death of an infant or young child that remains unexplained after a complete autopsy.

toddler   A child from infancy through 3 years of age.

tracheostomy tube   A tube inserted into the trachea in children who cannot breathe on their own; passes through the neck directly into the major airways.

Assessment in Action

Pediatric patients make up a small portion of EMS calls. It is easy to forget vital components of care when skills are not used. Refresher training is imperative to maintain knowledge and skills.

1. At which stage of development does a pediatric patient develop stranger anxiety?
   A. infant
   B. toddler
   C. preschool age
   D. school age

2. Child abuse may be defined as:
   A. emotional abuse.
   B. sexual abuse.
   C. neglect.
   D. all of the above.

3. The medical practice devoted to the young is known as:
   A. geriatrics.
   B. podiatry.
   C. pediatrics.
   D. hemotology.

4. Why are head injuries common in children?
   A. their tendency to fall a lot
   B. the size of their feet
   C. their lack of muscular coordination
   D. the size of the head

5. The _____ dictates the amount of air inspired for children.
   A. intercostal muscles
   B. retractions
   C. diaphragm
   D. length of the trachea

6. _____ results from disorganized electrical activity in the brain.
   A. Meningitis
   B. Seizures
   C. Lethargy
   D. Increased intracranial pressure

Challenging Questions

7. Explain the anatomical differences between a child and an adult that affect pediatric airway management techniques.

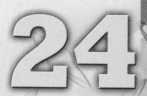

24

Pediatric Assessment and Management

You are the Provider 1

You are on scene on a Saturday morning with a 3-year-old girl who is "feeling bad". Her mother tells you that she will not eat or drink this morning and she says her throat hurts. She also has a cough. She is lying on the sofa watching cartoons.

Initial Assessment	Recording Time: 0 Minutes
Appearance	Pale
Level of consciousness	Alert
Airway	Open and clear
Breathing	A little fast and shallow
Circulation	Radial pulses present

1. How should you approach the patient?
2. What questions should you ask the mother?

Pediatric Assessment and Management

There are many causes of emergencies in infants and children. Although you might not be able to identify the exact cause, you must be able to intervene appropriately. You will face some special challenges in caring for sick and injured children. First and foremost is the ability to assess the needs of infants and children. Other challenges will include managing the child's airway, ventilation, and the care of injuries.

This chapter discusses the importance of assessment and setting priorities when dealing with children. Discussion of procedures for opening and maintaining the airway in infants and children follows, including placement of airway adjuncts and use of oxygen delivery devices, including bag-mask ventilation. The causes and management of airway obstruction from foreign objects are covered next. We also review management of cardiac arrest and of trauma, seizures, altered level of consciousness, poisoning, meningitis, shock, and dehydration.

EMT-Bs who are calm when caring for adults often find themselves anxious when dealing with critically ill or injured infants or children. However, treatment of children is the same as that of adults in most emergency situations. Once you understand the differences in anatomy between children and adults and learn to recognize signs of respiratory distress in children, you will find it easier to approach even the youngest patients in a relaxed, professional manner.

Because a young child might not be able to speak, your assessment of his or her condition must be based in large part on what you can see and hear yourself.

In addition, families may be helpful in providing vital information about an accident or illness. You should include families in the assessment and, whenever possible, include them in all decisions about care and transportation.

Scene Size-up

As with any EMS call, the scene size-up begins by ensuring that you and your partner have taken the appropriate body substance isolation precautions. As soon as you arrive at the scene, look for hazards or potential threats. Resist the temptation to hastily access the patient because you know it is a child. Personal safety must always remain your priority.

As you enter the scene, note the position in which the child is found. Observe the area for clues to the mechanism of injury (MOI) or nature of illness; these observations will help guide your assessment and management priorities.

Note the presence of pills, medicine bottles, or household chemicals that would suggest possible ingestion by the child. If the child has been injured—a motor vehicle crash, fall, or pedestrian incident—carefully observe the scene or vehicle (if involved) for clues to the potential severity of the child's injuries.

You must not discount the possibility of child abuse. Conflicting information from the parents or caregivers, bruises or other injuries not consistent with the MOI described, or injuries not consistent with the child's age and developmental abilities should increase your index of suspicion for abuse.

Initial Assessment

Many components of the pediatric initial assessment can be accomplished by simple observation when you enter the scene or room. As with adults, the objective of the initial assessment is to identify and treat immediate or potential threats to life.

General Impression

The initial assessment begins as you form a general impression of the child's condition and of the environment. Determining a chief complaint, often expressed as what the parent is most concerned about, may help to focus your attention toward potential life-threatening problems. Also note the degree of interaction between the parent or caregiver and the child; ask the parent or caregiver if the child is acting normally. Determine whether the child recognizes the parent or

Technology

Interactivities

Vocabulary Explorer

Anatomy Review

Web Links

Online Review Manual

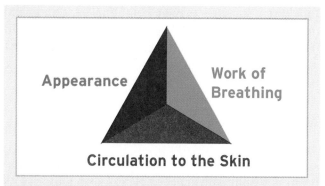

Figure 24-1 The three components of the pediatric assessment triangle (PAT) include appearance, work of breathing, and circulation to the skin.

Table 24-1 The AVPU Scale

Alert: Normal interactiveness for age
Verbal
■ Appropriate: Responds to name
■ Inappropriate: Nonspecific or confused
Painful
■ Appropriate: Withdraws from pain
■ Inappropriate: Sound or movement without purpose or localization of pain
Unresponsive: No response to any stimulus

caregiver; failure to do so is an ominous sign and indicates a very sick child.

Pediatric Assessment Triangle

The pediatric assessment triangle (PAT) is a structured assessment tool that allows you to rapidly form a general impression of the pediatric patient's condition without touching him or her. The intent is to provide a first glance assessment to identify the general category of the child's physiologic problem and to establish urgency for treatment and/or transport. The PAT is a visual assessment of the child before performing a hands-on assessment.

The PAT consists of three elements: appearance (muscle tone and mental status), work of breathing, and circulation to the skin Figure 24-1 ▲.

Appearance

Evaluating the child's appearance involves noting the level of consciousness or interactiveness and muscle tone—signs that will provide you with information about the adequacy of the child's cerebral perfusion and overall function of the central nervous system.

Much of the information about the child's level of consciousness can be obtained by using the PAT. In addition, you can evaluate the child's level of consciousness by using the AVPU scale, modified as necessary for the child's age Table 24-1 ▶.

An infant or child with a normal level of consciousness will act appropriately for his or her age, exhibiting good muscle tone and maintaining good eye contact. An abnormal level of consciousness is characterized by age-inappropriate behavior or lack of interaction, poor muscle tone, or poor eye contact with the caregiver or EMS personnel.

Work of Breathing

A child's work of breathing increases as the body attempts to compensate for abnormalities in oxygenation and ventilation. Increased work of breathing often manifests as tachypnea (increased respiratory rate), retractions of the intercostal muscles or sternum Figure 24-2 ▼, or the way the child positions himself or herself.

Circulation to the Skin

An important sign of perfusion is circulation to the skin. When cardiac output falls, the body, through vasoconstriction, shunts blood from areas of lesser need (such as the skin) to areas of greater need (such as the brain, heart, and kidneys).

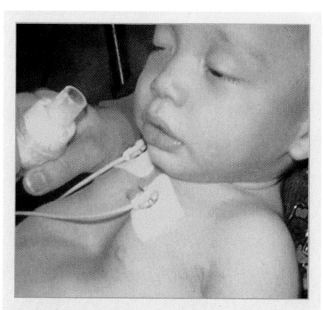

Figure 24-2 Retractions of the intercostals muscles or sternum indicate increased work of breathing.

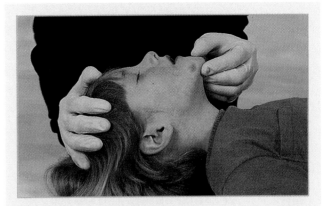

Figure 24-4 Use the head tilt–chin lift maneuver to open the airway of a child without trauma.

Pallor of the skin and mucous membranes may be seen in compensated shock; it may also be a sign of hypoxia or _anemia_. Mottling is caused by constriction of peripheral blood vessels and is another sign of poor perfusion (Figure 24-3 ▾). _Cyanosis_ reflects a decreased level of oxygen in the blood. Cyanosis is a late sign of respiratory failure or shock; absence of discoloration, however, does not rule out these conditions. Never wait for the development of cyanosis before administering oxygen!

Airway, Breathing, and Circulation

After forming your general impression of the child using the PAT, perform a hands-on assessment of the child's vital functions—airway, breathing, and circulation—and treat any immediate or potential threats to life. As previously discussed, although your assessment of a child may require some modification based on patient age, the overall assessment flow is essentially the same as for adults.

Airway Assessment

If the infant or child's airway is open and the patient can maintain it (as is often the case in conscious patients), you can proceed with assessing the adequacy of respirations. However, if the child is unresponsive or has difficulty keeping the airway clear, you must ensure that the airway is properly positioned and that it is clear of mucus, vomitus, blood, and foreign bodies.

If trauma has been ruled out, open the child's airway with the head tilt–chin lift maneuver (Figure 24-4 ▴). If the MOI suggests a possible head or neck injury, use the jaw-thrust maneuver to open the airway (Figure 24-5 ▾). Remember, maintaining the airway takes priority over spinal stabilization. Use a head tilt–chin lift maneuver if unable to keep the airway open with a jaw-thrust.

Positioning the airway correctly is critical in pediatric emergency care. Position the airway in a _sniffing position_, which may require the placement of a folded sheet or towel behind the head or shoulders (Figure 24-6 ▸). When the head is bent back (hyperextended) or forward (flexed), the airway may become obstructed because of kinking of the trachea.

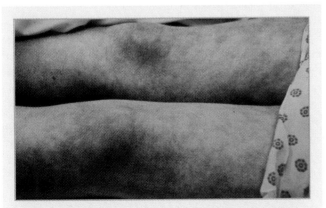

Figure 24-3 Mottling of the skin indicates poor perfusion and is the result of constriction of peripheral blood vessels.

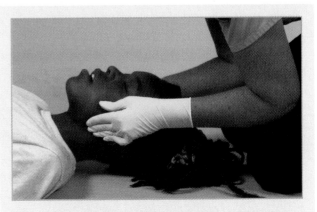

Figure 24-5 Use the jaw-thrust maneuver in a child with possible spinal injury.

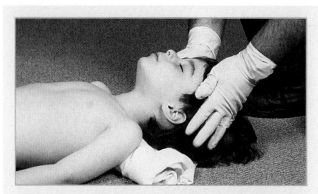

Figure 24-6 The airway should be placed in a neutral position to keep the tracheas from kinking when the head is flexed or hyperextended.

Make sure the child's airway is open and clear. Next, establish whether the child can maintain his or her own airway spontaneously (without the use of airway adjuncts) or whether adjuncts will be necessary to maintain airway patency.

Breathing Assessment

Assess a child's breathing by using the look, listen, and feel technique, noting the degree of air movement at the nose and mouth and determining whether the chest is rising adequately. In infants, belly breathing is considered adequate owing to the soft pliable bones of the chest and the strong muscular diaphragm.

If the child is conscious and not in need of immediate intervention (such as suctioning or assisted ventilation), assessing respirations is usually easier with the child sitting on the caregiver's lap. Listen for abnormal respiratory sounds (Table 24-2 ▼), and note any signs of increased respiratory effort.

Table 24-2 Abnormal Respiratory Sounds

- **Stridor:** High-pitched inspiratory sound: indicates a partial upper airway obstruction (such as in croup or from a foreign body)
- **Wheezing:** High- or low-pitched sound heard usually during expiration; indicates a partial lower airway obstruction (such as in asthma or bronchiolitis)
- Grunting: An "uh" sound heard during exhalation; reflects the child's attempt to keep the alveoli open; indicates inadequate oxygenation
- **Absent breath sounds (despite increased work of breathing):** Indicates a complete upper or lower airway obstruction (such as foreign body, severe asthma, or pneumothorax)

When observing a child's respiratory effort, note any signs of increased work of breathing, including the following:

- Accessory muscle use: Contractions of the muscles above the clavicles (supraclavicular)
- Retractions: Drawing in of the muscles between the ribs (intercostal retractions) or of the sternum during inspiration
- Head bobbing: The head lifts and tilts back during inspiration, then moves forward during expiration
- Nasal flaring: The nostrils widen; usually seen during inspiration
- Tachypnea: Increased respiratory rate

As the child begins to tire, respirations often become weak and ineffective and the accessory muscles become less prominent during breathing. Bradypnea, a decrease in the respiratory rate, is an ominous sign and indicates impending respiratory arrest. Do not mistake the slowing of respirations for a sign of improvement; it usually indicates that the child's condition has deteriorated. You must be prepared to begin ventilatory assistance.

Circulatory Assessment

When assessing circulation, you must determine whether the child has a pulse, is bleeding, or is in shock. Remember, infants and children can tolerate only small amounts of blood loss before circulatory compromise occurs. Assess and control any active bleeding early in your assessment.

Pulses may be difficult to palpate if they are weak, very fast, or very slow. In infants, palpate the brachial pulse or femoral pulse. In children older than 1 year, palpate the carotid pulse. Note the rate and quality of the pulse: Is it weak or strong? Is it normal, slow, or fast? Strong central pulses usually indicate that the child is not hypotensive; however, this does not rule out the possibility of compensated shock. Weak or absent peripheral pulses indicate decreased perfusion. The absence of a central pulse (that is, brachial or femoral in infants, carotid in older children) indicates the need for CPR.

Tachycardia may be an early sign of hypoxia or shock, but it may also reflect less serious conditions such as fever, anxiety, pain, and excitement. Like respiratory rate and effort, heart rate should be interpreted within the context of the overall history, PAT, and the entire initial assessment.

When hypoxia or shock becomes critical, bradycardia occurs. As with slowing respirations, bradycardia in a child is an ominous sign and often indicates impending cardiopulmonary arrest.

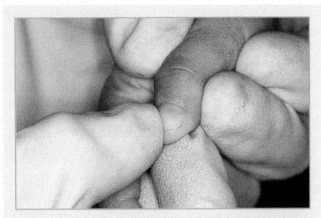

Figure 24-7 Estimate the capillary refill time by squeezing the end of a finger or toe for several seconds until the nailbed blanches. Normal color should return within 2 seconds after you let go.

Feel the skin for temperature and moisture at the same time you assess the child's pulse. Is the skin warm and dry or cold and clammy? Estimate the <u>capillary refill time (CRT)</u> by squeezing the end of a finger or toe for several seconds and then observing the return of blood to the area Figure 24-7 ▲ . Color should return in less than 2 seconds after you release the finger or toe. The CRT is used to assess <u>end-organ perfusion</u>. It is most reliable in children younger than 6 years; however, factors such as cold temperatures may affect the CRT.

Transport Decision

After you have completed the initial assessment and initiated any treatment, you must make the decision to initiate immediate transport or stay on scene for additional assessment and treatment. If the child is in stable condition, you may elect to perform a focused history and physical exam at the scene.

Immediate transport is indicated if the scene is unsafe for the child. You should also provide rapid transport if a significant MOI was involved, the child has any problems with the ABCs, or the child has significant pain.

If the child's condition is urgent, perform a rapid assessment and initiate immediate transport. Additional assessment and treatment can be performed en route. If the child's condition is nonurgent, perform a focused history and physical exam at the scene, provide additional treatment as needed, and then transport.

Transportation

Children weighing less than 40 lb should be transported in a car seat as long as the situation allows. Many types of seats are available. A seat should be chosen to fit the appropriate weight of the child and should meet the current applicable standards set by your governing agency. There are only a few locations to place a car seat in an ambulance. Seats are designed to be forward-facing or rear-facing; they cannot be mounted sideways on a bench seat. Seats should not be mounted in the front of an ambulance, especially if the ambulance is equipped with airbags. To mount a car seat to the stretcher, place the head of the cot in an upright position. Place the seat so it is against the back of the cot. Secure one of the cot straps from the upper portion of the cot through the seat belt positions on the seat, and strap it tightly to the cot. Repeat on the lower portion of the cot. Push the seat into the cot tightly, and retighten the straps.

To secure a seat to the captain's chair, follow the seat manufacturer's instructions. Remember that children younger than 1 year must be transported in a rear-facing position owing to the lack of mature neck muscles.

In some situations, it is not appropriate to secure a child in a car seat, for example if the child has to be immobilized on a long board or requires splinting that does not fit in the seat. A child in unstable condition who requires airway or ventilatory support should be positioned to maximize meeting the airway and ventilatory requirements.

Transition Phase

If the child's condition does not require immediate transport, the <u>transition phase</u> can allow the infant or child to become familiar with you and your equipment. This will help to alleviate the child's anxiety, allowing you to perform a more thorough and accurate assessment.

Remember that sick or injured children are afraid and do not understand why you are there and what you are doing. As a result, they are less likely than adults to trust you. The transition phase will facilitate the trust-building process between you and the child.

■ Focused History and Physical Exam

A focused history and physical exam of a child should be performed at the scene, unless his or her condition dictates immediate transport. The purpose of the focused history and physical exam is to obtain additional, specific information about the child's illness or injury. This portion of your assessment includes performing a physical exam (rapid or focused), obtaining vital signs, and interviewing the patient or guardian about the patient's medical history. The order of these three portions of the assessment will vary according to whether the child is a medical patient (responsive or unresponsive) or a trauma patient (with significant or nonsignificant MOI).

Focused Physical Exam

The focused physical exam should be performed on all children without life-threatening illnesses or injuries who do not require a rapid assessment (for example, responsive children for whom obtaining a medical history will guide you in your physical exam or trauma patients with a nonsignificant MOI). Focus your assessment on the area(s) of the body affected by the illness or injury.

Young children should be assessed starting at the feet and ending at the head; older children can be assessed using the head-to-toe approach, as with adults. The extent of the physical exam will depend on the situation and may include the following:

- Pupils
  - Note the size, equality, and reactivity of the pupils to light.
- Capillary refill (in children younger than 6 years)
  - Normal CRT should be less than 2 seconds.
  - As discussed earlier, assess CRT by blanching the finger or toenail beds; the soles of the feet may also be used.

- Cold temperatures will increase CRT, making it a less reliable sign.
- Level of hydration
  - Assess skin turgor, noting the presence of tenting.
  - In infants, note whether the fontanels are sunken or flat.
  - Ask the parent or caregiver how many diapers the infant has soiled during the last 24 hours.
  - Determine whether the child is producing tears when crying; note the condition of the mouth. Is the oral mucosa moist or dry?

Rapid Physical Exam

A rapid physical exam should be used when pediatric patients have potentially life-threatening or hidden injuries (unresponsive medical patients or trauma patients with a significant MOI). It should be performed quickly, and then vital signs and history should be obtained. Identifying these problems early can help prepare your patient for transport or identify the need for ALS providers.

Pediatric Vital Signs

During your assessment, you should obtain a complete set of baseline vital signs, including pulse; skin

You are the Provider 2

The mother tells you that her daughter was treated a little over a week ago for an upper respiratory infection. She finished her prescribed medication and then started feeling bad again yesterday.

You form a general impression as you approach the patient. She is alert but listless. She notices you, but does not attempt to move away or speak. Because her airway and respirations appear to be adequate, you decide to do a toe to head assessment.

The mother called 9-1-1 today because the patient is so lethargic and just "not acting right". She has also had febrile seizures in the past and the mother did not want to take a chance.

Vital Signs	Recording Time: 2 Minutes
Skin	Pale, warm to touch
Pulse	136 beats/min, regular
Oxygen saturation	96% while breathing room air
Respirations	28 breaths/min, slightly shallow

3. What should you ask about her previous infection?
4. How should you administer oxygen?
5. Why is her pulse rate so fast?

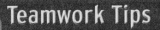

Teamwork Tips

One rescuer should focus on building a rapport with the child during the assessment while the second rescuer concentrates on acquiring needed supplies and assisting as needed.

color, temperature, and condition; blood pressure; respirations; and pupils. Guidelines used to assess adult circulatory status—heart rate and blood pressure—have important limitations in children. First, normal heart rates vary with age in children. Second, blood pressure is usually not assessed in children younger than 3 years; it offers little information about the child's circulatory status and is usually difficult to obtain. In these patients, assessment of the skin is a better indication of circulatory status.

It is important to use appropriately sized equipment when assessing a child's vital signs. To obtain an accurate reading of a child's blood pressure, you must use a cuff that covers two thirds of the patient's upper arm. A blood pressure cuff that is too small may give you a falsely high reading, whereas a cuff that is too large may give you a falsely low reading.

Respiratory rates may be difficult to interpret. A rapid respiratory rate may simply reflect high fever, anxiety, pain, or excitement. A normal rate, on the other hand, may occur in a child who has been breathing rapidly with increased work of breathing for some time and is now becoming tired. In infants and children younger than 3 years, evaluate respirations by assessing the rise and fall of the abdomen. Assess the pulse rate by counting for at least 1 minute, noting its

quality and regularity. Pulse oximetry can also be used to monitor the patient's status.

Note that normal vital signs in pediatric patients vary with the age of the child (Table 24-3 ▾). Remember that your approach to taking vital signs also varies with the age of the child. Be gentle, talk to the child, assess respirations and then pulse, and assess blood pressure last. Warm your stethoscope on your hands or a cloth before placing it on the skin. You may also want to let the child hold the equipment or stethoscope first, which may help to reduce the child's anxiety.

Evaluate pupils with a penlight. The response of pupils is a good indication of how well the brain is functioning, particularly when trauma has occurred. Be sure to compare the size of each pupil with the other.

SAMPLE History

Your approach to the history will depend on the age of the patient. Historical information from young children will need to be obtained from the parent or caregiver. When dealing with a school-age child or young adolescent, you will usually be able to obtain most of the information from the patient.

Information about sexual activity, the possibility of pregnancy, or the use of illicit drugs or alcohol should be obtained from an adolescent patient in private. Most adolescents will be reluctant to provide this information in the presence of their parents. When asking such questions, assure the adolescent that this information is important and is needed to provide the most appropriate care.

Asking the parent or child about the immediate illness or injury should be based on the child's chief complaint. Together with an evaluation of the child's medical

Table 24-3 Vital Signs by Age

Age	Respirations (breaths/min)	Pulse (beats/min)	Systolic Blood Pressure (mm Hg)
Neonate: 0 to 1 mo	30 to 60	90 to 180	50 to 70
Infant: 1 mo to 1 y	25 to 50	100 to 160	70 to 95
Toddler: 1 to 3 y	20 to 30	90 to 150	80 to 100
Preschool age: 3 to 6 y	20 to 25	80 to 140	80 to 100
School age: 6 to 12 y	15 to 20	70 to 120	80 to 110
Adolescent: 12 to 18 y	12 to 16	60 to 100	90 to 110
Older than 18 y	12 to 20	60 to 100	90 to 140

history, this may provide clues to the underlying illness or injury and other conditions that may exist.

When interviewing a parent or older child about the chief complaint, obtain the following pertinent information:

- Nature of the illness or injury
- How long the patient has been sick or injured
- Presence of fever
- Effects of the illness or injury on the child's behavior
- Change in bowel or bladder habits
- Presence of vomiting or diarrhea
- Frequency of urination

When obtaining information about the child's medical history, use SAMPLE to inquire whether the child is currently under the care of a physician, has any chronic illnesses, takes any medications on a regular basis, or has any known drug allergies.

If the caregiver is unable to accompany you to the hospital, get a name and phone number so the staff can call if there are questions. This might be the case when you respond to a daycare facility or babysitter's location. Care may be delayed if this information is not available.

Detailed Physical Exam

Pediatric patients often require constant intervention and observation en route to the hospital. In these situ-ations, or when priority problems require your atten-tion, a detailed exam may not be necessary. However, in many situations, pediatric patients should have a thorough, detailed physical exam, looking over their complete body for signs and symptoms of problems. This is particularly true of patients experiencing trauma from a significant MOI when subtle signs of injury may be present.

Ongoing Assessment

Reassess the child's condition as the situation dic-tates—every 15 minutes for a child in stable condition and at least every 5 minutes for a child in unstable condition.

The physiologic safeguards in infants and chil-dren can decompensate with alarming unpredictabil-ity; therefore, continually monitor respiratory effort, skin color and condition, and level of consciousness or interactiveness. If the child's condition deteriorates, immediately repeat the initial assessment and adjust your treatment accordingly.

The Pediatric Airway

Positioning the Airway

Correct positioning of the airway is critical in pedi-atric emergency care. Always position the airway in

You are the Provider 3

The patient is compliant with your assessment and you note that she feels somewhat warm to the touch. She tolerates blow-by oxygen as long as the mother holds it. The mother tells you her daughter has been coughing up yellow-greeenish phlegm for 2 days. As you lift the girl's shirt you note some slight intercostal retractions.

The mother has made an appointment with the doctor, but since it is Saturday she will not be able to see him until Monday. The patient has had acetaminophen twice today for the fever.

Reassessment	Recording Time: 5 Minutes
Pulse	136 beats/min, irregular
Capillary refill time	<2 seconds
Respirations	28 breaths/min, not quite as shallow as earlier
Breath sounds	Rales bilaterally
Pulse oximetry	97% with blow-by oxygen

6. What else could you do to make the patient feel more comfortable?
7. What does the productive cough indicate?
8. How should she be transported?
9. Should you examine her airway and throat? Why or why not?

a neutral sniffing position. This accomplishes two goals at once, keeping the trachea from kinking and maintaining the proper alignment should you have to immobilize the spine. If the child has been involved in trauma or trauma is suspected, use the jaw-thrust maneuver to open the airway. Remember to place the patient on a firm surface. Fold a small towel to a thickness of approximately 1" and place it under the patient's shoulders and back to maintain the airway in the sniffing position.

Airway Adjuncts

In children with inadequate ventilation, you should use an airway adjunct to maintain an open airway. Placing the adjuncts correctly starts with choosing the appropriately sized equipment (Table 24-4 ▼).

Oropharyngeal Airway

An oropharyngeal airway should be used for pediatric patients who are unconscious and in possible respiratory failure. This adjunct should not be used in conscious patients or those who have a gag reflex.

Patients with a gag reflex do not tolerate an oropharyngeal airway. In addition, this adjunct should not be used in children who may have ingested a caustic or petroleum-based product because it may induce vomiting. (Skill Drill 24-1 ▶) reviews the steps for inserting an oropharyngeal airway in a child:

1. **Determine the appropriately sized airway** by measuring from the corner of the patient's mouth to the earlobe or by using the length-based pediatric resuscitation tape.
2. **Place the airway next to the face** with the flange at the level of the central incisors and the bite block segment parallel to the hard palate. The tip of the airway should reach the angle of the jaw (**Step ①**).
3. **Position the patient's airway.** If the emergency is medical, use the head tilt–chin lift technique, avoiding hyperextension. Place a towel under the patient's shoulders. If the MOI indicates possible head or spine injuries, use the jaw-thrust maneuver and provide in-line spinal stabilization (**Step ②**).

Table 24-4 Pediatric Equipment: Getting the Size Right

The best way to identify the appropriately sized equipment for a pediatric patient is to use the pediatric resuscitation tape measure, which can determine weight and height in patients weighing up to 75 lb (34 kg) (Figure 24-8 ▶). The proper sequence for using the tape is as follows:

1. Place the patient supine on a flat surface.
2. Lay the tape next to the patient with the multicolored side up.
3. Place the red end of the tape at the top of the patient's head.
4. Place one hand with its side down on top of the patient's head, covering the red box at the end of the tape.
5. Starting from the patient's head, run the side of your free hand down the tape.
6. Stretch the tape out the full length of the child, stopping at the heel. If the child is longer than the tape, stop here and use the appropriate adult technique.
7. Place your free hand, side down, at the bottom of the child's heel.
8. Note the color or letter block and weight range on the edge of the tape where your hand is. Say the color or letter out loud.

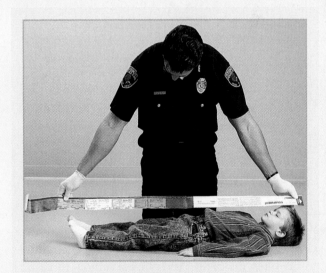

Figure 24-8 Use of a pediatric resuscitation tape measure is one way to identify the correct size for airway adjuncts.

9. Select the appropriately sized equipment by matching the color or letter on the tape to the color or letter on the equipment.

Skill Drill 24-1 — Inserting an Oropharyngeal Airway in a Child

1. Determine the appropriately sized airway. Confirm the correct size visually, by placing it next to the patient's face.

2. Position the patient's airway with the appropriate method.

3. Open the mouth. Insert the airway until the flange rests against the lips. Reassess the airway.

4. **Open the mouth** by applying pressure on the chin with your thumb.

5. **Insert the airway** by depressing the tongue with a tongue blade applied to the base of the tongue and inserting the airway directly over the tongue blade. If a tongue blade is not available, point the airway tip toward the roof of the mouth to depress the tongue. Gently rotate the airway into position as it passes through the mouth toward the curve of the tongue. Insert the airway until the flange rests against the lips.

6. **Reassess the airway** after insertion (**Step 3**). Take care to avoid injuring the hard palate as you insert the airway. Rough insertion can cause bleeding, which can aggravate airway problems and may even cause vomiting.

Nasopharyngeal Airway

A nasopharyngeal airway is usually well tolerated and is not as likely as the oropharyngeal airway to cause vomiting. Unlike the oropharyngeal airway, the nasopharyngeal airway is used for conscious patients or for patients with altered levels of consciousness. It is rarely used in infants younger than 1 year.

A nasopharyngeal airway should not be used in patients with nasal obstruction or head trauma (possible basal skull fracture) or in patients with moderate to severe head trauma because this adjunct could increase intracranial pressure. Review the steps in

Skill Drill 24-2 ▶ to insert a nasopharyngeal airway in a child:

1. **Determine the appropriately sized airway.** The external diameter of the airway should not be larger than the diameter of the nares.

2. **Place the airway next to the patient's face** to make sure the length is correct. The airway should extend from the tip of the nose to the tragus, the small cartilaginous projection in front of the opening of the ear.

3. **Position the patient's airway** using the techniques described for the oropharyngeal airway (**Step 1**).

4. **Lubricate the airway** with a water-soluble lubricant.

5. **Insert the tip into the right nostril** with the bevel pointing toward the septum, or central divider in the nose (**Step 2**).

6. **Carefully move the tip forward, following the roof of the mouth,** until the flange rests against the outside of the nostril (**Step 3**). If you are inserting the airway on the left side, insert the tip into the left nostril upside down, with the bevel pointing toward the septum. Move the airway forward slowly about 1" until you feel a slight resistance, and then rotate the airway 180°.

7. **Reassess the airway** after insertion.

An airway with a small diameter may easily become obstructed by mucus, blood, vomitus, or the

Skill Drill   24-2   Inserting a Nasopharyngeal Airway in a Child

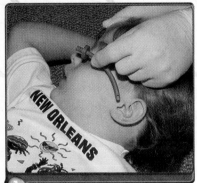

1 Determine the correct airway size by comparing its diameter to the opening of the nostril (naris). Place the airway next to the patient's face to confirm correct length. Position the airway.

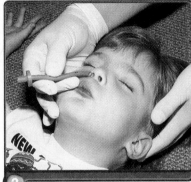

2 Lubricate the airway. Insert the tip into the right nostril with the bevel pointing toward the septum.

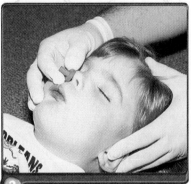

3 Carefully move the tip forward until the flange rests against the outside of the nostril. Reassess the airway.

soft tissues of the pharynx. If the airway is too long, it may stimulate the vagus nerve and slow the heart rate or enter the esophagus, causing gastric distention. Inserting the airway in responsive patients may cause a spasm of the larynx and result in vomiting. Nasopharyngeal airways should not be used when patients have facial trauma because the airway may tear soft tissues and cause bleeding into the airway.

Assisting Ventilation and Oxygenation

After opening the airway, you should assess the patient's ventilation status. Look, listen, and feel for breathing. Remember to observe chest rise in older children and abdominal rise in younger children and infants. Skin condition indicates the amount of oxygen getting to the organs of the body. Patients who have pale, mottled, or blue skin may have an inadequate level of oxygen in their blood. All trauma patients should receive oxygen.

■ Oxygen Delivery Devices

In treating infants and children who require oxygen, you have several options:

- A nonrebreathing mask at 10 to 12 L/min provides up to 90% oxygen concentration.
- The blow-by technique at 6 L/min provides more than 21% oxygen concentration.

- A nasal cannula at 2 to 6 L/min provides 24% to 44% oxygen concentration.
- A bag-mask device (with oxygen reservoir) at 10 to 15 L/min provides over 90% oxygen concentration.

Children need enough air delivered for adequate gas exchange in the lungs. Using a nonrebreathing mask, a nasal cannula, or a simple face mask is indicated only for patients who have adequate respirations and/or tidal volumes. The <u>tidal volume</u> is the amount of air that is delivered to the lungs and airways in one inhalation.

Nonrebreathing Mask

A nonrebreathing mask delivers up to 90% oxygen to the patient and allows the patient to exhale all carbon dioxide without rebreathing it. To apply a nonrebreathing mask:

1. **Select the appropriately sized pediatric nonrebreathing mask.** The mask should extend from the bridge of the nose to the cleft of the chin.
2. **Connect the tubing** to an oxygen source set at 10 to 12 L/min.
3. **Adjust oxygen flow** as needed to match the patient's respiratory rate and depth. The reservoir bag should neither deflate completely nor fill to bulging during the respiratory cycle.

Blow-by Technique

The blow-by technique does not provide a high concentration of oxygen but is better than no oxygen at all. To administer blow-by oxygen:

1. **Place oxygen tubing through a small hole in the bottom of a 6- to 8-oz paper cup.** A cup is a familiar object that is less likely to frighten young children than an oxygen mask. You may be able to use an oxygen mask with an older child. If a cup is not available, hold the end of the oxygen tubing to the child's face so the oxygen flows across the mouth and nose.
2. **Connect tubing to an oxygen source** set at 6 L/min.
3. **Hold the cup approximately 1" to 2" away from the child's nose and mouth.**

Nasal Cannula

Some patients prefer this adjunct, whereas others find it uncomfortable. When using a nasal cannula for a child, be sure to choose the appropriately sized cannula (Figure 24-9 ▾). The prongs should not fill the nostrils entirely. Set the oxygen flow rate to 2 to 6 L/min.

Bag-mask Ventilation

Bag-mask ventilation is indicated for patients who have respirations that are too slow or too fast to provide an adequate volume of inhaled oxygen, who are

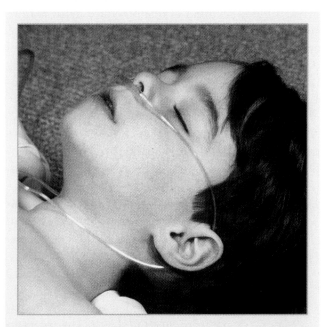

Figure 24-9 The prongs of a pediatric nasal cannula should not fill the nares entirely.

> ### ⚠ Pediatric Needs
>
> One of the problems associated with abdominal injuries in children is the presence of air in the stomach. Children, especially those who have had a traumatic injury, tend to swallow air. Air in the stomach can cause distention and interfere with your assessment. Air can also accumulate in the stomach with artificial ventilation, making it less effective. This is one of the reasons for using the jaw-thrust maneuver to position the airway, as it decreases the amount of air accumulating in the stomach.

unresponsive, or who do not respond in a purposeful way to painful stimuli.

Errors in technique—providing too much volume with each breath, squeezing the bag too forcefully, or ventilating at too fast a rate—can result in gastric distention. An inadequate mask seal or improper head position can lead to hypoventilation or hypoxia.

One-rescuer Bag-mask Ventilation

Review the steps for one-rescuer bag-mask ventilation in Skill Drill 24-3 ▶ :

1. **Open the airway,** and insert the appropriate airway adjunct (**Step ①**).
2. **Position the mask on the patient's face** by using the E-C grip. Form a C with the thumb and index finger along the mask while the other three fingers form an E along the mandible. With infants and toddlers, support the jaw with only your third finger. Be careful not to compress the area under the chin because you may push the tongue into the back of the mouth and block the airway. Keep your fingers on the lower jaw.
3. **Make sure the mask forms an airtight seal** on the face. Use the E-C technique to hold the mask in position while you lift the jaw to hold the airway open (**Step ②**).
4. **Squeeze the bag** to deliver ventilations at the appropriate rate. For children and infants, ventilate once every 3 to 5 seconds, or 12 to 20 times a minute.
5. **Allow 1 second per ventilation,** providing adequate time for exhalation by using the phrase "squeeze, release, release" (**Step ③**).

Skill Drill 24-3   One-rescuer Bag-mask Ventilation on a Child

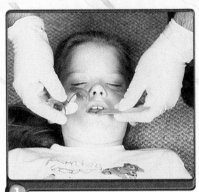

1 Open the airway and insert the appropriate airway adjunct.

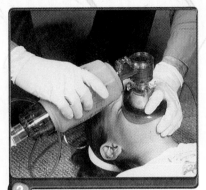

2 Hold the mask on the patient's face with a one-handed head tilt-chin lift technique (E-C grip). Ensure a good mask-face seal while maintaining the airway.

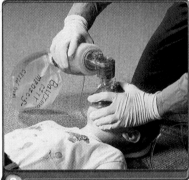

3 Squeeze the bag 12 to 20 times a minute for infants and children. Ventilations should be delivered over 1 second. Allow adequate time for exhalation.

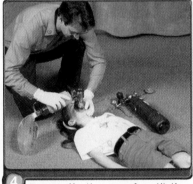

4 Assess effectiveness of ventilation by watching for equal chest rise and fall.

6. **Assess effectiveness** of ventilation by watching for equal rise and fall of the chest (**Step 4**).

Two-rescuer Bag-mask Ventilation

For two-person bag-mask ventilation, one rescuer holds the mask to the patient's face and maintains the position of the head. The second rescuer ventilates the patient. This technique is usually more effective in maintaining a tight seal.

■ Airway Obstruction

Children, especially those younger than 5 years, can (and do) obstruct their airway with any object they can fit into their mouth: hot dogs, balloons, grapes, or coins. In cases of trauma, a child's teeth may have been

dislodged into the airway. Blood, vomitus, or other secretions can also cause partial or complete obstruction.

Airway obstructions can also be caused by infections, including pneumonia, croup, and epiglottitis Figure 24-10 ▶ . Croup is an infection of the airway below the level of the vocal cords, usually caused by a virus. Epiglottitis is an inflammation of the soft tissue in the area above the vocal cords that is usually caused by an infection. Infection should be considered as a possible cause of airway obstruction if a child has congestion, fever, drooling, and cold symptoms. Provide rapid transport for children with these signs and symptoms. Without special equipment and training, attempts to clear an airway that is blocked because of inflammation or infection can increase the obstruction.

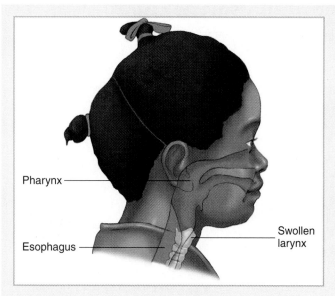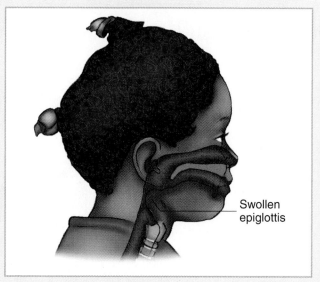

Figure 24-10 Epiglottitis is inflammation, usually due to an infection, that can cause airway obstruction in children.

Signs and Symptoms

Obstruction by a foreign object may involve the upper or the lower airway. Signs and symptoms frequently associated with an upper airway obstruction include decreased or absent breath sounds and stridor. <u>Stridor</u>, a high-pitched noise heard mainly on inspiration, is usually caused by swelling of the area surrounding the vocal cords or by an upper airway obstruction.

Signs and symptoms of a lower airway obstruction include <u>wheezing</u> and/or crackles. <u>Crackles</u> are caused by the flow of air through liquid, present in the air pouches and smaller airways in the lungs. Crackles sounds like the blowing of bubbles through a straw in a glass filled with liquid.

Emergency Medical Care

Treatment of a child with an airway obstruction must begin immediately. If the child is conscious and you are certain there is a foreign body in the airway—that is, if someone actually saw the object go into the child's mouth—encourage the child to cough to clear the airway. Abdominal thrusts are recommended to relieve a complete (severe) airway obstruction in a responsive child. If the object in the airway does not completely block the flow of air, the child may be able to breathe adequately without intervention. If the obstruction is mild (partial), do not intervene except to provide supplemental oxygen (if tolerated), and provide reassurance **Figure 24-11 ▶**. Allow the child to

remain in whatever position is most comfortable, and monitor his or her condition.

If you see signs of complete or severe airway obstruction, you must attempt to clear the airway at once. The signs to assess for include the following:

- Ineffective cough (no sound) or no cough at all
- Inability to speak or cry
- Poor or no air exchange, unable to move any air

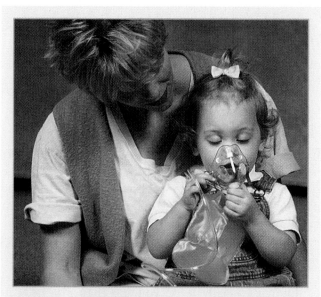

Figure 24-11 If a child has a partial airway obstruction, do not intervene except to give supplemental oxygen and allow the child to remain in whatever position is most comfortable.

- Increasing respiratory difficulty, with stridor
- Cyanosis
- Loss of consciousness

Management of Airway Obstruction in a Child

Abdominal thrusts are recommended to relieve an airway obstruction in a child who is responsive. These thrusts increase the pressure in the chest, creating an artificial cough that may force a foreign body from the airway.

Follow these steps to remove a foreign body obstruction from a conscious child who is in a standing or sitting position Figure 24-12 ▼:

1. **Stand or kneel on one knee behind the child,** and wrap your arms around the child's waist. Prepare to give abdominal thrusts by placing your fist just above the patient's navel and well below the lower tip of the sternum. Place your other hand over that fist.
2. **Deliver rapid, distinct abdominal thrusts** in an upward direction. Be careful to avoid applying force to the lower rib cage or sternum. Repeat the thrusts until the child expels the foreign body or loses consciousness.

If you manage to clear the airway obstruction in an unconscious child but he or she still has no spontaneous breathing or circulation, perform CPR.

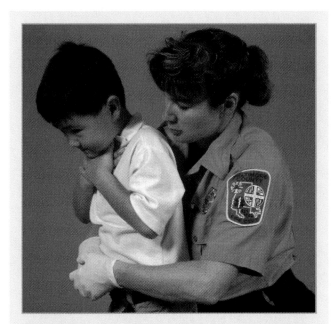

Figure 24-12 To perform an abdominal thrust in a child, kneel behind the child, wrap your arms around his or her body, and place your fist just above the navel and well below the lower tip of the sternum.

If a responsive child who was choking becomes unresponsive, gently lower the child to the ground. Open the airway and look in the back of the throat for the object. If you can see the object, carefully remove it with your fingers. Never perform blind finger sweeps in any patient—regardless of age—as doing so may push the object farther into the airway.

Assess the child for signs of adequate breathing; if adequate breathing is not present, attempt to deliver a ventilation. If the first ventilation does not cause visible chest rise, reopen the airway reattempt to ventilate. If both ventilation attempts fail to produce visible chest rise, immediately begin CPR, starting with chest compressions. Compressions are performed regardless of whether a pulse is present in a child who is choking. Remember that with two-person CPR, the compression/ventilation ratio is 15:2. If you are alone, deliver 30 compressions to 2 ventilations. Each time you open the airway to ventilate, look in the back of the throat for the object. Remove it if you see it, and reassess the child's condition.

Management of Airway Obstruction in an Infant

Abdominal thrusts are not recommended for infants because of the risk of injury to the immature organs of the abdomen. Instead, use back slaps and chest thrusts to try to clear a severe airway obstruction in an infant, as follows Figure 24-13 ▶:

1. **Hold the infant face down,** with the body resting on your forearm. Support the infant's jaw and face with your hand, and keep the head lower than the rest of the body.
2. **Deliver five back slaps** between the shoulder blades with the heel of your hand. Use enough force to expel the object.
3. **Place your free hand behind the infant's head and back,** and bring the infant upright on your thigh, sandwiching the infant's body between your two hands and arms. The infant's head should remain below the level of the body.
4. **Give five quick chest thrusts** in the same location and manner as chest compressions, using two fingers placed on the lower half of the sternum. For larger infants, or if you have small hands, you can perform this step by placing the infant in your lap and turning the infant's whole body as a unit between back slaps and chest thrusts.
5. **Check the airway.** If you can see the foreign body, remove it. If not, repeat the cycles of back slaps

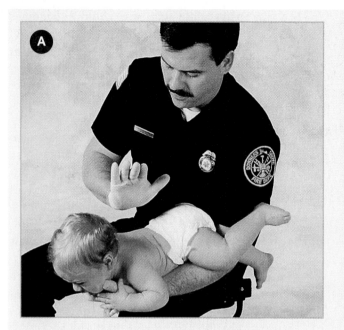
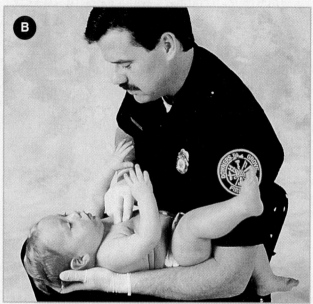

Figure 24-13 Managing airway obstruction in an infant. **A.** Hold the infant face down with the body resting on your forearm. Support the jaw and face with your hand, and keep the head lower than the rest of the body. Give the infant five back slaps between the shoulder blades, using the heel of your hand. **B.** Give the infant five quick chest thrusts, using two fingers placed on the lower half of the sternum.

and chest thrusts until the object is expelled or until the infant loses consciousness.

6. **If the infant is still unconscious after removal of the object,** check for circulation and perform CPR if necessary.

■ Neonatal Resuscitation

At birth, most infants require resuscitation measures that stimulate them to breathe air and stimulate the circulation of blood (Table 24-5 ▶). These measures include positioning of the airway, drying, warming, suctioning, and tactile stimulation. Here are some tips to help you maximize the effects of the measures:

- Position the infant on his or her back with the head down and the neck slightly extended. Place a towel or blanket under the infant's shoulders to help maintain this position. Alternatively, you can place the infant on his or her side, which will facilitate drainage of fluid from the mouth and nose.
- Suction the mouth and then nose using a bulb syringe or suction device with an 8F or 10F catheter. Suction both sides of the back of the mouth, where secretions tend to collect, but avoid deep suctioning of the mouth and throat; this can cause the heart rate to slow. Aim

blow-by oxygen at the infant's mouth and nose during resuscitation.

- In addition to drying the infant's head, back, and body vigorously with dry towels, you may rub the infant's back and slap the soles of his or her feet.

Table 24-5 Rescue Measures for a Neonate Who Is Not Breathing	
Assess and support	■ Temperature (warm and dry) ■ Airway (position and suction) ■ Breathing (stimulate to cry) ■ Circulation (heart rate and color)
BLS interventions	■ Dry and warm the infant. ■ Clear the airway with a bulb syringe. ■ Stimulate the infant if he or she is unresponsive. ■ Perform bag-mask ventilation of the neonate if needed. This is seldom required. ■ Perform chest compressions if there is no pulse or if the pulse is less than 60 beats/min.

Table 24-6 Additional Neonatal Resuscitation Efforts

If the Heart Rate Is . . .	More Than 100 Beats/Min	60 to 100 Beats/Min	Fewer Than 60 Beats/Min
Do this:	Keep the neonate warm.	Begin assisted bag-mask ventilation with 100% oxygen.	Begin assisted bag-mask ventilation with 100% oxygen.
	Transport the neonate.	Reassess the neonate every 30 seconds until heart rate and respirations are normal.	Begin chest compressions. Call for ALS backup. If the heart rate does not increase, medication and ALS will be needed.
	Assess the neonate continuously.	Continue to reassess the infant. Call for ALS backup. Keep the neonate warm.	Reassess the neonate every 30 seconds until heart rate and respiration are normal.

- When a neonate is in distress, you should be properly equipped for resuscitation measures. All ambulances should have the following equipment and supplies for neonatal resuscitation:
  - A bulb syringe
  - Clean, dry towels
  - An infant blanket
  - A bag-mask device (450 mL capacity)
  - Clear masks in infant and premature infant sizes
  - Two umbilical clamps
  - Sterile 4 × 4 gauze
  - A stocking cap
  - An oxygen source with tubing

Additional Resuscitation Efforts

Observe the infant for spontaneous respirations, skin color, and movement of the extremities. If the respiratory effort appears appropriate, evaluate the heart rate by palpating the pulse at the base of the umbilical cord or at the brachial artery. The heart rate is the most important measure in determining the need for further resuscitation Table 24-6 ▲ .

If chest compressions are required, give them at a rate of 120 beats/min using the hand-encircling technique or the two-finger technique. Coordinate chest compression with ventilation at a ratio of 3:1.

■ Basic Life Support Review

Because most children have healthy hearts, sudden cardiac arrest is rare. More commonly, children have cardiopulmonary arrest because of respiratory or circulatory failure due to illness or injury. For this reason, the airway and breathing are the focus of pediatric basic life support (BLS) Table 24-7 ▶ . For purposes of pediatric BLS, an infant is defined as up to 1 year of age and a child as 1 year until the onset of puberty (12 to 14 years of age).

Respiratory problems leading to cardiopulmonary arrest in children can have a number of different causes, including the following:

- Injury—blunt and penetrating
- Infections of the respiratory tract or another organ system
- A foreign body in the airway
- Near drowning
- Electrocution
- Poisoning or drug overdose
- Sudden infant death syndrome (SIDS)

Determining Responsiveness

Never shake a child to determine whether he or she is responsive, especially if there is a possible neck or back injury. Instead, gently tap the child on the

You are the Provider 4

The mother holds the patient and continues to give her the blow-by oxygen en route to the emergency department. In the emergency department, the patient is given a breathing treatment to loosen the mucous in her lungs and another prescription for antibiotics. She is allowed to go home with the agreement to follow up with her physician on Monday morning.

Table 24-7 Review of Pediatric BLS

Action	Infants Younger Than 1 Year	Children Between Age 1 and Puberty
Airway	Head tilt–chin lift maneuver; jaw thrust if spinal injury is suspected	Head tilt–chin lift maneuver; jaw thrust if spinal injury is suspected
Breathing		
Initial	Two breaths at a rate of 1 second/breath (Use a bag-mask ventilation, if available, with oxygen.)	Two breaths at a rate of 1 second/breath (Use bag-mask ventilation, if available, with oxygen.)
Subsequent	12 to 20 breaths/min	12 to 20 breaths/min
Circulation		
Pulse check	Brachial artery	Carotid artery
Compression area	Just below nipple line on sternum	Center of sternum between nipples
Compression method	Two fingers or two thumbs and encircled hands for two-person CPR	Heel of hand with/other hand on top or one hand for small patients
Compression depth	1/3 to 1/2 depth of chest	1/3 to 1/2 depth of chest
Compression rate	100/min	100/min
Compression/ventilation ratio	30:2 for one-person CPR 15:2 for two-person CPR	30:2 for one-person CPR 15:2 for two-person CPR
Foreign body obstruction	Back slaps and chest thrusts	Abdominal thrusts

shoulder, and speak loudly. If a child is responsive but struggling to breathe, allow him or her to remain in whatever position is most comfortable.

Airway

Because children often put toys and other objects, as well as food, in their mouths, foreign body obstruction of the upper airway is common. The steps for removing a foreign object are reviewed earlier in this chapter. You must make sure that the upper airway is open when dealing with pediatric respiratory emergencies or cardiopulmonary arrest. If the child is unconscious and lying in a supine position, the airway may become obstructed when the tongue and throat muscles relax and the tongue falls backward.

If the child is unconscious but breathing adequately, place him or her on one side or the other in the recovery position, in which the upper leg is flexed and bent forward for stabilization and the head is positioned to allow drainage of saliva or vomitus Figure 24-14 ▶ . Do not use this position if you suspect a spinal injury unless you can secure the child to a backboard that can be tilted to the side.

The two common techniques for manually opening the airway in an unresponsive child are the head tilt–chin lift maneuver and the jaw-thrust maneuver.

If head and spine trauma are suspected, you should use a jaw thrust to open the airway. If you are unable to maintain the airway with a jaw thrust, use the head tilt–chin lift maneuver to open the airway.

Remember that the head of an infant or young child is disproportionately large in comparison with the chest and shoulders. As a result, when a child is lying flat on his or her back, especially on a backboard, the head will bend forward onto the upper chest, which can potentially obstruct the upper airway. To avoid this possibility, place a wedge of padding under the upper part of the chest and the shoulders.

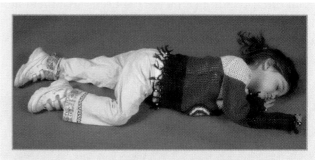

Figure 24-14 A child who is unconscious but breathing adequately should be placed in the recovery position to allow saliva or vomitus to drain from the mouth.

Breathing

Once the airway is open, determine whether the child is breathing spontaneously, using the look, listen, and feel technique. If an infant or small child is breathing, provide immediate transport. A child who is in respiratory distress should be allowed to stay in whatever position is most comfortable.

If an infant or child is not breathing, provide rescue breathing while keeping the airway open. If you are using mouth-to-mouth resuscitation with an infant, place your mouth over the infant's mouth and nose to create a seal. If you are providing bag-mask ventilation in an infant, use the properly sized mask and the technique described earlier.

In an older child and when two rescuers are available, use your thumb and index finger to apply cricoid pressure (the Sellick maneuver). This will decrease the risk of gastric distention and aspiration of vomitus.

In a child with a tracheostomy tube, remove the mask from the bag-valve device and connect it directly to the tracheostomy tube to ventilate the child. If a bag-mask device is unavailable, a pocket mask or barrier device over the tracheostomy site can be used. Place your hand firmly over the child's mouth and nose to prevent the artificial breaths from leaking out of the upper airway.

Circulation

Once you have opened the airway and provided two rescue breaths, you must determine the child's circulatory status. Check the pulse in a carotid artery in an older child and in the brachial artery in young children and infants. You should begin compressions if there is no pulse or the pulse is less than 60 beats/min with signs of poor perfusion. Palpating the pulse in an infant or child can be difficult; take at least 5 seconds but no more than 10 seconds to find the pulse.

For chest compressions to be effective, the patient should be placed on a firm, flat surface with the head at the same level as the body. If you need to carry an infant while providing CPR, your forearm and hand can serve as the flat surface. Follow these steps to perform infant chest compressions Skill Drill 24-4 ▾ :

1. **Place the infant on a firm surface,** using one hand to keep the head in an open airway position. You can also use a pad or wedge under the shoulders and upper body to keep the head from tilting forward.
2. Imagine a line drawn between the nipples. **Place two fingers on the sternum, just below the nipple line** (**Step** ①).
3. **Using two fingers, compress the sternum** about one third to one half the depth of the chest. Compress the chest at a rate of 100 compressions/min.

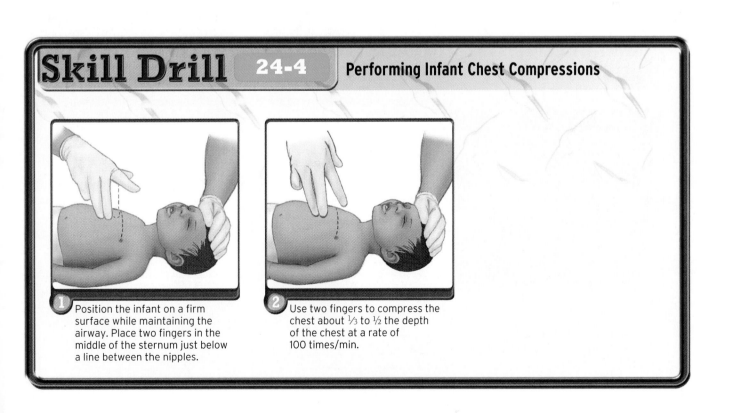

Skill Drill   24-4   Performing Infant Chest Compressions

① Position the infant on a firm surface while maintaining the airway. Place two fingers in the middle of the sternum just below a line between the nipples.

② Use two fingers to compress the chest about ⅓ to ½ the depth of the chest at a rate of 100 times/min.

4. **After each compression, allow the chest to fully re-coil back to its normal position.** Allow equal time for compression and relaxation of the chest (**Step ②**).

Coordinate effective compressions (push hard and fast) with ventilations in a 15:2 ratio for two-person CPR and a 30:2 ratio for one-person CPR. You should make every effort possible to minimize interruptions in the delivery of chest compressions. Make sure the infant's chest rises with each ventilation. If the chest does not rise or rises only a little, reposition the airway with a chin lift. Reassess the infant for signs of spontaneous breathing or pulses after 2 minutes (about five cycles of CPR). With two-person CPR, you

should also switch positions at this 2-minute interval, but limit the interruption to the chest compressions being delivered.

Skill Drill 24-5 ▾ shows the steps for performing CPR in children between 1 year and puberty:

1. **Place the child on a firm surface,** and use one hand to maintain the head in a tilted-back position (**Step ①**).
2. **Place the heel of your hand on the center of the sternum between the nipples.** Use one hand for a small child and two hands, if needed, for a larger child (**Step ②**).
3. **Compress the chest** about one third to one half its total depth. Compress the chest at a rate of

Skill Drill 24-5 Performing CPR on a Child

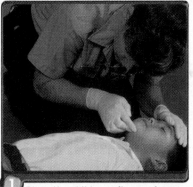

① Place the child on a firm surface, and open the airway.

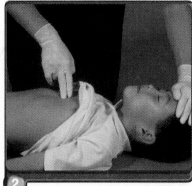

② Place the heel of your hand on the center of the sternum between the nipples. Use one hand for a small child and two hands, if needed, for a larger child.

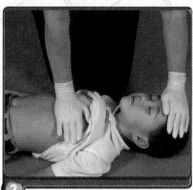

③ Compress the chest about one third to one half its total depth. Compress the chest at a rate of 100 compressions/min, allowing the chest to fully recoil with each compression. Coordinate effective compressions with ventilations in a ratio of 15:2 for two-person CPR or 30:2 for one-person CPR.

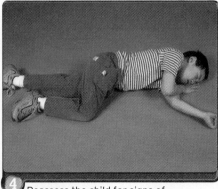

④ Reassess the child for signs of spontaneous breathing and pulse after 2 minutes or five cycles of CPR. If the child resumes effective breathing, place him or her in the recovery position.

100 compressions/min, allowing the chest to fully recoil with each compression. Compression and relaxation should be about the same duration.

4. **Coordinate rapid compressions and ventilations** in a 15:2 ratio for two-person CPR (30:2 for one-person CPR), making sure the chest rises with each ventilation. Deliver each ventilation over a period of 1 second (**Step ③**).

5. **Reassess the child** for signs of spontaneous breathing and pulse after 2 minutes or five cycles of CPR.

6. **If the child resumes effective breathing,** place him or her in the recovery position (**Step ④**).

Remember, if the child has reached puberty or is the size of an adult, use the adult CPR sequence, including the use of the automatic external defibrillator (AED).

AED Use in Children

Owing to the success of the AED programs for adults, pediatric AEDs have been developed and are becoming more accessible in the community. If your service uses an AED with a pediatric dose-reduction system and pediatric defibrillation pads, you should be familiar with the local protocols. During CPR, the AED should be applied to children (over 1 year of age) after the first two minutes of CPR have been completed. As discussed earlier, cardiac arrest in children is usually due to respiratory causes, and oxygenation is vitally important. After the first 2 minutes of CPR, the AED should be used to deliver shocks in the same manner as with an adult patient. It is important to note that if you do not have pediatric-sized defibrillation pads and a pediatric dose-reduction system, you should use a regular AED on children older than 1 year of age. AEDs are not recommended for use in infants less than 1 year of age.

■ Cardiopulmonary Arrest

Cardiac arrest in infants and children is most often associated with respiratory failure and respiratory arrest. Children are affected differently from adults when it comes to decreasing oxygen concentrations. An adult becomes hypoxic, and the heart becomes irritable and sudden cardiac death occurs. This is often in the form of ventricular fibrillation and is the reason that an AED is the treatment of choice. Children, on the other hand, become hypoxic and their heart rate slows, becoming more and more bradycardic. The heart will

beat slower and become weaker with each beat until no pulse is felt. The survival rate after cardiac arrest in the prehospital setting is about 5%. However, the survival rate after respiratory arrest is about 75%. Therefore, a child who is breathing very poorly with a slowing heart rate must be ventilated with high concentrations of oxygen early to try to oxygenate the heart before cardiac arrest occurs.

■ Pediatric Trauma

Anatomic differences between pediatric and adult patients make children more prone to injury. The trauma assessment of a child follows the same format as for an adult. Once the MOI has been determined and the ABCs have been addressed, you must determine whether to use a focused or head-to-toe exam. Remember that young children cannot be specific about location or severity of pain, so a complete head-to-toe exam is usually necessary.

When beginning the exam, determine the age of the child. Infants, toddlers, and preschool-age children do not like to be touched. If possible, the exam should start from the toes and move toward the head, leaving any noticeably injured areas for last. Starting at the core may make the child more upset and less likely to assist with your exam.

The head is injured most often and is the most likely injury to cause death. The child's head is large compared with the body, and most multisystem trauma will involve the head. During your assessment, concentrate on keeping the airway open. Keep reassessing the child, and monitor the vital signs often. Hyperventilation of a head-injured child should be avoided.

Cervical spine injury is more prevalent in children than in adults owing to the weaker muscles of the neck. This is one of the reasons that children younger than 1 year should always be in a rear-facing car seat when being transported. Careful immobilization should be used to maintain a neutral head and neck position.

Immobilization

Immobilization is necessary for all children who have possible head or spinal injuries. Review the steps for immobilizing a child in **Skill Drill 24-6 ▶**:

1. **Maintain the child's head in a neutral position** by placing a towel under the shoulders and torso (**Step ①**).

2. **Place an appropriately sized cervical collar on the patient** (**Step ②**).

Skill Drill 24-6   Immobilizing a Child

1 Use a towel under the back, from the shoulders to the hips, to maintain the head in a neutral position.

2 Apply an appropriately sized cervical collar.

3 Log roll the child onto the immobilization device.

4 Secure the torso first.

5 Secure the head.

6 Ensure that the child is strapped in properly.

3. **Carefully log roll the child** onto the immobilization device (**Step ③**).
4. **Secure the patient's torso** to the immobilization device first (**Step ④**).
5. **Secure the child's head** to the immobilization device (**Step ⑤**).
6. **Complete immobilization** by ensuring that the child is secured properly (**Step ⑥**).

Immobilization can be difficult owing to the child's body proportions. Young children require padding under the torso to maintain a neutral position. At around 8 to 10 years of age, children no longer require padding underneath the torso to create a neutral position; they can simply lie supine on the board. Because a child's body is narrower than an adult's, padding will be required along the sides for the

child to be properly secured on an adult-sized long board.

Some infants will be in a car seat when you assess them. If the child has stable vital signs and minimal injury and the car seat is visibly undamaged, the child can be left in the seat and secured within it for transportation. If the child is in unstable condition or has injuries or the car seat is visibly damaged, the child must be removed from the car seat for you to properly assess, treat, immobilize, and transport.

Ideally, a cervical collar would be used when immobilizing an infant or toddler in a car seat; however, in most cases, an appropriately sized cervical collar will not be available. In this case, place rolled towels on either side of the head to prevent side-to-side movement. Do not place a towel in the shape of an upside-down "U" over the child's head; this may press down on the head and compromise the airway and spinal cord. The steps for immobilizing an infant in a car seat follow (Skill Drill 24-7 ▾):

1. **Carefully stabilize the infant's head in a neutral position.** Leave all car seat straps in place (**Step ①**).
2. **Place an appropriately sized cervical collar** on the patient if available. Otherwise, place rolled towels or padding alongside the infant to fill the spaces between the infant and the car seat (**Step ②**).
3. **Carefully secure the padding,** using tape to keep it in place (**Step ③**).
4. **Secure the car seat to the stretcher** (**Step ④**).

Review these steps to immobilize an infant out of a car seat (Skill Drill 24-8 ▶):

1. **Carefully stabilize the infant's head in a neutral position,** and lay the seat down in a reclined position on a hard surface (**Step ①**).
2. **Position a pediatric board or other similar device** between the patient and the surface on which the infant is resting (**Step ②**).
3. **Carefully slide the infant into position** on the board (**Step ③**).
4. **Make sure the infant's head is in a neutral position** by placing a towel under the infant's shoulders (**Step ④**).
5. **Secure the torso first,** and place padding to fill any voids (**Step ⑤**).
6. **Secure the infant's head** to the board (**Step ⑥**).

Skill Drill 24-7   Immobilizing an Infant in a Car Seat

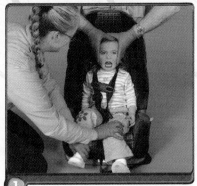

① Carefully stabilize the infant's head in a neutral position.

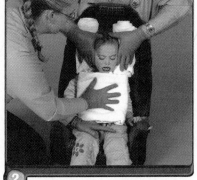

② Place an appropriately sized cervical collar on the patient if available. Otherwise, place rolled towels or padding alongside the patient.

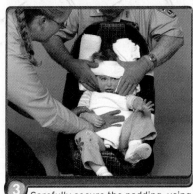

③ Carefully secure the padding, using tape to keep it in place.

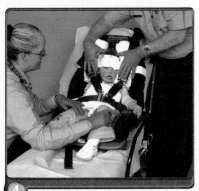

④ Secure the car seat to the stretcher.

Skill Drill   24-8   Immobilizing an Infant Out of a Car Seat

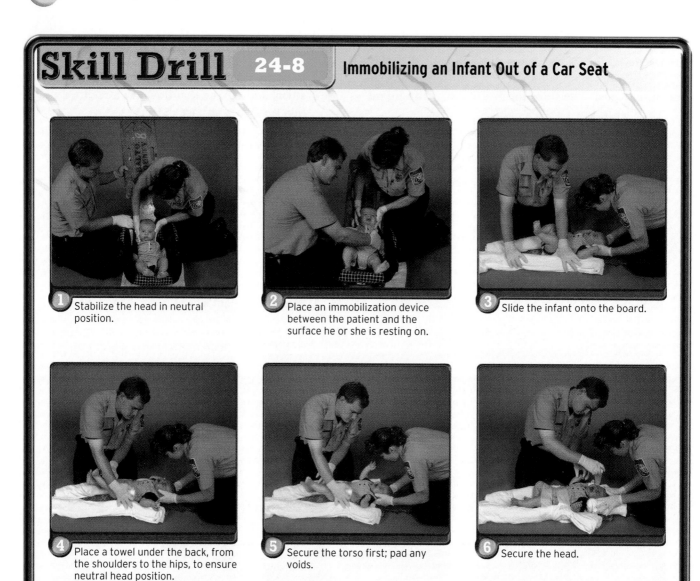

1. Stabilize the head in neutral position.

2. Place an immobilization device between the patient and the surface he or she is resting on.

3. Slide the infant onto the board.

4. Place a towel under the back, from the shoulders to the hips, to ensure neutral head position.

5. Secure the torso first; pad any voids.

6. Secure the head.

Management of Pediatric Injuries

Extremity injuries in children are generally managed in the same manner as those in adults. Painful, deformed limbs with evidence of broken bones should be splinted. Specialized splinting equipment, such as a traction splint for fractures of the femur, should be used only if it fits the child. You should not attempt to use adult immobilization devices for a child unless the child is large enough to properly fit in the device.

■ Pediatric Medical Emergencies

Like the pediatric trauma assessment, the pediatric medical assessment follows the same pathways as in the adult, with emphasis on the differences in the pediatric patient. Some medical complaints merit additional discussion.

Respiratory Emergencies

In the early stages of respiratory distress or failure, respirations may be too slow or too fast for the patient's age. Keep reference charts handy for normal vital signs for pediatric patients. Respirations exceeding 60 breaths/min are a sign of a problem. In most cases, you should begin to assist ventilation immediately, even if the child appears to be breathing adequately. But remember, you are treating the child, not the numbers. A child breathing 60 breaths/min who is playing happily does not need assisted ventilation;

a child breathing 60 breaths/min who is lying unconscious on the floor does.

Signs and Symptoms

In the early stages of respiratory distress, you may note changes in the child's behavior, such as combativeness, restlessness, and anxiety. As the body attempts to maximize the amount of air going into the lungs, the work of breathing increases. Signs and symptoms of increased work of breathing include the following:

- Nasal flaring as the body tries to increase the size of the airway
- Grunting respirations as the body attempts to keep the alveoli expanded at the end of expiration
- Wheezing, stridor, or other abnormal airway sounds
- Accessory (intercostal) muscle use (Remember, in young children, the diaphragm is the major muscle of ventilation.)
- Retractions, or movements of the child's flexible rib cage
- The tripod position; in older children, maximizes the airway

As the child's condition progresses to possible respiratory failure, efforts to breathe decrease; the chest rises less with inspiration. The body has used up its available energy stores and cannot continue to support the extra work of breathing under these conditions. At this point, cyanosis may develop (a late sign). Remember that not all children become cyanotic.

Changes in behavior will also occur. The patient may experience periods of apnea (absence of breathing). As the lack of oxygen becomes more serious, the heart muscle itself becomes hypoxic and the rate slows. This leads to bradycardia, a condition in which the heart rate is less than 60 beats/min in children or less than 80 beats/min in neonates. Bradycardia is almost always related to a lack of oxygen and is an ominous sign in pediatric patients. If the heart rate is fast, you need to continue your assessment to determine the cause. If the heart rate is slow or absent, you must intervene immediately. Without aggressive airway management, bradycardia may quickly progress to cardiopulmonary arrest.

Respiratory failure can be due to airway obstruction, trauma, problems with the nervous system, dehydration (often caused by vomiting and diarrhea), or metabolic disturbances. Regardless of the cause, your

Documentation Tips

Along with the respiratory rate, include any signs of distress or accessory muscle use (such as respirations - 42 and shallow with nasal flaring and intercostal retractions).

first step is always to focus on ensuring adequate oxygenation and ventilation. Never forget that a child's condition can progress from respiratory distress to respiratory failure at any time. For this reason, you must reassess children frequently.

Emergency Medical Care

A child or infant in respiratory distress or possible respiratory failure needs supplemental oxygen. Remember, anxiety, agitation, and crying may increase the effort or work of breathing, so use whichever method seems least upsetting to the child—mask, blow-by, or nasal cannula. You may need to be creative and distract the child with games, a toy, or talking.

Allow the child to remain in a comfortable position. For a small child, this may mean sitting on the caregiver's lap. Give nothing by mouth, in case the child's condition deteriorates suddenly. If the patient's condition has progressed to respiratory failure, you must begin assisted ventilation immediately and continue to provide supplemental oxygen.

Shock

Shock is a condition that develops when the circulatory system is unable to deliver a sufficient amount of blood to the organs of the body, resulting in organ failure and, eventually, cardiopulmonary arrest. In children, shock is rarely due to a primary cardiac event, such as a heart attack. The most common causes of shock in children include the following:

- Traumatic injury with blood loss (especially abdominal)
- Dehydration due to diarrhea and vomiting
- Severe infection
- Neurologic injury such as severe head trauma
- A severe allergic reaction to an insect bite or allergy (anaphylaxis)
- Diseases of the heart
- A collapsed lung (pneumothorax)
- Blood, fluid, or inflammation around the heart (cardiac tamponade or pericarditis)

Infants and children have less blood circulating in their bodies than adults do, so the loss of even a small volume of fluid or blood may lead to shock. Pediatric patients also respond differently than do adults to fluid loss. They may respond by an increased heart rate, increased respirations, and vasoconstriction (evidenced by pale or blue skin). You must be able to recognize the signs of shock in infants and children.

Loss of more than 25% of the blood volume significantly increases the risk of shock. Signs of shock in children are the following:

- Tachycardia
- Poor capillary refill
- Mental status changes

Begin by assessing the ABCs and treating immediately. Children in shock often have increased respirations but do not have a fall in blood pressure until shock is severe.

In assessing circulation, you should pay particular attention to the following:

Pulse. Assess the rate and the quality of the pulse. A weak, "thready" pulse is a sign that there is a problem. The appropriate rate depends on age; a rate of more than 160 beats/min suggests shock.

Skin signs. Assess the temperature and moisture on the hands and feet. How does this compare with the temperature of the skin on the trunk of the body? Is the skin dry and warm or cold and clammy?

CRT. Squeeze a finger or toe for several seconds until the skin blanches, then release it. Does the fingertip return to its normal color within 2 seconds, or is the return of color delayed?

Color. Assess the patient's skin color. Is it pink, pale, ashen, or blue?

Blood pressure is the most difficult vital sign to measure in pediatric patients. The cuff must be the proper size—two thirds the length of the upper arm. The value for normal blood pressure is also age-specific. Remember that blood pressure may be normal in compensated shock. Low blood pressure is a sign of decompensated shock, a serious condition that requires care an ALS team can provide.

Part of your assessment should include talking with the parents or caregivers to determine when the signs and symptoms first appeared and whether any of the following has occurred:

- Decrease in urine output (With infants, are there fewer than 6 to 10 wet diapers?)
- Absence of tears, even when the child is crying
- Changes in level of consciousness and behavior

Time should not be wasted in field procedures. Ensure that the airway is open, prepare to ventilate, control

bleeding, and give supplemental oxygen. Continue to monitor airway and breathing. Position the patient with the head lower than the feet by elevating the feet with blankets. Keep the patient warm with blankets and by turning up the heat in the patient compartment. Provide immediate transport, and continue monitoring vital signs en route. Contact ALS backup as needed. Allow a caregiver to accompany the child whenever possible.

Seizures

Seizures in children may appear in several different ways, including shaking of the whole body or movement in just a single arm or leg. Seizures can also appear as lip smacking, eye blinking, or staring off into space. In a true seizure, movements cannot be stopped on command or by holding an extremity.

Altered mental status and/or the inability of others to stop a movement or range of movements in the affected limb are common to all seizures. Some patients may feel pins and needles, hear sounds, and see hallucinations. In all but absence seizures, a postictal period of extreme fatigue or unresponsiveness occurs after the seizure for anywhere from a few minutes to several hours. During this time, the patient may appear sleepy and/or confused and is not able to interact appropriately. A short period of seizure activity (less than 30 minutes) is not in itself harmful to the patient. After 30 to 45 minutes, however, the brain may run low on energy stores, and continued activity can be harmful. Status epilepticus is a continuous seizure or multiple seizures without a return to consciousness for 30 minutes or more.

If you can identify the cause of the seizure, you will be better able to monitor the patient for potential complications associated with the underlying problem. In particular, be alert to the presence of medications, possible poisons, and indications of abuse or neglect.

Febrile Seizures

Febrile seizures are common in children between the ages of 6 months and 6 years. Most pediatric seizures are due to fever alone. These seizures typically occur on the first day of a febrile illness, are characterized by generalized tonic-clonic seizure activity, and last less than 15 minutes with a short postictal phase or none at all. They may be a sign of a more serious problem, such as meningitis. Obtain a history from the caregivers because the child may have had a previous febrile seizure.

If you are called to care for a child who has had a febrile seizure, you often will find that the patient is awake, alert, and fully interactive when you arrive. Keep in mind that a persistent fever can lead to another seizure. Carefully assess the ABCs, begin cooling measures with tepid (not cold) water, and provide prompt transport; all children with febrile seizures need to be examined in the hospital setting.

Emergency Medical Care

Although medical management of seizures in the hospital setting may vary according to cause, your assessment and management of the patients remain essentially the same. First, ensure that the scene is safe for you, your partner, and the patient. Next, perform an initial assessment, focusing on the ABCs. If possible, obtain a brief history from the caregivers about previous serious illnesses or seizures and current medication or trauma.

Securing and protecting the airway are your priorities. To avoid obstruction from the tongue falling back into the airway, place a child who is having a seizure or who is in a postictal state in the recovery position if you can do so without having to use extreme force against the seizure activity. In the case of trauma, place the head in a neutral in-line position and ensure that the cervical spine is protected. Be ready to use suction to prevent aspiration of stomach contents, blood, or vomitus. Do not place your fingers in the mouth of a patient who is having a seizure.

A patient who is having a seizure or in a postictal state may not be breathing adequately. Assessing the rate and depth of respirations in this situation can be difficult but is essential. Patients may have shallow, rapid breathing or may have occasional deep respirations. Signs that a patient is not breathing adequately include the following:

- Very slow respirations
- Very shallow breaths
- Bluish tint to lips or pale lips
- Snoring respirations caused by the tongue blocking the airway

Deliver oxygen by mask, blow-by, or nasal cannula. If there are no signs of improvement, begin bag-mask ventilation with appropriately sized equipment.

In patients experiencing a seizure, adequate blood pressure and pulse rate usually are maintained unless the seizure is caused by an underlying circulatory or neurologic problem or trauma, including bleeding, heart problems, or brain injury. Nevertheless, you must evaluate the pulse and blood pressure and reevaluate them. Once the ABCs have been addressed, assessment and management should proceed. If the patient is seizing, note the type of movement and position of the eyes because this information may help hospital staff make a diagnosis. If there is a fever, begin cooling measures such as removing clothing and placing towels moistened with tepid water on the child. A child with febrile seizures can have another seizure if the temperature remains high. Do not use alcohol or cold water to cool a patient. Make sure the patient is protected from hitting the sides of the stretcher or nearby equipment. Take any medications or possible poisons at the scene to the hospital with the patient. If the patient is in status epilepticus, call for ALS backup.

Dehydration

Dehydration can be described as mild, moderate, or severe. The severity of dehydration can be gauged by looking at several clues Table 24-8 ▾ . For example, an infant with mild dehydration may have dry lips and

Table 24-8 Vital Signs and Symptoms of Dehydration

	Mild Dehydration	Moderate Dehydration	Severe Dehydration
Pulse	Normal	Increased	Increased; 160+ signals impending shock
Level of activity	Normal or slowed	Slowed	Variable, weak to unresponsive
Urine output	Decreased	Decreased	No output
Skin	Normal	Cool, mottled; poor turgor	Cool, clammy; poor turgor; delayed CRT
Mouth	Decreased saliva	Dry mucous membranes	Dry mucous membranes
Eyes	Normal	Tears	Sunken eyes
Anterior fontanel	Normal to sunken	Sunken	Very sunken
Level of consciousness	Normal	Altered	Altered; lethargic
Blood pressure	Normal	Normal	Normal to low when shock sets in

gums, decreased saliva, and fewer wet diapers throughout the day. As the dehydration grows more severe, the lips and gums may become very dry, the eyes may look sunken, and the infant may be sleepy and/or irritable, refusing feedings. The skin may be loose and have no elasticity; this condition is called poor skin turgor Figure 24-15 ▶ . Infants may also have sunken fontanels.

Young children can compensate for fluid losses by decreasing blood flow to the extremities and directing it to vital organs such as the brain and heart. Children who are moderately to severely dehydrated may have mottled, cool, clammy skin and delayed CRT. Respirations will usually be increased. Remember that the blood pressure may remain normal.

Emergency medical care should include carefully assessing the ABCs and obtaining baseline vital signs. However, if the dehydration is severe, ALS backup may be necessary so that intravenous access can be

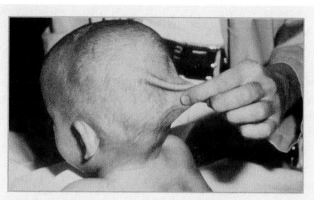

Figure 24-15 An infant with dehydration may exhibit "tenting" or poor skin turgor.

obtained and rehydration can begin. All children with signs and symptoms of moderate to severe dehydration should be transported to the emergency department.

You are the Provider   Summary

Managing a child in an emergency situation can be very trying. Children compensate well and then can go downhill fast. Anticipate problems early and treat aggressively when dealing with pediatrics.

1. **How should you approach the patient?**
   Gather a general impression as you approach the patient. Make specific note of the airway and breathing. If the patient is breathing sufficiently, use a toe-to-head assessment to lessen any anxiety.

2. **What questions should you ask the mother?**
   Does the child have any medical problems?
   Does she take any medications?
   How long has this been going on?
   Has the mother given her anything for this?
   Is she coughing anything up? Is so, what color is it?
   Has she had any difficulty breathing?
   Has she had any other pain?

3. **What should you ask about her previous infection?**
   What were the signs and symptoms she was experiencing at that time? What was the diagnosis? What did the doctor say? What type of medication was she taking?

4. **How should you administer oxygen?**
   Any way she will tolerate it. Blow-by might be the best choice.

5. **Why is her heart rate so fast?**
   It is within normal limits for a 3-year-old child. It may be at the upper end because she may be a little dehydrated.

6. **What else could you do to make her feel more comfortable?**
   Let Mom hold her. Give her a favorite toy to take with her. Let her hold and look at your equipment as you are using it.

7. **What does the productive cough indicate?**
   Possible infection.

8. **How should she be transported?**
   In a position of comfort—probably in Mom's lap. This is not an emergency transport, but she should be monitored closely for any changes.

9. **Should you examine her airway/throat? Why or why not?**
   No. Even though she does not present with the classic signs, she could have epiglottitis. Any manipulation or aggravation of the airway, even from crying, could cause a laryngospasm that completely occludes her airway.

Prep Kit

Ready for Review

- Use a pediatric resuscitation tape measure to determine the appropriately sized equipment for children.
- Use the pediatric assessment triangle (PAT) to obtain a general impression of the infant's or child's condition.
- In treating possible respiratory failure in a child, always position the airway in a neutral position.
- Appropriate oxygen delivery devices include the blow-by technique at 6 L/min, a nonrebreathing mask at 10 to 12 L/min, and a bag-mask device at 10 to 15 L/min.
- Provide bag-mask ventilation for a child whose breathing and tidal volume are inadequate and who has an altered level of consciousness.
- The three keys to successful use of bag-mask ventilation in a child are: (1) have the appropriate equipment in the right size; (2) maintain a good face-to-mask seal; and (3) ventilate at the appropriate rate and volume— 12 to 20 breaths/min for an infant or child, 1 second per ventilation. Squeeze gently, and stop squeezing as the chest wall begins to rise; use the phrase "squeeze, release, release" to maintain a proper rhythm.
- Children younger than 5 years often obstruct their upper and lower airways with a variety of foreign objects.
- If the child with a mild airway obstruction is conscious, encourage him or her to cough to clear the airway.
- If the child is unresponsive, you should first open the airway and perform a finger sweep only if you can see an object. Never perform blind finger sweeps in infants or children with an airway obstruction.
- In treating an unresponsive child with a severe airway obstruction, attempt to ventilate and start CPR. Look in the back of the throat each time you stop compressions to ventilate. Remove the object if you can see it.
- In a conscious child who is sitting or standing, apply abdominal thrusts from behind. Continue to perform abdominal thrusts until the obstruction is relieved or the child loses consciousness.
- Signs of shock in children are tachycardia, poor CRT, and mental status changes. You must be very alert for signs of shock in children because their conditions decompensate rapidly.
- Febrile seizures are common in children between the ages of 6 months and 6 years. Most pediatric seizures are due to fever alone. Carefully assess the ABCs, begin cooling measures, and provide prompt transport.
- The most common cause of dehydration in children is vomiting and diarrhea. Life-threatening diarrhea can develop in an infant in hours. You can determine whether a child's dehydration is mild, moderate, or severe by assessing the child's urine output, level of activity, mental status, skin tone, and pulse.
- If the child is unresponsive but breathing adequately, place him or her in the recovery position unless you suspect a spinal injury. Use the head tilt–chin lift or jaw-thrust maneuver to open the airway in a child who is unresponsive and not breathing.
- If a child is not breathing, provide rescue breathing while keeping the airway open. Ventilate infants and children at a rate of 12 to 20 times per minute with each ventilation being delivered over 1 second.
- To provide CPR in an infant, compress the chest at a rate of 100 compressions/min; use two fingers, and compress the lower half of the sternum to a depth that is one half to one third the depth of the chest.
- In children, compress the chest at a rate of 100 times per minute. Use the heel of one hand (two hands for older children) on the sternum at the nipple line. Compress the chest one half to one third the depth of the chest.
- Whenever giving CPR, your efforts should revolve around limiting the interruptions of chest compressions being delivered.

Vital Vocabulary

anemia A deficiency of red blood cells or hemoglobin.

apnea Absence of breathing.

AVPU scale Used to assess level of consciousness; recorded as being alert, verbally responsive, responsive to pain, or unresponsive.

bradycardia A heart rate of less than 60 beats/min in children or less than 80 beats/min in infants.

bradypnea Slow respiratory rate; ominous sign in a child that indicates impending respiratory arrest.

capillary refill time (CRT) The amount of time that it takes for blood to return to the capillary bed after applying pressure to the skin or nail bed; indicates the status of end-organ perfusion; reliable in children younger than 6 years.

central pulses The pulses that are closest to the core (central) part of the body where the vital organs are located; the carotid, femoral, and apical pulses.

crackles A crackling breath sound caused by the flow of air through liquid in the lungs; a sign of lower airway obstruction.

Technology

- Interactivities
- Vocabulary Explorer
- Anatomy Review
- Web Links
- Online Review Manual

croup Infection of the airway below the level of the vocal cords, usually caused by a virus.

cyanosis A blue discoloration of the skin and mucous membranes; indicates a decreased level of oxygen in the blood.

end-organ perfusion The status of perfusion to the vital organs of the body; determined by assessing capillary refill time (CRT).

epiglottitis Inflammation of the soft tissue in the area above the vocal cords, usually due to an infection.

grunting An "uh" sound heard during exhalation; reflects the child's attempt to keep the alveoli open; a sign of increased work of breathing.

head bobbing The head lifts and tilts back during inspiration, then moves forward during expiration; a sign of increased work of breathing.

nasal flaring Widening of the nares during inspiration; commonly seen in infants; indicates increased work of breathing.

pediatric assessment triangle (PAT) A structured assessment tool that allows you to rapidly form a general impression of the infant or child without touching him or her; consists of assessing appearance, work of breathing, and circulation to the skin.

pediatric resuscitation tape A tape used to estimate an infant's or a child's weight on the basis of length; appropriate drug doses and equipment sizes are listed on the tape.

retractions Drawing in of the intercostal muscles and sternum during inspiration; a sign of increased work of breathing.

sniffing position Optimum neutral head position for an uninjured child who requires airway management.

stridor A high-pitched breath sound heard mainly on inspiration that is a sign of upper airway obstruction.

tachypnea Increased respiratory rate.

tenting A condition in which the skin remains elevated after being pulled gently; indicates dehydration.

tidal volume The amount of air that is delivered to the lungs and airways in one inhalation.

transition phase A period that allows an infant or a child to become familiar with you and your equipment; only appropriate if the child's condition is stable.

tripod position An abnormal position to keep the airway open; it involves leaning forward onto two arms stretched forward.

wheezing A whistling breath sound caused by air traveling through narrowed air passages within the bronchioles; a sign of lower airway obstruction.

work of breathing An indicator of oxygenation and ventilation; reflects the child's attempt to compensate for hypoxia.

Assessment in Action

Assessment and care of children often requires a creative approach. Remember that pediatric patients are not simply "little adults" and must be treated based on age as well as assessment findings.

1. A child in respiratory distress needs oxygen by _____.
   A. nonrebreather mask
   B. the least upsetting method
   C. bag-mask
   D. nasal cannula

2. Seizure activity can appear as _____.
   A. lip smacking
   B. shaking of the entire body
   C. staring into space
   D. all of the above

3. Which of the following is a contraindication for the use of a nasopharyngeal airway?
   A. broken teeth
   B. nasal flaring
   C. head trauma
   D. unresponsiveness

4. Where should you check for a pulse in an infant?
   A. popliteal
   B. radial
   C. carotid
   D. brachial

5. _____ helps to keep the alveoli inflated at the end of expiration.
   A. Coughing
   B. Hiccuping
   C. Grunting
   D. Nasal flaring

6. The most likely injury to cause death in a pediatric patient is a _____ injury.
   A. thorax
   B. head
   C. abdominal
   D. pelvic

Challenging Questions

7. What determines whether or not a child should be removed from a car seat and immobilized in another fashion?

25

Geriatric Emergencies

You are the Provider 1

You are called to a residence for an elderly woman who lives alone and is not feeling well. As you enter the residence you find her sitting in a recliner. She has bruises all over her arms and states that she has "thin skin." Her house is neat and tidy, but your partner trips over a loose rug in the entryway.

Initial Assessment	Recording Time: 0 Minutes
Appearance	Pale
Level of consciousness	Alert and oriented
Airway	Open and clear
Breathing	Normal
Circulation	Radial pulses present, irregular

1. What aspect of aging would explain the bruising of her arms?
2. The assessment of the house falls under which part of the GEMS diamond?
3. To what part of the GEMS diamond does the fact that she lives alone refer?

Geriatrics

Geriatric patients are people who are older than 65 years. In this chapter, we use 65 years as the threshold age to be consistent with the definition used by other medical groups and governmental agencies.

According to US Census Data, almost 35 million people are older than 65 years. It is projected that by the year 2020, the geriatric population will be greater than 54 million. This is a very significant evolutionary trend for EMT-Bs because older people are major users of the EMS and health care systems in general. These calls may be difficult for you because the "classic" presentation of medical conditions common in younger patients may be altered. An acute myocardial infarction may present as jaw or neck pain, and some older patients may not experience chest pain at all. Their aging bodies can mask serious medical conditions. Older patients frequently have chronic medical problems and may be taking numerous medications for their illnesses. Providing effective treatment for this growing number of patients requires that all EMT-Bs understand the issues related to aging and that they modify some of their assessment and treatment approaches to deal with this age group.

A large percentage of your patient contacts involve older people. Lifesaving interventions for geriatric patients may include reviewing the home environment to ensure that safe and livable conditions exist, providing information on preventing falls, and making referrals to appropriate social services agencies when needed. EMT-Bs who respond to the homes of geriatric patients are in an ideal position to provide not only immediate help to patients, but also key information to others in the health care and social services systems. Often, simple preventive measures can help older people avoid further injury, costly medical treatment, and death.

This chapter also reviews some of the specialized equipment that is commonly found in the home. Implants such as vascular access devices (VADs), dialysis access devices, tracheostomies, feeding tubes, and ventricular shunts are discussed.

Communication and Older Adults

Good communication is essential to successful assessment and treatment of older patients. Many things make communicating with older patients challenging. The aging process brings about changes in vision, hearing, taste, smell, and touch. Also, there are changes in communication abilities that accompany aging and dementia and other diseases. Although these symptoms can be frustrating, they are considered normal parts of aging.

Communication Techniques

Your first words can gain or lose the patient's trust. Speak respectfully when you introduce yourself. If you know the patient's name, use it. Older people may be insulted if you use their first name. If they suggest that you call them by their first name, it is fine to do so. If you do not know their first name, use "Sir" or "Ma'am." Do not use "Hon," "Dearie," or "Grandma." Use short words, and ask only one question at a time. In general, when interviewing an older patient, the following techniques should be used:

- Identify yourself. Do not assume an older patient knows who you are.
- Be aware of how you present yourself. Avoid showing frustration and impatience through body language.
- Look directly at the patient.
- Speak slowly and distinctly.
- Explain what you are going to do before you do it. Use simple terms to explain the use of medical equipment and procedures, avoiding medical jargon and slang.
- Listen to the answer the patient gives you.
- Show the patient respect. Never use the patient's first name without his or her permission.
- Do not assume that all older patients are hard of hearing. Ask the patient if he or she can

Technology

Interactivities

Vocabulary Explorer

Anatomy Review

Web Links

Online Review Manual

Refresher.EMSzone.com

hear you and verify by asking him or her to tell you his or her understanding of what you just said.

- Do not talk about the patient in front of him or her; to do so gives the impression that the patient has no say in decision making. This is easy to forget when the patient has impaired cognitive (thought) processes or has difficulty communicating.
- Be patient.

As for patients of any age, older patients have more difficulty communicating clearly when they are stressed by an emergency or a personal crisis.

The GEMS Diamond

When you are dispatched to care for older patients, it is important to remember certain key concepts. The GEMS diamond Table 25-1 ▾ was created to help you remember what is different about older patients. The GEMS diamond is not intended to be a format for the approach to geriatric patients, nor is it intended to replace the ABCs of care. Instead, it serves as an acronym for the issues to be considered when assessing every older patient.

"G" of the GEMS diamond stands for "geriatric." When responding to an emergency involving an older

---

Table 25-1 The GEMS Diamond

G   Geriatric Patients

- Present atypically.
- Deserve respect.
- Experience normal changes with age

E   Environmental Assessment

- Check the physical condition of the patient's home: Is the exterior of the home in need of repair? Is the home secure?
- Check for hazardous conditions that may be present (for example, poor wiring, rotted floors, unventilated gas heaters, broken window glass, clutter that prevents adequate egress).
- Are smoke detectors present and working?
- Is the home too hot or too cold?
- Is there an odor of feces or urine in the home? Is bedding soiled or urine-soaked?
- Is food present in the home? Is it adequate and unspoiled?
- Are liquor bottles present? If so, are they lying empty?
- If the patient has a disability, are appropriate assistive devices (for example, a wheelchair or walker) present?
- Does the patient have access to a telephone?
- Are medications out of date or unmarked, or are prescriptions for the same or similar medications from many physicians?
- If living with others, is the patient confined to one part of the home?
- If the patient is residing in a nursing facility, does the care appear to be adequate to meet the patient's needs?

M   Medical Assessment

- Older patients tend to have a variety of medical problems, making assessment more complex. Keep this in mind in all cases—both trauma and medical. A trauma patient may have an underlying medical condition that could have caused or may be exacerbated by the injury.
- Obtaining a medical history is important in older patients, regardless of the chief complaint.
- Initial assessment
- Ongoing assessment

S   Social Assessment

- Assess activities of daily living (eating, dressing, bathing, toileting).
- Are these activities being provided for the patient? If so, by whom?
- Are there delays in obtaining food, medication, or other necessary items? The patient may complain of this, or the environment may suggest this.
- If in an institutional setting, is the patient able to feed himself or herself? If not, is food still sitting on the food tray? Has the patient been lying in his or her own urine or feces for prolonged periods?
- Does the patient have a social network? Does the patient have a mechanism to interact socially with others on a daily basis?

patient, you should consider that older patients are different from younger patients and may not present with the same signs and symptoms as younger patients do.

"E" of the GEMS diamond stands for an environmental assessment. Assessment of the environment can help give clues to the patient's condition or the cause of the emergency. Is the home too hot or too cold? Is the home well kept and secure? Are there hazardous conditions? Preventive care is also very important for a geriatric patient who may not carefully study the environment or may not realize where risks exist.

"M" of the GEMS diamond stands for medical assessment. Older patients tend to have a variety of medical problems and may be taking numerous prescription, over-the-counter (OTC), and herbal medications. Obtaining a thorough medical history is very important in older patients.

"S" stands for social assessment. Older people may have a shrinking social network because of the death of a spouse, family members, and friends. Older people may also need assistance with activities of daily living, such as dressing and eating. There are numerous social agencies that are readily available to help geriatric patients. Consider obtaining information pamphlets about some of the agencies for older people in your area. If you have these brochures with you and encounter a person in need, you can provide this valuable information. Social agencies that deal with the older population are happy to share a listing of the services they provide.

Leading Causes of Death

The leading causes of death in the geriatric population include heart disease, cancer, stroke, chronic obstructive pulmonary disease and other respiratory illnesses, diabetes, and trauma. The physiologic aging of older people makes them more vulnerable than younger people to the effects of disease and injury. In addition, acute illness and trauma are more likely to involve organ systems beyond those initially involved. For example, in a geriatric patient who has fallen and fractured a hip, pneumonia may develop during recovery.

Physiologic Changes That Accompany Age

As a person gets older, the body experiences physiologic changes. In general, a 65-year-old person cannot

expect to have the same degree of physical performance as when he or she was 30 years old. By the time a person reaches 65 years, the amount of total body water and the number of body cells has decreased by as much as 30%. Generally, after age 30, organ systems begin to deteriorate at a rate of roughly 1% per year. However, aging does not necessarily mean that a person will experience disease.

Common stereotypes about older people include the presence of mental confusion, illness, a sedentary lifestyle, and immobility. Although these perceptions are common, they are usually far from the norm. Older people can stay fit and be active, even though they will not be able to perform at the same level as they did in their youth. Most older people lead active lives, participating in the community and in sports, and they are generally healthy despite the aging process.

Skin

As we get older, our skin becomes thinner and wrinkled. Collagen, a protein that is the chief component of connective tissue and bones, and elastin, a protein that helps to make the skin pliable, are lost as we age. The layer of fat under the skin also becomes thinner. As the elasticity of the skin declines, bruising becomes more common because the skin can tear more easily. Without the elasticity of the skin and the cushioning that the fat provides, the skin does not constrict and stop the bleeding as quickly when it is injured. This causes more and larger bruises after minimal trauma. There are also fewer sweat glands, so older skin tends to feel dry. Another problem that affects the skin is pressure ulcers, sometimes referred to as bedsores. Pressure ulcers form when the patient is lying in the same position for a long time. The pressure from the weight of the body cuts off the blood flow to the area of skin. With no blood flow to the skin, a sore develops. These sores can develop in as little as 45 minutes.

Senses

The pupils of the eyes begin to lose the ability to handle changes in light and require more time to adjust. This can make driving and walking more hazardous Figure 25-1 ▶ . Lighting changes can cause problems of visual acuity and depth perception. Cataracts, clouding of the lenses or their surrounding membranes, interfere with vision and make it difficult to distinguish colors and see clearly, increasing the likelihood of falls

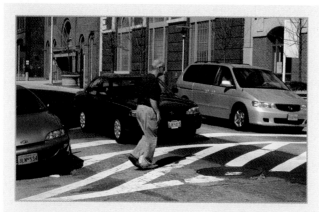

Figure 25-1 Changes in vision, hearing, posture, and motor ability predispose older people to a greater risk of being struck by a vehicle.

and accidents and accounting for some mistakes in taking medications. Hearing is the sensory change that affects the most people. Changes in the inner ear make hearing high-frequency sounds difficult. Changes in the ear can also cause problems with balance and make falls more likely. Changes in appetite may occur because of a decrease in the number of taste buds. The sense of touch lessens from loss of the end nerve fibers. This loss, in conjunction with the slowing of the peripheral nervous system, can create situations in which an older person can be injured. For example, an older person may be slow to react when touching something hot. This delayed response could result in a burn.

Respiratory System

Although the alveoli in an older person's lung tissue become enlarged, their elasticity decreases, making it harder to expel used air. This change in lung tissue quality is comparable to a balloon that has been expanded and then deflated; the balloon loses some of its ability to contract to its original state after inflation. The lack of elasticity results in a decreased ability to exchange oxygen and carbon dioxide. The body's chemoreceptors, which monitor the changes in oxygen and carbon dioxide levels in the blood, slow with age. This can present as lower pulse oximetry readings, even in healthy people. A decrease in the number of cilia that line the bronchial tree lessens the ability to cough and, therefore, increases the chances of infection. Patients lose muscle mass in the chest and may get less help from muscles in the chest wall when they have trouble breathing.

Cardiovascular System

Cardiac output is a measure of the workload of the heart. We normally compensate for an increased demand on the cardiovascular system by increasing our heart rate, increasing the contraction of the heart, and constricting the blood vessels to nonvital organs. Aging decreases the body's ability to speed up contractions, to increase contraction strength, and to constrict blood vessels because of stiffer vessels. Many geriatric patients are at risk for <u>atherosclerosis</u>, an accumulation of fatty material in the arteries. It is a form of arteriosclerosis. Major complications of atherosclerosis include myocardial infarction and stroke. The presence of <u>arteriosclerosis</u>, a disease that causes the arteries to thicken, harden, and calcify, makes stroke, heart disease, hypertension, and bowel infarction more likely. Older people are also at an increased risk for <u>aneurysm</u>, an abnormal, blood-filled dilation of the wall of a blood vessel. Severe blood loss can occur when an aneurysm bursts.

Renal System

Kidney function in older people declines from 20% to 50% because of a decrease in the number of nephrons. The kidneys are important in eliminating certain medications from a person's system. With a decrease in renal function, levels of medications may rise, creating the impression of an overdose. Electrolyte disturbances are also more likely to occur with the lowered filtering of the blood, which can often be the cause of altered mental status in older people.

Nervous System

The number of brain cells in some areas may decrease by as much as 45%. By age 85 years, a 10% reduction in brain weight can result in increased risk of head trauma. Short-term memory impairment, a decrease in the ability to perform psychomotor skills, and slower reflex times are normal in the aging process. This decline may make assessment of older patients challenging. Previous injury or illnesses that are not associated with the current problem may also alter the assessment findings. It is important to compare older patients' current status with their normal abilities.

Musculoskeletal System

The disks between the vertebrae begin to narrow, and a decrease in height of between 2" and 3" may occur. A decrease in the amount of muscle mass often results in less strength, and fractures are more likely because of a decrease in bone density (osteoporosis). Posture also changes; flexion at the neck and a forward bending of the shoulders may produce a condition called <u>kyphosis</u> (also called "humpback," "hunchback," or "Pott curvature"), making immobilization of geriatric patients more challenging Figure 25-2 ▼.

Gastrointestinal System

A decrease in the volume of saliva and gastric juices causes a dry mouth, making it harder to chew and begin to digest foods. A slowing of the intestinal tract may cause constipation or fecal impaction. Decreased liver function makes it harder to detoxify the blood and eliminate substances such as medications and alcohol. This change can make it difficult for patients

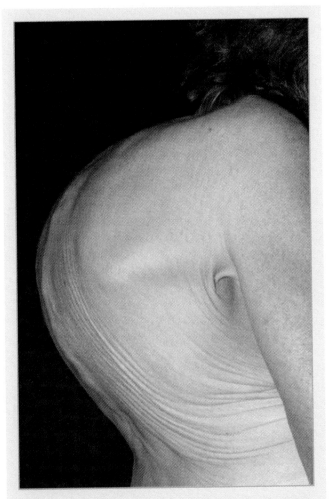

Figure 25-2 Kyphosis, in which the back becomes hunched, often develops in older people.

and their physicians to find the appropriate dosage for new medications.

■ Polypharmacy

Older people account for one eighth of the population but use one quarter of the prescribed medications and one third of the OTC medications sold in the United States. Many medications have interactions or counteractions when taken together. Polypharmacy refers to the use of multiple prescription drugs by one patient, causing the potential for negative effects such as overdosing or drug interaction.

Many patients have more than one physician, such as a family physician for everyday care, a cardiologist for the heart, and an endocrinologist for the treatment of diabetes, all of whom may prescribe medications for the patient. But what if the patient does not tell each physician about all of the medications he or she takes? The patient may not remember the medications one doctor prescribed or may not want to tell one doctor about seeing another.

Other sources of medications include OTC medicines such as aspirin, antacids, cough syrups, and decongestants. Herbal remedies can also interact with prescribed and OTC medications. You must be aware of the implications of medication issues when caring for geriatric patients. Complete assessment of a patient includes obtaining a medication history.

■ Impact of Aging on Trauma

You must consider the body's decreasing ability to tolerate injury when you are assessing and caring for a geriatric patient. An isolated hip fracture in a healthy 25-year-old adult is rarely associated with overall decline. However, the same injury in an 85-year-old patient can produce a wide-ranging, systemic impact that results in deterioration, shock, and hypoxia. Although an injury may be considered isolated and not alarming in most adults, an older patient's overall physical condition may lessen the body's ability to compensate for the effects of even simple injuries. In younger patients, the ability to increase heart rate, constrict blood vessels, and breathe faster and deeper helps compensate for injuries. The aging body has a heart that can no longer beat faster, vessels that cannot constrict owing to atherosclerosis, and lungs that do not exchange oxygen as well.

Documentation Tips

Document all medications that the patient is taking. Don't forget to include over-the-counter medications and herbal remedies. Gather these medications to take to the hospital with the patient as well.

Falls and Trauma

A medical condition such as fainting, a cardiac rhythm disturbance, or a medication interaction may lead to a fall that injures the patient. Whenever you assess a geriatric patient who has fallen, it is important to find out why the fall occurred. Was the patient dizzy before the fall? Does the patient remember the fall? Did a fainting episode cause the fall and injury, or did the patient trip on something or lose balance? Sometimes, a recent history of starting or stopping blood pressure medication is enough to cause a patient to become dizzy and fall. Consider that the fall may have been caused by a medical condition, and look carefully for clues from the patient, bystanders, and the environment. Although the trauma sustained from the fall can be serious, you should also consider that if a medical condition caused the fall, it might continue to be an issue. When you respond to a motor vehicle crash, be alert to the possibility that a medical emergency may have caused the accident, especially in single vehicle collisions with no apparent cause.

Because brain tissue shrinks with age, older patients are more likely to sustain closed head injuries, such as subdural hematomas. These hematomas can go unnoticed because the blood has a void to fill before it produces pressure in the skull showing the familiar signs of head trauma.

As a result of bone loss from <u>osteoporosis</u>, a generalized bone disease that is commonly associated with postmenopausal women, older patients of both sexes are prone to fractures, especially in areas such as the hip. With age, the spine stiffens as a result of shrinkage of disk spaces, and vertebrae become brittle. Compression fractures of the spine are more likely to occur.

Because of the amount of flexion that occurs in the spinal column, hip, or knee of older patients, the use of conventional splints and backboards to immobilize the patient may be difficult or impossible unless a lot of padding is used. What is considered a normal anatomic position for children and adults might be abnormal for some geriatric trauma patients. You should try to determine the patient's baseline condition and what was normal for the patient before the accident. Trying to force a patient with pronounced joint flexion into "normal" anatomic position can be painful for the patient and frustrating for you and should

You are the Provider 2

Your partner rolls up the rug and places it out of the way to avoid a fall hazard for the patient. He takes her vital signs while you talk to her.

After several attempts at trying to learn the patient's medical history, you realize that she is hard of hearing. You do learn that she had a syncopal episode earlier today and that she has not been feeling well for several days.

Vital Signs	Recording Time: 2 Minutes
Skin	Pale, dry
Pulse	96 beats/min, irregular
Blood pressure	138/64 mm Hg
Respirations	18 breaths/min, slightly shallow

4. What are possible causes of the syncopal episode?
5. What can you do to help with the communication problem?
6. What questions should you ask about the syncopal episode?

Documentation Tips

When treating a patient who has fallen, always include the following in your PCR:

- Why did the fall occur?
- Was the patient dizzy before the fall?
- Did the patient have a syncopal episode?
- Did the patient trip over something?

never be done. Some devices, such as traction splints, simply do not work on patients with flexed hips and knees. Splinting devices such as vacuum mattresses that conform to body contours may be a good choice for immobilization.

Impact of Aging on Medical Emergencies

Syncope

You should always assume that syncope, or fainting, in an older patient is a life-threatening problem until proven otherwise. Syncope is often caused by an interruption of blood flow to the brain. Syncope has many causes, some of which are significant and others not. Regardless, an older person who has a syncopal episode should be transported to determine the cause of the syncope. Table 25-2 ▶ lists possible causes of syncope in geriatric patients.

Table 25-2 Possible Causes of Syncope in Geriatric Patients

Arrhythmias and heart attack	The heart is beating too fast or too slowly, the cardiac output drops, and blood flow to the brain is interrupted. A heart attack can also cause syncope.
Vascular and circulatory volume changes	Medication interactions can cause venous pooling and vasodilation, widening of a blood vessel, which results in a drop in blood pressure and inadequate blood flow to the brain. Another cause of syncope can be a drop in blood volume because of hidden bleeding from a condition such as an aneurysm.
Neurologic cause	A transient ischemic attack or a "brain attack" can sometimes mimic syncope.

Heart Attack

The classic symptoms of a heart attack are often not present in geriatric patients. As many as one third of older patients have "silent" heart attacks in which the usual chest pain is not present. Table 25-3 ▼ reviews the signs and symptoms that are commonly noted in geriatric patients who are experiencing a heart attack.

Table 25-3 Common Signs and Symptoms of Heart Attack in Geriatric Patients

Dyspnea	Dyspnea, the feeling of shortness of breath or difficulty breathing, is a common complaint in geriatric patients and is sometimes associated with heart attack. It is often combines with other symptoms, such as nausea, weakness, and sweating. Chest pain associated with angina typically has an onset during periods of stress or exertion. In geriatric patients, chest pain is often not present, but exertional dyspnea is. As the disease progresses, dyspnea may occur without exertion. Dyspnea in older people can be the equivalent of chest pain in younger patients who are having angina or a heart attack. In addition, congestive heart failure and acute pulmonary edema may result from the silent heart attack.
A weak feeling	Weakness can have many causes; however, you should suspect a heart attack in a patient with a sudden onset of weakness. Weakness is often associated with sweating.
Syncope, confusion, altered mental status	Syncope can have many causes, and in geriatric patients, none of these causes should be presumed to be minor. Major life-threatening causes of syncope are often cardiac in origin. Altered mental status is usually a sign of poor blood supply to the brain, often from cardiac arrhythmia and heart attack.

Acute Abdomen

Because of an aging nervous system, abdominal complaints in geriatric patients are difficult to assess. A number of life-threatening abdominal problems are common in older patients. In the field, the one real threat from abdominal complaints is blood loss, which can lead to shock and death. Abdominal aortic aneurysm (AAA) is one of the most rapidly fatal conditions. An AAA tends to develop in people who have a history of hypertension and atherosclerosis. The walls of the aorta weaken, and blood begins to leak into the layers of the vessel, causing the aorta to bulge like a bubble on a tire. If enough blood is lost into the vessel wall itself, shock occurs. If the wall bursts, fatal blood loss rapidly occurs. When the problem is found early, there is a chance to repair the vessel before rupture and fatal blood loss occur.

A patient with an AAA most commonly reports abdominal pain radiating through to the back with occasional flank pain. If the AAA becomes large enough, it can be felt as a pulsating mass just above and slightly to the left of the navel during your physical examination. Occasionally, the AAA causes a decrease in blood flow to one of the legs, and the patient complains of some discomfort in the affected extremity. Assessment may also reveal diminished or absent pulses in the extremity. Compensated shock (early shock) and decompensated shock (late shock) as a result of blood loss are common occurrences. Because of a decrease in blood volume and decreased blood flow to the brain, the patient may experience syncope. You should treat the patient for shock and provide prompt transport to the hospital.

Another cause of abdominal pain and shock is gastrointestinal bleeding, which can occur for a variety of reasons. A common sign is the vomiting of blood or material that looks like coffee grounds. Bleeding that travels through the lower digestive tract usually manifests as black or tarry stools, whereas frank red blood usually means a local source of bleeding, such as hemorrhoids. A patient with gastrointestinal bleeding may experience weakness, dizziness, or syncope. Bleeding in the gastrointestinal system can be life threatening because of the potential for blood loss and shock.

Bowel obstructions occur frequently in the geriatric population. The gastrointestinal tract slows with aging, and the patient can experience problems having bowel movements. When these patients go into the bathroom and are straining to have a bowel movement, they can stimulate the vagus nerve and produce a reaction called vasovagal attack, in which the heart rate drops dramatically and the patient becomes dizzy or passes out. The patient will usually be in stable condition on your arrival but requires transport to rule out other conditions.

Altered Mental Status

Because of our stereotypical perceptions about older people, we may expect them to forget names or not be able to remember events or learn new things. However, these types of changes in mental status are not part of the normal aging process. They may be part of a slow deterioration in the patient's condition or a disease of rapid onset, neither of which is normal. To determine the onset of this change in mental status, you must compare the patient's ability to function with that of the recent past. This will help to establish a baseline and give some perspective on the onset of the change. The two terms that are often used to describe a change in mental status are *delirium* and *dementia.*

Delirium is a change in mental status that is marked by the inability to focus, think logically, and maintain attention. Acute anxiety may be present in addition to the other symptoms. Usually, memory remains mostly intact. Delirium is commonly marked by acute or recent onset and is a red flag for a new health problem. Delirium may be caused by tumors, fever, or drug or alcohol intoxication or withdrawal. Delirium can be a result of metabolic causes as well. Any time a patient has an acute onset of this type of behavior, you should rapidly assess the patient and treat for hypoxia, hypovolemia, and hypoglycemia.

Delirium has a rapid onset and usually is curable if identified early. Dementia is the slow onset of progressive disorientation, shortened attention span, and loss of cognitive function. Dementia develops slowly over a period of years rather than a few days. Alzheimer disease, cerebrovascular accidents, and genetic factors may cause dementia. Dementia is usually considered irreversible and can be the result of many neurologic diseases. The patient's history and determination of function in the recent past are key factors in determining the baseline.

■ Impact of Aging on Psychiatric Emergencies

For the majority of older people, the later years represent fulfillment and satisfaction with a lifetime of accomplishments. For some older adults, however, later life is characterized by physical pain, psychological distress, doubts about the significance of life's accomplishments, financial concerns, loss of loved ones, dissatisfaction with living conditions, and seemingly unbearable disability. When these factors lead to hopelessness and depression, even suicide is a possible outcome.

Depression

Depression is a common, often debilitating psychiatric disorder experienced by approximately 2 million older American adults. Older adults residing in skilled nursing facilities are even more likely to be depressed. Depression is diagnosed three times more commonly in women than in men. In contrast with the normal emotional experiences of sadness, grief, loss, and temporary bad moods, depression is extreme and persistent and can interfere significantly with an older adult's ability to function. It is impossible to predict which older adults will have depression, but studies indicate that substance abuse, isolation, prescription medication use, and chronic medical conditions all contribute to the onset of significant depression. Treatment of severe depression in older adults usually consists of psychological counseling, medication, or a combination of both. For many older adults, simply reestablishing relationships with the community or with family is enough to lessen the severity of the illness.

Suicide

Older men have the highest suicide rate of any age group in the United States. Equally concerning is the fact that older persons who attempt suicide choose much more lethal means than younger victims and generally have diminished recuperative capacity to survive an attempt. Suicide can happen in any family, regardless of socioeconomic class, culture, race, or religious affiliation. Some common predisposing events and conditions include death of a loved one, physical illness, depression and hopelessness, alcohol abuse and dependence, and loss of meaningful life roles.

Only a small percentage of these patients pursue medical treatment for psychological issues. Not only do many fail to seek care, but they also frequently deny the problem when asked about it. It is vital that all members of the health care team be aware of the issues and take appropriate steps to ensure patient safety and initiate effective treatment.

■ Advance Directives

Many people today are making use of advance directives, specific legal papers that direct relatives and caregivers about what kind of medical treatment may be given to patients who cannot speak for themselves. An advance directive is also commonly called a living will. Mentally competent adults and emancipated minors have the right to consent to or decline treatment, provided they are competent to do so. The definition of competence is often debated, but a person who is older than 18 years, alert, not intoxicated, and understands the consequences of his or her decision is generally deemed competent. Patients who are unconscious or in a medical crisis are not able to inform medical personnel about their wishes to consent to or decline treatment.

Advance directives may also take the form of "do not resuscitate" (DNR) orders. A DNR order gives you permission to not attempt resuscitation for a patient in cardiac arrest. However, for a DNR order to be valid, in general, the patient's medical problems must be clearly stated, and the form must be signed by the patient or legal guardian and by one or more physicians. In most states, the form must be dated within the preceding 12 months. Even in the presence of a DNR order, you are still obligated to provide supportive measures that may include oxygen delivery, pain relief, and comfort when you can. Learn and become familiar with your state laws regarding this issue.

A health care power of attorney is an advance directive that is exercised by a person who has been authorized by the patient to make medical decisions for the patient. Be sure to follow your service's protocol when faced with any advance directive.

Dealing with advance directives has become more common for EMS providers because more individuals are electing to use hospice services and spend their final days at home. Although advance directives may be in place, family members or caregivers who are faced with the final moments of life or when the patient's condition worsens often become alarmed and call 9-1-1. Family members and caregivers may then become upset when you take resuscitative action and begin transportation to the hospital.

Another common situation is the transportation of patients from nursing facilities. Specific guidelines vary from state to state; however, you should consider the following general guidelines:

- Patients have the right to refuse treatment, including resuscitative efforts, provided that they are able to communicate their wishes.
- A DNR order is valid in a health care facility only if it is in the form of a written order by a physician.
- You should periodically review state and local protocols and legislation regarding advance directives.
- When you are in doubt or when there are no written orders, you should attempt to resuscitate the patient.

It is absolutely essential that every EMS provider be familiar with state regulations regarding advance directives. Every service should also provide additional training on the actions you should take when presented with advance directives. When in doubt, your best course of action is to take resuscitative action that is appropriate to the situation and to practice sound medical treatment.

■ Elder Abuse

Reports and complaints of abuse, neglect, and other related problems among the nation's older population are on the rise. Elder abuse is defined as any action on the part of an older individual's family member, caregiver, or other associated person that takes advantage of the older individual's person, property, or emotional state. Elder abuse is also called "granny beating" and "parent battering."

The exact extent of elder abuse is not known for several reasons, including the following:

- Elder abuse is a problem that has been largely hidden from society.
- The definitions of abuse and neglect among the geriatric population vary.
- Victims of elder abuse are often hesitant to report the problem to law enforcement agencies or human and social welfare personnel.

A parent who feels ashamed or guilty because he or she raised the abuser is a typical victim of elder abuse. The abused person may also feel traumatized by the situation or be afraid that the abuser will try to get back at him or her. In some areas of the country, there is a lack of formal reporting mechanisms, and some states lack statutory provisions that require that elder abuse be reported.

The physical and emotional signs of abuse, such as rape, spouse beating, or nutritional deprivation, are often overlooked or not accurately identified. Older women in particular are not likely to report incidents of sexual assault. Patients with sensory deficits, senility, and other forms of altered mental status, such as drug-induced depression, may not be able to report abuse.

Elder abuse occurs most often in women older than 75 years. The abused person is often frail with multiple chronic medical conditions, has dementia, and may have an impaired sleep cycle, sleepwalking, and periods of shouting at others. The person may be incontinent and in general is dependent on others for activities of daily living.

Abusers of older people are often products of child abuse themselves, and the abuse that is inflicted on the older person may be retaliatory. Most of these abusers are not trained in the particular care that older people require and have little relief time from the constant care demands of their own family, children, and spouse. Their lives are now complicated by the constant, demanding needs of the older person they have to care for.

The abuser may also have marked fatigue, be unemployed with financial difficulties, and abuse one or more substances. With a careful eye, you can recognize the clues to these stressful situations and help guide the family toward programs in their community that are geared to helping the whole family. Programs such as adult daycare, Meals on Wheels, and many local individualized programs help decrease the stress on the family and lower the chances of abuse.

Abuse is not restricted to the home; environments such as nursing, convalescent, and continuing care centers are also sites where older people sustain physical, psychological, and pharmacologic harm.

Assessment of Elder Abuse

While assessing the patient, you should try to obtain an explanation of what happened. You should suspect abuse when answers to questions about what caused the injury are vague or avoided.

You must also suspect abuse when you are given unbelievable answers from the patient, the possible abuser, or a significant witness. You should be suspicious if you think "Does this make sense?" or "Do I really believe this story?" while reviewing the patient's history. If you see burns, especially cigarette burns or any type of bruising or burns that have a specific pattern, you should suspect abuse. EMS providers may be the first health care providers to observe the signs of possible abuse. Information that may be important in assessing possible abuse includes the following:

- Repeated visits to the emergency department or clinic
- A history of being accident-prone
- Soft-tissue injuries
- Unbelievable or vague explanations of injuries
- Psychosomatic complaints
- Chronic pain
- Self-destructive behavior
- Eating and sleep disorders
- Depression or a lack of energy
- Substance and/or sexual abuse

You should remember that many patients who are being abused are so afraid of retribution that they make false statements. A geriatric patient who is being abused by family members may lie about the origin of abuse for fear of being thrown out of the home. In other cases of elder abuse, sensory deprivation or dementia may hinder adequate explanation.

In addition to the lifesaving care that you can provide the patient, your examination of the patient can help to reduce further trauma from abuse through its very identification. Repeated abuse can lead to a high risk of death. A preventive measure in reducing additional maltreatment of the patient is identification of the abuse by emergency medical providers Table 25-4 ▶ .

Table 25-4 Categories of Elder Abuse

Physical	■ Assault
	■ Neglect
	■ Dietary deprivation
	■ Poor maintenance of home
	■ Poor personal hygiene
Psychological	■ Neglect
	■ Verbal
	■ Treating the person as an infant
	■ Deprivation of sensory stimulation
Financial	■ Theft of valuables
	■ Embezzlement

Signs of Physical Abuse

Signs of abuse may be obvious or subtle. Inflicted bruises are usually found on the buttocks and lower back, genitals and inner thighs, cheeks or earlobes, upper lip and inside the mouth, and neck. Pressure bruises caused by the human hand may be identified by oval grab marks, pinch marks, or handprints. Human bites are typically inflicted on the upper extremities and can cause lacerations and infection. You should inspect the patient's ears for indications of

You are the Provider 3

Your partner applies oxygen via a nonrebreathing mask at 15 L/min. The patient tells him where she keeps her medications and he goes to the kitchen to retrieve them.

After assisting her with her hearing aid, the patient tells you that she is 84 years old and has a history of high blood pressure, "sugar" problems, high cholesterol, and had a heart attack two years ago. She has not had a "spell" like this in quite a while, and cannot remember what the doctor told her when it happened before.

Reassessment	Recording Time: 5 Minutes
Pulse	96 beats/min, irregular
Blood pressure	138/64 mm Hg
Respirations	18 breaths/min, not quite as shallow
Breath sounds	Clear bilaterally
Pulse oximetry	96% on oxygen via nonrebreathing mask

7. Based on her medical history, what do you think was the cause of her syncope?
8. What in her history would contribute to this condition?
9. Should she be transported? Why or why not?

twisting, pulling, or pinching or evidence of frequent blows to the outer ears. You should also investigate multiple bruises in various states of healing by asking the patient and reviewing the patient's activities of daily living.

Burns are a common form of abuse. Typical abuse from burns is caused by contact with cigarettes, matches, heated metal, forced immersion in hot liquids, chemicals, and electrical power sources.

It may be difficult to see failure to thrive in an older patient who has been abused. You should observe the patient's weight and try to determine whether the patient appears undernourished or has been unable to gain weight in the current environment. Does the patient have an increased appetite? Has medication been withheld? Is money being withheld so the patient cannot buy food or medicine? You should also check for signs of neglect, such as evidence of a lack of hygiene, poor dental hygiene, poor temperature regulation, or lack of reasonable amenities in the home.

You must regard injuries to the genitals or rectum with no reported trauma as evidence of sexual abuse in any patient. Geriatric patients with altered mental status may not be able to report sexual abuse.

■ Special-needs Patients

The field of medicine is constantly evolving. Patients with unusual diseases and disabling conditions are living longer and doing so outside traditional care facilities. Technological advances are enabling people with special needs to transfer home from the hospital sooner.

Suddenly being confronted with strange technological equipment and medical devices can be confusing and can interfere with patient care. Being prepared for such events can be as simple as being aware of people with special needs in your community and being familiar with those needs. Having a basic understanding of the medical equipment and devices that patients with special needs use will give you the confidence you need to provide quality patient care.

When responding to a patient with special needs, the families or caregivers often know more about the special problems of that particular patient than you do. When in doubt, ask what you can do to help most.

One of the most intimidating factors in responding to special-needs patients is the array of specialized devices and equipment that may be present. This may include vascular access devices, dialysis access sites, tracheostomies, ventilators, feeding tubes, and ventricular shunts. It is helpful to know about these things before an emergency situation occurs.

Vascular Access Devices

Vascular access devices (VADs) enable rapid access to the venous system. Many patients with cancer, chronic diseases, or conditions that require frequent access to venous circulation are fitted with these specialized catheters, which are inserted into the central circulation where they remain for weeks or months. VADs are often referred to as central lines, implanted ports, or peripherally inserted central catheters (PICC or PIC lines). Central lines and implanted ports tunnel under the skin to the vein. The distal tip of the line rests in the superior vena cava. PICC lines are small and do not tunnel under the skin; they are typically inserted through peripheral veins in the arms or legs. VADs are usually found on either side of the chest wall but may also be in an arm. In children, the neck and thigh are additional sites. There may be one, two, or three ports coming from a common catheter. Implanted ports are placed entirely under the skin with no exposed part, only a palpable bump under the skin, usually in the chest or abdominal wall.

If the port is exposed, it is important to keep the area as clean as possible and covered to avoid the chance of the line being accidentally pulled out of place. One common emergency involving VADs is bleeding from the site. Bleeding can be controlled by direct pressure. If a cap is dislodged, crimp the tubing by folding it over, to prevent air from entering, and replace the cap. If the patient needs to be transported and the tubing is attached to a pump, have the caregiver or family member disconnect the tubing for you. Consider contacting medical control if you are uncertain how to manage a particular device.

Dialysis Access Sites

There are various reasons the kidneys may not function correctly. Regardless of the reason, dialysis, a method of clearing toxins from the blood, may be necessary. There are two types, peritoneal dialysis and hemodialysis.

Peritoneal dialysis, a method using the abdominal capillaries to clear toxins, uses an implanted abdominal catheter for access. Dialysis fluid is fed through the catheter into the abdominal cavity where it is allowed

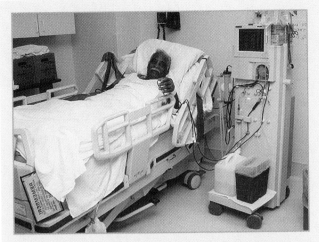

Figure 25-3 Hemodialysis involves shunting the patient's blood through a dialysis machine.

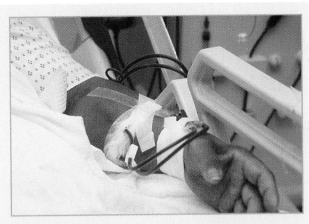

Figure 25-4 Access sites for hemodialysis may be internal, such as a fistula or graft.

to circulate for several hours before it is drained off. The process of exchanging fluid takes 45 minutes to an hour and is repeated 4 to 6 times a day. During the time the fluid is allowed to circulate through the abdomen, the catheter is clamped and secured by a dressing. It is important to avoid pulling and tugging the catheter. Common emergencies include infection at the site that may result in peritonitis, a painful and dangerous infection of the lining of the abdomen.

Hemodialysis, cleansing of toxins through the blood, involves shunting the patient's blood through a dialysis machine (Figure 25-3 ▲). Once the blood has been cleansed, it is returned to the patient. This process takes several hours and is usually done three times a week. Access sites are usually on the forearms but may also be on the thigh. The sites may be external, such as a shunt, or internal, such as a fistula or graft (Figure 25-4 ▶). The most common type is a fistula, created by establishing an opening in an artery and an adjacent vein. The high pressure arterial system causes the vein to dilate and bulge. The bulging vein is used for the dialysis process. Grafts are used less often today because of the success of fistulas and VADs.

The most important principle to remember about a dialysis access site is to protect it from any type of trauma. These sites are particularly prone to clot formation, irritation of the vessels, and infection. For these reasons, do not take a blood pressure in an arm with a dialysis access site.

The most likely emergency involving hemodialysis sites is bleeding. Because access involves an arterial source, loss of blood can be extreme. Prolonged direct pressure is usually required to control the bleeding.

Tracheostomies and Ventilators

A tracheostomy is a surgical opening created to aid in breathing or to be used when sustained ventilatory support is needed (Figure 25-5 ▶). Patients may require a tracheostomy for many reasons: trauma to the face or respiratory centers, paralysis of the respiratory muscles, tumors, soft-tissue swelling, inability to expel secretions, pulmonary conditions requiring prolonged mechanical ventilation, or, in the case of children, immature respiratory centers. Modern tracheostomy tubes are made of flexible materials that are comfortable and have few associated risks. The tubes may be of single or double construction and come with or without cuffs (Figure 25-6 ▶). Cuffed tubes

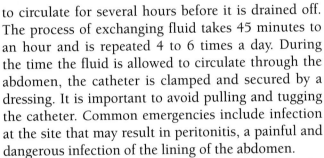

You are the Provider 4

You and your partner assist her onto the stretcher after assuring that she did not fall. She is transported to the local emergency department where she is treated for angina and sent for a heart catheterization and angioplasty. She also received two stents. The doctor tells her that she probably would have had a major heart attack had she waited to seek treatment.

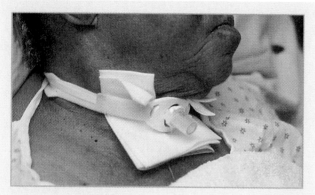

Figure 25-5 A tracheostomy.

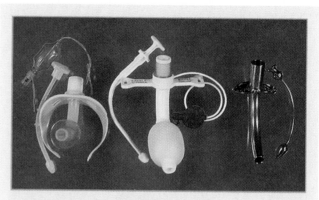

Figure 25-6 Tracheostomy tubes.

are more common for adults, and uncuffed tubes are more likely to be seen in children. A double tube has an inner cannula that is designed to be easily removed and cleaned or replaced if necessary to maintain good air exchange. The inner cannula must be in place for effective bag-mask ventilation. There are also special tracheostomy tubes that allow for speaking. These tubes must also have the inner cannula in place for effective bag-mask ventilation.

Management of emergencies that involve patients with tracheostomy tubes requires a good assessment and the skills necessary to maintain an open airway and provide adequate oxygen exchange. The most common complications include obstruction, dislodgment, and infection. Obstruction is usually caused by mucus. When mucus obstructs a double tube and suction is ineffective, the inner cannula should be removed and rinsed with sterile water or saline. Suction is vital for children with respiratory difficulty. Use a soft-tip suction catheter small enough to fit through the tracheostomy tube. If you do not have one, the family or caregiver should have suction tubes of the correct size.

Signs of dislodgment include mild to severe respiratory distress. The area may appear puffy with a crackling sensation (crepitus) noted on palpation. The patient will require supplemental oxygen and ventilatory support. Infection can result in pneumonia, which will also require ventilatory support.

Some patients with a tracheostomy require constant ventilatory support. You may be called because of actual or potential ventilator problems. The caregiver or family member is most familiar with the machine and should be asked to disconnect it for you. Immediate bag-mask ventilation and supplemental oxygen should be provided.

Feeding Tubes

Adequate nutrition depends on the ability to swallow and absorb nutrients. Patients who are unable to swallow or who have had significant trauma, tumors, or surgical procedures on the mouth or esophagus may need <u>enteral</u> feedings. Enteral feedings are those given via the stomach or intestines. Gastric, gastrostomy, and jejunostomy tubes are the usual methods for providing nutrition on a long-term basis.

Gastric tubes are usually inserted through the nose to the stomach or upper intestine. The tube may be attached to a container within a backpack to provide almost constant water and nutrition. It is important not to pull on the tube or dislodge it. Gastric tubes are typically used only for short-term nutritional support.

Gastrostomy tubes are surgically placed in the abdominal wall and pass through it into the stomach. The tube may extend out from the skin and is sutured in place and covered by a dressing. The tube may have a "button" device at skin level, which allows for attachment of a safety cap after the feeding tube is removed.

Jejunostomy tubes are placed through the abdominal wall directly into the small intestine. Like gastrostomy tubes, jejunostomy tubes are typically sutured in place and covered with a dressing. Feeding through a jejunostomy tube is associated with a lower risk of regurgitation and aspiration than feeding through a gastrostomy tube in patients who are unable to protect their upper airways or who have swallowing difficulties.

Complications with feeding tubes include accidental removal or displacement. Unless the tube has been inserted through the nose or mouth, displacement is not an emergency. Displacement of a nasogastric or orogastric tube can be an emergency if feeding solution is still being administered or has already resulted in aspiration. In this case, treat the respiratory distress and transport. Immediately stop administration of any feeding through the tube.

Ventricular Shunts

A ventricular shunt (also called a CSF shunt) is a tube that extends from the ventricles of the brain to the chest or abdomen and is designed to drain excess cerebrospinal fluid (CSF). You may be able to feel the tubing under the skin behind the ear or on the side of the neck. Many ventricular shunts also have a small reservoir with a one-way valve located on the outside of the skull just under the skin. It forms an easily palpated bulge that the caregiver or family member may refer to as a pump. Do not manipulate this pump unless you are directed to do so by medical control and your local protocol permits.

The most common complications with this type of shunt are obstruction and infection. Obstruction causes increased intracranial pressure with headaches, irritability, visual disturbances, altered mental status, vomiting, seizures, bradycardia with hypertension, and irregular respirations. Infection can cause similar signs and symptoms as well as fever. In case of obstruction or infection, manage the patient's airway, give high-concentration oxygen, and provide ventilatory support as needed. Provide rapid transport and consider calling for ALS backup.

You are the Provider Summary

Understanding the aging process is key to treating geriatric patients. Special care and handling is required for optimal outcome in any situation involving an elderly person. Continuing education is important for all providers.

1. **What aspect of aging would explain the bruising on her arms?**
   As we age, the skin becomes thinner and wrinkled, collagen is lost, the fat layer under the skin becomes thinner, and the skin cannot constrict and stop bleeding as quickly as in younger individuals.

2. **The assessment of the house falls under which part of the GEMS diamond?**
   "E" stands for environment. The environment can give many clues to the patient's well-being and care.

3. **What part of the GEMS diamond refers to the fact that she lives alone?**
   "S" stands for social assessment. This refers to the patient's social network of family members, friends, etc.

4. **What are possible causes of the syncopal episode?**
   Arrhythmias and heart attack, vascular and volume changes, neurologic causes.

5. **What can you do to improve the communication?**
   Stand on the side on which she hears best.
   Speak slowly and clearly.
   Do not yell.
   If she has a hearing aid, assist her in putting it in.

6. **What questions should you ask about the syncopal episode?**
   Has this ever happened before?
   If so, did she see a doctor?
   What did the doctor tell her about her condition?
   Did she fall?
   Does she know how long the episode may have lasted?

7. **Based on her medical history, what do you think was the cause of her syncope?**
   Possible cardiac arrhythmia or precursor to a heart attack.

8. **What in her history would contribute to this condition?**
   She has a history of an MI plus she has high cholesterol. Major complications of elevated cholesterol include myocardial infarction and stroke.

9. **Should she be transported? Why or why not?**
   Yes. It is not normal for a patient to "pass out." Even though she has complained of no other problems, she still needs to be evaluated. She could be having a silent MI.

Prep Kit

Ready for Review

- Management of geriatric patients can present you with many challenges that are not seen with younger patients and with a host of different problems that may be difficult and frustrating to solve.
- The GEMS diamond is a tool to help remember key concepts when assessing geriatric patients.
  - G stands for geriatric: older patients present atypically.
  - E is for environment: be aware of the patient's living environment.
  - M reminds you that older patients usually have more medical problems (and medications), so medical history is important.
  - S emphasizes the social aspects of the patient's life and the importance of the patient's social network.
- The health problems of the older population are multifaceted. Frequent barriers to communication can be expected.
- The leading causes of death in older people include heart disease, cancer, stroke, cardiopulmonary disease, respiratory illnesses, diabetes, and trauma.
- Physiologic changes that accompany aging include the following:
  - Changes in skin quality
  - Weakening of the senses
  - Decrease in respiratory system function
  - Compromised cardiac and renal function
  - Decline in nervous system function
  - Decrease in muscle and bone mass
  - Decrease in gastrointestinal system function
- These changes affect the body's ability to isolate simple trauma and may influence how other medical emergencies present.
- Polypharmacy refers to taking many medications or taking too many medications. Complete assessment of a patient must include obtaining a medication history.
- To determine the onset of altered mental status, compare the patient's ability to function with that of the recent past. Delirium and dementia are the two terms often used to describe a change in mental status.

- Advance directives, or living wills, specify what kind of medical treatment may be given to patients who cannot speak for themselves. Every EMT-B should be familiar with his or her state regulations regarding advance directives.
- The exact extent of elder abuse is not known because many patients do not report it.
- Abusers are often family members who must care for the older person in addition to caring for their own spouses and children. Elder abuse also occurs in nursing, convalescent, and continuing care centers.
- Elder abuse can be gruesome, vulgar, and barbaric. Your responsibility is to provide lifesaving care to the patient and try to reduce additional abuse through identification of the problem.
- There are many patients at home with advanced technological equipment to manage their medical conditions.
- Vascular access devices (VADs) allow for rapid access to the vascular system for patients with cancer, chronic diseases, and conditions that require frequent access to vascular circulation.
- VADs are often referred to as central lines, implanted ports, or PICC lines.
- A common emergency with VADs is bleeding from the site. Control bleeding with direct pressure.
- Dialysis is a method of clearing toxins from the blood. Protect dialysis sites from trauma. Control bleeding with direct pressure.
- A tracheostomy is a surgical opening to aid in breathing or to be used when sustained ventilatory support is needed.
- The most common complications with tracheostomies include obstruction, dislodgment, and infection.
- Patients who are unable to swallow or who have had significant trauma, tumors, or surgical procedures on the mouth or esophagus may require a feeding tube.
- Complications with feeding tubes include accidental removal or displacement and aspiration of gastric contents into the lungs.

Vital Vocabulary

abdominal aortic aneurysm (AAA) A condition in which the walls of the aorta in the abdomen weaken and blood leaks into the layers of the vessel, causing it to bulge.

advance directives Written documentation that specifies medical treatment for a competent patient should the patient become unable to make decisions; also called living wills.

aneurysm A swelling or enlargement of a part of an artery, resulting from weakening of the arterial wall.

arteriosclerosis A disease that is characterized by hardening, thickening, and calcification of the arterial walls.

atherosclerosis A form of arteriosclerosis in which cholesterol and other fatty substances build up inside the walls of blood vessels, forming plaque, which eventually leads to partial or complete blockage of blood flow and the formation of clots that can break off and embolize.

cataracts Clouding of the lens of the eye or its surrounding transparent membranes.

central lines Venous access devices that are tunneled under the skin to access a major vein; the port is usually located in the chest wall and is outside the skin.

delirium A change in mental status marked by the inability to focus, think logically, and maintain attention.

dementia The slow onset of progressive disorientation, shortened attention span, and loss of cognitive function.

dialysis A method of clearing the blood of toxins.

elder abuse Any action on the part of an older person's family member, caregiver, or other associated person that takes advantage of the older individual's person, property, or emotional state; also called granny beating and parent battering.

enteral Pertaining to the stomach or intestines.

fistula In dialysis, a surgical opening connecting an artery and a vein.

graft In dialysis, an artificial tube used to connect two ends of vessels; often used for vascular access for hemodialysis.

hemodialysis A method of dialysis that shunts the patient's blood through a dialysis machine and then returns the cleansed blood to the patient.

implanted ports Vascular access devices that tunnel under the skin to the vein.

kyphosis A forward bending of the back caused by an abnormal increase in the curvature of the spine.

osteoporosis A generalized bone disease, commonly associated with postmenopausal women, in which there is a reduction in the amount of bone mass, leading to fractures after minimal trauma in either sex.

peripherally inserted central catheters (PICC or PIC lines) A small catheter that accesses a major vein from a peripheral vein, usually in the arm or leg.

peritoneal dialysis A method of dialysis that uses the peritoneal membrane and abdominal capillaries to cleanse the blood of toxins.

syncope A fainting spell or transient loss of consciousness, often caused by an interruption of blood flow to the brain.

tracheostomy A surgical opening in the trachea to aid in breathing or for use when sustained ventilatory support is needed.

vascular access devices (VADs) Devices that enable rapid access to the vascular system.

ventricular shunt A tube that extends from the ventricles of the brain to the chest or abdomen, designed to drain excess cerebrospinal fluid (CSF); also called a CSF shunt.

Assessment in Action

Geriatric patients present with a variety of special needs.
Familiarize yourself with various devices you may come in contact with and maintain a good working knowledge of how aging affects the body.

1. _____ causes hardening of the arteries.
   A. Atherosclerosis
   B. Arteriosclerosis
   C. An aneurysm
   D. An embolism

2. The "M" of the GEMS diamond stands for medical assessment. This includes evaluating _____.
   A. prescription medications
   B. over-the-counter medications
   C. herbal remedies
   D. all of the above

3. A _____ is designed to drain excess cerebrospinal fluid.
   A. gastrostomy tube
   B. tracheostomy
   C. ventricular shunt
   D. fistula

4. _____ is commonly marked by acute onset.
   A. Alzheimer's
   B. Dementia
   C. Depression
   D. Delirium

5. As many as _____ of older patients have "silent" heart attacks.
   A. $1/5$
   B. $1/2$
   C. $1/3$
   D. $3/4$

6. A _____ is a surgical opening for breathing.
   A. fistula
   B. tracheostomy
   C. graft
   D. gastrostomy

Challenging Questions

7. Explain the difference between an *advance directive* and a *DNR*.

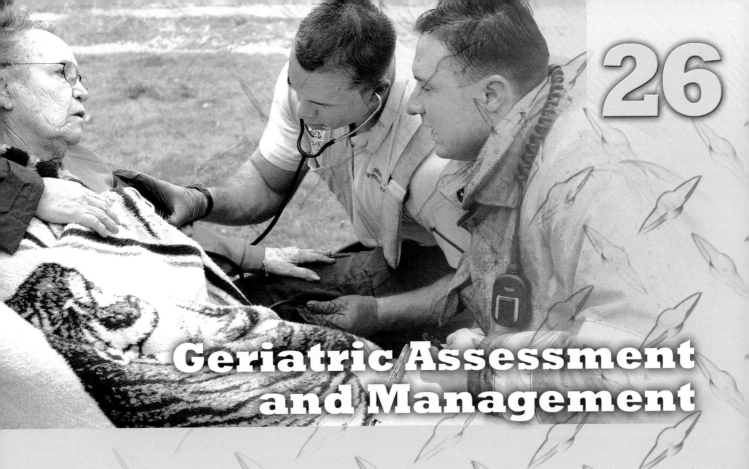

26

Geriatric Assessment and Management

You are the Provider 1

You and your partner have just entered a residence where an elderly woman called 9-1-1 complaining of shortness of breath. The door to the home was locked and fire department personnel were called to gain access. The patient lives alone and needs a walker to get around.

Initial Assessment	Recording Time: 0 Minutes
Appearance	Pale, diaphoretic
Level of consciousness	Alert and oriented
Airway	Open and clear
Breathing	A little fast and shallow
Circulation	Radial pulses present, irregular, weak

1. What should you notice as you enter the residence?
2. What is your first priority?
3. How will you use the extra help?

Geriatric Assessment and Management

Assessing older patients uses the same basic approach as for other patients. The steps are scene size-up, initial assessment, focused history and physical exam, detailed physical exam, and ongoing assessment. Certain parts of your exam may require you to modify your approach so you are more aware of the conditions around you that may affect geriatric patients. The condition of a geriatric patient may be worse than indicated by the patient's current signs and symptoms. Remember that injuries and conditions in geriatric patients often have a more significant effect than they would in younger patients.

Assessing an Older Patient

A useful tool to use when assessing geriatric patients is the GEMS diamond. It is designed to help you remember to look for clues that can make a big difference for geriatric patients.

Scene Size-up

Geriatric calls are more frequent than calls for other age groups and, often, the information that dispatch receives is vague. The "G" in the GEMS diamond is for geriatric concerns. Consider carefully the potential nature of illnesses and mechanisms of injury (MOIs) as reported in your dispatch information.

As you approach any scene, you must be keenly aware of the environment and the reason you were called. The "E" of the GEMS diamond is for the environment. When you arrive at a patient's residence,

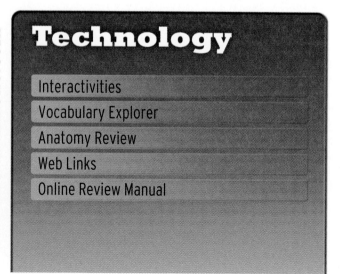
EMT-B Safety

Look for hazards such as loose rugs or other obstacles that may present a danger to the patient or rescuers. Prevent falls by tacking down throw rugs with nails or double-sided tape.

you should look for important clues to determine not only your safety, but also that of the occupant. The environment can provide a great deal of important information if you know what to look for. Look for hazards, such as steep stairs, missing handrails, inadequate lighting, or other things that could cause a fall. Another aspect to consider in the geriatric environment is the overall appearance of the home. Determine whether there is evidence of adequate food, water, heat, lights, and ventilation. Is the home clean? Many older patients may have a hard time physically keeping up with the cleaning or financially keeping food or heat in their home. The general condition of the home may give you important clues.

Your assessment of the scene will continue even after you begin the assessment of the patient. Activities of daily living such as the ability to move around, talk on the telephone, prepare and eat meals, perform basic cleaning skills, and attend to personal hygiene are essential for continued health in all people. For older people, normal aging or a disease process may make activities of daily living difficult and cause a cascade of problems.

Initial Assessment

General Impression

The sequence of the initial assessment is the same for pediatric, adult, and geriatric patients. Begin with a general impression, including determining the chief complaint and the patient's level of consciousness (LOC). A geriatric patient's chief complaint may be an exacerbation of a chronic problem. Because it is something the patient has always had to deal with, the patient may have waited until the problem is worse than usual. At other times, very subtle and simple complaints may indicate very serious problems.

The "S" in the GEMS diamond stands for social situation. We all need a network of people around us for ongoing socialization and to help in times of need. However, as we age and outlive friends and family, our social network may become smaller. When an older patient has fewer people to interact with, he or she may call on EMS for complaints that seem trivial to us but significant to him or her.

Use the AVPU scale to determine a patient's LOC. However, do not make assumptions about an older patient's LOC. Never assume that an altered mental status is normal. Altered mental status indicates some level of brain dysfunction and is a serious problem. The best rule of thumb is always to compare the patient's current LOC or ability to function with the level or ability before the problem began. Do not assume that confusion or unresponsiveness is normal behavior for anyone. In many cases, you may have to rely on a family member or caregiver to help establish the patient's baseline **Figure 26-1 ▶**.

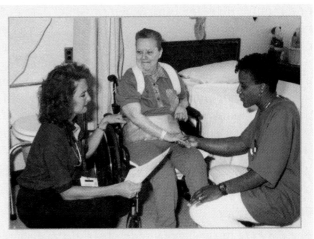

Figure 26-1 Interview family members, friends, and caregivers as part of your assessment of a geriatric patient.

Airway, Breathing, and Circulation

During the initial assessment, you will assess the patient's ABCs. If a life-threatening condition exists, you will have to perform emergency treatment before continuing your assessment. If the airway is inadequate, manage it with positioning and airway adjuncts as necessary. Ensure that breathing is adequate, apply oxygen, evaluate for bleeding, and treat for shock.

Transport Decision

The initial assessment sets the tone and helps you decide whether the patient requires rapid treatment and transport. In most cases, you will have time to stay on scene to properly assess and manage the patient. Use your assessment to determine the best way to package and transport. When possible, take the patient to the hospital of his or her choice. This will allow continuity of care if the patient has been there before and can decrease the anxiety of the patient. Allow the patient to assume a position of comfort. This may be upright for respiratory distress calls or legs raised for a patient with low blood pressure.

Focused History and Physical Exam

The focused history and physical exam of a geriatric patient should be performed en route to the hospital

You are the Provider 2

You note that the house is neat and tidy. It is a little cool, but the patient is dressed warmly. You notice that she appears somewhat fatigued and she was not able to get up on her own to open the door.

Vital Signs	Recording Time: 2 Minutes
Skin	Pale, diaphoretic
Pulse	104 beats/min, irregular
Blood pressure	112/98 mm Hg
Respirations	20 breaths/min, slightly shallow

4. What type of oxygen does she need? Why?
5. What should you ask about her dyspnea?
6. What should you ask about other symptoms?

to minimize time on scene, when possible. The purpose of the focused history and physical exam is to obtain additional, specific information about the patient's illness or injury. This portion of your assessment includes performing a physical exam (rapid or focused), obtaining vital signs, and interviewing the patient or family members about the patient's medical history. The order of these three portions of the assessment varies if the older patient is a medical patient (responsive or unresponsive) or a trauma patient (with significant or nonsignificant MOI).

SAMPLE History

The patient's history is one of the best tools you have when assessing an older patient. To obtain an accurate history, patience and good communication skills are essential. An older patient's diminished sight, hearing, and speaking ability may hamper communication. If possible, take a few moments to have the patient put in dentures or a hearing aid and put on glasses. All of these items can help the patient communicate with you more effectively.

Communicating With an Older Patient

When speaking with an older patient, bend down so that you are eye-to-eye with the patient. Be sure that the patient can see your face. Patients who have difficulty hearing will often look for clues in the speaker's facial expressions to assist in understanding the subject matter. Turn on a light if you are in a dimly lit room. Turn off televisions or radios. Use a normal tone of voice, especially if the patient is wearing a hearing aid. A loud tone may actually cause sound distortion in the hearing aid and make communication worse. Ask as many open-ended questions as possible, and use closed-ended questions to clarify points. It is better to ask an open-ended question such as "Please tell me about the pain you are feeling," rather than a closed-ended one such as "Is the pain sharp or dull?" While taking the history, write down any key points on a notepad so that you do not ask the same question repeatedly because you forgot the answer. After interviewing the patient, ask family members or caregivers to clarify what you just learned from the patient. Be careful not to offend the patient. Taking a few minutes to obtain an accurate history saves time in the long run by providing information on which appropriate decisions can be based.

An inadequate or inappropriate history-gathering technique can hamper communications. You must be able to gain a patient's confidence, which is best ac-

complished by treating the patient with respect; taking a slow, deliberate approach; and explaining what you are doing. Avoid being overly familiar with the patient, and do not use first names or nicknames unless the patient asks you to.

Often when there are multiple responders, everyone asks questions at the same time. This technique may result in obtaining a haphazard history regardless of the patient's age. For geriatric patients who may have communication or perceptual problems, it makes obtaining a thorough SAMPLE history almost impossible. In addition, many people are reluctant to discuss their problems in front of a crowd. Be sure to have one EMT-B obtain the patient's history, one question at a time, providing as much privacy as possible **Figure 26-2 ▾**.

Older patients have often had similar episodes and can compare the current situation with one in the past. In geriatric patients, a condition will often present in episodes that will progressively worsen with time. There are also conditions that can change the symptoms experienced by the patient. A diabetic patient may not have pain from a cardiac event because of the loss of nerve cells over time from the diabetes.

The "M" in the GEMS diamond stands for medical history and medications. During your SAMPLE history, you will evaluate the medical history and current medications. These will have an important part in the assessment of geriatric patients.

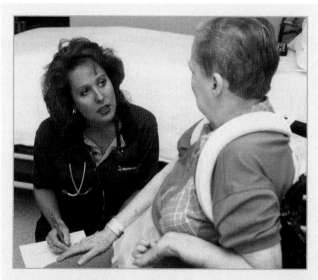

Figure 26-2 A slow, deliberate approach to the patient history, with one EMT-B asking the questions, is generally the best strategy for assessing a geriatric patient.

Medication Use

Medications can become a significant problem for older patients. The average patient older than 65 years will be taking four or more medications and be using over-the-counter (OTC) medications as well. Polypharmacy means that a patient takes multiple medications.

If time allows, review all of the medications that are prescribed for the patient. Ask the patient whether he or she takes all of the medications. Often the patient may stop taking a medication because of the side effects without talking with the doctor. For example, blood pressure medication may cause the patient to feel dizzy. The patient does not like the feeling and stops taking the medication. The effect is that the blood pressure rises and can lead to a medical emergency.

Look for medications that have been started or stopped during the last 2 weeks. Medications that have been used by the patient for a while are not likely to become a sudden problem. However, starting a new medication or suddenly stopping a medication can have significant effects on the body. Ask the patient whether he or she has taken any other medications. Patients may take the medication prescribed for their spouse or family member if they think they have the same symptoms. Also ask about OTC medications, such as aspirin and herbal supplements such as ginkgo biloba. These OTC medications may seem harmless to the patient but may interact with prescribed medications. The patient's medications should be collected and taken to the hospital with the patient.

Focused Physical Exam

The chief complaint and the medical history will help guide you in performing a focused physical exam. A focused physical exam is performed on conscious medical patients or trauma patients with a limited MOI. It allows you to focus on specific problems that may need more clarification. Because of the complexity of the conditions of geriatric patients and the vagueness of complaints, you should consider broadening your physical exam to include more areas rather than fewer. This may better help separate chronic problems from more acute problems.

Rapid Physical Exam

A rapid physical exam is typically performed before obtaining the vital signs and history. The goal is to identify hidden threats not picked up in the initial assessment. This rapid head-to-toe assessment is performed on unresponsive medical patients and patients with a more significant MOI. Remember, though, that the geriatric body is more fragile than a younger body. It will take a lesser MOI to produce significant injuries. For this reason, you should consider a rapid head-to-toe exam for most geriatric trauma

You are the Provider 3

One fire fighter applies a nonrebreathing mask at 15 L/min while the other helps your partner bring in the stretcher. You ask the patient about her history and she tells you that she has high blood pressure and non-insulin-dependent (type 2) diabetes. She has taken her medicine as prescribed today and ate her normal breakfast 2 hours ago.

She describes a pressure in her chest just behind her sternum and tells you that it has been going on for about 45 minutes. She has been feeling faint off and on. She is also a little nauseated.

Reassessment	Recording Time: 5 Minutes
Pulse	108 beats/min, irregular
Blood pressure	112/98 mm Hg
Respirations	20 breaths/min, not quite as shallow
Breath sounds	Clear bilaterally
Pulse oximetry	95% with oxygen via nonrebreathing mask

7. What do you think is going on?
8. What treatment does she need?
9. How should she be transported?

patients before obtaining vital signs and a SAMPLE history.

Baseline Vital Signs

Normal vital signs will change with age. Irregularity of the pulse becomes more prevalent as patients age. Blood pressure increases slightly because the blood vessels have been partially blocked due to atherosclerosis. After a person reaches 65 years, the increase in systolic pressure is usually only 1 mm Hg per year. Keep in mind that many medications used to treat arrhythmias and hypertension may prevent an increased pulse rate when needed. For example, a patient with low blood pressure and a pulse rate of 84 beats/min may be in serious shock. The rate, rhythm, and quality of respirations vary depending on the health of the patient's respiratory system. Pupils are also slower to react to light, and pupil checks can be complicated by cataracts or previous eye surgeries.

Detailed Physical Exam

Of all the patients you will care for, geriatric patients are patients who should have a detailed physical exam in most situations. The changes that occur because of aging alter how the patient experiences pain. Chronic changes can mask acute problems, and acute problems may be mistaken for chronic problems. The vagueness of complaints may prevent the identification of serious problems. A thorough, detailed exam from head to toe, when correlated with the history and vital signs, can help identify potential conditions.

Ongoing Assessment

Priority patients require frequent reassessment, and geriatric patients are no different. Because many older patients are unable to compensate as well for loss of oxygenation or blood, it is very important to record vital signs every 5 minutes. Talking with the patient is a good way to monitor the LOC.

■ Common Complaints of Older Patients

Common chief complaints of older patients include the following: shortness of breath; chest pain; dizziness or weakness; fever; trauma; falls; generalized pain; and nausea, vomiting, and diarrhea. Altered mental status also is a common problem. The complaints that deserve special attention in older patients are described in the following sections on trauma and medical emergencies.

■ Geriatric Trauma

Mechanism of Injury

Falls are the leading cause of trauma, death, and disability in older people. Most patients survive, but a significant number require hospitalization. Motor vehicle trauma is the second leading cause of trauma death in the geriatric population. A geriatric patient is five times more likely than a younger patient to be fatally injured in a car crash, even though excessive speed is rarely a cause in the older age group. Pedestrian accidents and burns are also common MOIs in geriatric patients.

Trauma in older people can be complicated by medical conditions. Often the cause of trauma is related to a medical condition, such as the patient becoming dizzy and then falling. Try to determine whether the patient had a medical complaint before the trauma.

Trauma Assessment

The priorities in the rapid trauma assessment do not change with older patients. However, there are several confounding factors that warrant review. When assessing the patient's mental status, remember that older patients may have medical conditions, such as Alzheimer disease or previous strokes, that may hinder your assessment. Make your judgment based on the patient's baseline status when possible. Many older patients have had some type of dental work done over their lifespan. Dentures, bridges, and dental implants may all become loosened following a traumatic event. Check the airway carefully for signs of loose or broken teeth. Older patients have decreased ability to increase the volume and rate of breathing to compensate for hypoperfusion. Carefully assess the patient to determine whether breathing is adequate. Assessment of pulses can be complicated by previous injuries or decreased circulation owing to medical problems. Many older patients have changes in their circulation as they age. **Table 26-1 ▶** lists changes associated with aging that may affect your physical exam of the patient. After completing your exam, be sure to obtain vital signs and complete a SAMPLE history. Because an older patient does not compensate well for trauma, small changes in the blood pressure or pulse can indicate a shift in how well the patient is compensating for trauma.

Injuries to the Spine

Injuries to the spine are a frequent problem in older people. Spinal injuries may be broadly classified as

Table 26-1 Changes Associated With Aging That May Affect the Exam

Part of the Body	Changes Possible With Aging	How to Examine
Pupils	May have cataracts, scars from surgery, or blindness (one or both sides)	Report what you see. It is not always as important to name the condition as it is to note a change.
Neck and back	Kyphosis (the curve in the upper back and neck formed by normal aging)	Note DCAP-BTLS (Deformities, Contusions, Abrasions, Punctures/Penetrations, Burns, Tenderness, Lacerations, and Swelling), and position a cervical collar when needed. Extra padding will be required to complete the immobilization. Use of a vacuum mattress or an inflatable pad on a long board can help fill the voids left by the changing shape.
Chest	Changes in lung sounds possibly due to previous medical conditions such as congestive heart failure or chronic obstructive pulmonary disease; chest wall more brittle in older patients	Listen to lung sounds early and reassess them periodically to help identify a problem. High-concentration oxygen is always indicated with patients in respiratory distress. Examine the chest for symmetry; look for broken ribs.
Abdomen	Abdomen senses less pain	Be careful to look for signs of trauma if the mechanism indicates, even if a patient is not complaining of pain.
Extremities	Decreased sensation due to lessened pain receptors and a slower nervous system; decreased circulation to the distal points	Examination of the extremities can be complicated by several factors, including previous injuries or surgeries that have left deformities. Try to determine whether the signs are new or old. Record your assessment as you find it to provide information for decision making.

stable or unstable. A stable spinal injury is one that has a low risk for leading to permanent neurologic deficit or structural deformity. An unstable spinal injury is one that has a high risk of permanent neurologic deficit or structural deformity. The injuries that older patients often incur while performing normal daily activities are most commonly stable ones, whereas unstable injuries tend to be the result of a significant trauma, such as falls from a substantial height or motor vehicle crashes.

Injuries to the upper cervical spine may be potentially lethal because the nerves innervating the diaphragm originate here. An injury at this level or higher may lead to death because of inability to breathe. Many cervical spine injuries in older patients result from hyperextension of the neck as the result of a fall or striking the head on the windshield during a motor vehicle crash. Because of the presence of arthritis, relatively small hyperextension injuries can cause the spinal cord to be squeezed, leading to a condition known as <u>central cord syndrome</u>. Central cord syndrome results in weak or absent motor function,

which is more pronounced in the upper extremities than the lower extremities. Although this type of spinal cord injury usually does not cause permanent deficits, recovery may take several months or even years.

Osteoporosis in the thoracic and lumbar spine contributes to a high rate of injury in this area in the older population. Three types of fractures are common in the thoracolumbar region: compression fractures, burst fractures, and seat belt–type injuries. Compression fractures are stable injuries in which often only the anterior third of the vertebra is collapsed. This type of fracture often results from minimal trauma, from simply bending over, rising from a chair, or sitting down forcefully. This is by far the most common type of spinal fracture seen in the older population. Burst fractures typically result from a higher energy mechanism such as a motor vehicle crash or fall from substantial height. These fractures are unstable and may lead to neurologic injury secondary to shifting of the vertebrae with damage to the spinal cord. Seat belt–type fractures involve flexion, and there is a distraction component (energy being dispersed in opposite directions) that causes a fracture through the entire vertebral body and bony arch. This type of injury typically results from an ejection or occurs in people wearing only a lap belt without a shoulder harness.

Injuries to the spinal cord are usually associated with neurologic deficits, which may be complete or incomplete. An example of an incomplete injury is central cord syndrome. Patients with incomplete spinal cord injuries may recover function over time, whereas those with a complete spinal cord injury are not likely to regain function.

As with all patients, prompt spinal immobilization is an effective method of reducing further damage to the spinal cord and preserving neurologic function. Often, patients may be found in positions in which the neck or body is not in the neutral position, such as the head being rotated to one side. To facilitate the application of a cervical collar, you should slowly return the head to the midline. At no time should these attempts continue if the patient develops changes in neurologic status or complains of increasing pain. If these complaints develop, the head should be secured in the position in which it is found by using blankets and tape to prevent further movement.

Older patients present several unique challenges to EMS providers when treating spinal injuries. To immobilize patients with kyphosis, several blankets and pillows or vacuum splints may be required to provide support to the head and upper back **Skill Drill 26-1 ▶**.

1. **Apply and maintain cervical stabilization.** Assess distal functions in all extremities (**Step ①**).
2. **Apply a cervical collar.** If a collar does not fit, do not attempt to straighten the patient's neck (**Step ②**).
3. **Rescuers kneel on one side of the patient** and place hands on the far side of the patient (**Step ③**).
4. On command, **rescuers roll the patient toward themselves and quickly examine the patient's back** (**Step ④**).
5. **Slide the backboard under the patient, and roll the patient onto the board** (**Step ⑤**).

6. **Pad the void space produced by the kyphotic spine** with pillows and blankets. The pillows and blankets should be as wide as the backboard to allow for effective immobilization and support. Place rolled towels or foam padding onto the surface of the backboard next to the patient's head (**Step ⑥**).
7. **Secure the torso to the backboard** with straps (**Step ⑦**).
8. **Secure the patient's head** and padding to the backboard with 2" tape. Apply the tape across the forehead and cervical collar to prevent the padding from becoming dislodged. (**Step ⑧**).

Head Injuries

Older patients who have signs or symptoms of a significant head injury should be assumed to have sustained a substantial injury even if neurologically intact at the time of exam. In addition, patients who have sustained even minor-appearing head injuries and who are taking anticoagulants (blood thinners) should be suspected of having a brain injury. In these situations, patients may need persuading to seek medical treatment because they may feel completely normal and may not believe medical treatment is necessary. When a patient refuses care yet has a high risk of brain injury, relatives or neighbors should be instructed to watch for subtle changes in neurologic status that could indicate deterioration in the patient's condition.

Prehospital treatment of older head-injured patients should be aimed at maintaining maximum oxygen delivery to the brain. Patients who have signs of head injury and no evidence of hypotension or shock may also benefit from a slight elevation of the head. This position may help reduce intracranial pressure and increase cerebral perfusion pressure.

Injuries to the Pelvis

Pelvic fractures in older patients often occur as the result of a combination of decreased bone strength due to osteoporosis and a low-energy mechanism such as

You are the Provider 4

The patient is placed on the stretcher in a position of comfort and transported to the closest emergency department with a cardiac unit. She is diagnosed as having a myocardial infarction and started on "clot-busting" medications. She is taken for surgery and spends a week in the cardiac intensive care. Once released, she is moved to a rehabilitation center with hopes of returning home at the end of the month.

Skill Drill 26-1 Immobilizing a Patient With Kyphosis on a Long Backboard

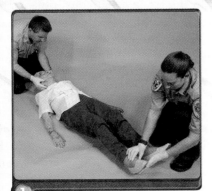

1. Apply and maintain cervical stabilization. Assess distal functions in all extremities.

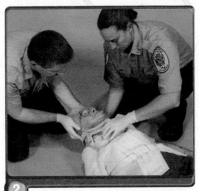

2. Apply a cervical collar. If a collar does not fit, do not attempt to straighten the patient's neck.

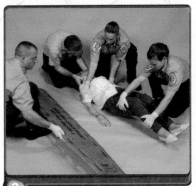

3. Rescuers kneel on one side of the patient and place hands on the far side of the patient.

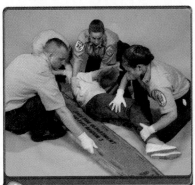

4. On command, rescuers roll the patient toward themselves and quickly examine the patient's back.

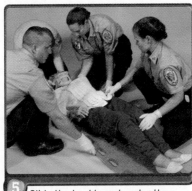

5. Slide the backboard under the patient and roll the patient onto the board.

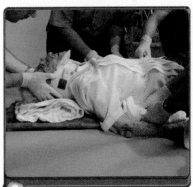

6. Pad the void space below the kyphotic region of the spine with pillows and blankets. Place rolled towels or foam padding onto the surface of the backboard next to the patient's head.

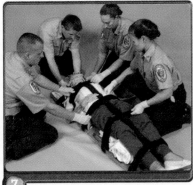

7. Secure the torso to the backboard with straps.

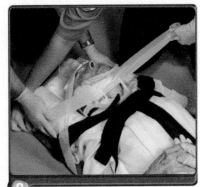

8. Secure the patient's head and padding to the backboard. Immobilize the rest of the body as usual.

Teamwork Tips

A patient who presents with kyphosis or other spinal deformity should be immobilized very carefully to prevent further pain or injury. One rescuer should support the patient in a comfortable position while maintaining c-spine alignment while the second rescuer uses any available material to pad all voids. If a c-collar will not fit, use rolled towels around the head and neck for stabilization.

a fall from a standing position. Pelvic fractures often present as hip or buttock pain. More serious high-energy fractures can pose a significant threat to life. Injuries of this type can be seen in a patient who has fallen from a significant height, been involved in a high-speed motor vehicle crash, or been struck by a car. This type of injury may result in fractures in two places in the pelvis with displacement of a segment of the pelvic ring (pelvic ring disruption). Pelvic ring disruption can lead to hemorrhage from the blood vessels that pass through the pelvis or to injury to the bladder, intestines, or lumbosacral nerve plexus. Older patients are less able than younger patients to tolerate the blood loss or other organ system injuries that are commonly associated with high-energy pelvic ring disruption.

The acetabulum is another site in the pelvis that may be injured as the result of high-energy trauma in older people. Injuries to the acetabulum can occur as the result of the knee being driven into the dashboard or ground with the head of the femur driven through the acetabulum. Owing to diminished bone strength, older patients are at a higher risk for this type of injury from lower energy mechanisms than would be required to cause a similar injury in younger patients.

Hip Fractures

One common debilitating musculoskeletal injury that occurs in older patients is a hip fracture. A hip fracture is a fracture of the head, neck, or proximal portion of the femur. Following a hip fracture, patients often have decreased mobility and independence and can require prolonged rehabilitation, which can be physically and emotionally challenging for the patient and his or her family. Despite the advances made in treatment, a large number of older people will have permanent impairment and nearly 20% die within the 12 months after injury.

Fractures of the hip should be treated by splinting the injured extremity with a blanket roll or long board splints. Fractures of the hip do not necessarily require the use of traction splints. The purposes of the blanket roll are to maintain the leg in a static position so that further injury does not occur and to help control pain **Skill Drill 26-2 ▶**.

1. **Assess pulse and motor and sensory function of the extremity.** Cover open wounds with dry, sterile dressings, and apply direct pressure, if necessary (**Step ①**).
2. **Place the patient on a scoop stretcher or long backboard** by log-rolling the patient onto the uninjured leg while having another provider support the injured extremity (**Step ②**).
3. While continuing to support the injured extremity in its deformed position, your partner should **place a blanket roll between the patient's legs (Step ③**).
4. **Place blankets and pillows under the injured extremity** to provide support to the fracture site in the deformed position (**Step ④**).
5. **Secure both legs and the padding to the backboard** with at least three cravats or straps (**Step ⑤**).
6. **Reassess pulse and motor and sensory function** (**Step ⑥**).

■ Geriatric Medical Emergencies

Determining the chief complaint of older patients can be challenging. Often, geriatric patients have multiple complaints from multiple conditions. Asking patients what problem bothers them the most today can help them focus on a single problem. The patient may complain of foot and ankle pain, but your examination reveals that the legs are swollen because of congestive heart failure. This patient may always be somewhat short of breath, and today may be only slightly different.

Remember that pain sensation may be diminished in older patients owing to the aging of the nervous system. Do not let this lead you to underestimate the severity of the patient's condition. In addition, fear of or the desire to avoid hospitalization often causes patients to understate or minimize symptoms.

Cardiovascular Emergencies

Because many older patients do not have the crushing chest pain that is experienced by younger patients, a common complaint of an older patient when experiencing a myocardial infarction (MI) is difficulty breathing. Older patients may also complain of

Skill Drill 26-2   Splinting a Hip Fracture

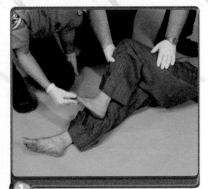

1 Assess pulse, motor, and sensory function. Cover wounds with dry, sterile dressings. Apply direct pressure if necessary.

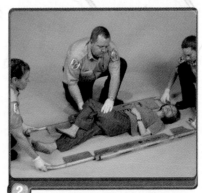

2 Place patient onto a scoop stretcher or long backboard by logrolling onto uninjured leg while provider supports injured extremity.

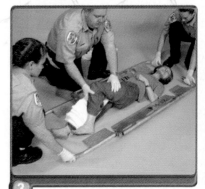

3 Continue to support the injured extremity while another provider places a blanket roll between the patient's legs.

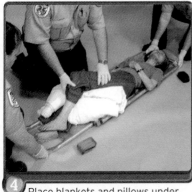

4 Place blankets and pillows under the injured extremity.

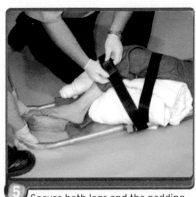

5 Secure both legs and the padding to the backboard with at least three cravats or straps.

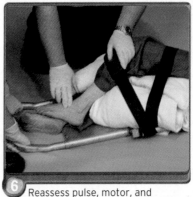

6 Reassess pulse, motor, and sensory function.

a toothache, arm pain, or back pain. This lack of usual symptoms can make cardiac emergencies more difficult to detect. It is often better to ask about chest discomfort rather than pain. Ask the patient whether he or she has experienced this before, and then ask how this is different. If the patient tells you that he or she felt this same way during a previous heart attack, it is a good bet that this may be another one.

Shortness of Breath

Shortness of breath, or dyspnea, can be related to many causes. The causes of dyspnea include asthma, chronic obstructive pulmonary disease, congestive heart failure, and pneumonia. However, an MI, bleeding, or even hyperglycemia can cause the patient to feel short of breath. To assess patients with shortness of breath, you must look at the entire picture. Complete the SAMPLE history and the physical exam. Assess the patient's work of breathing, including lung sounds, retractions, sitting in a tripod position, and cyanosis. If the patient becomes short of breath with activity, did the distress occur with the same amount of activity or with less activity than before? Does the patient sleep propped up on pillows? All patients experiencing shortness of breath should receive oxygen.

Syncope

Sudden unconsciousness (syncope) or the feeling of almost passing out (near syncope) can occur for many reasons in older people. Simple causes such as standing up too fast or straining to have a bowel movement while constipated can cause an older patient to faint. More deadly causes of syncope include an MI or hypoglycemia. The assessment for syncope includes a SAMPLE history and physical exam. During your history taking, ask what was happening before the syncope occurred. Also try taking the blood pressure while the patient is lying flat, seated, and standing. Drops in systolic blood pressure of more than 10 mm Hg can indicate problems in circulating volume, including dehydration.

Altered Mental Status

Acute onset of altered mental status is not normal for a patient of any age. Even patients with Alzheimer disease should not have sudden changes in their mental status. Changes indicate a problem in supplying the brain with the nutrition it needs. Infection, hypoglycemia, hypoxia, hypotension, cerebrovascular accident (stroke), trauma, seizures, medication interactions, electrolyte imbalances, and psychotic episodes can all affect how the brain functions. Most sudden changes are caused by a reversible condition. Evaluate and treat for hypoxia or hypoglycemia if present.

Acute Abdomen

In older patients, the nervous system response to pain in the abdomen is decreased. When an older patient complains of abdominal pain, it is usually a more serious event than in a younger patient. Ask whether the patient has had a change in bowel movements. The slowing of the gastrointestinal system in older people can cause constipation or bleeding. When palpating the abdomen, look for a pulsating mass, indicating an abdominal aortic aneurysm, found most commonly in patients older than 70 years.

Septicemia and Infectious Disease

Infections in an older person can be severe and dangerous. Septicemia is the disease state that results from the presence of microorganisms or their toxic products in the bloodstream. Septicemia (also often referred to as *sepsis*) is a serious problem that every EMS provider should know how to recognize and treat. Use appropriate body substance isolation precautions when you think a patient may have an infection. Think of septicemia whenever you see a hot, flushed patient who also has tachycardia and an increased respiratory rate. Symptoms of infection may be present, such as fever, chills, cough, or burning with urination. Often the infection will cause altered mental status. Think septic shock when hypotension is also present.

■ Response to Nursing and Skilled Care Facilities

Responding to a nursing home or skilled care facility is common for EMS providers. Before you provide transport for the patient, you should obtain the following critical information from the nursing staff:

- What is the patient's chief complaint today?
- What initial problem caused the patient to be admitted to the facility?

To determine the nature of the problem, you will usually have to compare the patient's present condition with his or her condition before onset of the symptoms. Ask the staff about the patient's mobility, activities of daily living, and ability to speak. This information will help to paint a picture of the patient's baseline condition.

Many facilities that are transferring patients will include a transfer record that includes the patient's history, medication lists and dosages, allergies, previous diagnoses, and vital signs. These records provide essential information and save time, especially when the patient cannot speak for himself or herself. Be sure to obtain this from the staff before leaving for the hospital.

You are the Provider Summary

Geriatric patients often present with different signs and symptoms from those experienced by average adults. You must be alert to small changes in vital signs along with unusual presentations of illness. Early recognition of distress and rapid transport may mean the difference between life and death.

1. **What should you notice as you enter the residence?**
   What does the residence look like? Is it clean? Is the temperature appropriate? Is the patient dressed appropriately? Are there hazards to the patient?

2. **What is your first priority?**
   ABCs. She is complaining of dyspnea, so oxygen should be applied as soon as possible.

3. **How will you use the extra help?**
   Ask the fire fighters to gather the patient's medications, bring in the stretcher, assist in lifting the patient, etc.

4. **What type of oxygen does she need? Why?**
   You should give oxygen by nonrebreathing mask. She is alert, and her rate and depth are okay for now. However, her airway should be closely monitored and you should be prepared to ventilate her if needed.

5. **What should you ask about her dyspnea?**
   How does she feel? How long has it been going on? Is she having any pain? What is her degree of distress? Has this happened before? If so, what did the doctor do then? Does anything make it better or worse?

6. **What should you ask about other symptoms?**
   Is she having any other problems? Does she feel any pain, pressure, or discomfort? Has anything changed? Does anything make any of it better or worse?

7. **What do you think is going on?**
   She is probably having a myocardial infarction.

8. **What treatment does she need?**
   High flow oxygen and rapid transport to the closest, most appropriate facility.

9. **How should she be transported?**
   She should be placed in a position of comfort and transported immediately.

Prep Kit

Ready for Review

- Although assessment of geriatric patients involves the same basic approach as that for any other patient, you should be more suspicious about the severity of the patient's condition and more aware of the environment.
- Injuries and medical conditions may be more significant or severe than what is indicated by the existing signs and symptoms. The injuries and conditions that are found will have a more profound effect than they would in a younger patient.
- In addition to the critical needs that an underlying medical problem may cause, the condition of an older patient is more unstable than that of a younger patient, and there is an increased possibility for sudden, rapid deterioration in the patient's condition.
- To obtain an accurate history for geriatric patients, patience and good communication skills are essential. A slow, deliberate approach to the patient history, with one EMT-B asking questions, is generally the best strategy.
- Polypharmacy and changes in medications can cause serious problems for geriatric patients.
- Common complaints of older patients include shortness of breath; chest pain; dizziness or weakness; fever; trauma; falls; generalized pain; and nausea, vomiting, and diarrhea. Altered mental status also is a common problem.

- The priorities in rapid trauma assessment do not change with older patients, although several factors, such as altered mental status and other physiologic changes associated with aging, should be considered as you conduct your assessment.
- Conditions such as cardiovascular emergencies, dyspnea, syncope, altered mental status, sepsis, and acute abdomen may present differently in older patients than in younger patients.
- When responding to nursing and skilled care facilities, you should determine the patient's chief complaint on that day and what initial problem caused the patient to be admitted to the facility.

Vital Vocabulary

acetabulum The depression on the lateral pelvis where its three component bones join, in which the femoral head fits snugly.

central cord syndrome A form of incomplete spinal cord injury in which some of the signals from the brain to the body are not received; results in weak or absent motor function, which is more pronounced in the upper extremities than the lower extremities.

polypharmacy Simultaneous use of many medications.

septicemia The disease state that results from the presence of microorganisms or their toxic products in the bloodstream.

Technology

- Interactivities
- Vocabulary Explorer
- Anatomy Review
- Web Links
- Online Review Manual

Assessment in Action

Geriatric patients often present differently than average adults and may have special needs for immobilization and care. Recognizing these differences can improve patient care and outcome.

1. _____ fractures are the most common spine fractures in geriatrics.
   - **A.** Osteoporatic
   - **B.** Compression
   - **C.** Hyperextension
   - **D.** Flexion

2. Common complaints associated with a myocardial infarction include:
   - **A.** toothache.
   - **B.** back pain.
   - **C.** dyspnea.
   - **D.** all of the above.

3. Most sudden changes in mental status are _____.
   - **A.** traumatic
   - **B.** irreversible
   - **C.** reversible
   - **D.** the result of seizure activity

4. Which of the following can affect brain function?
   - **A.** seizures
   - **B.** hypotension
   - **C.** medication interactions
   - **D.** All of the above

5. The "E" of the GEMS diamond is assessed during the _____.
   - **A.** scene size-up
   - **B.** initial assessment
   - **C.** focused history and physical
   - **D.** reassessment

6. When communicating with an older person who has difficulty hearing, you should _____.
   - **A.** turn on a light
   - **B.** turn off televisions
   - **C.** use a normal tone of voice
   - **D.** all of the above

Challenging Questions

7. To assess geriatric patients with shortness of breath you must look at the entire picture. How should this patient be assessed?

8. What are the signs and symptoms of septicemia?

Advanced Skills

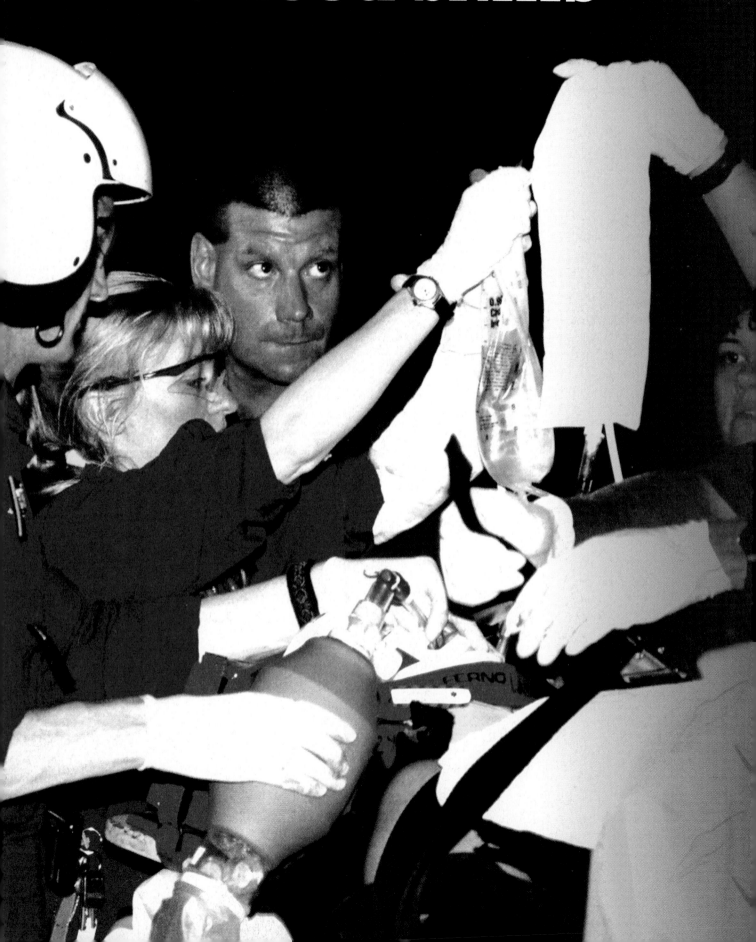

7

Section

27

Advanced Airway Management

You are the Provider 1

You and your partner, a paramedic, are called to a cardiac arrest. The patient is a 67-year-old man who has a history of cardiac problems. He had a pacer/defibrillator implanted four years ago and has been having chest pain frequently over the last week. His wife tells you that he was not feeling well this morning and did not eat his breakfast or take his medication.

Initial Assessment	Recording Time: 0 Minutes
Appearance	Pale
Level of consciousness	Unresponsive
Airway	Fluid in the airway
Breathing	Apneic
Circulation	Pulseless

1. What is the first step in treating this patient?
2. Can you use an AED on this patient?
3. When should you attempt a definitive airway?

Advanced Airway Management

The single most important manipulative skill you will use as an EMT-B is establishing and maintaining a patient's airway. The vast majority of conscious patients with an intact gag reflex can maintain their own airway. Most conscious patients may only need oxygen and close monitoring for any changes. Patients with an altered mental status may require an oropharyngeal or nasopharyngeal airway and suctioning. However, patients who are unresponsive and not breathing on their own will fare better with advanced airway techniques. The purpose of advanced airway management is to provide better airway protection and improve ventilation by using a tube to create a direct channel to the trachea. Endotracheal (ET) intubation is a difficult skill to master and requires additional training for EMT-Bs. Blind intubation using a lighted stylet is another technique for establishing ET tube placement. Additional options include using a multilumen airway or a laryngeal mask airway (LMA). All of these techniques require additional training, appropriate approval for their use, and medical oversight.

The chapter begins with a brief review of basic airway management skills, gastric tubes, and the Sellick maneuver. The rest of the chapter reviews ET intubation, the use of a lighted stylet, multilumen airway devices, and the LMA.

Basic Airway Management

You should always assess the airway first in an injured or ill patient. This rule applies to the basic and advanced levels of airway management. Advanced airway techniques begin only after proper basic airway management has been completed.

The first step in airway management is opening a patient's airway. You should use the head tilt–chin lift maneuver in a patient with no suspected spinal injury and the jaw-thrust maneuver in a patient you suspect has a spinal injury. After you have opened the airway, you should assess the airway and evaluate the need for suctioning.

After the airway has been cleared, you need to determine whether the patient needs an airway adjunct. The basic airway adjuncts that are already available to you are oropharyngeal and nasopharyngeal airways. The more advanced airway adjuncts that may be available to you, with approval of your medical director, will be discussed in this chapter.

Gastric Tubes

Patients who have gastric distention or are vomiting are especially challenging to manage. You must use basic suctioning techniques to prevent aspiration in a patient who is vomiting. Patients with gastric distention are prone to vomiting; therefore, you should consider using a gastric tube for these patients.

A gastric tube is an advanced airway adjunct that provides a channel directly into a patient's stomach, allowing for the removal of gas, blood, and toxins or to instill medications and nutrition. In the field, you will use a gastric tube primarily to decompress the stomach of a patient with gastric distention. Gastric distention is most common in children during artificial ventilation but is also seen in adults.

There are two types of gastric tubes: nasogastric tubes, which are inserted through the nose, and orogastric tubes, which are inserted through the mouth. A nasogastric tube is contraindicated in a patient with major facial, head, or spinal trauma. In these patients, an orogastric tube is safer. A nasogastric tube can cause nasal trauma with bleeding, or it can accidentally be passed into the trachea, interfering with the airway and ventilation. In a patient with a basal skull fracture, a nasogastric tube can accidentally be passed into the brain.

Inserting a gastric tube can activate a patient's gag reflex, causing vomiting and aspiration. Clearly, inserting a gastric tube is a delicate task that should be performed according to local EMS protocol and medical direction only. Special care is called for if the patient has head, spinal, or major facial trauma.

Technology

- Interactivities
- Vocabulary Explorer
- Anatomy Review
- Web Links
- Online Review Manual

You will need the following equipment for gastric tube insertion:

- Properly sized tubes
  - Newborn and infant, 8F
  - Toddler and preschool, 10F
  - School-age child, 12F
  - Adolescent, 14F to 16F
  - Adult, 16F to 18F
- Catheter-tipped 60-mL syringe
- Water-soluble lubricant
- Emesis container
- Tape
- Stethoscope
- Suctioning unit and catheters

Once you have prepared and assembled the proper equipment, use the following procedure to insert a gastric tube:

1. **Measure the tube** from the tip of the nose, to the earlobe, to the epigastric area below the xiphoid process. (If you are using an orogastric tube, measure from the teeth to the angle of the jaw and down to the epigastric area.) Mark the measured length on the tube with a piece of tape, or note the number on the tube.
2. **Lubricate the distal end of the tube** with a water-soluble lubricant.
3. **Place the patient in the proper position.** If you do not suspect a spinal injury, place the patient supine, with the head flexed so the chin rests on the chest.
4. **Pass the tube along the nasal floor** (or, for an orogastric tube, over the tongue to the back of the throat) until you reach the tape marker.
5. **Confirm proper tube placement** by aspirating stomach contents with the syringe or injecting 30 to 50 mL of air into the tube and listening for gurgling over the stomach with the stethoscope.
6. **Aspirate air and stomach contents** with the syringe, once placement is confirmed, to decompress the stomach, or attach to on-board suction. Follow local protocols concerning the type of suction to use (intermittent or continuous).
7. **Secure the tube** in place with tape.

■ The Sellick Maneuver

Intubating an unresponsive patient who has no gag reflex may cause vomiting and aspiration, which can ultimately damage airway tissues and block the lower airway passages. A procedure called the Sellick maneuver, or cricoid pressure can be helpful in avoiding these complications in the field.

The cricoid cartilage, located just below the thyroid cartilage (Adam's apple), is a rigid, ring-shaped structure that completely encircles the larynx at the top of the trachea. It can be difficult to locate in infants, children, and small adults. The depression between the thyroid cartilage and the cricoid cartilage is called the cricothyroid membrane. The esophagus is much softer than the trachea and does not have rings of cartilage to hold it open. It is normally closed, opening only as we eat or drink. By applying pressure on the cricoid cartilage, you can squeeze the esophagus shut and, thus, prevent solids and fluids from leaving the esophagus and eventually being aspirated into the larynx and trachea. When performing this maneuver, be sure to correctly identify anatomic landmarks to avoid damaging other structures or inadvertently obstructing the airway.

To perform the Sellick Maneuver (cricoid pressure), review the steps in Skill Drill 27-1 ▶ :

1. **With the patient's neck slightly extended** (only if there is no suspicion of spinal injury), visualize the cricoid cartilage, just below the thyroid cartilage (Adam's apple) (**Step 1**).
2. **Confirm location of the cricoid cartilage** by palpating with the tip of your index finger (**Step 2**).
3. **Place a thumb and index finger on either side of the midline of the cricoid cartilage.** Apply firm, but not excessive, posterior pressure on the cricoid cartilage to compress and shut off the esophagus behind it. Too much pressure could collapse the larynx. Maintain this pressure until the patient is intubated (**Step 3**).

■ ET Intubation

Endotracheal intubation is the insertion of a tube into the trachea to maintain the airway. This can be done through the mouth (called orotracheal intubation) or through the nose (called nasotracheal intubation). In either case, the tube passes directly through the larynx between the vocal cords and then into the trachea.

As an EMT-B, you will only be intubating patients who are unresponsive with no gag reflex or in cardiac arrest. You should not immediately intubate a patient who is unresponsive or in cardiac arrest. First, you should open the airway with the appropriate BLS maneuver, clear the airway, and provide bag-mask

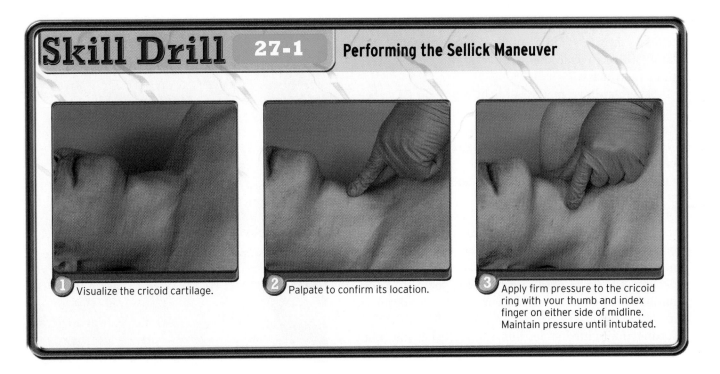

Skill Drill   27-1   Performing the Sellick Maneuver

1. Visualize the cricoid cartilage.

2. Palpate to confirm its location.

3. Apply firm pressure to the cricoid ring with your thumb and index finger on either side of midline. Maintain pressure until intubated.

ventilation. You should then consider ET intubation based on your local protocols. Because of the time that it takes to properly prepare intubation equipment, you must always secure the patient's airway with basic methods first because they are much quicker to perform and effective in many situations when properly performed.

Orotracheal Intubation

Orotracheal intubation is the most effective way to control a patient's airway and has many advantages over other airway management techniques Table 27-1 ▶. It is indicated for patients who cannot protect their own airways as a result of unconsciousness or cardiac arrest. It is also used for patients who need prolonged artificial ventilation, are unresponsive to painful stimuli, or have no gag reflex or ability to cough.

Teamwork Tips

Assist an ALS provider who is attempting to intubate a difficult patient by applying the Sellick maneuver. This moves the trachea posteriorly to allow for better visualization.

Equipment

You should assemble all the equipment that you will need before starting the procedure and while the patient is being preoxygenated with bag-mask

Table 27-1 Advantages of Orotracheal Intubation

- Completely controls and protects the airway
- Delivers better minute volume without the difficulty of maintaining an adequate mask seal, as is needed with a BVM device. (The minute volume is the volume of air cycled through the alveoli in 1 minute.)
- May be left in place for several days if prolonged ventilation is required
- Prevents gastric distention, which means less risk of regurgitation of stomach contents and greater opportunity for good tidal volume
- Minimizes the risk of aspiration of stomach contents into the respiratory system because a balloon seals off the trachea
- Allows for direct access to the trachea for suctioning
- Allows for the delivery of high volumes of oxygen at higher than normal pressures
- Provides a route for administration of certain medications (only if other medication routes are not available)

ventilation. You will be working in proximity to the patient's airway, so the minimum body substance isolation (BSI) precautions include gloves, eye protection, and a mask.

There are two methods for inserting an ET tube. Both use ET tubes with slight differences in equipment. The visualized technique uses a laryngoscope, which enables visualization of the vocal cords to manually place the ET tube between the vocal cords and into the trachea. The blind technique uses a <u>lighted stylet</u>. The light at the end of the stylet is extremely bright. The light can be visualized on the outside of the body when placed in the trachea. The light cannot be seen if it is placed in the esophagus (there is too much tissue for the light to penetrate to the outside). Because the vocal cords are normally located in the midline of the neck, a light seen in the sternal notch is below the vocal cords and in the trachea. After inserting the lighted stylet into the ET tube, the tube is then inserted into the airway, with the light as a guide.

The equipment for visualized and blind ET intubation is basically the same with the exception of the insertion-visualization device. The following is a list of equipment needed:

- BSI equipment
- Properly sized ET tube
- Laryngoscope handle and blade (visualized technique)
- Stylet (visualized technique) or lighted stylet (blind technique)
- 10-mL syringe
- Oxygen, with a device for bag-mask ventilation before and after intubation
- A suctioning unit with rigid and soft-tip catheters
- Magill forceps
- Towels for raising the patient's head and/or shoulders
- A stethoscope
- Water-soluble lubricant for the ET tube
- A commercial securing device
- A secondary confirmation device

You must check your equipment daily to ensure that it is all available and to be certain that it is properly assembled and working, especially before you try to intubate a patient.

Laryngoscope

The purpose of a <u>laryngoscope</u> is to sweep the tongue out of the way and align the airway so that you can

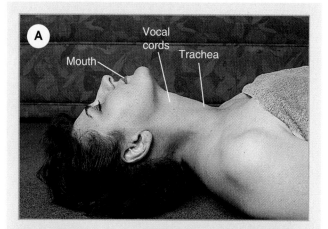

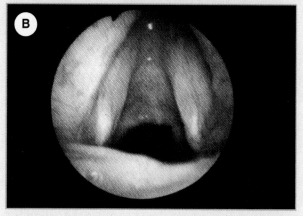

Figure 27-1 A. You must see the vocal cords to pass an ET tube through them. The vocal cords are located in the upper airway at the entrance to the larynx. **B.** A view of the vocal cords.

see the vocal cords and pass the ET tube through them 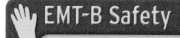 .

The handle of the laryngoscope contains batteries to provide power to the light and has a locking bar to connect the handle to the blade. Blades are curved or straight and range in size from 0 to 4 Figure 27-2 ▶ .

The two blade designs function differently to align the structures so that you can visualize the vocal cords. The curved (Macintosh) blade is inserted just in front of the epiglottis, into the <u>vallecula</u> (the space

EMT-B Safety

Visualization of the vocal cords requires the EMT to be in close proximity to the patient's airway. Always wear goggles or a face shield when attempting an intubation.

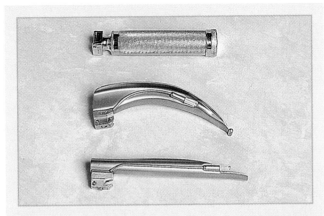

Figure 27-2 Laryngoscope blades can be curved or straight and come in different sizes.

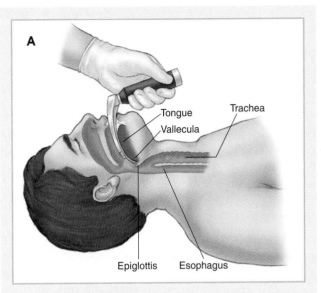

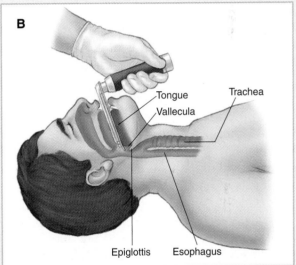

Figure 27-3 A. Insert a curved blade just in front of the epiglottis into the vallecula. **B.** Insert a straight blade past the epiglottis.

between the base of the tongue and the epiglottis), allowing you to see the glottic opening and vocal cords Figure 27-3 A ▶. The straight (Miller) blade is inserted past the epiglottis Figure 27-3 B ▶. Because its broader base and flange provide better displacement of the tongue, a curved blade is preferred for use in older children. A straight blade, which actually lifts the epiglottis out of the way to allow for visualization of the glottic opening and vocal cords, is preferred for use in infants. You should practice intubation with curved and straight blades so that you will feel comfortable using both techniques in a real patient situation.

A notch on the blade locks onto the locking bar of the handle. Because adequate lighting is essential for you to visualize the epiglottis and vocal cords, the light source is near the tip of the blade. You can activate the light by lifting the blade away from the handle until it locks at a right angle. The light should be bright white and tight. However, the bulb will not come on if the blade is not attached properly, the bulb is burned out or loose, or the batteries in the handle are dead. Always carry extra batteries for the handle and extra light bulbs in assorted sizes for each blade.

Lighted Stylet

The lighted stylet comes in one size that fits all adult and many pediatric ET tubes. The lighted stylet consists of a malleable metal wand with a light source at one end and a handle with an energy source at the other. The wand is designed to provide stiffness and shaping to the tube. Once an ET tube is threaded onto the wand, the handle will have a locking device to secure the proximal end of the ET tube Figure 27-4 ▶. This prevents the

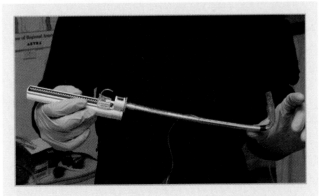

Figure 27-4 A lighted stylet used in conjunction with an ET tube.

ET tube from moving before insertion and the stylet from protruding beyond the end of the ET tube.

ET Tubes

Endotracheal tubes come in many sizes, and the size is specified by the measurement of the inside diameter of the tube. Sizes range from 2.5 to 9 mm. The length of the ET tube is marked on the outside of the tube in centimeters. The overall length of a tube for an adult is usually 33 cm. The following are general guidelines to use when intubating an average-sized adult patient:

- The centimeter markings on the outside of the tube will usually indicate that it is 15 cm to the vocal cords, 20 to 21 cm to the sternal notch, and 25 cm to the carina.
- You can mark the length for placement of the ET tube by looking at where the tube lines up with the teeth on an intubated patient. This tube-to-teeth mark is usually at around 22 cm. Once the patient is intubated, you should monitor the centimeter marking at the patient's teeth because this will determine whether the tube has moved from its original position.

The proper size of tube for adult men ranges from 7.5 to 8.5 mm; for adult women, it ranges from 6.5 to 8.0 mm **Figure 27-5 ▼**. For most efficient use of the tube, use the largest-diameter ET tube that you can. A good rule of thumb is to always have a 7.5-mm ET tube on hand; this size tube will fit most men and women. However, you should carry a complete selection of tube sizes in the unit to ensure that no matter what size you choose, you have one tube smaller and one tube larger, in case you need it.

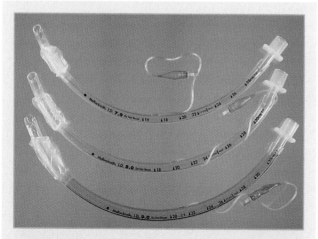

Figure 27-5 Endotracheal tubes that are used for adults generally range from 6.5 to 8.5 mm. Note the centimeter markings.

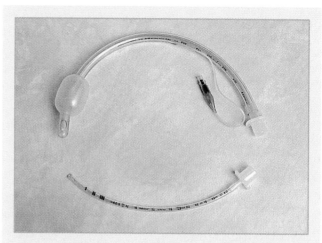

Figure 27-6 The components of the adult ET tube include a 15/22-mm adapter that attaches to a ventilating device, a pilot balloon, the tube, a balloon cuff (shown inflated), and Murphy's eye. The pediatric tube shown at the bottom includes an adapter and Murphy's eye at the uncuffed distal end of the tube.

Components of an ET tube include a standard 15/22-mm adapter, which attaches to any ventilation device, such as for bag-mask ventilation or a mechanical ventilator **Figure 27-6 ▲**. A pilot balloon is attached to the tube to indicate how well the balloon cuff at the distal end of the ET tube is inflated. The cuff at the end of the tube holds about 10 mL of air. The small hole at the distal end of the tube across from the bevel end, called Murphy's eye, helps to prevent tube obstruction by secretions.

For children, it is best to have a chart or length-based tape device to help you with sizing the ET tube. Generally, for newborns and small infants, the proper tube size ranges from 3.0 to 3.5 mm; for infants up to 1 year, it is 4.0 mm. You may also follow a formula for sizing tubes in children. You can calculate tube size in children by adding 16 to the child's age and then dividing by 4. Another method is to select a tube that roughly equals the size of the diameter of the patient's little finger across the nail bed. No matter what size you decide to use, you should also have one tube larger and one tube smaller available.

For children older than 8 years and with adults, you will use cuffed tubes. However, in younger children, the circular narrowing of the trachea at the level of the cricoid cartilage functions as a cuff. Uncuffed tubes are used for children younger than 8 years. Always watch the tube pass through the vocal cords in a child (as well as in an adult) to make sure that the tip of the ET tube is in the proper position.

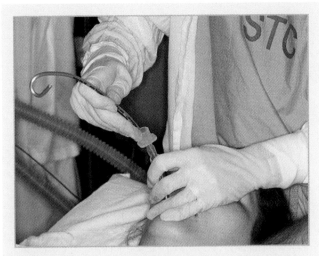

Figure 27-7 A wire stylet, which adds rigidity and shape to the tube, must be removed after tube placement.

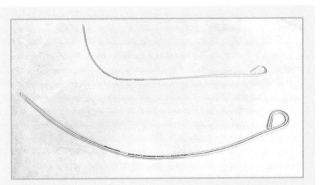

Figure 27-8 Bend the tip of the stylet into a hockey stick shape for a pediatric patient, as shown at the top. Bend the stylet to form a gentle curve for an adult patient, as shown at the bottom.

Stylet

A plastic-coated wire called a <u>stylet</u> may be inserted into the ET tube to add rigidity and shape to the tube Figure 27-7 ▲ . You should bend the tip of the stylet to form a gentle curve in adults. Because the pediatric airway is more angular and less aligned than the adult airway, you should bend the tip of the stylet into a hockey stick shape for use in an infant or child Figure 27-8 ▶ . You should also apply a little water-soluble lubricant to the distal end of the tube to make it easier to insert and to the end of the stylet to make it easier to remove once the tube is in place.

Do not insert the stylet past Murphy's eye because it could puncture or lacerate delicate airway tissues

Figure 27-9 ▶ . A good rule of thumb is to keep the stylet ¼" proximal to the cuff in adults and 1" from the end of the tube in infants and children. Before you attempt intubation, you should always confirm that the stylet is not sticking out past the end of the ET tube.

These principles are also followed for the lighted stylet. The lighted stylet may or may not be disposable, depending on the manufacturer. Because the light source is in the handle, make sure you have replacement handles or batteries available.

Syringe

You will use the 10-mL syringe to test for air leaks in the ET tube before intubation. You will use it again after the ET tube is in place to inflate the cuff and provide a seal inside the trachea to prevent aspiration.

You are the Provider 2

The fire department has taken over compressions and ventilations. The cardiac monitor is attached and the rhythm is not shockable. Your partner is attempting to gain IV access while you check the equipment for intubation.

Vital Signs	Recording Time: 2 Minutes
Skin	Pale, slightly cool
Pulse	Pulseless
Pupils	Slightly dilated
Respirations	Apneic

4. What equipment is needed to perform an intubation?
5. What is the Sellick maneuver?
6. What size tube should this patient require?

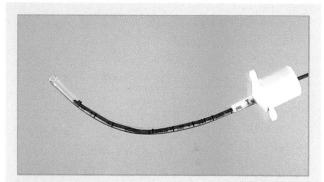

Figure 27-9 Do not insert the stylet past Murphy's eye because it could damage airway tissues. Keep the stylet ¼" proximal to the cuff in the adult tube and 1" from the end of the pediatric tube.

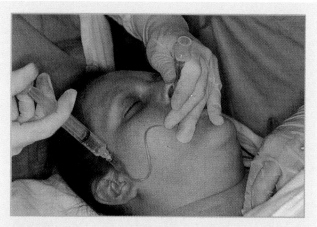

Figure 27-10 Inflate the cuff with 5 to 10 mL of air, and then immediately remove the syringe from the pilot balloon to prevent air from leaking back into the syringe.

Take the following steps to use the syringe properly:

1. As you are assembling and checking your equipment before intubation, pull back on the plunger of the syringe to the 7- to 8-mL mark to **fill the syringe with the amount of air that is needed to inflate the cuff.**
2. **Attach the syringe to the pilot balloon,** and test the cuff by inflating it with 5 to 10 mL of air.
3. **Deflate the cuff** after you have confirmed that there are no air leaks.
4. With the syringe still attached, **remove the air from the cuff** by pulling back on the plunger to the 10-mL mark. Be sure that the syringe remains attached to the pilot balloon with the plunger pulled back to the 10-mL mark.

After the ET tube has been properly inserted in the patient, you will inflate the cuff with 5 to 10 mL of air and then immediately remove the syringe from the pilot balloon to prevent air from leaking back into the syringe Figure 27-10 ▶ .

Other Equipment

You must also have a device available to secure the ET tube in place. A commercial securing device may be more effective than tape. There are many manufacturers of securing devices; you should become familiar with the device used in your system Figure 27-11 ▶ .

Tape could also be used as a backup system to a commercial device. Medical control may also advise you to use an oral airway or similar device in intubated patients to prevent them from biting down on the tube. In addition, you will need the following equipment:

- Oxygen
- A suctioning unit
- A device for bag-mask ventilation
- Magill forceps (can be used to help guide the tube in the visualized technique)
- Towels for raising the patient's head or shoulders if necessary
- Secondary confirmation device
- Cervical collar and backboard

You will need to use bag-mask ventilation to preoxygenate the patient before attempting intubation. The suctioning unit should be readily available to clear any fluid or particles from the mouth Figure 27-12 ▶ . Use a rigid, large-bore suction catheter to clear the mouth before intubation. Once the patient

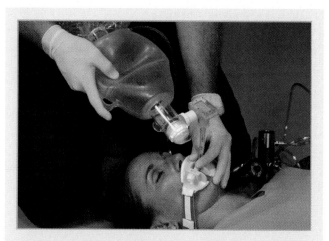

Figure 27-11 Secure the ET tube in place with a commercial device or tape, depending on your system's protocol.

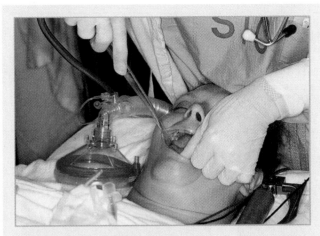
Figure 27-12 Suction any fluid or particles from the mouth before any attempt to intubate.

is intubated, you might need to use a French catheter to suction fluids from inside the ET tube.

The Intubation Procedure
Visualized (Oral) Intubation

You may intubate only if authorized to do so by off-line or online medical control, according to your local protocols. Once you have made the decision to intubate, you must act quickly, carefully, and efficiently. If environmental light is too bright and you are using a lighted stylet, move the patient to your ambulance or another place where ambient light can be controlled. Be sure to follow BSI precautions, including the use of gloves, eye protection, and a mask. You should not use more than 30 seconds in an attempt to intubate a patient. The 30-second time limit begins when you stop ventilation and insert the laryngoscope blade or the lighted stylet into the patient's mouth; it ends when the ET tube has been properly placed and ventilation has begun again. If you are not successful in placing the ET tube, stop, withdraw the tube, hyperventilate the patient, and try again according to your local protocols.

Intubation is a multiple-person task, especially in a situation involving cardiac arrest and use of an automated external defibrillator, or AED. Remember that defibrillation with an AED and limiting the interruption of chest compressions are priorities in a cardiac arrest. Intubating a patient who is in cardiac arrest should occur only after indicated shocks and one or two rounds (2 minutes per round) of CPR.

Review the steps in **Skill Drill 27-2** to perform visualized orotracheal intubation:

1. **Open the patient's airway,** and clear the airway of any foreign material. Be sure to use BSI precautions.

2. **Insert an oropharyngeal airway,** and preoxygenate the patient by using bag-mask ventilation (**Step 1**).

3. **As your partner ventilates the patient,** you should quickly assemble and test your equipment. Verify that the bulb on the laryngoscope or lighted stylet is working, select the proper size of tube, and make sure the ET tube cuff has no leaks. If you are using a nonlighted stylet, insert it in the ET tube. Lubricate the tube and stylet as needed (**Step 2**).

4. **Confirm that the patient has been properly preoxygenated.** Stop ventilating the patient, and remove the oral airway if it is in place.

5. If another EMT-B is available, have him or her **perform the Sellick maneuver** to improve visualization of the vocal cords or positioning of the lighted stylet. Maintain pressure on the cricoid cartilage until the ET tube cuff is inflated.

6. **Position the patient's head and neck** to allow for the best visualization of the vocal cords. When you are using the laryngoscope, place towels under the patient's shoulders, if necessary, to raise the head for a better view of the vocal cords. When you are using the lighted stylet, grasping the tongue and jaw and pulling upward will aid in insertion (**Step 3**).

7. **To intubate a patient you suspect has a spinal cord injury,** you should make sure that your partner maintains manual in-line stabilization of the head and neck in the neutral position while you attempt the intubation. You might need to lie on your stomach or straddle the patient's head while leaning back to visualize the vocal cords adequately (**Step 4**).

8. **Grasp the laryngoscope handle in your left hand.** Make sure the blade is locked into place and the bulb is illuminated. Open the patient's mouth, and gently place the blade in the right side of the patient's mouth, then move it toward the center of the mouth, sweeping the tongue to the left. The tongue must be displaced for you to visualize the vocal cords. Visualize the epiglottis. Advance a curved blade along the base of the tongue until its tip rests at the vallecula; advance a straight blade along the base of the tongue until you see it catch the epiglottis. Lift

Skill Drill 27-2   Performing Orotracheal Intubation

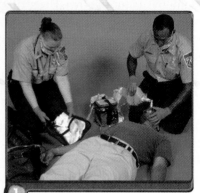

1 Open and clear the airway. Insert an oropharyngeal airway, and preoxygenate with a bag-mask device.

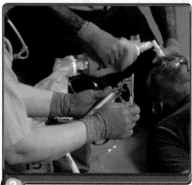

2 Assemble and test intubation equipment as your partner continues to ventilate.

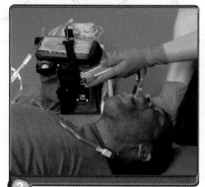

3 Confirm adequate preoxygenation, and remove the oral airway. If available, have another rescuer perform the Sellick maneuver to improve visualization of the cords. Use the head tilt–chin lift maneuver to position a nontrauma patient for insertion of the laryngoscope.

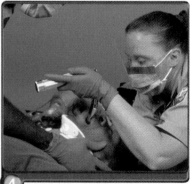

4 In a trauma patient, maintain the cervical spine in-line and neutral as your partner lies down or straddles the patient's head to visualize the vocal cords.

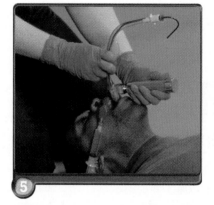

5 Insert the laryngoscope from the right side of the mouth, and move the tongue to the left. Lift the laryngoscope away from the posterior pharynx to visualize the vocal cords. Do not pry or use the teeth as a fulcrum. Insert the ET tube from the right side until the ET tube cuff passes through the vocal cords. Remove the laryngoscope and stylet. Hold the tube carefully until it is secured.

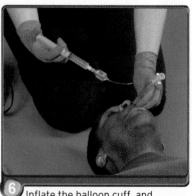

6 Inflate the balloon cuff, and remove the syringe as your partner prepares to ventilate.

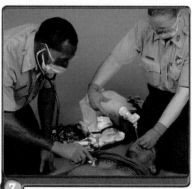

7 Begin ventilating, and confirm placement of the ET tube by listening over the stomach and both lungs. Also confirm placement with an end-tidal carbon dioxide detector or EDD, if available.

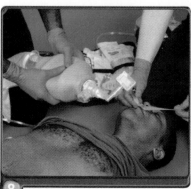

8 Secure the tube, and continue to ventilate. Note and record depth of insertion (centimeter marking at the teeth), and reconfirm position after each time you move the patient.

the laryngoscope away from the posterior pharynx so that you can see the vocal cords. The lifting force is directed straight up, parallel to the long axis of the laryngoscope handle, not back toward the patient's head. It should feel as if you are picking up the patient's head by the jaw. To avoid breaking the patient's teeth or lacerating the lips, never use the blade as a lever or fulcrum against the upper teeth. Do not lose sight of the vocal cords at any time after you have visualized them. Proper placement of the ET tube depends on your visualization of the tube as it is placed between the vocal cords.

9. **Insert the ET tube** with your right hand, keeping the vocal cords and the tip of the tube in sight at all times. Do not advance the ET tube down the center of the laryngoscope blade, or your view of the vocal cords will be obstructed. Advance the tube from the right side of the patient's mouth. Watch the uninflated cuff on the tube as it passes through the vocal cords, then advance the ET tube until the cuff is just past the vocal cords. Note and document the centimeter markings on the outside of the ET tube at the level of the teeth. Once the tube has been inserted through the vocal cords into the trachea, gently remove the laryngoscope and stylet, if a stylet was used. **Do not let go of the ET tube until it is secured (Step ⑤).**

10. **Inflate the cuff** on the end of the tube with 5 to 10 mL of air. Gently squeeze the pilot balloon cuff to verify the amount of air you should use. The pilot balloon should be full but easily compressed between your fingers. Immediately detach the syringe so that the air in the cuff will not empty back into it (**Step ⑥**).

11. **You or your partner** (whoever is not holding the ET tube in place) **should begin ventilating the patient** with a device for bag-mask ventilation attached to the ET tube. Confirm placement of the ET tube. Listen with a stethoscope over the stomach and then both lungs as the patient is being ventilated. You should be able to hear equal breath sounds over the right and left lung fields and no sounds over the stomach. Listen at the sternal notch in children. You should see both sides of the chest rise and fall with each ventilation. This is especially important in children because breath sounds in children may be misleading. You may hear them even if the tube

is in the esophagus. You should not be able to hear breath sounds in the stomach.

Proper confirmation of ET tube placement is essential. If you did not actually visualize the ET tube passing through the vocal cords, you may have placed the ET tube in the esophagus rather than in the trachea, which can prove fatal for the patient. The actual visualization of the ET tube as it passes through the vocal cords is the best way to confirm proper placement.

It is recommended that you use a secondary method of confirming proper tube placement. There are several devices available—esophageal detector devices, <u>end-tidal carbon dioxide detectors</u> (sometimes abbreviated as $ETCO_2$ detectors, and including colorimetric detectors), and portable capnography monitors.

Esophageal detector devices are designed to connect directly to the ET tube once the patient has been intubated. Two common devices use a syringe with plunger or a bulb syringe design. The device works by attempting to withdraw air from the ET tube. If the tube is properly placed, air will freely withdraw through the syringe or will inflate the bulb because the trachea will not collapse around the end of the ET tube (Figure 27-13 ▾). However, if the ET tube is in the esophagus, the soft tissues of the esophagus will collapse around the end of the tube and there will be noticeable resistance to

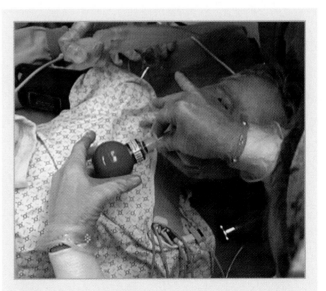

Figure 27-13 If the ET tube is in the trachea, air will freely inflate the bulb of the esophageal detector device.

the withdrawal of air through the syringe or plunger or to the inflation of the bulb.

End-tidal carbon dioxide detectors and capnography monitors sense the amount of carbon dioxide during the exhalation phase. Patients in respiratory and/or cardiac arrest will not be producing carbon dioxide. Therefore, you cannot get an accurate reading until you have restored effective ventilation and circulation to the patient.

One example of an end-tidal carbon dioxide detector is a disposable plastic indicator with chemically treated paper that changes from purple to yellow in the presence of carbon dioxide (usually takes several ventilations to obtain a reading) **Figure 27-14 ▾**. The device connects between the ET tube and the device for bag-mask ventilation. Secondary confirmation is made by verifying the appropriate color change. If carbon dioxide is present, it will change the color of the indicator to yellow. If the ET tube is in the esophagus, ventilation will not produce any carbon dioxide and there will be no color change on the indicator (may change to tan, but generally will stay purple).

Capnography monitors can also be used for secondary confirmation of ET tube placement. These devices monitor for the presence of carbon dioxide through an adapter that connects between the ET tube and the device for bag-mask ventilation. During ventilation, the amount of carbon dioxide present is displayed as a number

or as a positive waveform on the monitor. Positive waveforms and/or carbon dioxide readings provide secondary confirmation of proper placement. If the ET tube is in the esophagus, waveforms and readings will not be present.

Remember that these are all devices used as secondary confirmation of ET tube placement. The devices do not give a 100% guarantee that the tube is in the correct location. Your primary confirmation is direct visualization of the tube passing through the vocal cords, auscultating good bilateral breath sounds (no epigastric sounds), and seeing the patient's chest rise and fall with each ventilation (**Step 7**).

12. **Once you have confirmed placement,** secure the ET tube in place with the device and technique that have been approved by your medical director.

Remember that even when placed properly, the ET tube will move if it is not secured. For this reason, you must never let go of the ET tube until it is secured. Even then, you must continuously check the tube to make sure it is secure and in the correct place. Check the centimeter marking on the ET tube at the teeth and assess it frequently for tube movement. Also, frequently reassess the epigastrium and breath sounds and your secondary confirmation methods. It is recommended that the head be immobilized and that cervical collars be placed on patients who are intubated (even if there is no trauma) to avoid unnecessary movement of the head during transport. Excessive head movement is thought to contribute to dislodgment of initially properly placed ET tubes. Continue to ventilate the patient at an age-appropriate rate. Also, again, remember to note the distance the tube has been inserted by frequently reassessing the centimeter marking on the tube at the teeth. Be sure to reassess breath sounds and equal expansion of both sides of the chest each time you move the patient (**Step 8**).

Complications

Endotracheal intubation is a difficult skill to master. If intubation takes longer than 30 seconds, the resulting delay in oxygenation may lead to brain damage. EMS providers need a great deal of expert instruction and practice to master this skill. The benefits and potential complications of ET intubation are summarized in **Table 27-2 ▸**.

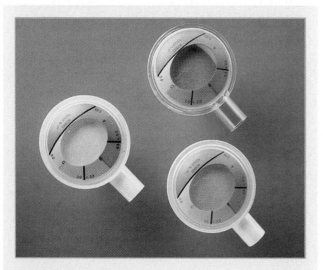

Figure 27-14 Color change on end-tidal carbon dioxide detectors can assist you in determining the location of the ET tube.

Table 27-2 Benefits and Complications of ET Intubation

Benefits	Complications
Provides complete protection of airway	Intubation of the right mainstem bronchus
Can be left in for long periods	Intubation of the esophagus, resulting in hypoxia
Delivers better oxygen concentration than a BVM device	Aggravation of a spinal injury
Prevents gastric distention and aspiration	More than 30 seconds to intubate can result in increased hypoxia
Allows for deep suctioning of the trachea	Vomiting and/or tube removal can result in aspiration
Allows for administration of certain medications	Soft-tissue trauma
	Mechanical failure
	Patient intolerance
	Decrease in heart rate

Intubating the Right Mainstem Bronchus

This is the most common error made during intubation. If you push or accidentally slip the tube in too far, the ET tube will pass into the right mainstem bronchus because it is shorter and straighter than the left mainstem bronchus. In this position, you will be ventilating only the right lung and will hear breath sounds only on the right side. To correct this, deflate the cuff and pull the ET tube back about 1 cm. Listen again for bilateral breath sounds. Make sure you do not completely remove the ET tube.

Intubating the Esophagus

This often occurs when you insert the ET tube without first seeing the vocal cords or without seeing the light in the midline when using a lighted stylet. As a result, the ET tube is inserted into the esophagus rather than the trachea. The result is rapid inflation of the patient's stomach rather than ventilation of the lungs. If not immediately recognized and corrected, the patient will die. To avoid this, carefully watch the ET tube as it passes through the vocal cords, or monitor the midline position of the lighted stylet. Next, auscultate over the epigastrium and over both lung fields. Watch for the rise and fall of the chest. If there is any doubt, pull out the ET tube, ventilate the patient, and reattempt the intubation. Be sure that you follow the protocol established by your medical director for the number of attempts that you are allowed when intubating a patient. If you are unsuccessful after two attempts, consider using an alternative airway device such as an LMA or a Combitube, or

You are the Provider 3

The patient's endotracheal tube is secured and confirmed via breath sounds and a commercial device. Your partner secures the IV and reassesses the cardiac monitor only to find the patient in asystole. He follows local protocols for drug administration. The patient is loaded into the ambulance and you move up front to drive. Two fire fighters ride in to assist with CPR.

Reassessment	Recording Time: 5 Minutes
Pulse	Pulseless
Blood pressure	-0-
Respirations	Apneic
Breath sounds	Clear bilaterally via ET tube
Pupils	Dilated bilaterally

7. Why should you mark the length of the ET tube?
8. What is your first indication of correct tube placement?
9. What is the most common error that is made during intubation?

insert an oral airway and ventilate with a bag-mask device.

Increased Hypoxia: Taking Too Long to Intubate

Do not take longer than 30 seconds trying to intubate, or the patient will become more hypoxic. Your partner or another member of the team should actually time the intubation. If you cannot complete the procedure within 30 seconds, you should stop and provide bag-mask ventilation and 100% oxygen for 2 to 3 minutes before trying again. Ask a third EMT-B to perform the Sellick maneuver so that you can see the vocal cords more clearly. If after two tries the tube cannot be passed, try another airway technique, or ask another qualified rescuer to try. If the patient is difficult to intubate, you should not waste time in the field. Use another airway adjunct, and provide immediate transport.

Patient Vomiting

A patient who is not totally unresponsive may begin to gag or try to remove the tube. Gagging may cause the patient to vomit and aspirate stomach contents. To avoid this, always check for a gag reflex before intubation, such as by flicking the patient's eyelashes. Patients who tolerate an oral airway do not have an intact gag reflex and may need intubation. You should always have a suctioning unit ready in case the patient vomits during the intubation procedure. Trying to insert an ET tube through the vocal cords can cause a spasm of the cords, or <u>laryngospasm</u>. If this occurs, stop intubating, and provide bag-mask ventilation.

Soft-Tissue Trauma

The laryngoscope and the tip of the ET tube can injure the lips, teeth, tongue, gums, and other airway structures. When used as a lever, the laryngoscope blade can easily break teeth, and pushing a tube blindly through the vocal cords can lacerate the soft tissues in the airway. Careful attention to your technique will minimize the risk of these complications.

Mechanical Failure

You may hear or feel air coming from the oropharynx when ventilating the patient. In an adult, this means that the cuff does not have enough air in it or that it has been torn and is leaking. If this occurs and ventilation is inadequate, you must get more air into the cuff (check the pilot balloon) or replace the tube. In a child, an air leak means that the uncuffed tube is too small or the child is large enough to need a cuffed tube.

EMT-B Safety

After an advanced airway (eg, ET tube, multi-lumen airway, LMA) has been inserted, two rescuers should no longer perform "cycles" of CPR. There should be no pause in compressions to deliver ventilations. The person performing chest compressions continues to do so at a rate of 100/min, and the person ventilating the patient should deliver 1 breath every 6 to 8 seconds (8 to 10 breaths/min).

Patient Intolerant of the ET Tube

Because of the reversal of hypoxia from direct oxygenation, a patient may regain a gag reflex or regain consciousness and try to remove the ET tube. Before removing the tube (<u>extubation</u>) in these circumstances, you should determine that the patient can obey commands. If he or she can, ensure that the suctioning unit is nearby and turned on. Then deflate the cuff, and carefully withdraw the ET tube as the patient exhales. Sometimes you may have to ask the patient to cough. Provide immediate suctioning if the patient vomits, then reassess the airway and administer supplemental oxygen. Always consult medical control before removing the ET tube. Generally, the only reason to extubate a patient in the field is if the patient is unreasonably intolerant of the tube. Be aware that conscious patients are at high risk for laryngospasm immediately following extubation.

Decrease in Heart Rate

Be sure to monitor the patient's vital signs carefully and continuously, particularly the heart rate. In children, it is important to check heart rate and skin color. With ET intubation, the heart rate may decrease when the airway has been stimulated. Use of a straight blade is recommended when intubating small children because it does not stimulate the airway as much as the curved blade.

■ Multilumen Airways

In addition to ET intubation, <u>multilumen airway</u> are other advanced airway devices that may be available to you. Depending on local protocol and your medical director, you may be trained in their use. The benefits and disadvantages of using multilumen airways are listed in Table 27-3 ▶.

Table 27-3 Benefits and Disadvantages of Multilumen Airways

Benefits	Disadvantages
Ease of proper placement	Loses effectiveness (cuff malfunction)
No mask seal necessary	Requires deeply comatose patient
Requires minimal skill and practice to maintain	Requires constant balloon observation
Easily used in spinal injury patients	Cannot be used on patients shorter than 5' tall
May be inserted blindly	Requires great care in listening for breath sounds
Protects the airway from upper airway secretions	Large balloon is easily broken and tends to push the PtL out of the mouth when inflated

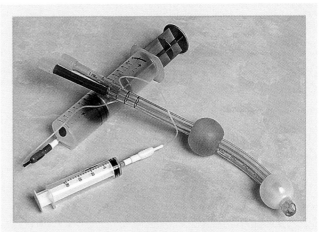

Figure 27-15 The ETC consists of a double-lumen tube and two balloon cuffs. The blue lumen is the primary ventilation port, and the clear lumen is the ventilation port if the tube is placed in the trachea.

The multilumen airways, which are inserted without direct visualization of the vocal cords, have been designed to provide lung ventilation when placed in the trachea or the esophagus, making them much easier to insert than an ET tube. We will review two of these adjuncts, the Esophageal Tracheal Combitube (ETC) and the pharyngeotracheal lumen airway (PtL). Remember that you must be trained and authorized to use these devices.

Esophageal Tracheal Combitube

The Esophageal Tracheal Combitube (ETC) consists of a double-lumen tube and two balloon cuffs Figure 27-15 ▶. The blue lumen (No. 1) is the primary ventilation port when the tube is inserted in the esophagus. The clear lumen (No. 2) is the ventilation port if the tube is placed in the trachea. The clear cuff at the tip of the tube (distal cuff) seals off the esophagus or the trachea; the larger, flesh-colored cuff near the midway point seals off the oropharynx and naso-

pharynx. A blue pilot balloon and a white pilot balloon correspond to the flesh-colored and distal cuffs. Two syringes are also included in the kit. The ETC is a single-use item and must be discarded after use.

The ETC is inserted blindly. If the tube happens to go into the trachea, ventilation is provided directly to the lungs. If the tube goes into the esophagus, as occurs most often, ventilation can still be provided to the patient Figure 27-16 ▶. You do not need to maintain a constant face mask seal with either placement. Instead, the ETC forms a seal in the oropharynx by an inflated cuff in the oropharynx, so you can ventilate the trachea via a tube, rather than a mask. This ease of ventilation is an advantage of the ETC.

Contraindications

Contraindications for the Combitube include the following:

- Conscious or semiconscious patients with a gag reflex
- Children younger than 16 years
- Adults shorter than 5' tall
- Patients who have ingested a caustic substance
- Patients who have a known esophageal disease

You are the Provider 4

The patient is still in asystole upon arrival at the emergency department. He has been down for approximately 30 minutes. The physician on staff reassesses the patient and calls the code.

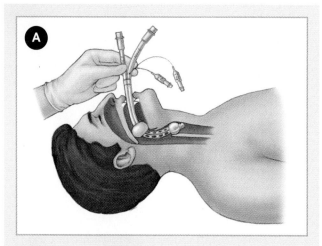

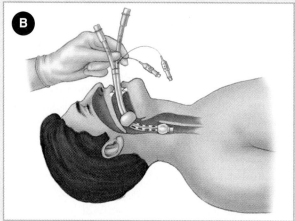

Figure 27-16 A. If the ETC is inserted into the trachea, it functions as an ET tube with ventilation provided directly into the trachea. **B.** If the ETC is inserted into the esophagus, ventilation can still be provided to the patient.

Inserting the ETC

As with ET intubation, you must act quickly and carefully use the ETC.

The steps for insertion of the ETC are as follows:

1. **Assemble and check** your equipment, which should include the ETC kit with syringes, water soluble lubricant, suction unit, device for bag-mask ventilation, and oxygen.

2. **Apply a water-soluble lubricant** to the ETC.

3. **Position the patient.** Open the patient's mouth, and make sure it is clear. Remove the oral airway if one has been inserted. Note that with an unconscious patient who may have a spinal injury, you must maintain the neck in a neutral, in-line position during insertion of the ETC.

4. **Preoxygenate the patient with 100% oxygen** using bag-mask ventilation.

5. **Lift the lower jaw and tongue** away from the posterior pharynx by inserting your thumb deep into the patient's mouth and grasping the tongue and lower jaw between your thumb and index finger.

6. **Gently guide the ETC** along the base of the tongue and into the airway. Hold the ETC so that it curves in the same direction as the natural curvature of the pharynx. Insert the tip into the mouth, and advance it carefully along the tongue. Do not use force. If you meet resistance, pull back and redirect the ETC. When the ETC is at the proper depth, the teeth will be between the heavy black lines.

7. **Inflate the blue pilot balloon** (and flesh-colored cuff) with the predrawn 100-mL blue-tipped syringe. Once the cuff is inflated and the pilot balloon is tense, immediately inflate the white pilot balloon (and the distal cuff) with the smaller, predrawn 15-mL syringe. The ETC usually will move forward a bit.

8. **Ventilate the patient** through the blue (No. 1) tube with bag-mask ventilation.

9. **Confirm the placement** of the tube. If the chest rises and falls and you hear breath sounds, the ETC is in the esophagus. When this is the case, continue to ventilate through the blue (No. 1) tube. If the chest does not rise and fall, and you do not hear breath sounds, the ETC is in the trachea. In this case, apply the device for bag-mask ventilation to the shorter, clear tube (No. 2), and ventilate the patient through it. Listen for breath sounds in all lung fields and over the stomach to verify that proper placement has occurred.

10. **Continuously monitor the patient.** Watch for balloon cuff leaks by carefully squeezing the pilot balloon. Use the syringes to keep the balloon cuffs properly inflated. Balloon cuffs may be torn by broken teeth, dentures, and bones.

Removing the ETC

Removal of the ETC airway is fairly simple. If the patient will no longer tolerate the ETC, you should remove it. Remember that the patient will likely vomit when the ETC is removed, so you must have a suctioning unit readily available. Be sure to turn the patient on his or her side to keep the airway clear of vomitus. When you are ready, simply deflate both balloon cuffs, and gently remove the tube.

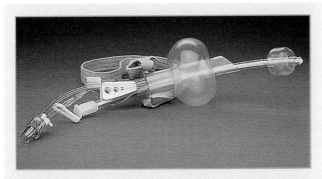

Figure 27-17 The PtL consists of two tubes, two balloon cuffs, a bite block, and a neck-retaining strap.

Pharyngeotracheal Lumen Airway

The pharyngeotracheal lumen airway (PtL) consists of two tubes, two balloon cuffs, a bite block, and a neck-retaining strap   Figure 27-17 ▲ . The long, clear (No. 3) tube contains a stylet and a low-pressure balloon cuff near its tip. The stylet is left in as a plug if the tube is placed in the esophagus but is removed if the tube ends up in the trachea. In either case, the balloon cuff prevents gastric contents from entering the lungs when the cuff is inflated.

The No. 3 tube passes through the larger-diameter, green (No. 2) tube. The No. 2 tube has a large balloon cuff designed to seal the oropharynx. This allows air to pass through it and into the trachea (if the No. 3 tube is placed in the esophagus) and prevents blood and debris from entering the airway from above. The balloon cuff in the No. 2 tube functions as the mask seal. The No. 1 tube is connected to these balloon cuffs to assist with inflation of these important airway seals.

The PtL is designed to be inserted blindly into the oropharynx and esophagus, but you must be trained and authorized to use it. If the tube happens to go into the trachea when blindly inserted, it will function like an ET tube. If the long tube goes into the esophagus, you can still provide adequate ventilation to the patient   Figure 27-18 ▶ . With the PtL, you need not maintain a constant face mask seal. The PtL forms an inflated cuff seal in the oropharynx, and the trachea may be ventilated via a tube rather than a mask.

Contraindications

You should not attempt to use the PtL in the following individuals:

- Conscious or semiconscious patients with a gag reflex

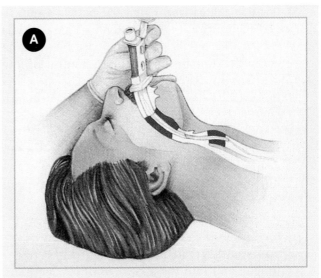

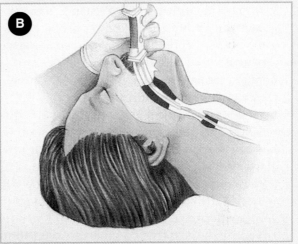

Figure 27-18 The PtL is inserted blindly into the oropharynx. **A.** If the PtL is inserted into the trachea, it functions as an ET tube with ventilation provided directly into the trachea. **B.** If the PtL is inserted into the esophagus, ventilation can still be provided to the patient.

- Children younger than 14 years
- Adults shorter than 5' tall
- Patients who have ingested a caustic substance
- Patients who have a known esophageal disease

Inserting the PtL

Take the following steps to insert the PtL:

1. **Assemble and check** your equipment, which should include a PtL with syringes, water-soluble lubricant, suctioning unit with suction catheters, a device for bag-mask ventilation, and oxygen.
2. **Lubricate the tube** on the PtL with a water-soluble lubricant.

3. **Position the patient.** Open the patient's mouth and make sure it is clear. Remove the oral airway if one has been inserted. With a trauma patient, maintain the neck in a neutral in-line position during insertion of the PtL.

4. **Preoxygenate the patient** with 100% oxygen with bag-mask ventilation.

5. **Lift the lower jaw and tongue** away from the posterior pharynx by inserting your thumb deep into the patient's mouth and grasping the tongue and lower jaw between your thumb and index finger.

6. **Hold the PtL** so that it curves in the same direction as the natural curvature of the pharynx. Gently guide the PtL along the base of the tongue and into the airway until the teeth are against the teeth strap. If resistance is met, pull back and redirect the PtL. When the PtL is at the proper depth, place the neck strap over the patient's head and tighten.

7. **Inflate the balloon cuffs** with the No. 1 tube. Be sure to close the white cap.

8. **Ventilate the patient** through the short, green No. 2 tube, and then listen for breath sounds.

9. **If you see the chest rise and hear equal breath sounds,** the No. 3 tube is in the esophagus, and you should ventilate the patient with the No. 2 tube. If the chest does not rise and fall and you do not hear equal breath sounds, the No. 3 tube is likely in the trachea. In this case, you should remove the stylet from the No. 3 tube and ventilate the patient using the No. 3 tube.

10. **Verify that the patient is receiving adequate ventilation** by listening to the lungs on both sides of the chest and over the stomach as you provide bag-mask ventilation.

11. **Continuously monitor the patient.** Watch for balloon cuff leaks, and use inlet tube No. 1 to keep the balloon cuffs properly inflated. Jagged, broken teeth, dentures, and bones can easily tear balloon cuffs, so you must use special care if the patient has facial trauma.

Removing the PtL

Removing the PtL is a simple procedure. You should remove the PtL if the patient will no longer tolerate it. The patient will likely vomit when the PtL is removed, so you must keep a suctioning unit readily available. Turn the patient to one side to help keep the airway clear of vomitus. When you are ready to remove the PtL, simply deflate the balloon cuffs and gently remove the tube.

■ Laryngeal Mask Airway

The laryngeal mask airway (LMA) was originally developed for use in the operating room. Use of the LMA has been expanded to the prehospital field, especially as an alternative for BLS providers.

The LMA consists of two parts: the tube and the mask or cuff. The device is made of silicone and is available in reusable (after proper sterilization) and disposable types. After blind insertion, the device molds and seals itself around the laryngeal opening by inflation of the mask. The epiglottis is contained within the mask or cuff. The device comes in seven sizes and can be used for children and adults
Table 27-4 ▾.

Use of the device requires training with a manikin. Proponents advocate additional training in an operating room with anesthetized patients to become familiar with the anatomic variations that cannot be duplicated by a manikin. This type of training helps avoid malpositioning. Malpositioning may occur when the device is located somewhere other than over the laryngeal opening or when the device is "folded over" and caught on top of the epiglottis. Malpositions can sometimes be managed by repositioning the patient's head, readjusting the LMA position, or adjusting the amount of air in the cuff. When in doubt, remove the device, ventilate the patient, and start over.

Contraindications

There are potential contraindications to use of the device. When positive-pressure ventilation with high

TABLE 27-4 LMA Sizes		
LMA Size	Patient's Weight or Size	Maximum Air in Mask (mL)
1	<5 kg (11 lb)	4
1.5	5 to 10 kg (11 to 22 lb)	7
2	10 to 20 kg (22 to 44 lb)	10
2.5	20 to 30 kg (44 to 66 lb)	14
3	30 kg (66 lb) to small adult	20
4	Adult	30
5	Large adult	40

airway pressures is required (as for a patient with asthma or chronic obstructive pulmonary disease), the mask may leak. Active vomiting may dislodge the device. Large esophageal tumors may prevent effectiveness of the LMA.

Inserting the LMA

Ensure that the patient has no gag reflex, then follow the steps in ▶ Skill Drill 27-3 ▶ to insert the LMA:

1. **Assemble and check** the proper equipment:
   - BSI equipment
   - LMA and syringe (check the cuff and valve)
   - Water-soluble lubricant
   - Suctioning unit with suctioning catheters
   - Device for bag-mask ventilation and oxygen (**Step ①**)

2. **Open the patient's airway,** and clear it of foreign material. Insert an oropharyngeal airway.

3. **Preoxygenate the patient** with bag-mask ventilation at the appropriate rate, depending on the age of the patient (20 to 24 breaths/min is typical for adults).

4. **Select the appropriate LMA size** as your partner ventilates the patient, and verify that the mask has no leaks. Fully deflate the mask and lubricate it (**Step ②**).

5. **Position the LMA for insertion** with the mask down, holding it like a pen (**Step ③**).

6. **Remove the oropharyngeal airway,** and, keeping the patient's neck flexed and the mouth open, begin to insert the mask (**Step ④**).

7. **When the widest part of the mask** is past the teeth, use your index finger to maintain a continuous forward pressure, sliding the LMA over the hard palate and soft palate into the hypopharynx until definite resistance is felt (**Step ⑤**).

8. **While removing your index finger,** gently press down on the tube with the other hand to prevent the LMA from being pulled out of place (**Step ⑥**).

9. **After ensuring that the black line on the LMA** is facing the upper lip, inflate the mask without holding the tube. Short outward movement is normal (**Step ⑦**).

10. **Confirm placement of the LMA** by listening over the stomach and lungs. You should hear equal breath sounds and see equal chest rise and fall; epigastric sounds should not be heard. Combativeness in a previously unconscious, unresponsive patient indicates that ventilations are successful and the patient has received adequate oxygen. Once this happens, the LMA must be removed immediately.

11. **Once you have verified tube placement,** insert a bite block, such as an oropharyngeal airway, and secure the tube in place with tape or a commercial device. As with other devices, if this device is not properly secured, it will dislodge, preventing oxygen from entering the lungs (**Step ⑧**).

Skill Drill 27-3 Using an LMA

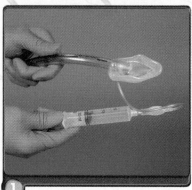

1 Assemble and check equipment.

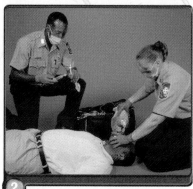

2 Open the airway, insert an oropharyngeal airway, and preoxygenate the patient. Choose the tube size, check the mask for leaks, and deflate and lubricate it.

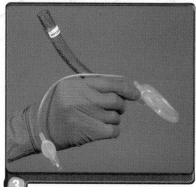

3 Grasp the tube, and position it for insertion, mask down.

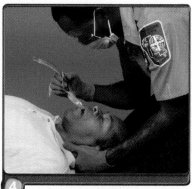

4 Remove the oral airway, and begin to insert the mask.

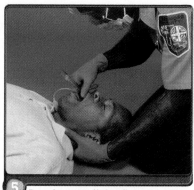

5 By using your index finger, push the mask up onto the hard palate and advance it until you feel resistance.

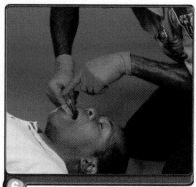

6 Use the other hand to stabilize the tube as you remove your index finger.

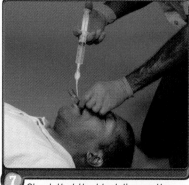

7 Check that the black line on the tube faces the upper lip, then inflate the tube without holding it.

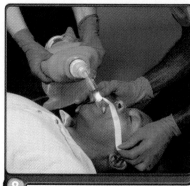

8 Confirm tube placement by listening over the stomach and lungs and with a secondary confirmation device. Insert a bite block, and secure the LMA.

You are the Provider   Summary

Not every call results in a positive outcome; however, airway is the first priority in treating any patient. Proficiency on your part may make all the difference. Practice intubation frequently on manikins so that you are prepared when you are called upon in the field.

1. What is the first step in treating this patient?
Suction the airway.

2. Can you use an AED on this patient?
Yes. The pads should not be placed over the site of the pacemaker.

3. When should you attempt a definitive airway?
As soon as possible after indicated shocks and one or two rounds of CPR. With an endotracheal tube in place, an ALS provider can administer drugs via the ET tube if no IV is established.

4. What equipment is needed to perform an intubation?
- BSI equipment
- Properly sized ET tube
- Laryngoscope handle and blade
- Stylet
- 10-mL syringe
- Oxygen with bag-mask device
- Suction unit and suction catheters
- Magill forceps
- Towels
- Stethoscope
- Water-soluble lubricant
- Commercial securing device or tape
- Secondary confirmation device

5. What is the Sellick maneuver?
Pressure applied to the cricoid cartilage. It serves the purpose of squeezing the esophagus shut and helping to prevent solids and liquids from leaving the esophagus and being aspirated into the trachea. It also helps to place the trachea in a better position for the rescuer who is trying to intubate when the trachea is very anterior.

6. What size tube should this patient require?
The proper-sized tube for an adult man ranges from 7.5 to 8.5 mm. For most efficient use of the tube, use the largest-diameter ET tube that you can.

7. Why should you mark the length of the ET tube?
Once the patient is intubated, you should monitor the centimeter marking at the patient's teeth because this will determine whether the tube has moved from its original position.

8. What is your first indication of correct tube placement?
Visualizing the cuff passing through the vocal cords.

9. What is the most common error that is made during intubation?
Intubating the right mainstem bronchus. If you push or accidentally slip the tube in too far, the ET tube will pass into the right mainstem bronchus because it is shorter and straighter than the left mainstem bronchus.

Prep Kit

Ready for Review

- Gastric tubes provide a channel directly into a patient's stomach, allowing for the removal of gas, blood, and toxins and for the administration of medications and nutrition. In the field, gastric tubes are most commonly used to decompress the stomach of a patient with gastric distention.
- There are two types of gastric tubes: nasogastric tubes and orogastric tubes. An orogastric tube, which is inserted through the mouth, is safer and easier to use. A nasogastric tube, which is inserted through the nose, can cause nasal trauma with bleeding and, in patients with a skull fracture, can be passed accidentally into the brain. Either type of tube can be passed accidentally into the trachea.
- Insertion of a gastric tube is a delicate task that should be performed only according to local EMS protocol.
- Special care should be taken when inserting a gastric tube in a patient who has head, spinal, or major facial trauma.
- Oral intubation is needed for patients who are unconscious, unresponsive, or in cardiac arrest.
- Orotracheal intubation controls and protects the airway and may be used long term if necessary. It also permits direct access to the trachea for suctioning, the delivery of high volumes of oxygen at higher than normal pressures, and the administration of certain medications.
- There are two techniques for insertion of an ET tube: using a laryngoscope and using a lighted stylet.
- Complications of ET intubation include intubation of the right mainstem bronchus or the esophagus, increased hypoxia because of taking too long to intubate, causing soft-tissue trauma, mechanical failure, and a decrease in heart rate. A patient who regains consciousness may vomit and/or try to remove the tube.
- A patient who has been intubated must be monitored continuously to evaluate the heart rate (especially in children) and lung sounds. In addition, movement of the patient can dislodge the ET tube. Always reassess breath sounds after any patient movement.
- The Esophageal Tracheal Combitube, the pharyngeotracheal lumen airway, and the laryngeal mask airway are inserted blindly and are easier to insert than an ET tube. However, you must be trained and authorized to use these devices.

Technology

- Interactivities
- Vocabulary Explorer
- Anatomy Review
- Web Links
- Online Review Manual

Vital Vocabulary

cricoid cartilage   A rigid, ring-shaped structure that completely encircles the larynx at the top of the trachea.

cricoid pressure   A technique that is used with intubation in which pressure is applied on either side of the cricoid cartilage to prevent gastric distention and aspiration and allow better visualization of vocal cords; also called the Sellick maneuver.

decompress   To release from pressure or compression.

end-tidal carbon dioxide detectors   Plastic, disposable indicators that signal by color change when an ET tube is in the proper place.

endotracheal intubation   Insertion of an endotracheal (ET) tube directly through the larynx between the vocal cords and into the trachea to maintain and protect an airway.

Esophageal Tracheal Combitube (ETC)   A multilumen airway that consists of a single, dual-lumen tube with two cuffs.

extubation   Removal of a tube after it has been placed.

gastric tube   An advanced airway adjunct that provides a channel directly into a patient's stomach for the removal of gas, blood, or toxins, or the instillation of medications and nutrition.

laryngeal mask airway (LMA)   An advanced airway device that is blindly inserted into the mouth to isolate the larynx for direct ventilation; consists of a tube and a mask or cuff that inflates to seal around the laryngeal opening.

laryngoscope   An instrument used to give a direct view of the patient's vocal cords during endotracheal intubation.

laryngospasm   Spasm of the larynx and surrounding structures.

lighted stylet   An instrument used to aid in blind insertion of an endotracheal tube.

multilumen airways   Advanced airway devices, such as the Esophageal Tracheal Combitube and the pharyngeotracheal lumen airway, that have multiple tubes to aid in ventilation, and will work whether placed in the trachea or esophagus.

nasotracheal intubation   Endotracheal intubation through the nose.

orotracheal intubation   Endotracheal intubation through the mouth.

pharyngeotracheal lumen airway (PtL)   A multilumen airway that consists of two tubes, two masks, and a bite block.

Sellick maneuver   A technique that is used with intubation in which pressure is applied on either side of the cricoid cartilage to prevent gastric distention and aspiration and allow better visualization of vocal cords; also called cricoid pressure.

stylet   A plastic-coated wire that gives added rigidity and shape to the endotracheal tube.

vallecula   The space between the base of the tongue and the epiglottis; receives the tip of a curved laryngoscope blade during endotracheal intubation.

Assessment in Action

You must be familiar with equipment, procedures, and anatomical landmarks in order to effectively perform advanced airway management. Establishing and maintaining a patient's airway is the single most important manipulative skill you will use as an EMT-B.

1. The _____ is located just below the Adam's apple.
   A. thyroid cartilage
   B. cricoid cartilage
   C. carina
   D. epiglottis

2. A nasogastric tube is contraindicated in a patient with major trauma to the _____.
   A. face
   B. head
   C. spine
   D. all of the above

3. The _____ is the space between the base of the tongue and the epiglottis.
   A. carina
   B. hyoid
   C. vallecula
   D. pyriform fossae

4. A _____ adds rigidity to an endotracheal tube.
   A. laryngoscope
   B. Miller blade
   C. distal cuff
   D. stylet

5. A _____ is an advanced airway that provides a channel directly into the patient's stomach.
   A. oropharyngeal airway
   B. nasopharyngeal airway
   C. gastric tube
   D. combitube

6. An LMA should not be used in which situation(s)?
   A. when there are esophageal tumors
   B. when there is vomiting
   C. when high airway pressures are required
   D. all of the above

Challenging Questions

7. What are the contraindications for the use of the Combitube?

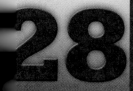

Assisting with IV Therapy

You are the Provider 1

You are assisting your EMT-I partner in starting an IV on a 57-year-old man who is complaining of abdominal pain with nausea and vomiting. He has been sick for 2 days and presents with skin tenting, making him a difficult stick.

Initial Assessment	Recording Time: 3 Minutes
Appearance	Pale, diaphoretic
Level of consciousness	Alert and oriented
Airway	Open and clear
Breathing	Normal
Circulation	Radial pulses present, a little tachycardic

1. What are your considerations for starting an IV on this patient?
2. What size IV catheter should you use?
3. What type of administration set will you use?

Introduction

This chapter is a review of assisting an advanced life support (ALS) provider in setting up the equipment necessary to gain intravenous (IV) access. We will review the equipment used and how to recognize potential complications of IV therapy.

IV Techniques and Administration

The most important thing to remember about IV techniques and fluid administration is to keep the IV equipment sterile. Planning ahead will help prevent mental and procedural errors while inserting an IV needle or catheter.

One way to ensure proper technique is to develop a routine to follow as you assemble the appropriate equipment. A routine will help you keep track of your equipment and the steps necessary to complete successful IV administration.

Equipment Assembly

To avoid delays or the possibility of IV site contamination, gather and prepare all of the equipment before the IV attempt. Table 28-1 ▶ lists a logical sequence of steps for assembling the equipment.

Choosing an IV Solution

In the prehospital setting, the choice of IV solution is limited to the <u>isotonic crystalloids</u>, normal saline (also called NS) and lactated Ringer's (also called LR) solutions. D_5W (5% dextrose in water) is commonly used as for administering medication.

Each IV solution bag is wrapped in a protective sterile plastic bag and is guaranteed to remain sterile

---

TABLE 28-1 EMT-B Steps in Assembling IV Equipment

1. Get your gloves on! BSI precautions cannot be emphasized strongly enough.
2. Obtain the solution requested by your ALS partner—check the bag for clarity, expiration date, and correct solution.
3. Choose an appropriate administration set for the patient.
4. Obtain the catheter requested by your ALS partner. Have a couple of catheters ready for insertion.
5. Spike the bag by inserting the administration set into the port in the fluid bag.
6. Allow fluid to pass through the administration set to completely displace all of the air in the tubing.
7. Tear tape for securing the IV site.
8. Open an alcohol wipe.
9. Have 4" × 4" pieces of gauze ready for catching blood.
10. After your ALS partner has inserted the catheter, adequately dispose of sharps.
11. Hook up the IV tubing, and adjust the flow.

---

until the posted expiration date. Once the protective wrap is torn and removed, the IV solution has a shelf life of 24 hours. The bottom of each IV bag has two ports: an injection port for medication and an <u>access port</u> for connecting the administration set Figure 28-1 ▼. The sterile access port is protected by a

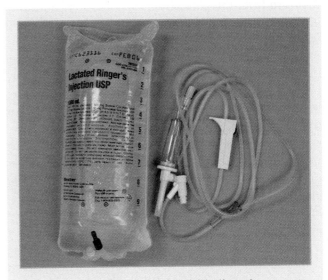

Figure 28-1 An IV bag with an administration set.

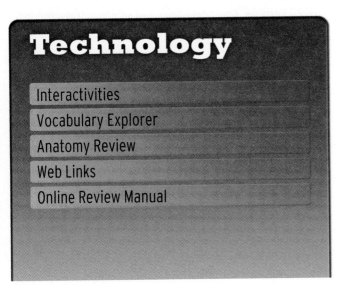

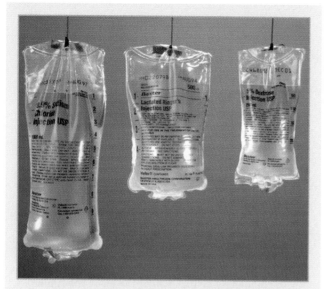

Figure 28-2 Examples of different IV bag sizes

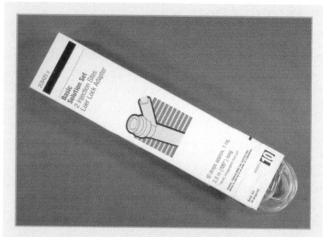

Figure 28-3 The number visible on the drip set refers to the number of drops it takes for a milliliter of fluid to pass though the orifice and into the drip chamber.

removable pigtail. Once this is removed, the bag must be used immediately or discarded.

Bags of IV solution come in different fluid volumes (Figure 28-2 ▲). In the prehospital setting, the IV bags are usually 1,000 mL or 500 mL. The smaller volumes (250 mL and 100 mL) usually are bags of D₅W and are used for mixing and administering medication.

Choosing an Administration Set

An <u>administration set</u> moves fluid from the IV bag into the patient's vascular system. As with IV solution bags, IV administration sets are sterile as long as they remain in their protective packaging. Once they are removed from the packaging, their sterility cannot be guaranteed. Each IV administration set has a <u>piercing spike</u> protected by a plastic cover. Again, once the piercing spike is exposed and the seal surrounding the cap is broken, the set must be used immediately or discarded.

There are different sizes of administration sets for different situations and patients. Most <u>drip sets</u> have a number visible on the package (Figure 28-3 ▶), which indicates the number of drops it takes for a milliliter of fluid to pass through the orifice and into the <u>drip chamber</u>. Drip sets commonly used in the prehospital environment come in two primary sizes: microdrip and macrodrip. A <u>microdrip set</u> allows 60 gtt (drops)/mL through the small, needlelike orifice inside the drip chamber. Microdrip sets are ideal for medication administration or pediatric fluid delivery because it is easy to control their fluid flow. A <u>macrodrip set</u> allows

10 to 15 gtt/mL through a large opening between the piercing spike and the drip chamber. Macrodrip sets are best used for rapid fluid replacement but can also be used for maintenance and <u>keep-the-vein-open (KVO) IV setup</u> or <u>to-keep-open (TKO) IV setup</u>.

Preparing an Administration Set

After choosing the IV administration set and the IV solution bag, verify the expiration date of the solution and check for solution clarity. Review the steps in Skill Drill 28-1 ▶ for spiking an IV bag.

1. **Remove the rubber pigtail** found on the end of the IV bag by pulling on it. The bag is still sealed and will not leak until the piercing spike of the IV administration set punctures this port.
2. **Remove the protective cover** from the piercing spike (remember, this spike is sterile!) (**Step ①**).
3. **Slide the spike into the IV bag port** until you see fluid enter the drip chamber (**Step ②**).
4. **Allow the solution to run freely** through the drip chamber and into the tubing to prime the line and flush the air out of the tubing (**Step ③**).
5. **Twist the protective cover** on the opposite end of the IV tubing to allow air to escape. Carefully remove the cover without breaching sterility. Let the fluid flow until air bubbles are removed from the line before turning the roller clamp wheel to stop the flow (**Step ④**). Replace the cover.
6. **Check the drip chamber;** it should be only half filled. The fluid level must be visible to

Skill Drill   28-1   Spiking the Bag

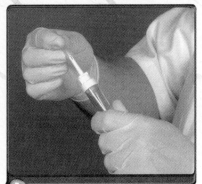

1 Remove the rubber pigtail found on the end of the IV bag by pulling on it. Remove the protective cover from the piercing spike.

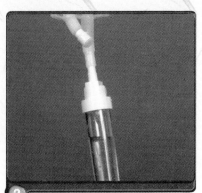

2 Slide the spike into the IV bag port until you see fluid enter the drip chamber.

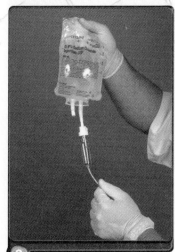

3 Allow the solution to run freely through the drip chamber and into the tubing to prime the line and flush the air out of the tubing.

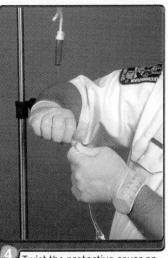

4 Twist the protective cover on the opposite end of the IV tubing to allow air to escape. Remove the cover. Let the fluid flow until air bubbles are removed from the line before turning the roller clamp wheel to stop the flow. Replace the cover.

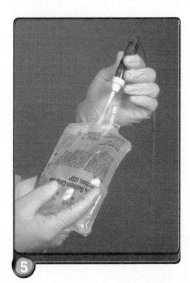

5 Check the drip chamber; it should be only half filled. If the fluid level is too low, squeeze the chamber until it fills; if the chamber is too full, invert the bag and the chamber and squeeze the chamber to empty the fluid back into the bag. Hang the bag in the appropriate location with the end of the IV tubing easily accessible.

calculate drip rates. If the fluid level is too low; squeeze the chamber until it fills; if the chamber is too full, invert the bag and the chamber and squeeze the chamber to empty the fluid back into the bag (**Step ⑤**).

7. Hang the bag in the appropriate location with the end of the IV tubing easily accessible.

Catheters

In IV therapy, a <u>catheter</u> is a hollow, plastic tube surrounding a needle that is inserted into a vein to keep the vein open **Figure 28-4 ▶**. The most common types of catheters found in the prehospital setting are <u>over-the-needle catheters</u> and <u>butterfly catheters</u> **Figure 28-5 ▶**. Advanced life support providers select

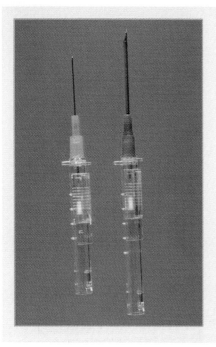

Figure 28-4 Over-the-needle catheters are commonly used in the prehospital environment.

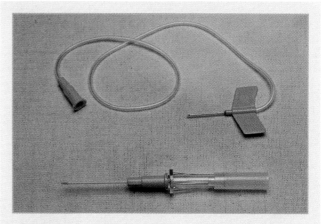

Figure 28-5 A butterfly catheter (top) and an over-the-needle catheter (bottom).

the catheter based on the purpose of the IV (fluid therapy versus medication administration), the age of the patient, and the location for the IV.

Catheters are sized by their diameter and referred to by the <u>gauge</u> of the catheter. A larger-diameter catheter corresponds to a smaller gauge. Thus, a 14-gauge catheter has a greater diameter than a 22-gauge catheter. With larger-diameter catheters, more fluid can be delivered into the vein faster.

Securing the Line

Once the catheter is in position and the IV is flowing properly, the site must be secured. Tape the area so that the catheter and tubing are securely anchored in case of a sudden pull on the line Figure 28-6 ▶. You should tear the tape before the IV catheter is inserted, because you will need one hand to stabilize the site while you tape the IV catheter and tubing. Double back the tubing to create a loop that will act as a shock absorber if the line is pulled accidentally. Avoid circumferential taping around any extremity because circumferential taping can act like a constricting band and stop circulation.

You are the Provider 2

You and your partner attempt to start an IV in the patient's left dorsal hand only to have blood pool in the tissue around the site. You remove the catheter and properly cover the site. A second attempt is made in the left forearm. This time you are able to feed the catheter into the vein and attach the IV fluid. After opening up the fluid, you note that is some puffiness around the IV site that does not appear to be bleeding.

Vital Signs	Recording Time: 5 Minutes
Skin	Pale, diaphoretic
Pulse	108 beats/min, irregular
Blood pressure	126/74 mm Hg
Respirations	20 breaths/min

4. Why was the second site in the forearm?
5. Why is there puffiness around the IV site when fluid is administered?
6. What should you do next?

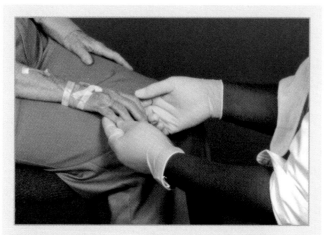

Figure 28-6 Tape the area so that the catheter and tubing are securely anchored.

■ Alternative IV Sites and Techniques

A <u>saline lock</u> is a way to maintain an active IV site without having to run fluids through the vein. This access device is used primarily for patients who do not need additional fluids but may need rapid medication delivery. A saline lock is attached to the end of an IV catheter and filled with approximately 2 mL of normal saline to keep blood from clotting at the end of the catheter (Figure 28-7 ▶). Saline remains in the port without entering the vein.

An <u>intraosseous (IO) needle</u> is used for emergency venous access in pediatric patients when immediate IV access is difficult or impossible. Often the children are experiencing a life-threatening situation such as cardiac arrest, status epilepticus, or progressive shock. The IO needle is inserted in the proximal tibia with a rigid, boring IV catheter, commonly known as a <u>Jamshidi needle</u> (Figure 28-8 ▶). This double needle, consisting of a solid boring needle inside a sharpened hollow needle, is pushed into the bone with a screwing, twisting action.

<u>External jugular IVs</u> provide venous access through the external jugular veins of the neck. These

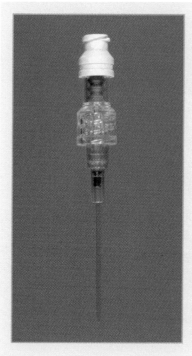

Figure 28-7 A saline lock is attached to the end of an IV catheter and filled with approximately 2 mL of normal saline.

are the same veins used to assess jugular vein distention. The vein is compressed by placing a finger on the vein above the clavicle, causing the vein to fill.

The catheter is inserted into the vein in the same manner as any other IV catheter, except the insertion point is very specific. The catheter is inserted midway between the angle of the jaw and the midclavicular line, with the catheter pointed toward the shoulder on the same side as the puncture site (Figure 28-9 ▶). These punctures are difficult because the veins are surrounded by a very tough, fibrous sheath that makes access difficult. Understanding the procedure is important because you may need to assist.

📝 Documentation Tips

Document the size of the IV catheter, the site, the type of fluid and flow rate, and any complications encountered.

Example: 20g IV L AC c NS @ 100 mL/hour

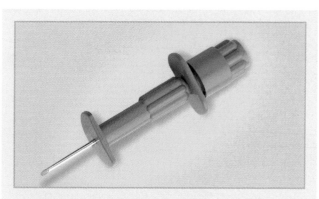

Figure 28-8 An intraosseous (IO) needle is used for emergency venous access in pediatric patients when immediate IV access is difficult or impossible.

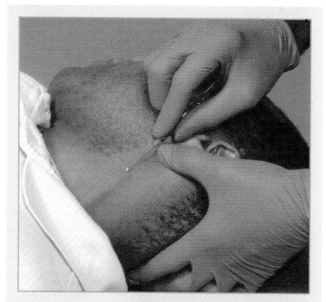

Figure 28-9 The external jugular IV requires a very specific insertion site midway between the angle of the jaw and the midclavicular line with the catheter pointed toward the shoulder on the same side as the puncture.

◼ Possible Complications of IV Therapy

Peripheral IV insertion carries risks. The problems associated with IV administration can be categorized as local reactions or systemic complications. <u>Local reactions</u> include problems like infiltration and phlebitis. <u>Systemic complications</u> include allergic reactions and circulatory overload.

Local IV Site Reactions

Most local reactions require that the IV catheter be removed and reinserted at an alternative site. Examples of common local reactions include infiltration, phlebitis, occlusion, vein irritation, and hematoma.

Infiltration

<u>Infiltration</u> is the escape of fluid into the surrounding tissue. This escape of fluid can cause a localized area of edema or simply swelling. Common causes of infiltration include the following:

- The IV catheter has passed completely through the vein and out the other side.
- The patient is moving excessively.
- The tape used to secure the area has become loose or dislodged.
- The catheter was inserted at too shallow an angle and has only entered the tissue surrounding the vein (more common with IV catheters in larger veins, such as those in the upper arm and neck).

The following are some of the signs and symptoms of infiltration:

- Edema at the catheter site
- Extremely slow IV flow despite use of a large catheter

You are the Provider 3

After removing the IV that has infiltrated, your partner looks for a site in the opposite extremity to no avail. The patient tells her that he has had surgery on that arm after a fracture and that there is usually not a vein available. She moves back to the left arm and is able to palpate a vein in the antecubital fossae. She is able to cannulate the vein and the IV is now flowing.

Reassessment	Recording Time: 7 Minutes
Pulse	112 beats/min, irregular
Blood pressure	126/78 mm Hg
Respirations	16 breaths/min
Breath sounds	Clear bilaterally
Pulse oximetry	98% while breathing room air

7. What should you watch for?
8. What is a catheter shear?
9. What should you watch for to avoid fluid overload?

- Patient complaint of tightness and pain around the IV site

To correct the infiltration, an ALS provider must remove the IV catheter and reinsert it at an alternative site. After this is done, you may apply direct pressure over the swollen area to reduce further swelling or bleeding into the tissue. Avoid wrapping tape around the extremity to apply direct pressure.

Phlebitis

Phlebitis is inflammation of the vein. Phlebitis is not usually seen with emergency prehospital patients, although you may encounter it in patients with IV drug abuse and in patients receiving IV therapy in a hospital outpatient treatment or home health care program. Often phlebitis is associated with fever, tenderness, and red streaking along the course of the associated vein. Some of the more common causes of phlebitis include localized irritation and infection from nonsterile equipment, prolonged IV therapy, and irritating IV solutions. If the phlebitis occurs, the ALS provider must discontinue and reestablish the IV therapy at another location, using new equipment.

Occlusion

In IV therapy, occlusion is the physical blockage of a vein or catheter. If the flow rate is not sufficient to keep fluid moving out of the catheter tip and if blood enters the catheter, a clot may form and occlude the flow. The first sign of a possible occlusion is a decreasing drip rate or the presence of blood in the IV tubing. Proximity to a valve is often the reason for this problem. Other causes can be related to patient movement that allows the line to become physically blocked, such as resting on the IV line or crossing the arms. Occlusion may also develop if the IV bag is nearly empty and the blood pressure overcomes the flow and causes blood to back up into the line.

Vein Irritation

Occasionally, a patient will experience vein irritation in reaction to the IV fluid. This is more common with IV medication administration and very uncommon with administration of pure IV fluids. Patients who have this problem often complain immediately that the IV is bothering them. It may tingle, sting, or itch. Note these complaints, and observe the patient closely in case a more serious allergic reaction develops.

The cause of venous irritation is usually excessively rapid infusion of an irritating solution. If

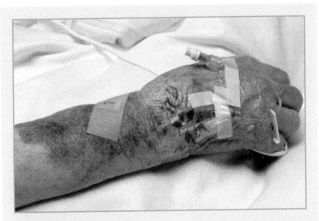

Figure 28-10 Hematomas can be caused by the improper removal of a catheter, resulting in the pooling of blood around the IV site, leading to tenderness and pain.

redness develops at the IV site with early phlebitis, the IV fluid should be discontinued. The ALS provider should reestablish a new IV site proximal to the site of the initial reaction using all new equipment.

Hematoma

A hematoma is an accumulation of blood in the tissues surrounding an IV site. Hematomas result from vein perforation or improper catheter removal, which allows blood to accumulate in the surrounding tissues. Blood can be seen rapidly pooling around the IV site, leading to tenderness and pain Figure 28-10 . Patients with a history of vascular diseases (such as in diabetes) or patients receiving certain drug therapies (such as corticosteroids) can have a predisposition to vein rupture or have a tendency toward rapid development of hematomas with IV insertion.

If a hematoma develops when IV catheter insertion is attempted, the procedure should stop. Direct pressure should be applied to help minimize bleeding. Application of ice may help. If a hematoma develops after a successful catheter insertion, evaluate the IV flow and the hematoma. This can be done by lowering the IV bag and watching for blood backup into the line. If the hematoma appears to be controlled and the flow is not affected, monitor the IV site and leave the line in place. If the hematoma develops as a result of discontinuing the IV, apply direct pressure to the site with a 4" × 4" gauze pad.

Systemic Complications

Systemic complications can evolve from reactions or complications associated with IV catheter insertion.

These complications can be life threatening and include allergic reactions, air embolus, catheter shear, circulatory overload, and vasovagal reactions.

Allergic Reactions

Allergic reactions to IV therapy are usually minor, but anaphylaxis is possible and must be treated aggressively. Allergic reactions can be related to an individual's unexpected sensitivity to an IV fluid or (much more commonly) to a medication. This sensitivity could be an unknown condition to the patient, so careful monitoring of the patient's condition is important.

Patient presentation depends on the extent of the reaction. Common signs and symptoms of an allergic reaction include itching, edema of face and hands, wheezing, shortness of breath, and urticaria.

If an allergic reaction occurs, the ALS provider should discontinue the IV fluid and remove the solution. Maintain an open airway, and monitor the ABCs and vital signs.

Air Embolus

Healthy adults can tolerate as much as 200 mL of air introduced into the circulatory system, but patients who are already ill or injured can be affected if any air is introduced. Properly flushing an IV line will help eliminate any potential of introducing air into a patient. IV bags are designed to collapse as they empty to help prevent this problem, but collapse does not always occur. Be sure to replace empty IV bags with full ones.

If your patient begins having respiratory distress, consider the possibility of an air embolus. Other signs and symptoms include cyanosis (even in the presence of high-flow oxygen), signs and symptoms of shock, loss of consciousness, and respiratory arrest.

Treat a patient with a suspected air embolus by placing the patient on his or her left side with the head down. Be prepared to ventilate the patient if he or she experiences increasing shortness of breath. Symptomatic air embolus is an extremely rare event and should be considered only after more common explanations for the patient's presenting symptoms have been excluded.

Catheter Shear

Catheter shear occurs when part of the catheter is pinched against the needle, and the needle slices through the catheter, creating a free-floating segment. This allows the catheter segment to travel through the circulatory system and possibly end up in the pulmonary circulation, causing a pulmonary embolus.

Treatment involves surgical removal of the sheared tip. Catheter hubs are radiopaque (that is, they will appear white in a radiograph) to aid in diagnosing this type of problem. This problem is caused by rethreading needles through catheters after they have been removed. To avoid this problem, a catheter should never be rethreaded back into a needle.

Patients who have experienced catheter shear present with sudden shortness of breath and possibly diminished breath sounds. The symptoms mimic those of an air embolus and can be treated the same way. Affected patients need continued IV access.

Circulatory Overload

An unmonitored IV bag can lead to circulatory overload. Healthy adults can handle as much as 2 to 3 extra liters of fluid without compromise. Problems occur when the patient has cardiac, pulmonary, or renal dysfunction. These types of conditions do not allow the patient to tolerate the additional demands associated with increased circulatory volume. The most common cause for circulatory overload in the prehospital setting is failure to readjust the drip rate after flushing an IV line immediately after insertion. Always monitor IV bags to ensure the proper drip rate.

Patient presentation includes shortness of breath, jugular vein distention, and increased blood pressure. Crackles are often heard when evaluating breath sounds. Acute peripheral edema can also indicate circulatory overload.

To treat a patient with circulatory overload, slow the IV rate to keep the vein open and raise the patient's head to ease respiratory distress. Administer high-flow oxygen, and monitor vital signs. Medical control should be contacted immediately.

Vasovagal Reactions

Some patients have anxiety concerning needles or in response to the sight of blood. Such anxiety may lead to a drop in blood pressure, and the patient may collapse. Patients can present with anxiety, diaphoresis, nausea, and syncopal episodes.

Treatment for a patient with a vasovagal reaction centers on treating for shock. Place the patient in the shock position, administer high flow oxygen, and monitor the vital signs.

Troubleshooting

Several factors can influence the IV flow rate. It is always helpful to perform the following checks after initiating IV fluid administration.

- **Check the IV fluid.** Thick, viscous fluids infuse slowly and may be diluted to help speed delivery. Cold fluids run slower than warm fluids. If possible, warm IV fluids should be administered during cold months.
- **Check the administration set.** Macrodrips are used for rapid fluid delivery, whereas microdrips are designed to deliver a more controlled flow.
- **Check the height of the IV bag.** The IV bag must be hung high enough to overcome the patient's own blood pressure. Hang the bag as high as possible.
- **Check the type of catheter used.** The wider the catheter (the smaller the gauge), the more fluid that can be delivered; 14 gauge is the widest, 27 gauge the narrowest.
- **Check the tourniquet.** A tourniquet or constricting band is used to start the IV. Accidentally leaving the constricting band on the patient's arm after establishing IV access can prevent the IV fluid from flowing at the proper rate.

Age-specific Considerations

Pediatric and geriatric patients have different medical needs from those of the general medical population, making it sometimes necessary to use other methods of assessment and treatment.

IV Therapy for Pediatric Patients

The same IV solutions and equipment as used for adults can be used for pediatric patients with a few exceptions. If an over-the-needle IV catheter is used, the 20-, 22-, 24-, or 26-gauge catheters are best for insertion **Figure 28-11 ▶**. Butterfly catheters are ideal for pediatric patients and can be placed in the same locations as over-the-needle catheters, as well as in visible scalp veins. Scalp veins are best used in infants. Intra-

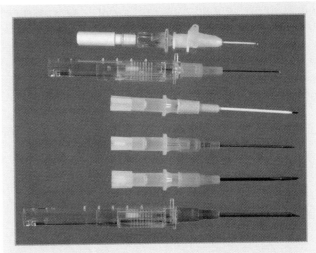
Figure 28-11 Note the difference in sizes of catheters.

osseous needles can be used for difficult and emergency fluid infusions. Stabilization is critical for these lines to maintain adequate flow. Once established, IO lines work as well as peripheral lines.

Fluid control for pediatric patients is important. Using a special type of microdrip set called a Volutrol IV allows you to fill the large drip chamber with a specific amount of fluid and administer only this amount to avoid fluid overload. The 100-mL calibrated drip chamber can be shut off from the IV bag.

IV Therapy for Geriatric Patients

Smaller catheters may be preferable for geriatric patients unless rapid fluid replacement is needed. Some

🖐 EMT-B Safety

All IV needles should be placed in the sharps container *immediately* after removal from the catheter to prevent an accidental needle stick.

You are the Provider 4

The patient is given a 20 mg/kg bolus of an isotonic crystalloid solution and is feeling a little better upon arrival at the emergency department. His IV has been slowed down to a KVO rate to prevent fluid overload. He is treated for a gastrointestinal virus in the ED and sent home with medication for nausea and diarrhea.

medications commonly used by older patients have the tendency to create fragile skin and veins. Often, simply puncturing the vein will cause a massive hematoma. The use of tape can lead to skin damage, so be careful when taping IV catheters and tubing on older patients.

The use of the smaller catheters (such as 20-, 22-, or 24-gauge catheters) may be more comfortable for the patient and can reduce the risk of extravasation. If fluid resuscitation is necessary, an appropriately sized catheter must be used.

Be careful when using macrodrips because they can allow rapid infusion of fluids, which may lead to edema if they are not monitored closely. With both geriatric and pediatric patients, fluid overload is a real possibility.

You are the Provider Summary

Initiating IVs requires a lot of practice to become proficient. Once you have stuck the patient unsuccessfully a couple of times, let someone else try. Everyone has off days, and some patients are extremely difficult to stick. In extreme cases, a physician may be needed to insert a central line.

1. What are your considerations for starting an IV on this patient?
Since he is dehydrated he will probably be difficult to stick. Even though he is not necessarily a geriatric patient, he may still have some of the qualities that make IVs more difficult.

2. What size IV catheter should you use?
An 18-gauge or 20-gauge should be used for a medical patient.

3. What type of administration set will you use?
A maxidrip (10-15 drop set); follow local protocol.

4. Why was the second site in the forearm?
Due to the way the veins branch off as you move further down the arm, you should never stick below a site that has already been stuck. Always start low and work your way up unless the patient is immediately critical. In this case (such as cardiac arrest) you should not start lower than the antecubital fossae.

5. Why is there puffiness around the IV site when fluid is administered?
The IV has infiltrated and fluid is escaping into the surrounding tissue.

6. What should you do next?
Stop the IV and attempt to start another either higher in the same extremity or in the opposite extremity.

7. What should you watch for?
Any infiltration, swelling or tenderness around the site, possible allergic reaction, and vein irritation.

8. What is a catheter shear?
Catheter shear occurs when part of the catheter is pinched against the needle, and the needle slices through the catheter, creating a free-floating segment. This allows the segment to travel through the circulatory system and possibly end up in the pulmonary circulation, causing a pulmonary embolus.

9. What should you watch for to avoid fluid overload?
Monitor the flow rate carefully and make note of any cardiac, pulmonary, or renal dysfunction. The signs of fluid overload are shortness of breath, JVD, rales, and increased blood pressure.

Prep Kit

Ready for Review

- Understanding the equipment used in IV access and knowing how to prepare it will help you to be a critical member of an ALS team.
- Anticipating your partner's needs and following a logical sequence of steps in assembling the equipment will help facilitate IV access.
- It is absolutely essential to take proper BSI precautions on any call involving IV therapy.
- In the prehospital setting, the choice of IV solution is usually limited to normal saline (NS) and lactated Ringer's (LR) solution.
- As an EMT-B, you can assist by preparing the equipment and supplies for IV therapy; checking the bag for clarity, expiration date, and correct solution; choosing the appropriate administration set; and spiking the bag.
- Once the IV is established, you should secure the site by taping the area.
- An administration set moves fluid from the IV bag into the patient's vascular system. Each IV administration set has a piercing spike protected by a plastic cover.
- Drip sets commonly used in the prehospital environment come in two primary sizes: microdrip and macrodrip. Microdrip sets allow 60 gtt/mL into the drip chamber. Macrodrip sets allow 10 to 15 gtt/mL into the drip chamber.
- A catheter is a hollow, laser-sharpened needle inside a hollow plastic tube inserted into a vein to keep the vein open. The most common type in the prehospital setting is the over-the-needle catheter.
- Alternative IV sites and techniques include saline locks, IO access, and external jugular IVs. A saline lock is attached to the end of an IV catheter and filled with approximately 2 mL of normal saline to keep blood from clotting at the end of the catheter. Access by the IO route is established in the proximal tibia with a rigid, boring IV catheter. External jugular IVs provide venous access through the external jugular veins of the neck.
- Possible complications of IV therapy include local reactions and systemic complications. Local reactions include infiltration, phlebitis, occlusion, vein irritation, and hematoma. Systemic complications include allergic reactions, air embolus, catheter shear, circulatory overload, and vasovagal reactions.
- If you encounter problems with the IV flowing effectively, potential causes are the fluid used, the administration set, the height of the bag, the type of catheter used, and the presence of a tourniquet.
- Pediatric and geriatric populations warrant specific attention. Different equipment and sites may be used for them. Older skin is more delicate and must be handled with care.

Vital Vocabulary

access port A sealed hub on an administration set designed for sterile access to the IV fluid.

administration set Tubing that connects to the IV bag access port and the catheter to deliver the IV fluid.

butterfly catheters Rigid, hollow, venous cannulation devices identified by plastic "wings" that act as anchoring points for securing the catheter.

catheter A flexible, hollow structure that drains or delivers fluids.

catheter shear The cutting of the catheter by the needle during improper rethreading of the catheter with the needle; the severed piece can then enter the circulatory system.

drip chamber The area of the administration set where fluid accumulates so that the drip rate can be determined and the tubing remains filled with fluid.

drip sets Another name for administration sets.

external jugular IV The IV access established in the external jugular vein of the neck.

gauge A measure of the interior diameter of the catheter. It is inversely proportional to the true diameter of the catheter.

infiltration The escape of fluid into the surrounding tissue.

intraosseous (IO) needle A rigid, boring catheter placed into a bone to provide IV fluids.

isotonic crystalloids The main type of fluids used in the prehospital setting for fluid replacement because of the ability to support blood pressure by remaining within the vascular compartment.

Jamshidi needle A type of intraosseous double needle consisting of a solid, boring needle inside a sharpened hollow needle.

keep-the-vein-open (KVO) IV setup A phrase that refers to the flow rate of a maintenance IV line established for prophylactic access.

local reactions Mild to moderate reactions to an irritant without systemic consequence.

macrodrip set An administration set named for the large orifice between the piercing spike and the drip

Technology

Interactivities

Vocabulary Explorer

Anatomy Review

Web Links

Online Review Manual

Refresher.EMSzone.com

chamber; allows for rapid fluid flow into the vascular system.

microdrip set An administration set named for the small orifice between the piercing spike and the drip chamber; allows for carefully controlled fluid flow and is ideally suited for medication administration.

occlusion Blockage, usually of a tubular structure such as a blood vessel.

over-the-needle catheters The prehospital standard for IV cannulation; consist of a hollow tube over a laser-sharpened, steel needle.

phlebitis Inflammation of a vein; often associated with a clot in the vein.

piercing spike The hard, sharpened plastic spike on the end of the administration set designed to pierce the sterile membrane of the IV bag.

saline lock A special type of IV apparatus, also called buff cap, heparin cap, and heparin lock.

systemic complications Moderate to severe complications affecting the systems of the body; after administration of medications, the reaction might be systemic.

to-keep-open (TKO) IV setup A phrase that refers to the flow rate of a maintenance IV line established for prophylactic access.

vasovagal reaction Sudden hypotension and fainting associated with traumatic or medical events.

Assessment in Action

Intravenous therapy plays a major role in ALS treatment of those who are ill or injured. As an EMT-B, you can be an invaluable member of the team through your knowledge and familiarity of procedures and equipment.

1. The escape of fluid into surrounding tissue is known as a(n) _____.
   - **A.** embolus
   - **B.** infiltration
   - **C.** hematoma
   - **D.** perforated vein

2. Possible complications of IV therapy include _____.
   - **A.** circulatory overload
   - **B.** infiltration
   - **C.** phlebitis
   - **D.** all of the above

3. An accumulation of blood in the tissue is known as a(n):
   - **A.** embolus.
   - **B.** infiltration.
   - **C.** hematoma.
   - **D.** perforated vein.

4. _____ needles are used for emergency venous access in pediatric patients.
   - **A.** Catheter
   - **B.** Over-the-needle
   - **C.** Butterfly
   - **D.** Intraosseous

5. What is the maximum amount of air introduced into the circulatory system that a healthy adult can tolerate?
   - **A.** 50 mL
   - **B.** 100 mL
   - **C.** 200 mL
   - **D.** 500 mL

6. Urticaria is a sign of:
   - **A.** air embolus.
   - **B.** allergic reaction.
   - **C.** phlebitis.
   - **D.** cardiac overload.

Challenging Questions

7. What are the signs and symptoms of an air embolus and what is the treatment?

Assisting with Cardiac Monitoring

You are the Provider 1

A 37-year-old man at a local office is complaining of his "heart running away." On arrival you find him sitting in his desk chair, pale and diaphoretic. He is also complaining of some nausea.

Initial Assessment	Recording Time: 0 Minutes
Appearance	Pale, diaphoretic
Level of consciousness	Alert and oriented
Airway	Open and clear
Breathing	A little fast and shallow
Circulation	Radials present, rapid

1. What are your priorities for this patient?
2. What questions should you ask about this episode?

Cardiac Monitoring

Within the past few years, a number of studies have examined the various aspects of the use of the 12-lead <u>ECG</u>, or electrocardiogram, in the prehospital setting. The evaluation and treatment of a patient experiencing the signs and symptoms of an acute myocardial infarction (AMI), or heart attack, has progressed to the point that use of a 12-lead ECG is rapidly becoming the norm when one considers the overall patient outcome. Early identification of an impending AMI allows the provider to alert the receiving hospital, which allows the hospital to prepare before receiving the patient. This can drastically reduce the time to definitive care (catheterization laboratory, or cath lab) and reduce overall cell death. Reduction in cell death means a more positive patient outcome.

The interpretation of a cardiac rhythm is not an EMT-B skill, but EMT-Bs can assist with electrode placement to prepare for <u>cardiac monitoring</u> by an ALS provider. Whether it be a 3-, 4-, or 12-lead system, it may also be helpful to be able to recognize a normal ECG tracing and become familiar with basic rhythm disturbances so that you can help identify many of the acute and chronic problems affecting the heart while learning the practice of ECG analyses.

The identification of cardiac conditions and correct management in the field requires that you have a good understanding of the basic anatomy and physi-

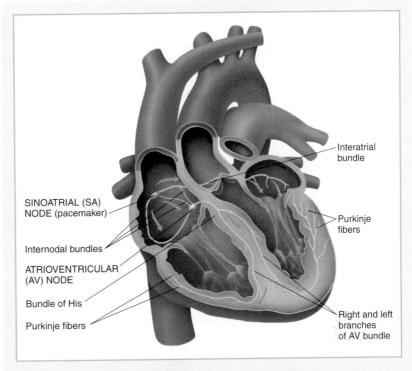

SINOATRIAL (SA) NODE (pacemaker)

Internodal bundles

ATRIOVENTRICULAR (AV) NODE

Bundle of His

Purkinje fibers

Interatrial bundle

Purkinje fibers

Right and left branches of AV bundle

Figure 29-1 The electrical conduction system of the heart.

ology of the heart and that you understand the basic terminology and techniques of cardiac monitoring.

Electrical Conduction System of the Heart

The heart contains a network of specialized tissue that is capable of conducting electrical current throughout the heart called the <u>electrical conduction system</u>. The flow of electrical current through this network causes contractions of the heart that produce pumping of blood.

When the heart is working normally, the electrical impulse moves through the electrical conduction system and produces a coordinated pumping contraction. If the heart is deprived of oxygen or is injured, its electrical system may not function and the heart may not continue to beat properly. Blood pressure decreases, and the patient may lose consciousness.

The Process of Electrical Conduction

The main function of the electrical conduction system is to create an electrical impulse and transmit it through the heart in an organized manner. Electrical conduction in the heart occurs through a pathway of

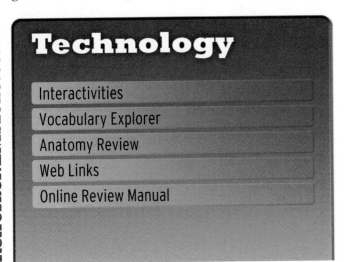

Technology

Interactivities

Vocabulary Explorer

Anatomy Review

Web Links

Online Review Manual

Refresher.EMSzone.com

special cells (Figure 29-1▲). This pathway contains the following components:

- The sinoatrial (SA) node, the heart's main pacemaker, which is located in the wall of the right atrium where it meets the superior vena cava
- Three internodal pathways: anterior, middle, and posterior, which transmit the pacing impulse from the SA node to the atrioventricular (AV) node
- The AV node, which transmits the impulse from the atria to the ventricles
- The bundle of His, which starts at the AV node and then splits into the right and left bundle branches; the only route of communication between the atria and the ventricles
- The left bundle, which travels through the interventricular septum and leads to the left face of the interventricular septum
- The right bundle, which leads to the right side of the interventricular septum
- The left anterior superior fascicle, which travels through the left ventricle to the Purkinje cells
- The left posterior fascicle, which is a fanlike structure leading to parts of the left ventricle
- The Purkinje system, which contains fibers that extend from the right bundle

For the heart to pump, one of the parts of the electrical conduction system needs to act as the heart's pacemaker. In a normally functioning heart, the SA node performs this function. It paces at a rate of 60 to 100 beats/min, with an average of 70 beats/min. Every cell in the conduction system is capable of setting the pace. However, the rate of each type of cell is slower than the cells that precede it. This means that the fastest pacer is the SA node, the next fastest is the AV node, and so on.

■ Electrodes and Waveforms

The ECG electrodes pick up the electrical activity of the heart occurring beneath them, and the ECG machine converts them to waveforms. When an electrical impulse is moving away from the electrode, the ECG machine converts it into a negative (downward) wave. When a wave moves toward an electrode, the ECG machine records a positive (upward) wave. When the electrode is somewhere in the middle, the ECG machine shows a positive wave for the amount of energy that is coming toward it and a negative wave for the amount going away from it. Therefore, if you see a change in the way the ECG waves look on the printout, it is an indication that something is changing in the way the impulse is being conducted in the heart.

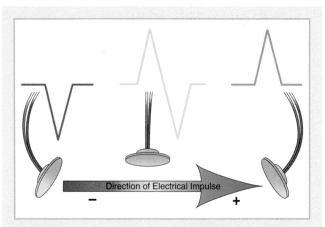

Figure 29-2 Three ECG patterns resulting from various lead placements.

The way an ECG looks depends on where the lead is placed (Figure 29-2▲). For example, if an electrical impulse is moving toward the patient's left side, a lead on the right arm will create negative a wave on the ECG, and a lead on the left arm will create a positive wave.

■ The ECG Complex

On the ECG, one complex represents one beat in the heart. The complex consists of several waves: the P, QRS, and T waves (Figure 29-3▼). These waves represent electrical activity in the heart. A segment is a specific portion of the complex. For example, the segment between the end of the P wave and the beginning of the Q wave is known as the P-R segment. An interval is the distance, measured as time, occurring between two cardiac events. The time between the beginning of the P wave and the beginning of the QRS

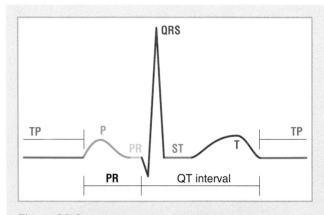

Figure 29-3 Basic components of the ECG complex.

complex is known as the P-R interval. Note that there is a P-R interval and a P-R segment.

ECG Paper

The paper on which an ECG is recorded contains a grid. As the ECG is recorded, the paper passes underneath the pen at a rate of 25 mm/sec. There is a relationship between the ECG grid and the ECG itself. Each little box on the ECG paper represents $\frac{1}{25}$ of a second, or 0.04 seconds. Each bigger box on the paper is composed of five smaller boxes, making each big box 5 × 0.04 seconds, or 0.20 seconds. Five big boxes equal 1 second. By knowing how much time each box on the grid represents, ALS providers can look for problematic waves or intervals that are slower or faster than normal.

Normal Sinus Rhythm

Sinus rhythm is a rhythm in which the SA node acts as the pacemaker. All of the P waves on the patient's ECG should be the same. A normal rate is from 60 to 100 beats/min. A rhythm strip with consistent P waves, consistent P-R intervals, and a regular heart rate between 60 and 100 beats/min is showing normal sinus rhythm Figure 29-4 ▶ .

The Formation of the ECG

This section shows how normal sinus rhythm looks when recorded by an ECG machine. While reviewing

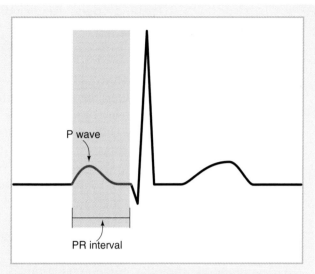

Figure 29-4 In all sinus rhythms, the P waves are identical.

this section, remember that production of the heart's rhythm is a continuous process. There is no actual period of rest or inactivity, and the cycle repeats over and over.

- The baseline is a period when the majority of the cardiac muscle is at rest Figure 29-5A ▶ .
- At this point, the SA node is firing and the electrical impulse is being transmitted through the internodal pathways to the AV node. Note that only a straight line exists so far on the ECG tracing Figure 29-5B ▶ .

You are the Provider 2

The patient tells you he has never experienced anything like this. His only medical history is high cholesterol and he is borderline hypertensive. He was working at his desk when the symptoms started. He has had a little pain, but it feels better right now. Your partner asks you to go ahead and apply oxygen and then bring in the 3-lead ECG cardiac monitor from the hall.

Vital Signs	Recording Time: 2 Minutes
Skin	Pale, diaphoretic
Pulse	116 beats/min, regular
Blood pressure	138/92 mm Hg
Respirations	18 breaths/min, deep

3. What type of oxygen does he need? Why?
4. What is the next step after applying oxygen?
5. What are the appropriate positions for the cardiac leads?

- The electrical activity in the right atria begins to create a P wave (Figure 29-5C ▶).
- The formation of the P wave is complete (Figure 29-5D ▶).
- The impulse has traveled through the bundle of His, right and left bundles, the fascicles, and the Purkinje system. As electrical activity occurs in the ventricles, the QRS complex begins to form (Figure 29-5E ▶).
- Electrical activity continues through the main portion of the left ventricle and gives rise to the large R wave depicted here (Figure 29-5F ▶).
- Electrical activity in the last part of the left ventricle is represented as the S wave or end portion of the QRS complex (Figure 29-5G ▶).
- At this point, the QRS complex is complete. Because the depolarization of the ventricles occurred using the normal electrical conduction system, the QRS complex should be normal in duration. The normal QRS interval is between 0.04 and 0.12 seconds (Figure 29-5H ▶).
- The formation of the T wave (Figure 29-5I ▶).
- The late part of the T wave (Figure 29-5J ▶).
- This is the final phase. The heart is relaxing. If the heart is functioning normally, the process listed here will repeat continuously (Figure 29-5K ▶).

■ Arrhythmias

An arrhythmia is an abnormal rhythm of the heart and is sometimes called a dysrhythmia. This section reviews common basic arrhythmias.

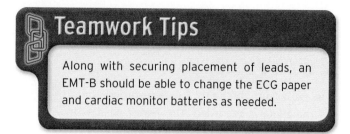

Teamwork Tips

Along with securing placement of leads, an EMT-B should be able to change the ECG paper and cardiac monitor batteries as needed.

Sinus Bradycardia

Bradycardia refers to a slow heart rate, usually less than 60 beats/min. Sinus bradycardia is a rhythm that has consistent P waves, consistent P-R intervals, and a regular heart rate that is less than 60 beats/min (Figure 29-6 ▼).

Most patients can tolerate heart rates between 50 and 60 beats/min without much difficulty. Sinus bradycardia typically becomes a problem when the heart rate drops to less than 50 beats/min. Under normal circumstances, however, heart rates as slow as the low 40s may be normal for very well-conditioned athletes and for some patients during sleep.

Sinus Tachycardia

Tachycardia refers to a fast heart rate, more than 100 beats/min. Sinus tachycardia is a rhythm that has consistent P waves, consistent P-R intervals, and a regular heart rate that is more than 100 beats/min (Figure 29-7 ▶).

Because tachycardia is the body's response to stress, it should not really be considered a pathologic rhythm. Cardiac output is maintained by the heart rate and stroke volume (amount of blood ejected by the heart during each mechanical contraction).

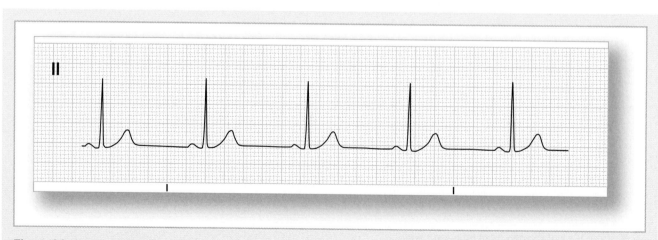

Figure 29-6 Sinus bradycardia.

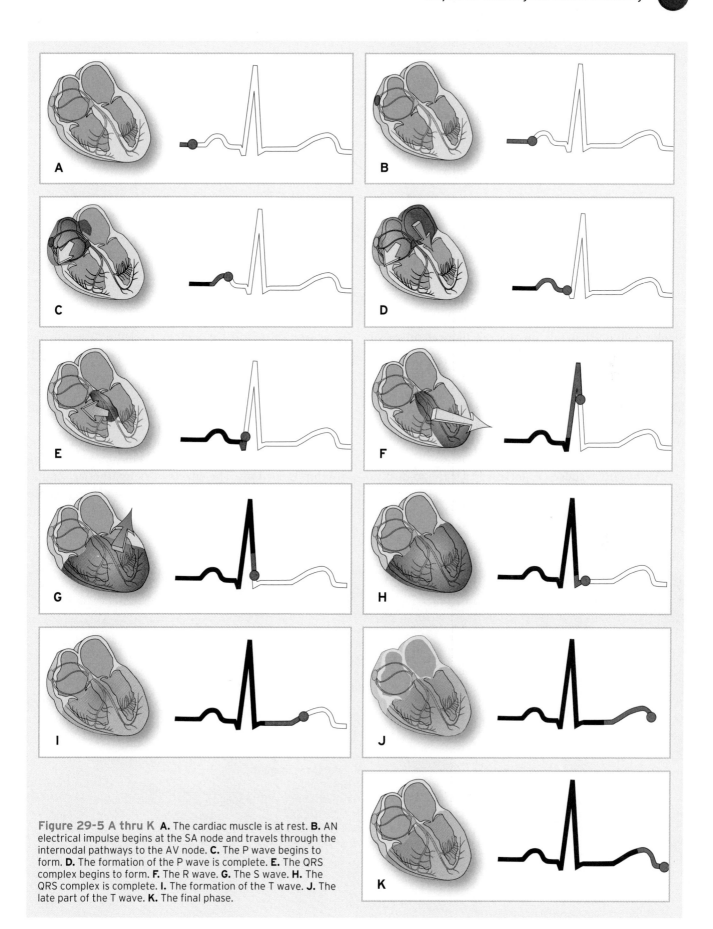

Figure 29-5 A thru K A. The cardiac muscle is at rest. **B.** AN electrical impulse begins at the SA node and travels through the internodal pathways to the AV node. **C.** The P wave begins to form. **D.** The formation of the P wave is complete. **E.** The QRS complex begins to form. **F.** The R wave. **G.** The S wave. **H.** The QRS complex is complete. **I.** The formation of the T wave. **J.** The late part of the T wave. **K.** The final phase.

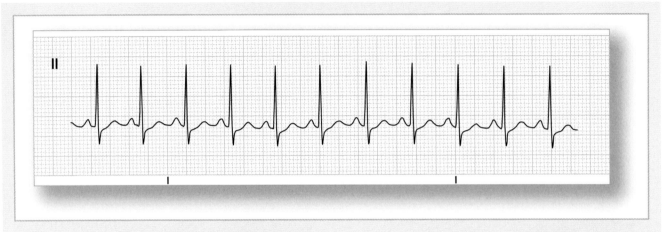

Figure 29-7 Sinus tachycardia.

Stroke volume depends on the mechanical filling of the heart and is a passive process and an active process. The heart passively fills when the AV valves open and the blood from the atria floods into the ventricular chambers. The atria actively overfill the ventricles when the atria mechanically contract. This pushes the remaining atrial contents into the already filled ventricles.

Tachycardia causes a decrease in cardiac output when the rate becomes so high that the stroke volume is affected. Tachycardia decreases the amount of passive filling time. In other words, as the amount of time needed to fill the ventricles decreases with increasing heart rates, the less the ventricles are filled, thereby decreasing cardiac output.

For any given patient, the heart rate is determined by a constant tug-of-war between the sympathetic and the parasympathetic divisions of the autonomic nervous system. If the parasympathetic dominates, the rhythm is slowed. If the sympathetic dominates, the rhythm is sped up. The effects of sympathetic stimulation can go beyond the rate; it can sometimes cause minor physiologic differences in the appearance of the QRS complex.

You are the Provider 3

The patient is placed on the stretcher in a position of comfort. You apply a nonrebreathing mask at 15 L/min and attach the leads of the cardiac monitor. As you are watching the rhythm you note a change. You recognize the components of a sinus rhythm that is just a little fast. While you are watching, the rate increases to 152 beats/min. The patient becomes a little more pale and diaphoretic. You load him into the ambulance and are en route to the hospital.

Reassessment	Recording Time: 5 Minutes
Pulse	152 beats/min, regular
Blood pressure	118/84 mm Hg
Respirations	20 breaths/min, a little shallow
Breath sounds	Clear bilaterally
Pulse oximetry	98% on oxygen via nonrebreathing mask

6. Why is his blood pressure decreased?
7. What is the patient's rhythm?
8. Is this considered a lethal rhythm?

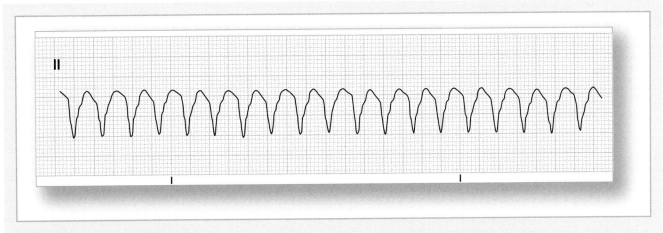

Figure 29-8 Ventricular tachycardia.

The heart rate in sinus tachycardia is more than 100 beats/min. Generally, it is between 101 and 160 beats/min in most patients. At this rate, the tachycardia itself does not pose significant problems. The heart rate in sinus tachycardia, however, can go up to 200 or even 220 beats/min in rare circumstances. At these rates, the rhythm can pose clinical and diagnostic challenges. In general, the maximum heart rate that can be considered normal for any individual patient is derived by using the following formula:

Maximum Heart Rate = 220 beats/min – Age (in years)

For example, a 20-year-old man has a maximum heart rate of 200 beats/min (220 beats/min – 20 years = 200 beats/min). Anything more than that level would be considered abnormal and would require further evaluation.

The maximum heart rate is usually reached during exercise or forced activity of some kind. Athletes and young people are able to tolerate the high levels without difficulty. Geriatric patients or patients with some cardiac pathology cannot tolerate levels near their maximum heart rate without some difficulty. Many people never get to their maximum levels because they have some disease in their electrical conduction system that limits the rate they can reach.

Ventricular Tachycardia

The most deadly arrhythmias include ventricular tachycardia, ventricular fibrillation, and asystole. Together, ventricular tachycardia and ventricular fibrillation account for more than 300,000 sudden cardiac deaths in the United States each year.

A basic definition of ventricular tachycardia is simply the presence of three or more abnormal ventricular complexes in a row with a rate of more than 100 beats/min `Figure 29-8 ▲`. The rate for ventricular tachycardia is between 100 and 200 beats/min, with the most common rates between 140 and 200 beats/min. Rates of more than 200 beats/min can occur, and when they do, the physical size and shape of the complexes slowly begin to blur with no discernible QRS, ST, or T waves. In fact, the complexes actually become unified in size and shape.

In general, ventricular tachycardia is a very regular rhythm. In about 10% of cases, there is slight irregularity, which causes a variation in the cadence of the complexes and usually is found if the rate is at the lower end of the range for ventricular tachycardia.

Ventricular Fibrillation

Ventricular fibrillation is a rapid, completely disorganized ventricular rhythm with chaotic characteristics. The electrocardiographic characteristics of this arrhythmia are undulations of varying shapes and sizes with no specific pattern and no discernable P, QRS, or T waves `Figure 29-9 ▶`.

The undulations occur anywhere from 150 to 500 times in a minute. Notice that we did not use the words "beats" to describe the undulations. This is because in ventricular fibrillation (V-fib), there is no organized beating of the heart.

Ventricular fibrillation can occur spontaneously in a patient with a normal heart. It is also common for ventricular tachycardia to deteriorate into ventricular fibrillation. However, the most common cause of the arrhythmia is an AMI. For many patients, this lethal

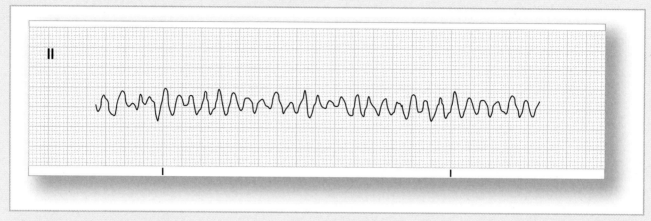

Figure 29-9 Ventricular fibrillation.

arrhythmia is the first sign of an early AMI. Together with ventricular tachycardia, these two arrhythmias account for more than 50% of deaths associated with coronary artery disease.

Ventricular fibrillation is a deadly arrhythmia and does not cease on its own. The only chance of survival is immediate treatment. Within only 10 to 20 seconds of cessation of cardiac output, life-threatening complications can begin. Immediate defibrillation is the most effective treatment for ventricular fibrillation.

Asystole

Asystole refers to the complete absence of any electrical cardiac activity. It looks like a straight or almost straight line on an ECG strip Figure 29-10 ▾ . There is a complete absence of any P, QRS, and T waves anywhere along the strip because no electrical activity is occurring.

The patient is clinically dead at this point. There is no electrical or mechanical activity. The decision about when to call or terminate resuscitation efforts depends on local protocol.

■ Assisting With Cardiac Monitoring

This section reviews the cardiac monitor and how to apply the leads. Depending on the patient and local protocols, the number of leads on your cardiac monitor may vary. You may have a 3-lead, 4-lead, or 12-lead system.

■ The 12-Lead System

Although most patients will need only three or four leads attached for standard ECGs, sometimes a

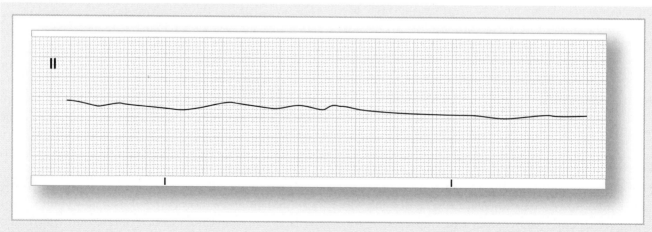

Figure 29-10 Asystole.

12-lead ECG is needed. The importance of obtaining a 12-lead ECG is for early identification of potential myocardial ischemia, or lack of oxygen to the heart's tissue, so that the cause can be appropriately treated and possibly reversed.

Even though obtaining a 12-lead ECG has distinct benefits, it is important to remember to always treat your patient first. If your patient is in severe distress, do not withhold treatment to obtain a 12-lead ECG.

There are some immediate advantages of 12-lead monitoring. An example is early identification of acute ischemia and the accurate identification of arrhythmias. Early identification and early treatment can lead to reperfusion of valuable cardiac muscle cells, preventing tissue death and reducing the potential for a life-threatening arrhythmia.

■ Lead Placement

A 4-lead ECG contains four leads. The electrodes are attached to wires (cables) that are attached to the cardiac monitor. These four leads are called the limb leads because they are placed on the patient's limbs or close to them 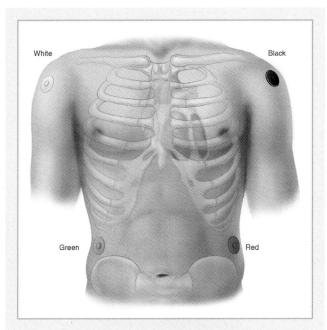. For a 4-lead ECG, the electrodes are placed with the white lead on the patient's right shoulder, the black lead on the patient's left shoulder, the green lead on the right side of the patient's abdomen, and the red lead on the left side of

the patient's abdomen. It does not matter if you place the arm leads on the shoulders or arms, as long as they are at least 10 cm from the heart. Likewise, for the abdominal or leg leads, it does not matter whether these are on the abdomen or legs, as long as they are at least 10 cm from the heart.

If your ECG monitor is a 3-lead ECG, electrode placement is the same as in a 4-lead system but will not have the green lead for placement.

When using a 12-lead ECG, electrodes are placed as shown in Figure 29-12. The limb leads are placed at least 10 cm from the heart. The chest leads, however, have to be placed exactly. Position the V_1 and V_2 leads on each side of the sternum at the fourth intercostal space. To locate this space, you must first find the angle of Louis. This is a hump located near the top third of the sternum. It is located next to the second rib. The space directly beneath it is the second intercostal space. Count down two more spaces to locate the fourth intercostal space. V_4 is at the fifth intercostal space in the midclavicular line. Follow the diagram in Figure 29-12 for the remaining positions.

Figure 29-11 4-lead electrode placement.

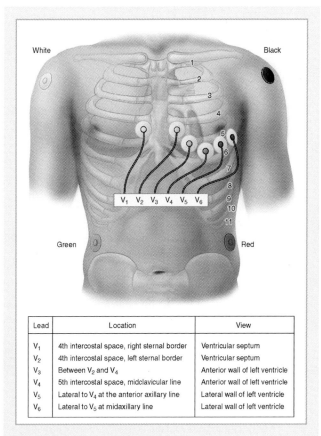

Lead	Location	View
V_1	4th intercostal space, right sternal border	Ventricular septum
V_2	4th intercostal space, left sternal border	Ventricular septum
V_3	Between V_2 and V_4	Anterior wall of left ventricle
V_4	5th intercostal space, midclavicular line	Anterior wall of left ventricle
V_5	Lateral to V_4 at the anterior axillary line	Lateral wall of left ventricle
V_6	Lateral to V_5 at midaxillary line	Lateral wall of left ventricle

Figure 29-12 12-lead electrode placement.

You are the Provider 4

The patient experiences a little pressure in his chest as his rate increases, but it subsides as the rate decreases. By the time you reach the emergency department his rate is down to 98 beats/min. He is feeling a little better and his blood pressure has increased slightly. He is diagnosed as having runs of sinus tachycardia. He is kept overnight for observation and given a prescription for a medication that will regulate his heart rate. He is back at work the following day.

Troubleshooting Lead Placement

It is very important to have direct skin contact when placing ECG electrodes. It may be difficult to place leads on patients in certain situations, for example if the patient's skin is diaphoretic (sweaty), oily, dirty, or hairy. Wipe and clean the patient's skin thoroughly with a towel. Using benzoin can help keep leads attached. If the patient's hair prevents attachment of the leads, use a razor to remove excess hair and then apply the leads.

You are the Provider Summary

Treatment for any cardiac complaint should include placing the patient in a position of comfort, applying high flow oxygen, placing the patient on the cardiac monitor, and if appropriate, assisting the patient with his or her nitroglycerin. The earlier dysrhythmia is recognized, the better the outcome for the patient.

1. **What are your priorities for this patient?**
   ABCs; recognize that this is a load-and-go patient.

2. **What questions should you ask about this episode?**
   Is he experiencing any pain?
   Does he have any medical problems?
   Has he ever had any cardiac problems?
   Does he have any shortness of breath?
   Is he experiencing any other symptoms?
   What was he doing when it started?
   Are there any provoking or palliating factors?

3. **What type of oxygen does he need? Why?**
   Any patient experiencing chest pain should have high flow oxygen. He has adequate tidal volume, so you should apply a nonrebreathing mask at 15 L/min.

4. **What is the next step after applying oxygen?**
   Apply the leads of the cardiac monitor.

5. **What are the appropriate positions for the cardiac leads?**
   White on the right shoulder, black on the left shoulder, red over the left upper quadrant of the abdomen.

6. **Why is his blood pressure decreased?**
   Tachycardia causes a decrease in cardiac output when the rate becomes so high that the stroke volume is affected. Tachycardia decreases the amount of passive filling time.

7. **What is the patient's rhythm?**
   Sinus tachycardia.

8. **Is this considered a lethal rhythm?**
   No. Because tachycardia is the body's response to stress, it should not really be considered a pathologic rhythm. However, any patient experiencing a cardiac episode should receive prompt treatment and transport.

Prep Kit

Ready for Review

- Cardiac monitoring is a skill that helps identify patients who are experiencing an AMI (a heart attack) and other dangerous abnormal heart rhythms. Time is of the essence in treating these patients.
- Cardiac monitoring is not an EMT-B skill, but your assistance can make the call run much more efficiently and smoothly, improving the patient's chances of survival.
- The flow of electrical current through the heart's electrical conduction system causes contractions of the heart. If the heart is deprived of oxygen or is injured, its electrical system may not function properly and the heart may not pump.
- Electrical conduction occurs through a pathway that includes the SA node, three internodal pathways, the AV node, the bundle of His, the left bundle, the right bundle, the left anterior superior fascicle, the left posterior fascicle, and the Purkinje system.
- An ECG machine converts electrical activity in the heart to waveforms.
- The ECG's appearance depends on where the leads are placed.
- The ECG is made of complexes. One complex represents one beat in the heart. The complex consists of the P, QRS, and T waves.
- The paper on which an ECG is recorded contains a grid that represents time.
- Normal sinus rhythm is a rhythm with a regular rate of 60 to 100 beats/min, consistent P waves, and consistent P-R intervals.
- An arrhythmia is an abnormal rhythm of the heart.
- Sinus bradycardia is a rhythm that has consistent P waves, consistent P-R intervals, and a regular heart rate that is less than 60 beats/min.
- Sinus tachycardia is a rhythm that has consistent P waves, consistent P-R intervals, and a regular heart rate that is more than 100 beats/min.
- The most deadly arrhythmias include ventricular tachycardia, ventricular fibrillation, and asystole.
- Ventricular tachycardia is the presence of three or more abnormal ventricular complexes in a row with a rate of more than 100 beats/min.
- Ventricular fibrillation is a rapid, completely disorganized ventricular rhythm with chaotic characteristics. It is deadly and requires immediate defibrillation.
- Asystole is the complete absence of any electrical cardiac activity and looks like a straight or almost straight line on an ECG strip.
- ECG monitors in the prehospital setting can be 3-lead, 4-lead, or 12-lead systems.
- When using a 3-lead ECG, the white lead should be placed on the patient's right shoulder, the black lead on the patient's left shoulder, and the red lead on the left side of the patient's abdomen.
- When using a 4-lead ECG, the white lead should be placed on the patient's right shoulder, the black lead on the patient's left shoulder, the green lead on the right side of the patient's abdomen, and the red lead on the left side of the patient's abdomen.
- When using a 12-lead ECG, the limb leads are placed in the same way as with a 4-lead ECG. The chest leads have to be placed exactly. Position the V_1 and V_2 leads on each side of the sternum at the fourth intercostal space.

Vital Vocabulary

3-lead ECG An ECG that uses three leads attached to the patient's skin.

4-lead ECG An ECG that uses four leads attached to the patient's skin; these include the limb leads.

12-lead ECG An ECG that uses 12 leads attached to the patient's skin; these include the limb leads and chest leads.

arrhythmia An abnormal rhythm of the heart, sometimes called a dysrhythmia.

asystole The complete absence of any electrical cardiac activity, appearing as a straight or almost straight line on an ECG strip.

cardiac monitoring The act of viewing the electrical activity of the heart through the use of an ECG machine or cardiac monitor.

chest leads The leads that are used only with a 12-lead ECG and must be placed exactly; includes leads V_1, V_2, V_3, V_4, V_5, and V_6.

ECG (electrocardiogram) an electronic tracing of the heart's electrical activity through leads, which originate in the electrocardiograph machine and contain electrodes that attach to the patient's chest and/or limbs.

electrical conduction system A network of special cells in the heart through which an electrical current flows, causing contractions of the heart that produce pumping of blood.

limb leads The four leads used with a 4-lead ECG; placed on or close to the right arm, left arm, right leg, and left leg.

Technology

- Interactivities
- Vocabulary Explorer
- Anatomy Review
- Web Links
- Online Review Manual

Refresher.EMSzone.com

normal sinus rhythm   A rhythm that has consistent P waves, consistent P-R intervals, and a regular heart rate between 60 and 100 beats/min.

sinus bradycardia   A rhythm that has consistent P waves, consistent P-R intervals, and a regular heart rate that is less than 60 beats/min.

sinus rhythm   A rhythm in which the SA node acts as the pacemaker.

sinus tachycardia   A rhythm that has consistent P waves, consistent P-R intervals, and a regular heart rate that is more than 100 beats/min.

ventricular fibrillation   A rapid, completely disorganized ventricular rhythm with chaotic characteristics, no specific pattern, and no discernable P, QRS, or T waves.

ventricular tachycardia   The presence of three or more abnormal ventricular complexes in a row with a rate of more than 100 beats/min.

Assessment in Action

Even though cardiac monitoring is not an EMT-B skill, the ability to help by attaching the monitor to the patient and recognizing abnormal rhythms can be invaluable to a paramedic when treating a critical patient. To be most proficient, you should have a good understanding of the basic anatomy and physiology of the heart, and understand the basic terminology and techniques of cardiac monitoring.

1. The intrinsic rate of the SA node is _____.
   - **A.** 60 to 100 beats/min
   - **B.** 40 to 60 beats/min
   - **C.** 20 to 40 beats/min
   - **D.** none of the above

2. Which of the following is correct for placement of ECG leads?
   - **A.** White lead on the right shoulder
   - **B.** Black lead on the left shoulder
   - **C.** Red lead on the left side of the abdomen
   - **D.** All of the above

3. The heart's main pacemaker is the _____.
   - **A.** Bundle of His
   - **B.** AV node
   - **C.** SA node
   - **D.** left ventricle

4. A _____ rhythm is one in which the SA node acts as pacemaker.
   - **A.** ventricular
   - **B.** junctional
   - **C.** internodal
   - **D.** sinus

5. _____ _____ is a chaotic rhythm with no discernible P, QRS, or T waves.
   - **A.** Ventricular tachycardia
   - **B.** Supraventricular tachycardia
   - **C.** Ventricular fibrillation
   - **D.** Atrial fibrillation

6. _____ is the amount of blood ejected with each beat.
   - **A.** Minute volume
   - **B.** Stroke volume
   - **C.** Cardiac output
   - **D.** Blood pressure

Challenging Questions

7. Trace the flow of electricity through the conduction system of the heart.

Index

NOTE: Page numbers with *f* indicate figures, and *t* indicate tables.

Photo Credits

Cover © Craig Jackson/IntheDarkPhotography.com; **Section Openers:** 1, © Chris Jensen; 5, © Craig Jackson/IntheDarkPhotograpy.com; 7, © Dan Myers; **Chapter 1:** Opener © Corbis; **Chapter 2:** 2-1 and 2-5 © Craig Jackson/IntheDarkPhotography.com; 2-6 © Jack Dagley Photography/ShutterStock, Inc.; 2-9a © NDP/Alamy Images; 2-9b © Fancy Photography/Veer; 2-10 © U.S. Department of Transportation; **Chapter 3:** Opener © Glen E. Ellman; 3-1 © Kenneth Murray/Photo Researchers, Inc.; 3-2 © Jack Dagley Photography/ShutterStock, Inc.; **Chapter 4:** 4-9a and b © Dr. P. Marazzi/Photo Researchers, Inc.; **Chapter 5:** Opener © Keith D. Cullom; 5-6b and 5-10 Courtesy of Laerdal Medical Corporation; **Chapter 6:** Opener © Craig Jackson/IntheDarkPhotography.com; 6-1 © Larry St. Pierre/ShutterStock, Inc.; 6-2 © Peter Willott, The St. Augustine Record/AP Photos; **Chapter 7:** 7-5 © Lawrence Migdale/Photo Researchers, Inc.; **Chapter 8:** 8-6 Courtesy of Dey, L. P.; **Chapter 13:** 13-1 Courtesy of Carol B. Guerrero; 13-2a Courtesy of Peggy Greb/USDA; 13-2b Courtesy of Daniel Wojcik/USDA; 13-5a Courtesy of Dey, L. P.; **Chapter 14:** Opener © Craig Jackson/IntheDarkPhotography.com; 14-1a Photographed by Kimberly Potvin; 14-1c © Jaimie Duplass/ShutterStock, Inc.; 14-1d © Cate Frost/ShutterStock, Inc; 14-2 © Glen E. Ellman; 14-4 © Oscar Knott/FogStock/Alamy Images; **Chapter 15:** Opener © Dennis Wetherhold, Jr.; **Chapter 16:** 16-2 © Craig Jackson/IntheDarkPhotography.com; **Chapter 17:** 17-7 Courtesy of David J. Burchfield, MD; **Chapter 18:** Opener © Dennis Wetherhold, Jr.; 18-1 © Shout Pictures/Custom Medical Stock Photo; 18-2 © Terry Dickson, Florida Times-Union/AP Photos; 18-3 Courtesy of Captain David Jackson, Saginaw Township Fire Department; 18-4 © Dr. E. Walker/Photo Researchers, Inc.; 18-6 and 18-7 © Dan Myers; **Chapter 19:** Opener © Steve L. Smith; **Chapter 20:** Opener © Dan Myers; **Chapter 21:** Opener © Craig Jackson/IntheDarkPhotography.com; 21-2 Photographed by Kimberly Potvin; 21-3 Courtesy of Rhonda Beck; 21-6 © English/Custom Medical Stock Photo; 21-10 Courtesy of Andrew N. Pollak, MD/University of Maryland School of Medicine; 21-13a © Suzanne Tucker/ShutterStock, Inc.; 21-19 and 21-22 © Charles Stewart & Associates; 21-23 © Dr. P. Marazzi/Photo Researchers, Inc.; 21-24 Courtesy of porkfork6/Flickr; **Chapter 22:** Opener © Craig Jackson/IntheDarkPhotography.com; 22-14 © Shout/Custom Medical Stock Photo; 22-15 © Eddie M. Sperling; **Chapter 23:** 23-2 © Eddie M. Sperling; 23-6 © Mediscan/Visuals Unlimited; 23-8a and b Courtesy of Ron Dieckmann, M. D.; 23-11 Courtesy of Cindy Bissell; **Chapter 24:** 24-2 and 24-3 Courtesy of Health Resources and Services Administration, Maternal and Child Health Bureau, Emergency Medical Services for Children Program; **Chapter 25:** 25-2 © Dr. P. Marazzi/Photo Researchers, Inc.; **Chapter 26:** Opener © Glen E. Ellman; **Chapter 27:** Opener © Keith D. Cullom; **Chapter 28:** Opener © Glen E. Ellman; 28-8 Courtesy of Cardinal Health; **Chapter 29:** Opener Courtesy of Philips Medical Systems. All rights reserved.; 29-2, 29-3, 29-4, 29-5a-k, 29-6, 29-7, 29-8, 29-9, and 29-10 From *Arrhythmia Recognition: The Art of Interpretation*, courtesy of Tomas B. Garcia, MD.